THYROID DISEASES

THYROID DISEASES

EDITED BY

FABRIZIO MONACO

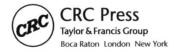

CRC Press
Taylor & Francis Group
Boca Raton London New York

CRC Press is an imprint of the
Taylor & Francis Group, an **informa** business

CRC Press
Taylor & Francis Group
6000 Broken Sound Parkway NW, Suite 300
Boca Raton, FL 33487-2742

First issued in paperback 2019

© 2012 by Taylor & Francis Group, LLC
CRC Press is an imprint of Taylor & Francis Group, an Informa business

No claim to original U.S. Government works

ISBN-13: 978-1-4398-6838-6 (hbk)
ISBN-13: 978-0-367-38130-1 (pbk)

Library of Congress Cataloging-in-Publication Data

Thyroid diseases / editor, Fabrizio Monaco.
    p. ; cm.
  Includes bibliographical references and index.
    Summary: "Covering cutting edge material on thyroid diseases including clinical presentation,
    diagnostic procedures, and therapeutic treatments, the author employs simple, concise
    language to offer a comprehensive examination of thyroid disorders. Each chapter incorporates
    a schematic layout with algorithms for diagnosis, treatment, and follow-up. Emphasizing
    subclinical and transient forms of hyper- and hypothyroidism and thyroid incidentalism, the
    author provides a description of frequently asked questions by patients and the appropriate
    practitioner responses for discussing the disorder and giving the pros and cons of the proposed
    treatment"--Provided by publisher.
  ISBN 978-1-4398-6838-6 (hardback : alk. paper)
  I. Monaco, Fabrizio.
  [DNLM: 1. Thyroid Diseases--diagnosis. 2. Thyroid Diseases--therapy. WK 200]

  616.4'4--dc23   2012010205

Visit the Taylor & Francis Web site at
http://www.taylorandfrancis.com

and the CRC Press Web site at
http://www.crcpress.com

This book is dedicated to:

Jack Robbins who taught me ethics in research,

Jean Roche who taught me that research is not merely discovering a phenomenon, but reaching out for truth,

Lidio Baschieri who made me fall in love with clinical medicine and taught me how to become a doctor,

and to Antonella, Gloria, and Olimpia, through whom I discovered how beautiful and joyful life is.

Contents

Foreword

This textbook edited by Fabrizio Monaco is an updated and outstanding overview of the etiology, pathophysiology, and clinical and instrumental diagnosis of thyroid disorders. It contains 31 homogeneous chapters written by well-known Italian experts in the field, all of whom bring to this book extensive clinical experience, both at the national and international levels. This book is a user-friendly and easy-to-consult reference for endocrinologists, general medicine physicians, specialists in other disciplines, and biologists and will also be useful for training physicians and medical students.

One of the primary aims of the authors was the quick identification of the core of each subject. Thus, a major focus was to make each subject easily understandable, thanks to the use of numerous tables and figures. In addition to the classical chapters on the subject, this text includes several chapters that are not commonly included in other treatises. They cover aspects of thyroid disease in the elderly and during pregnancy, iodine deficiency, antithyroid treatment, thyroid disruptors, and thyroid in the intensive care unit, thereby making this textbook unique.

This book is ideal for those who want to improve their knowledge of thyroid malfunctions and management of their patients. I have no doubt that this text will become a landmark in the medical and endocrinological literature, provide a fundamental source of information for clinicians in practice, and drive the need for researching new questions in basic and medical science.

Aldo Pinchera

Preface

Although many books about thyroid diseases were published in the past, no recent book details these diseases and dysfunctions didactically in a homogeneous and uniform way. In fact, every chapter of this book presents a didactic methodological exposition starting with definition of the dysfunction or disease, followed by epidemiology, etiopathogenesis, clinical features, first and second level tests for diagnosis, first and second line therapies, prognosis, and follow-up.

The recent recognized thyroid dysfunctions such as transient forms of hyper- and hypothyroidism, subclinical hyper- and hypothyroidism, thyroid dysfunction during gestation and postpartum, and the influence of iodine on the thyroid during pregnancy are treated as separate entities. The final chapters concern the importance of many drugs that modify thyroid function and thyroid disruptors that affect thyroid homeostasis. Special focus is on the bimodal and/or transient development of some thyroid diseases, the evolution of diagnosis, the priorities of therapies, and lifelong follow-up of patients. All the chapter authors pursued long periods of training in outstanding research laboratories and are active investigators and well known in the international arena.

The didactic and practical approach of this book should make it useful for practicing clinicians and those in training including medical students, medical and surgical residents, fellows in endocrinology and internal medicine, and clinicians in other areas of medicine.

The aim of this book is to transmit what the writers know. The reader is the judge of whether he or she learns. If this book meets with readers' approval, its goal will be reached. If not, readers' criticisms will stimulate further improvement and study.

Fabrizio Monaco

About the Editor

Fabrizio Monaco, M.D. was born in Rome. He earned an M.D. (cum laude) from the University of Rome, then completed specialization programs in endocrinology and internal medicine at the same university.

Dr. Monaco served as an investigator for the U.S. National Research Council from 1966 through 1986. He joined the University of Chieti-Pescara as a full professor of endocrinology and advanced to director of the Postgraduate School of Endocrinology and chief of the Section of Endocrinology of the Department of Medicine at the university.

Dr. Monaco's interest in thyroid physiology and disease led him to an international postdoctoral research fellowship at the U.S. National Institutes of Health. He also was the principal investigator for a number of U.S. Public Health Service research grants and taught and performed studies at a number of research and academic institutions throughout Europe and the United States.

Along with 98 publications in international journals, Dr. Monaco has written and edited a number of books on thyroid function and diseases. They include *Thyroid Diseases: Clinical Fundamentals and Therapy* (with M.A. Satta, B. Shapiro, and B. Troncone, 1993, CRC Press), *Terapia Endocrina e Metabolica*, 2nd edition (1993, Pensiero Scientifico Editore), *Linea Guida per la Diagnosi, la Terapia e il Controllo delle Malattie Endocrine e Metaboliche* (2000, Societa Editrice Europea), *Malattie della Tiroide* (2007, Societa Editrice Universo), *Principi di Terapia Endocrina e Metabolica* (2010, Societa Editrice Universo), and five editions of *Trattato di Endocrinologia Clinica* (1996–2011, Societa Editrice Universo).

Contributors

Laura Agate
Department of Endocrinology and
  Metabolism
University of Pisa
Pisa, Italy
laura.agate@virgilio.it

Luigi Bartalena
Department of Clinical and
  Experimental Medicine
University of Insubria
and
Endocrine Unit
Ospedale di Circolo
Varese, Italy
luigi.bartalena@uninsubria.it

Paolo Beck-Peccoz
Department of Medical Sciences
University of Milan
and
Endocrinology and Diabetology Unit
IRCCS Fondazione Cà Granda IRCCS
Ospedale Maggiore Policlinico
Milan, Italy
paolo.beckpeccoz@unimi.it

Salvatore Benvenga
Department of Clinical and
  Experimental Medicine and
  Pharmacology
University of Messina
and
Policlinico Gaetano Martino
Messina, Italy
s.benvenga@me.nettuno.it

Antonio Bianchi
Division of Endocrinology and
  Metabolic Diseases
Institute of Medical Pathology
Policlinico Gemelli
Catholic University
Rome, Italy
abianchi69@yahoo.it

Bernadette Biondi
Department of Clinical and Molecular
  Endocrinology and Oncology
University of Naples Federico II
Naples, Italy
bebiondi@unina.it; bebiondi@libero.it

Fausto Bogazzi
Department of Endocrinology
University of Pisa
Pisa, Italy
f.bogazzi@endoc.med.unipi.it

Ines Bucci
Section of Endocrinology, Urology,
  Nephrology, and Andrology
Department of Medicine and Sciences
  of Aging
G. d'Annunzio University of
  Chieti–Pescara
Chieti, Italy
email ibucci@unich.it

Irene Campi
Department of Medical Sciences
University of Milan
Milan, Italy
iren.campi@tiscali.it

Maria Grazia Castagna
Department of Internal Medicine,
    Endocrinology, Metabolism, and
    Biochemistry
University of Siena
Siena, Italy
m.g.castagna@ao-siena.toscana.it

Marco Centanni
Department of Science and Medico-
    Surgical Biotechnologies
Sapienza University of Rome
Rome, Italy
marco.centanni@uniroma1.it

Luca Chiovato
Unit of Internal Medicine and
    Endocrinology
University of Pavia
and
IRCCS Fondazione Salvatore Maugeri
Pavia, Italy
luca.chiovato@fsm.it

Susanna Carlotta Del Duca
Department of Science and Medico-
    Surgical Biotechnologies
Sapienza University of Rome
Rome, Italy
susanna.delduca@alice.it

Rossella Elisei
Department of Endocrinology and
    Metabolism
University of Pisa
Pisa, Italy
relisei@endoc.med.unipi.it

Cesidio Giuliani
Section of Endocrinology, Urology,
    Nephrology, and Andrology
Department of Medicine and Sciences
    of Aging
G. d'Annunzio University of
    Chieti–Pescara
Chieti, Italy
cgiulian@unich.it

Francesco Latrofa
Department of Endocrinology
University of Pisa
Pisa, Italy
latrofaf@libero.it

Serafino Lio
Endocrinology Unit
Department of Medicine
Ospedale Pompeo Tomitano
Oderzo, Italy
slio@ulss.tv.it

Enrico Macchia
Department of Endocrinology
University of Pisa
Pisa, Italy
enrico.macchia@med.unipi.it

Flavia Magri
Unit of Internal Medicine and
    Endocrinology
University of Pavia
and
IRCCS Fondazione Salvatore Maugeri
Pavia, Italy
flavia.magri@fsm.it

Stefano Mariotti
Department of Medical Sciences
University of Cagliari
and
Endocrine Unit
Azienda Ospedaliero-Universitaria di
    Cagliari
Cagliari, Italy
mariotti@medicina.unica.it

Enio Martino
Department of Endocrinology
University of Pisa
Pisa, Italy
enio.martino@med.unipi.it

Mariacarla Moleti
Department of Clinical and
    Experimental Medicine and
    Pharmacology
University of Messina
and
Policlinico Gaetano Martino
Messina, Italy

Eleonora Molinaro
Department of Endocrinology and
    Metabolism
University of Pisa
Pisa, Italy
elemoli@hotmail.com

Fabrizio Monaco
Section of Endocrinology, Urology,
    Nephrology, and Andrology
Department of Medicine and Sciences
    of Aging
G. d'Annunzio University of
    Chieti–Pescara
Chieti, Italy
hmonac@gmail.com; fmonaco@unich.it

Giorgio Napolitano
Section of Endocrinology, Urology,
    Nephrology, and Andrology
Department of Medicine and Sciences
    of Aging
G. d'Annunzio University of
    Chieti–Pescara
Chieti, Italy
gnapol@unich.it

Furio Pacini
Department of Internal Medicine,
    Endocrinology, Metabolism, and
    Biochemistry
University of Siena
Siena, Italy
pacini8@unisi.it

Giampaolo Papi
Department of Internal Medicine
Ospedale Ramazzini
Carpi, Italy
papigiampaolo@hotmail.com; info@
    infotiroide.it

Luca Persani
Department of Medical Sciences
University of Milan
and
IRCCS Istituto Auxologico Italiano
Milan, Italy
luca.persani@unimi.it

Alfredo Pontecorvi
Division of Endocrinology and
    Metabolic Diseases
Institute of Medical Pathology
Policlinico Gemelli
Catholic University
Rome, Italy
pontecorvi@rm.unicatt.it

Mario Rotondi
Unit of Internal Medicine and
    Endocrinology
University of Pavia
and
IRCCS Fondazione Salvatore Maugeri
Pavia, Italy
mario.rotondi@fsm.it

Rosaria M. Ruggeri
Department of Clinical and
    Experimental Medicine and
    Pharmacology
University of Messina
and
Policlinico Gaetano Martino
Messina, Italy
rmruggeri@unime.it

Maria Laura Tanda
Department of Clinical and
    Experimental Medicine
University of Insubria
and
Endocrine Unit
Ospedale di Circolo
Varese, Italy
maria.tanda@uninsubria.it

Luca Tomisti
Department of Endocrinology
University of Pisa
Pisa, Italy
lucatomisti@gmail.com

Francesco Trimarchi
Department of Clinical and
    Experimental Medicine and
    Pharmacology
University of Messina
and
Policlinico Gaetano Martino
Messina, Italy
trimarchi@unime.it

Francesco Vermiglio
Department of Clinical and
    Experimental Medicine and
    Pharmacology
University of Messina
and
Policlinico Gaetano Martino
Messina, Italy

Paolo Vitti
Department of Endocrinology
University of Pisa
Pisa, Italy
paolo.vitti@med.unipi.it

1 Suggestions for a New Classification of Thyroid Diseases

Fabrizio Monaco

CONTENTS

Key words: classification, clinical evolution, transient, persistent, subclinical, polar, hyperthyroidism, thyrotoxicosis.

1.1 INTRODUCTION

It has been recently suggested to revise the classification of thyroid diseases[1] after the only official classification reported in 1969 by the American Thyroid Association (ATA).[2] The ATA classification was based on two points: the presence of goiter and thyroid function.[2] Neither etiology, pathology, evaluation of the clinical evolution, nor the transitory, persistent, or permanent dysfunction of the thyroid gland was mentioned. Goiter, without specifying the dimension of the enlargement, was a basic point of the classification; the function was simply evaluated as nontoxic or toxic. The nontoxic forms included the normal function of the gland and its hypofunction.[2,3] At the end of its report, the ATA voted that the classification "… be reviewed periodically and revised as further knowledge might require."[2]

During the past 40 years, no revised classification nor updated nomenclature of thyroid diseases has been reported in spite of our greater understanding and knowledge of the molecular mechanisms underlying hormonogenesis and mechanisms of thyroid hormone actions.[4–9] We now know that hormonal dysfunction occurs both at the glandular and at the target tissue levels, more precisely at receptor and postreceptor level.[10] Genetic defects of thyroid hormonogenesis,[4,6] postpartum thyroiditis,[11] evolution of diffuse to nodular goiter,[12] and the complex effects of iodine on the function of endemic goiter have been identified.[13] Moreover, in the past 40 years, most countries started screening screen for congenital hypothyroidism so that the clinical consequences of this syndrome should disappear as a clinical entity throughout the world in the near future (see Chapter 11).

In recent decades, the clinical evolution of thyroid diseases has been studied exhaustively; we now know that the functional behaviors of several thyroid diseases change over time from hyper- to hypofunction or vice versa.[14–16] The change of thyroid function is of critical clinical importance, because it implies continuous follow-up with consequent updating of therapy. Moreover, the presence of goiter can be considered only a parameter of thyroid dysfunction since often a disease precedes goiter onset or vice versa. For example, drugs and environmental factors can affect thyroid function without modifying thyroid morphology (see Chapters 30 and 31). Today we know that many thyroid diseases occur without the presence of goiter, i.e., thyrotoxicosis factitia, postpartum thyroiditis, and even Graves' disease. The need to update the nomenclature of thyroid diseases was recognized in the last 30 years by identifying the importance of environmental factors and the reversibility and transient clinical evolution of several thyroid diseases.[17] Recently some internal medicine texts reported the newly identified thyroid diseases as special topics, taking into account the clinical evolution of thyroid diseases and the molecular mechanisms.[8,9] This chapter presents some suggestions for a new classification of thyroid diseases to stimulate the official Continental Thyroid Associations to revise the ATA classification of 1969.

1.2   THYROID FUNCTION

The function of the thyroid is critical in most thyroid diseases because it represents the basis for diagnosis and therapy. Euthyroidism, hyperthyroidism, and hypothyroidism identify normal, excessive, or defective thyroid hormone synthesis, release, and their presence in target tissue. These terms are no longer sufficient to distinguish whether the thyroid hormones derive from the thyroid function, the destruction of thyroid cells with release into circulation of thyroid hormones, iatrogenic causes, or target tissue abnormalities. Thus, the three terms should reflect normal, increased, or low levels of thyroid hormones both in the circulation and at the cellular level.

Euthyroidism means normal thyroid function and normal thyroid hormones in the circulation and at the cellular level. For example, diffuse and nodular goiter with normal circulating hormonal levels could be considered euthyroidism, and not nontoxic goiter, because hypothyroidism is not considered. Note that the so-called euthyroid diffuse and nodular goiter is likely to imply a relative partial hypofunction in many cases (see Chapter 2). Sporadic or endemic subgroupings are reserved for epidemiological (not functional) purposes.[1] Similarly, for diffuse toxic goiter or Basedow-Graves' disease, the words *goiter* and *toxic* should be omitted. Goiter is not always present and *toxic* should be replaced with *hyperthyroidism* to differentiate true thyroid hyperfunction from other forms of excessive thyroid hormones not caused by thyroid hyperfunction (see Chapter 21). This dysfunction could be defined by the names of the first authors who describe the diseases (e.g., Basedow and Graves) or with a term such as *autoimmune hyperthyroidism*, but any terminology needs an exhaustive discussion of experts.

Hyperthyroidism presupposes a clinical symptomatology due to excessive thyroid function. It is now compulsory to distinguish hyperthyroidism due to overproduction of thyroid hormones (see Chapter 18) or excess circulating hormones in the absence of thyroid hyperfunction from excessive e.g. intake, excess release of thyroid hormones, or syndromes of pituitary resistance to thyroid hormones (see Chapters 14 and 21). Use of the hyperthyroidism term should be restricted to excessive hormone production by the thyroid, whereas the term *thyrotoxicosis** is more appropriate in cases of excessive amounts of circulating thyroid hormones not overproduced by the gland.

Hypothyroidism is almost always due to the lack of thyroid hormone production. We now know that in the generalized and peripheral resistance to thyroid hormones, there is normal thyroid function, and the defect is in target organs at the receptor or postreceptor level (see Chapter 14).

1.3 CLINICAL EVOLUTION

The thyroid function evolves over time in several thyroid diseases. Diffuse goiter shows normal circulating hormonal levels for years; later becomes nodular,[12] and may evolve in hypothyroidism or hyperthyroidism, depending on iodine supply.[14,15] In autoimmune thyroid diseases like Basedow-Graves' disease and postpartum or Hashimoto's thyroiditis, the function can vary over time, depending on the presence of stimulating or blocking autoantibodies, environmental agents, or iodine supply (see Chapters 4 and 5). The natural history of Basedow-Graves' disease is characterized by remissions and exacerbations with 10 to 15% of patients progressing with time to hypothyroidism. Similarly postpartum or Hashimoto's thyroiditis remit or can progress to hyper-hypothyroidism showing transient periods of hypo-hyperthyroidism (see Chapters 15 and 22).

Therefore, it should be emphasized that most thyroid diseases are lifelong, that the subclinical forms are clearly recognized today, and that many dysfunctions are transient. Thus, thyroid dysfunction should be designated as *persistent* or *transient*. A transient disease lasts only a few months (less than 1 year) and spontaneously reverts to normal. It is important to consider not only the functional presentation, but also the evolution of many thyroid diseases as a function of time, because the change from hypo- to hyperfunction and vice versa, requires continuous follow-up and updated therapies.

Also the term *polar* could be considered to describe the frequent change of function during the evolution of the thyroid dysfunction.[18] Thus, I suggest the possibility of including the polar, transient, and persistent terms in an updated classification (Table 1.1).

Finally, I think that the Graves' ophthalmopathy term should be updated since the ocular complication is an orbital rather than an ocular disease. Perhaps a more

---

* The term *thyrotoxicosis* indicates clinical signs and symptoms secondary to the excessive presence of serum thyroid hormones. The term generally relates to the hyperfunction of the thyroid but also to the release into circulation of preformed hormones as in destructive thyroiditis or to excessive intake (surreptitious or iatrogenic) of thyroid hormones. Therefore, thyrotoxicosis can occur with and without hyperthyroidism.

TABLE 1.1
Classification of Thyroid Diseases

I. **Diseases characterized by euthyroidism**
  A. Euthyroid goiter[a]
  1. Diffuse
  2. Nodular
  3. Transient
  a. Physiological: menarche, pregnancy, menopause
  b. Iatrogenic: iodine excess or deficiency, antithyroid drugs, environmental or diet
  B. Tumors
  1. Benign (single nodule)
  2. Malignant
  a. Differentiated (papillary and follicular)
  b. Undifferentiated (anaplastic)
  c. Medullary
  C. Thyroiditis
  1. Acute thyroiditis
  2. Subacute thyroiditis (de Quervain's)[b]
  3. Chronic autoimmune thyroiditis or Hashimoto's disease[c]
  4. Postpartum and silent thyroiditis[c]
  5. Riedel's thyroiditis
  D. Thyroid incidentaloma

II. **Diseases characterized by hyperthyroidism**
  A. With thyroid gland hyperfunction
  1. Hyperthyroid goiter with thyroid-associated orbitopathy or Basedow-Graves' disease[d]
  2. Multinodular hyperthyroid goiter or Plummer's disease
  3. Autonomous nodule (prehyperthyroid and hyperthyroid or pretoxic and toxic)
  4. Rare forms: excessive exogenous iodine, hyperthyroidism due to Hashimoto's disease (Hashitoxicosis), postpartum thyroiditis (in hyperthyroid phase), pituitary resistance to thyroid hormones, TSH-secreting pituitary adenoma, chorionic gonadotropin-secreting tumor, adenoma or carcinoma (follicular) of the thyroid
  B. Thyrotoxicosis without thyroid gland hyperfunction
  1. Excessive, exogenous thyroid hormones (thyrotoxicosis factitia and iatrogenic)
  2. Postinflammatory or from destruction of thyroid
  3. Amiodarone- or iodine-induced[b]
  C. Subclinical hyperthyroidism
  D. Transient hyperthyroidism
  E. Thyroid crisis

III. **Thyroid-associated orbitopathy[c]**

IV. **Diseases characterized by hypothyroidism**
  A. With thyroid gland hypofunction
  1. Primary hypothyroidism
  a. Adult (iatrogenic; surgery, ^{131}I therapy, external radiotherapy, chronic autoimmune thyroiditis in hypothyroid phase); Graves' disease (end state); diffuse and nodular goiter; iodine deficiency[f]
  b. Neonatal congenital (ectopia, agenesis, dyshormonogenesis)

TABLE 1.1 (continued)
Classification of Thyroid Diseases

    2. Secondary: hypothalamic–pituitary or central hypothyroidism
    3. Dyshormonogenetic congenital goiter
  B. Without hypothyroidism
    1. Generalized and peripheral resistance to thyroid hormones (receptor and postreceptor defects)
  C. Subclinical hypothyroidism
  D. Transient hyperthyroidism
  E. Hypothyroid coma

[a] Goiter is an increase of thyroid volume (>40 mL, twice the normal volume of the adult thyroid) determined by ultrasound. It is insufficient to define goiter as indefinite enlargement of the thyroid (i.e., based only on clinical parameters) when imaging techniques allow detection of lesions as small as 2 mm.

[b] Subacute thyroiditis shows three clinical phases: initial hyperthyroidism due to thyroid destruction, a middle (euthyroid) phase, and a final end-stage hypothyroidism. Similarly amiodarone thyroiditis can show phases of hypo- and hyperthyroidism; the latter may be due to thyroid destruction or hyperfunction.

[c] Chronic autoimmune thyroiditis generally shows generally two clinical phases: a hyperthyroid phase due to iodine intake (Hashimoto's) or derepression of the immune system (postpartum and silent thyroiditis) followed by an end-stage hypothyroid phase. The euthyroid phase is asymptomatic and can last for decades.

[d] It is improper to define Basedow-Graves' disease as diffuse toxic goiter because goiter is absent in some forms and a goiter may change from diffuse to nodular.

[e] This definition is suggested as a replacement for "eye changes of Graves' disease" because eye changes can occur in many autoimmune thyroid diseases.

[f] In severe iodine deficiency, hypothyroidism can develop over the years due to progressive impairment of thyroid hormone biosynthesis or concurrent autoimmune thyroid disease. It has to be emphasized that frequent forms of hypothyroidism are iatrogenic; the forms due to chronic autoimmune thyroiditis cannot be accompanied by goiter in the atrophic variant.

appropriate definition could be *orbitopathy* (see Chapter 26). Moreover it should be remembered that the ocular complication is present more often in Graves' disease, but also appears in many autoimmune thyroid diseases associated with hypofunction and with euthyroidism.

1.4 CONCLUSION

More than 40 years have passed since the first classification of thyroid diseases. I strongly suggest that we revise the classification of thyroid diseases. Several disease entities, like postpartum thyroiditis and syndromes of resistance to thyroid hormones, are now well recognized. The clinical evolution influences the course of the disease with the recognition of subclinical, transient, and polar forms (Table 1.1).

When the publisher accepted my proposal to edit another book on thyroid diseases, I asked the coauthors to write the chapters included here. I did not ask or compel any authors to accept my proposed nomenclature. As a result all the coauthors used the nomenclature considered appropriate for the diseases described. As the reader can see, several coauthors, all scientists with international reputations, many from the same schools, and many who worked all over the world used different terms to define the same diseases.

This further strengthens my proposal that a common nomenclature and updated classification for thyroid diseases are needed. I therefore suggest that the Continental Thyroid Association (CTA), American Thyroid Association (ATA), European Thyroid Association (ETA), Asia and Oceania Thyroid Association (AOTA), and Latin American Thyroid Society (LATS) establish an ad hoc committee to review the classification in accord with the ATA's 1969 statement that "... the classification ... be reviewed periodically and revised as further knowledge might require."[2]

REFERENCES

1. Monaco, F. 2003. Classification of thyroid diseases: suggestions for a revision. *J Clin Endocrinol Metab* 88: 1428–1432.
2. Werner, S.C. 1969. Classification of thyroid diseases. Report of the Committee on Nomenclature of the American Thyroid Association. *J Clin Endocrinol Metab* 29: 860–862.
3. Werner, S.C. and Ingbar, S.H. 2005. *The Thyroid: A Fundamental and Clinical Text,* 9th ed., Braverman, L.E. and Utiger, R.D., Eds. Philadelphia: Lippincott Williams & Wilkins.
4. Wartofsky, L. 2001. The thyroid gland. In *Principles and Practice of Endocrinology and Metabolism*, 3rd Ed., Becker, K.L., Ed. Philadelphia: Lippincott Williams & Wilkins, 308–471.
5. Cooper, D.S. 2009. *Medical Management of Thyroid Disease,* 2nd ed. London: Informa Healthcare.
6. Kronenberg, H.M. et al., Eds. 2008. *Williams Textbook of Endocrinology*, 11th ed. Philadelphia: Saunders Elsevier.
7. De Groot, L.J. and Jameson, J.L., Eds. 2010. *Endocrinology*, 6th ed. Philadelphia: Saunders Elsevier.
8. Fauci, A.S. et al., Eds. 2008. *Harrison's Principles of Internal Medicine*, 17th ed. New York: McGraw Hill.
9. Goldman, L. and Ausiello, D., Eds. 2008. *Cecil Textbook of Medicine*, 23rd ed. Philadelphia: Saunders Elsevier.
10. Refetoff, S. and Usala, S.J. 1993. The syndromes of resistance to thyroid hormones. *Endocr Rev* 14: 348–399.
11. Amino, N. et al. 1982. High prevalence of transient postpartum thyrotoxicosis and hypothyroidism. *New Engl J Med* 306: 849–852.
12. Studer, H., Peter, H.J., and Gerber, H. 1989. Natural heterogeneity of thyroid cells: the basis for understanding thyroid function and nodular goiter growth. *Endocr Rev* 10: 125–113.
13. Delange, F. et al. 1998. *Elimination of Iodine Deficiency Disorders (IDD) in Central and Eastern Europe, the Commonwealth of Independent States, and the Baltic States*. WHO/Euro/NUT/98.1. Geneva: World Health Organization, 1–168.
14. Lamberg, B.A. et al. 1981. Spontaneous hypothyroidism after antithyroid treatment of hyperthyroid Graves' disease. *J Endocrinol Invest* 4: 399–402.
15. Wakakuri, N., Kubo, T., and Katagawa, M. 1985. Hyperthyroidism and primary hypothyroidism. *Arch Intern Med* 145: 1527–1528.

16. Amino, N. 1992. Postpartum thyroiditis. In *Thyroid Diseases: Clinical Fundamentals and Therapy,* Monaco F. et al., Eds. Boca Raton, FL: CRC Press, 239–249.
17. Robbins, J., Rall, J.E., and Gorden, P. 1980. The thyroid and iodine metabolism. In *Metabolic Control and Disease,* Bondy, P.K. and Rosenberg, L.E., Eds. Philadelphia: W.B. Saunders, 1325–1425.
18. Monaco, F. 1993. Classification of thyroid diseases. In *Thyroid Diseases: Clinical Fundamentals and Therapy,* Monaco F. et al., Eds. Boca Raton, FL: CRC Press, 3–11.

2 Diffuse and Nodular Goiter

Francesco Latrofa and Paolo Vitti

CONTENTS

Key words: iodine, iodine deficiency, iodine intake, familial goiter, sporadic goiter, functioning thyroid nodule, non-functioning thyroid nodule, thyroid hormones, TSH, thyroid autoantiboidies, calcitonin, thyroid ultrasound, thyroid scintigraphy, thyroid fine needle cytology, iodine prophylaxis, LT_4 therapy, radioiodine therapy, recombinant human TSH, thyroidectomy, percutaneous ethanol injection, laser thermal ablation.

2.1   INTRODUCTION

The term *goiter* refers to an enlarged thyroid gland in the absence of autoimmune thyroid diseases and thyroid cancer. The traditional classification of goiter typically includes the endemic, sporadic, and familiar forms. As a matter of fact, these three types are non-distinguishable from a clinical and pathological view because they differ only for the various influences on their development of endogenous and exogenous factors.

Goiter in the absence of thyroid nodules (diffuse goiter) is common and usually asymptomatic. In clinical practice, nodular goiter is more frequently encountered because it is more common in areas with iodine deficiency, frequently involves elderly people, and represents an evolution of the diffuse goiter that is more typical of youth. The nodular goiter may present with multiple distinct or coalescent nodules.

Thyroid nodules may be also single or dominant in the context of a goiter or isolated in a gland of normal size and exhibit different pathogenesis and pathology. They may be hyperfunctioning and then cause hyperthyroidism or non-functioning and cause pressure symptoms when they grow large enough. Although non-functioning nodules are rarely symptomatic, they require a diagnostic work-up to exclude the presence of a thyroid cancer. Thyroid cancer is the most frequent endocrine cancer, but is rarely a cause of death.

Nonetheless, due to the high prevalence of thyroid nodules, usually asymptomatic and discovered incidentally in the course of ultrasound (US) and computerized tomography (CT), the diagnostic procedures applied in thyroid nodular disease increased rapidly in recent years. As a result, several consensus statements and guidelines related to the best possible cost–benefits and valid approaches to the diagnostic evaluation of thyroid nodules have been published in recent years.

The prevalence of diffuse and nodular goiter is very dependent on the iodine nutrition of a population. The prevalence of thyroid nodules is also influenced by the dietary iodine dietary, but also depends on the method employed for diagnosis. Epidemiological studies based on thyroid palpation in iodine-sufficient areas have demonstrated a prevalence of 10% in women and 2% in men. In systematic studies, thyroid nodules, mostly non-palpable, can be identified by thyroid US in 20 to 50% of subjects. The prevalence of thyroid nodules is higher in women and increases after 60 years of age.

2.2 IODINE DEFICIENCY DISORDERS (IDD) AND ENDEMIC GOITER

2.2.1 Iodine Metabolism

The widespread most important cause of goiter is iodine deficiency. Iodine is essential for the synthesis of thyroid hormones and thus for mammalian life. While most iodide is found in the oceans, the amounts in potable water and vegetable (then animal) animal food are inadequate in many areas where glaciations removed it from surface soils. Endemic goiter is more common in mountainous regions, but it may be also present in coastal regions. More commonly affected are the extra-urban and especially rural populations that eat non-industrial local foods that are poor in iodine. Indeed, at present, economic status more than geographical location is the main determinant of the quality of food and its iodine content.

Foods of marine origin have high contents of iodine. Only a few populations, such as some inhabitants of the coastal regions of Japan who eat large amounts of seaweed exhibit high iodine intakes. However, because most foods and beverages contain low amounts of iodine, in the absence of iodine prophylaxis programs, iodine intake may be insufficient. In many countries salt, bread, and milk are fortified with iodine in efforts to eradicate iodine deficiency. Other sources of iodine are compounds used by industry and agriculture, supplements, disinfectants, and medicines. About 90% of iodine contained in food is absorbed, mainly in the stomach and duodenum. The absorbed iodide and that resulting from the peripheral metabolism of thyroid hormones and iodothyronines constitute the extrathyroidal pool of inorganic iodine in equilibrium with the thyroid and the kidneys.

The body of an adult contains approximately 20 mg of iodine and the thyroid concentrates 70 to 80% of the total iodine content through the sodium–iodine symporter (NIS) located on the basolateral surfaces of thyrocytes. On the apical surfaces of the thyrocytes, thyroperoxidase (TPO) catalyzes the synthesis of monoiodotyrosine (MIT) and diiodotyrosine (DIT). The coupling of two DITs produces T_4; the coupling of one MIT and one DIT to produces T_3. A normal adult utilizes ~80 µg/day of iodide to produce thyroid hormones. Ninety percent of the plasma iodine is excreted by the kidney and only a small amount in the feces.

When iodine intake is slightly insufficient (i.e., <100 μg/day), TSH induces a higher NIS expression with an increase of thyroid iodine uptake and preferential synthesis of T_3, thus allowing a normal content of intrathyroidal iodine. In chronic iodine deficiency, the thyroid content of iodine progressively decreases, the metabolic balance of iodine becomes negative, and goiter ensues.

Adequate iodine intake is particularly important during pregnancy to prevent the possible consequences of iodine deficiency in both the mother (goiter) and in the fetus (mental impairment). Pregnancy is associated with relevant changes in thyroid physiology (reviewed by Glinoer).[1] During early gestation, serum thyroxine-binding globulin (TBG) increases markedly under the influence of elevated estrogen concentration and the clearance of plasma iodine increases as a consequence of the higher glomerular filtration. Iodine deficiency induces a relative hypothyroxinemia in pregnancy that in turn stimulates TSH secretion, enhances thyroid stimulation, and increases thyroid volume in both the mother and the fetus (Table 2.1). At the end of the first trimester, a transient stimulation of thyroid by high levels of human chorionic gonadotropin (hCG) occurs. During the second half of gestation, the placental type 3 iodothyronine deiodinase increases the metabolism of maternal T_4. As a consequence, the maternal thyroid gland is required to increase its hormonal production through an increase of iodine uptake and a depletion of intrathyroidal stores. Later in gestation, the passage of iodine to the fetal placental unit is another cause of deprivation of maternal iodine.

For these reasons, as noted in European areas showing mild iodine deficiencies, increases of goiter formation during pregnancy are only partially reversible after delivery. In addition, iodine deficiency is correlated with a larger thyroid volume in newborns and therefore goiter formation may start during fetal thyroid development (Table 2.2; reviewed by Glinoer).[1]

TABLE 2.1

Regulation of Thyroid Function in Normal Pregnancy

High estrogen levels	Elevated human chorionic gonadotropin (hCG)	Transplacental passage and deiodination of thyroid hormones
↓	↓	
Increase in TBG levels	Peak hCG levels (end of first trimester)	
↓		
Transient decrease in free hormones	↓	
↓		
Rise in serum TSH concentrations		
↳	Stimulation effects on maternal thyroid gland	

TABLE 2.2
Iodine-Deficient Nutritional Status
in Pregnancy

Relative hypothyroxinemia, iodine deficiency
  in pregnancy
↓
Enhanced thyroidal stimulation
↓
Goiter formation

2.2.2 EPIDEMIOLOGY

When the main cause of a goiter is a deficient dietary iodine intake, it is classified as endemic and belongs to the spectrum of a group of related iodine deficiency disorders (IDDs); see Table 2.3. In 1990 only a few countries (United States, Canada, Switzerland, Australia, and some of the Scandinavian countries) were iodine sufficient. Asia, Africa, and Latin America were historically more prone to iodine deficiency, but recent extensive iodine prophylaxis through enrichment of salt for alimentary use (universal salt iodination or USI) has made most regions of these continents iodine sufficient.

The worldwide state of iodine nutrition was reviewed in 2008. The data were based on urinary iodine (UI) surveys performed between 1997 and 2006 in 41 countries and estimates obtained in 2003 in 89 countries; for 63 countries UI data were not available.[2] The data covered 92.4% of the world population aged 6 to 12 yrs and showed that 31.5% (264 million) of school-age children had insufficient iodine intakes (below 100 µg/L; Table 2.4). The lowest prevalence of ID was in the Americas (10.6%) where >90% of households consumed iodine-enriched salt.

Paradoxically, rich European countries lacking specific iodine prophylaxis programs remain mildly iodine deficient.[3,4] The prevalence of iodine deficiency in

---

TABLE 2.3
Iodine Deficiency Disorders

Age Group	Disorder
All ages	Goiter
Fetus and neonate	Abortion, stillbirth, perinatal and infant mortality, cretinism, hypothyroidism
Child and adolescent	Overt or subclinical hypothyroidism, impaired mental and physical development
Adult	Impaired mental function, toxic nodular goiter, increased occurrence of hypothyroidism, endemic mental retardation, decreased fertility rate

TABLE 2.4

Proportion of Population and Number of Individuals with Insufficient Iodine Intake by WHO Region, 2006

| | Insufficient iodine intake (UI <100 µg/L) | | | |
| | School-Age Children[a] | | General Population[b] | |
WHO Region	Proportion (%)	Total Number (millions)	Proportion (%)	Total Number (millions)
Africa	40.8	57.7	41.5	312.9
Americas	10.6	11.6	11.0	98.6
Southeast Asia	30.3	73.1	30.0	503.6
Europe	52.4	38.7	52.0	459.7
Eastern Mediterranean	48.8	43.3	47.2	259.3
Western Pacific	22.7	41.6	21.2	374.7
Total	31.5	263.7	30.6	2,000.0

[a] Aged 6 to 12 years.
[b] All age groups.

Europe has been reduced by 30% from 2003 to 2010 but 44% of school-age children still have insufficient iodine intake.[4] Although the United Kingdom was considered iodine sufficient for a long time, it was shown in 14- and 15-year-old school girls that the median UI was 80 µg/L.[5] In Italy, iodine deficiency was initially shown in the mountainous regions of the Alps, but subsequent epidemiological studies demonstrated its presence in all areas, particularly in southern and insular regions. Recently the status of iodine nutrition was assessed in southern Italian regions.[6] UI was randomly measured in 26,913 subjects, as part of the project titled "Eradication of Endemic Goiter and Iodine Deficiency Disorders in Southern Italy." UI was lower than 100 µg/L in 64.3% and lower than 50 µg/L in 34.9% of samples. Median UI in non-urban areas was significantly lower than in urban areas (69 versus 79 µg/L; p < 0.0001). No statistical differences were found among UI excretions of children residing in lowland, coastal, mountainous, and hilly areas.

2.2.3 IODINE DEFICIENCY AND MENTAL IMPAIRMENT

Goiter is the most common clinical manifestation of iodine deficiency, but another important consequence is defective development of the central nervous system that may lead to several impairments from mild cognitive defects to cretinism because brain development depends on thyroid hormones during fetal and early postnatal life. The frequency and severity of the neurological impairments are proportional to the magnitude of iodine deficiency.

The clinical manifestation caused by severe iodine deficiency is referred to as endemic cretinism. In its classical description, endemic cretinism includes neurological and myxedematous forms. The neurological type presents with severe mental retardation with squint, deaf mutism, motor spasticity, and goiter. The myxedematous form involves less severe mental retardation and more pronounced hypothyroid features including severe growth retardation, incomplete maturation of the features, dry and thickened skin, dry and sparse hair, and delayed sexual maturation.

In many instances, both sets of features were present in different severities in all subjects affected; some studies suggest that selenium deficiency combined with severe iodine deficiency can more specifically induce forms of atrophic rather than goitrous hypothyroidism. Selenium is normally present in high concentrations in the normal thyroid and is essential for selenoenzymes such as glutathione peroxidase (GPX) that acts as an antioxidant and type I 5′-deiodinase. The mechanism starts when iodine deficiency causes thyroid hyperstimulation by TSH that leads to increased production of H_2O_2 within the thyroid follicular cells; selenium deficiency also results in accumulation of H_2O_2 due to GPX deficit. Excess H_2O_2 can induce thyroid cell destruction and myxedematous cretinism. On the other hand, a deficiency of the selenoenzyme 5′-deiodinase causes decreased catabolism of T_4 to T_3 with increased availability of T_3 for the fetal brain and prevention of neurological deficits.

Cases of overt myxedematous, neurological, or mixed endemic cretinism are reported in areas of severe iodine deficiency such as Africa and Asia. However, in European countries characterized by slight to moderate iodine deficiency, large goiters and cretinism are no longer observed. However, several reports have described cases of neurological deficits (Table 2.5) or minor neuropsychological impairments. In Tuscany, neuropsychological performance was tested in 107 children living in a village characterized by mild iodine deficiency (UI = 64 µg/L) by a block design subtest of the Wechsler Intelligence Scale for Children and simple reaction times to visual stimuli. The results were compared with those obtained in children born and living in an iodine-sufficient area. The block design test results were not different for the two groups of children, while reaction times were significantly delayed in children living in the iodine-deficient village. These data indicate that mild iodine deficiency may impair the rate of motor response to perceptive stimuli even in the absence of general cognitive defects. Mild-to-moderate iodine deficiency was also

TABLE 2.5

Neuropsychological Defects in Infants and School Children Residing in Mildly to Moderately Iodine-Deficient Areas of Europe

Region	Tests	Findings	Authors
Spain	Locally adapted Bayley, McCarthy, Cattell	Lower psychomotor ability and mental development	Bleichrodt et al.
Sicily, Italy	Bender-Gestalt	Low percent integrative motor ability Neuromuscular and neurosensorial	Vermiglio et al.
Tuscany, Italy	Wechsler Raven	Low verbal IQ, perception, and motor ability	Fenzi et al.
Tuscany, Italy	Wechsler Intelligence Scale for Children	Low velocity of motor response to visual stimuli	Aghini-Lombardi et al.

TABLE 2.6

Recommended Nutrient Intake (RNI) for Iodine (μg/day)

Age or Population Group	RNI
Children 0 to 5 years	90
Children 6 to 12 years	120
Adults >12 years	150
Pregnancy	250
Lactation	250

Source: WHO, UNICEF, and ICCIID. 2007. *Assessment of Iodine Deficiency Disorders and Monitoring Their Elimination,* 3rd ed. Geneva.

shown to be associated with minor neurological deficits in Sicily and reduced motor skills in Spain.

2.2.4 IODINE REQUIREMENTS

Several studies established the iodine requirement at different ages and physiological conditions, although with some limitations. According to the World Health Organization/International Council for the Control of Iodine Deficiency Disorders (WHO/ICCIDD), the recommended nutrient intake for iodine is 90 μg/day in infants and children under 6 years of age, 120 μg/ day in children 6 to 12 years of age, and 150 μg/day in adults (Table 2.6). The recommended intake in adults does not seem to change with age. However, during pregnancy, the recommended intake increases to 250 μg/day as a consequence of the increased maternal production of thyroid hormones, iodine transfer to the fetus, and the increased renal clearance of iodine. The recommended intake in lactating women is 250 μg/day to compensate the iodine loss in breast milk.

2.2.4.1 Assessment of Iodine Intake

The methods for the assessment of iodine nutrition in populations are goiter prevalence, urinary iodine concentration (UI), serum TSH in newborns, and serum thyroglobulin (Tg); see Table 2.7.

Goiter can be measured by neck inspection and palpation or by thyroid ultrasonography. According to WHO/ICCIDD, grade 0 is a thyroid that is not palpable or visible, grade 1 is a goiter that is palpable but not visible when the neck is in the normal position, and grade 2 is a goiter that is clearly visible when the neck is in a normal position. Thyroid ultrasound is more sensitive and specific than palpation but requires valid references of thyroid volume data. Goiter surveys as indicators of iodine sufficiency are usually done in school-age children because the survey subjects are easily recruitable, and hopefully reflect the actual impact on humans

TABLE 2.7

Methods for Assessment of Iodine Nutrition in Populations

Goiter prevalence

Urinary iodine (UI) concentration

Serum TSH in newborns

Serum Tg

of iodine deficiency. It must be noted that enlarged thyroids in children who were iodine-deficient during the first years of life may not regress completely after introduction of salt iodization.

The WHO established a total goiter rate in school children to define the severity of iodine deficiency. Rates below 5.0% indicate iodine sufficiency; 5.0 to 19.9%, mild deficiency, 20.0 to 29.9%, moderate deficiency, and above 30.0%, severe deficiency. In addition, a reduction of goiter rate by ultrasound indicates that iodine deficiency has disappeared and thus a frequency of goiter under 5% in school children must be considered as a parameter of iodine sufficiency.[7]

Because more than 90% of dietary iodine is excreted in the urine, measurement of UI is a reliable index of recent dietary iodine intake. Its determination in a population is directly correlated with the frequency of goiter and the disorders of iodine deficiency. A UI level of <100 µg/L in school-age children indicates insufficient iodine intake; iodine deficiency is severe at <20 µg/L, moderate at 20 to 49 µg/L, and mild at UI 50 to 99 µg/L. An adequate UI value is 100 to 199 µg/L while a value >200 µg/L can induce thyrotoxicosis and other adverse effects in susceptible groups (Table 2.8).

TSH concentrations obtained during screening to detect congenital hypothyroidism in newborns is useful to assess iodine nutrition because an increase of fetal TSH is a mechanism that adapts to iodine deficiency. Indeed, iodine deficiency causes a shift toward higher TSH values in the neonatal screening of congenital hypothyroid-

TABLE 2.8

Epidemiological Criteria for Assessing Iodine Nutrition in Population Based on Median Range of UI in School-Age Children

UI (µg/L)	Iodine Intake	Iodine Nutrition
<20	Insufficient	Severe iodine deficiency
20 to 49	Insufficient	Moderate iodine deficiency
50 to 99	Insufficient	Mild iodine deficiency
100 to 199	Adequate	Optimum
>200	More than adequate	Risk of iodine-induced thyrotoxicosis
>300	Excessive	Risk of adverse health consequences

ism. A TSH value >5 mU/L in whole blood collected 3 to 4 days after birth in more of 3% of newborns indicates iodine deficiency in a population.[7]

Thyroglobulin (Tg) is the most abundant intrathyroidal protein. Serum Tg is higher in iodine-deficient than in iodine-sufficient areas as a consequence of TSH stimulation and the higher rate of goiter and falls quickly with iodine prophylaxis.

2.3 FAMILIAL OR DYSHORMONOGENETIC GOITER AND OTHER FORMS OF CONGENITAL GOITER

These goiters are covered in detail (see Chapter 13). Thyroid dyshormonogenesis accounts for 15 to 20% of cases of congenital primary hypothyroidism. The severe forms of dyshormonogenesis are associated with goiter in most patients. Defects of thyroid genes that cause loss of function of enzymes and other proteins involved in thyroid hormone synthesis (thyroid dyshormonogenesis) may induce hypothyroidism. As a result, TSH levels increase, causing hyperstimulation of the thyroid tissue with a consequent goiter that may be found at birth or can develop later.

Most forms of congenital hypothyroidism with goiter are inherited as autosomal recessive. These cases were characterized in the past by goiter and various degrees of cretinism. However, since most of these defects also induce hypothyroidism, they are now identified during neonatal screening for congenital hypothyroidism and treated early with L-thyroxine. Treatment prevents the development of goiter. However, the neonatal screening can miss some cases that can develop later in life, in concomitance with a higher need for thyroid hormone or a period of iodine deficiency. Congenital dyshormonogenetic goiter is reported in detail (see Chapter 15).

Thyroid dyshormonogenesis may be caused by defects of iodide organification [disorders of sodium–iodine symporter (NIS), Pendred syndrome (PDS), thyroperoxidase (TPO), dual oxidase 2 (DUOX2), and dual oxidase maturation factor 2 (DUOXA2)], defects of Tg synthesis, and defects of iodide recycling (iodotyrosine deiodinase or DHEAL1); see Table 2.9. NIS is implicated in trapping of iodine; PDS

TABLE 2.9

Congenital Disorders Associated with Goiter

Familial dyshormonogenetic goiter

    Defects of iodide organification

        Sodium–Iodine symporter (NIS)

        Pendren syndrome (PDS)

        Thyroperoxidase (TPO)

        H_2O_2 generation system (dual oxidase 2-DUOX2 and dual oxidase maturation factor 2- DUOXA2)

        Defects of thyroglobulin (Tg)

        Defects of iodide recycling (Iodotyrosine deiodinase 1 or DHEAL1)

    Mutations of TSH receptor

        Familial non-autoimmune hyperthyroidism

        Sporadic non-autoimmune hyperthyroidism

Thyroid hormone resistance

in the apical efflux of iodine; TPO, DUOX2, and DUOXA2 in organification and coupling of iodide; Tg is the substrate for TPO; and DHEAL1 is involved in intra-thyroidal iodine recycling.

Other forms of congenital thyroid defects associated with goiter include gain-of-function mutations of the TSH receptor (TSH-R) that cause autosomal dominant toxic thyroid hyperplasia or sporadic (neonatal) toxic thyroid hyperplasia. An additional cause of congenital goiter is the resistance of target tissues to thyroid hormones and this type is usually diagnosed later in life.

2.3.1 Defects of Sodium–Iodine Symporter

The sodium–iodine symporter (NIS) is an intrinsic membrane protein located in the basolateral membranes of thyrocytes and is responsible for the transport of iodine into cells. Its expression in the thyroid is a prerequisite for thyroid scintigraphy. NIS defects cause a variable clinical phenotype.[8] It may be diagnosed via neonatal screening for congenital hypothyroidism or during childhood or infancy for the presence of hypothyroidism and goiter. It is inherited as autosomal recessive and is clinically evident when both alleles are affected. The iodine intake influences the clinical expression of the defect. Thyroid volume and degree of hypothyroidism can be variable and can cause mental retardation.

Diagnostic criteria for NIS defects are: goiter with clinical or subclinical hypothyroidism; little if any uptake of iodine in the thyroid; and no concentrations of iodine in salivary glands and stomach (Table 2.10).

2.3.2 Pendred Syndrome (PDS)

PDS mediates exchanges of chloride with iodide and other anions and is expressed in the thyroid, the inner ear, the kidney, and the maternal side of the placenta. In the thyroid, it is located at the apical membranes of thyrocytes and appears to be involved in mediating iodide efflux into the follicular lumen. PDS is an autosomal recessive disease characterized by sensorineural deafness and hereditary goiter associated with euthyroidism or hypothyroidism and a partial defect in iodide organification.[9] Its incidence is estimated to be 10 in 100,000 individuals. A profound

TABLE 2.10
Diagnostic Tests for Familial Dyshormonogenetic Goiter

	Iodide Organification Defects	Tg Defects	Iodide Recycling Defects
TSH	↑	↑	↑
Thyroid volume	↑	↑	↑
Serum thyroid hormone	↓	↓	↓
Serum Tg	↑	Usually ↓	↑
Perchlorate test	↑ discharge (PDS, TPO, DUOX2, DUOXA2)	N	N

sensorineural deafness is the most relevant clinical sign. The thyroid may be of normal size or small or a large goiter may develop. Goiter usually develops during childhood. Patients with PDS develop hypothyroidism only when nutritional iodine intake is low. Patients from countries with high iodine intakes (Japan and Korea) are euthyroid, whereas those from iodine-deficient areas may present with congenital hypothyroidism.

Diagnosis is based on the demonstration of sensorineural defects associated with an iodine organification defect through a positive perchlorate (CLO_4^-) discharge test indicating normal iodine trapping and organification defect (Table 2.10).

2.3.3 Defects of Thyroperoxidase (TPO)

The TPO gene encodes for a 110-kDa (933 amino acids) glycosylated hemoprotein anchored in the apical plasma membranes of thyrocytes. TPO is responsible for oxidizing I^- into I^+, iodinating tyrosyl groups of Tg, forming 3-monoiodotyrosine (MIT) and 3,5-diodotyrosine (DIT), and binding one MIT and one DIT to form T_3 or two DIT to form T_4. H_2O_2 is the substrate for iodide organification. TPO defects are inherited in an autosomal recessive fashion. Currently 61 different mutations are reported, including missense (the most common), nonsense, and frameshift mutations.[10]

In the presence of a suspicious TPO defect, TPO activity is evaluated by a radioiodine uptake and a perchlorate test. After perchlorate administration, most of the iodide is released from the thyroid, indicating an iodide organification defect (Table 2.10).

2.3.4 Defects of Thyroidal H_2O_2 Generating System

TPO catalyzes iodination of Tg and subsequent oxidative coupling of iodinated tyrosyl residues to iodothyronines are rate-limited by the availability of hydrogen peroxidase (H_2O_2), which is the final electron acceptor. H_2O_2 is provided to TPO by the heterodimeric NADPH oxidase complex of dual oxidase 2 (DUOX2) and DUOX maturation factor 2 (DUOXA2) located at the apical plasma membranes. It is likely that the expressivity of defects of DUOX2 gene is influenced by iodine intake since increased iodine intake could lead to better utilization of H_2O_2.

The incidence of DUOX2 and DUOXA2 mutations in congenital hypothyroidism is unknown, but they are common in the subgroup of patients with partial iodide organification defects.[11] Mutations of DUOX2 and DUOXA2 have never been associated with goiter.

2.3.5 Defects of Thyroglobulin (Tg)

Tg is the most abundant protein of the thyroid and is secreted by the thyrocytes into the follicular lumen. After translation, posttranslational processes take place in the endoplasmic reticulum, Golgi apparatus. and follicular lumen. In the follicular lumen, several tyrosine residues are iodinated and certain iodinated residues are coupled to form T_4 and T_3. Each dimeric Tg molecule yields two molecules of T_4. In the presence of low iodine concentrations, the tyrosine residues implicated in hormonogenesis are the first to be iodinated. The newly secreted Tg molecules remain near the apical membranes of the thyrocytes for hormone formation, internalization, or degradation. Tg in the centers of the follicles forms aggregates, serving as iodine and hormone reservoirs. Tg interacts with several proteins on the apical membranes in the exocytosis and endocytosis processes. The immature molecules are recycled through the trans-Golgi compartments.

The prevalence of defects of the Tg gene is approximately 1 in 100,000 live births. Tg gene defects are inherited in an autosomal recessive manner and affected individuals are homozygous or compound heterozygous for mutations in the gene.[12]

The clinical picture of a patient with defects of the Tg gene is characterized by goiter, subclinical or clinical hypothyroidism, enhanced iodine trapping, and usually a negative perchlorate test (Table 2.10). A feature observed in most cases is an absolute or relative decrease in circulating Tg. However, in some defects of the Tg gene, truncated Tg proteins can be secreted and are sufficient for partial hormone synthesis.

2.3.6   Defects of Iodotyrosine Deiodinase (DHEAL1)

DHEAL1 is the main enzyme responsible for the deiodination of mono- and diiodotyrosines. The resulting iodide is used for further synthesis of thyroid hormones. The deficiency of iodothyrosine deiodinase does not affect thyroid hormone synthesis but induces a defect of the recycle of iodine in the thyroid and a urinary loss of iodothyrosine (the precursors of thyroid hormones) with a consequent loss of iodine that cannot be recovered by the thyroid. The increased levels of TSH, in turn, stimulate the thyroid, inducing goiter and increased leakage of iodotyrosine.

Phenotypes of the defects are variable, ranging from large goiters with hypothyroidism and cretinism to non-toxic goiters.[13] Some cases develop early in life and others are diagnosed at puberty or in adulthood. The type of inheritance is autosomal recessive. Individuals carrying heterozygous mutations may show goiter or hypothyroidism. The severity of the phenotype depends on the severity of the defect and on iodine supply.

Uptake and release of iodine and pertechnate are high and faster. Serum Tg is elevated (Table 2.10). The diagnosis is based on the diiodotyrosine test that requires the intramuscular or intravenous injection of radioiodine-labeled iodotyrosine and urine collection at intervals of a few hours.

2.3.7   Mutations of TSH-R: Familial Non-Autoimmune Hyperthyroidism and Sporadic Non-Autoimmune Hyperthyroidism

The TSH receptor (TSH-R) gene is located on chromosome 14 and encodes for a transmembrane receptor coupled to G proteins. Binding of TSH to the TSH-R leads via G proteins to activation of the adenylyl cyclase (AC) and phospholipase C (PLC) signalling pathways. Somatic mutations in the TSH-R or $G_{s\alpha}$ proteins constitutively activate the cAMP cascade and induce thyroid growth and hyperfunction.

Overt neonatal hyperthyroidism affects 1 out of 50,000 neonates. It is predominantly caused by the transplacental passage of maternal TSH-R autoantibodies with stimulating activity and disappears within the first 4 months of life. Mutations in the TSH-R or in the stimulatory G protein genes that cause a constitutive activation of the intracellular signalling cascade are more uncommon causes of neonatal non-autoimmune hyperthyroidism (NAH). These mutations can be inherited as autosomal dominant (familial NAH) or can occur as de novo mutations (sporadic NAH).

Since the first description, 17 constitutively activating TSH-R mutations have been described in 24 families with familial NAH.[14] Most patients were hyperthyroid, some with mild (subclinical) hyperthyroidism and others with a severe form. The age of onset ranges from the neonatal period to adulthood. Diffuse goiter is found in children; multinodular goiter is typical of older patients. Patients with the same mutation of the TSH-R gene may present with wide phenotypic variability and patients of the same family carrying the same mutation show large differences in the onset and severity of the disease.

After the first report, only a few cases of sporadic NAH have been described. The diagnosis should be suspected in a neonate with severe hyperthyroidism and goiter when the mother has no history of Graves' disease and the history is negative for familial NAH. The disease develops earlier and in a more severe form than familial NAH; patients present with fetal or neonatal hyperthyroidism that may be very severe. Low birth weight and premature birth are common. The thyroid size is also variable, with larger and multinodular goiters affecting older patients. As in familial NAH, the germline mutations were heterogyzous and genotype did not correlate with phenotype. The constitutive activity of the TSH-R is usually higher in sporadic than in familial NAH, inducing the more severe forms of hyperthyroidism and a younger age of onset. The mutations of the TSH-R found in the sporadic cases have been identified also in toxic adenomas.

Reported cases of congenital hyperthyroidism from mutations of the $G_{s\alpha}$ protein (Gsp mutations) have been associated with McCune-Albright syndrome and in some toxic adenomas and follicular carcinomas.

2.3.8 THYROID HORMONE RESISTANCE

Goiter is a common finding in patients with resistance to thyroid hormone, described in Chapter 16.

2.4 SPORADIC GOITER

Goiter encountered in patients living in iodine-sufficient areas is classified as sporadic and is the most common form in developed countries. In most patients, the etiology of sporadic goiter remains obscure although the interplays of various degrees of iodine deficiency and unspecified genetic factors are likely to play the main roles.

In regions where iodine deficiency is moderate or severe, the nutritional defect is the most relevant factor of induction of goiter. On the other hand, in areas of iodine sufficiency, patients with sporadic goiters often reveal a positive familial history, stressing the point that genetic factors, likely subtle forms of the same genetic defects described in the previous paragraph, are likely to play a role. The familial aggregation of goiters has been demonstrated in Greece and in other countries. In addition, in both endemic and non-endemic areas, female monozygotic twins show higher concordance rates for goiter than female dizygotic twins.

Linkage analysis has been employed to identify the genes involved in the development of goiter. The multinodular goiter 1 (MNG-1) locus on chromosome 14q31 was identified as a result of the investigation of a Canadian family. A second locus (MNG-2) was identified on the Xp22 region in a study of an Italian family characterized by an X-linked dominant pattern of inheritance. A subsequent genome-wide linkage analysis identified four novel candidate loci on chromosomes 2q, 3p, 7q, and 8p.[15] However, the identification of the factors involved in each patient is both hard to establish and also devoid of practical clinical implications.

In association with iodine deficiency, other exogenous factors can contribute to the development of goiter. Some elements that inhibit thyroid hormone synthesis (goitrogens) are contained in some natural foods (Table 2.11).[16] The substances contained in the seeds of Brassicaceae in association with iodine deficiency have been relevant to the pathogenesis of goiter in some African regions. The cyanogenic glucosides contained in cassava, lima beans, turnips, and sweet potatoes and the glucosinolates contained in cabbage, kale, broccoli, turnips, and rapeseed are metabolized to substances interfering with iodine uptake by the thyroid. The cassava, when not adequately cooked, releases cyanide that is metabolized to thiocyanate. Also cigarette smoking is associated with goiter formation due to the high thiocyanate content in cigarettes. Iodine nutrition in breast-fed infants has been shown to be impaired by maternal cigarette smoking. Flavonoids contained in soy may reduce TPO activity. Industrial pollutants known as endocrine disruptors, for example, nitrate, resorcinol, and perchlorate, that interfere with thyroid hormone synthesis have been identified.[17] Thyonamide and lithium are pharmacological goitrogen agents.

TABLE 2.11
Natural Goitrogens

Goitrogens	Agent	Action
Millet, soy beans	Flavonoids	Impairs thyroperoxidase
Cassava sweet potato, sorghum	Cyanogenic glucosides	Inhibits iodine thyroidally metabolized to thiocyanate uptake
Babassu coconut	Flavonoids	Inhibits thyroperoxidase
Cruciferous vegetables: cauliflower, broccoli, turnips, cabbage	Glucosinolates	Impairs thyroidal iodine uptake
Seaweed (kelp)	Iodine excess	Inhibits release of thyroid hormones
Malnutrition: iron	Vitamin A deficiency	Increases TSH stimulation
	Iron deficiency	Reduces TPO activity
Selenium	Selenium deficiency	Causes deiodinase deficiency; impairs thyroid hormone synthesis

Source: Medeiros-Neto, G. and Knobel, M. 2010. In *Endocrinology*. New York: Elsevier. With permission.

Iodine excess has also been described to be associated with goiter in susceptible individuals. Patients with Graves' disease and Hashimoto's thyroiditis may have subtle enzymatic deficits that cause failure to escape the block of iodine organification induced by excess iodine (Wolff-Chaikoff effect). Thus, a form of endemic goiter can be induced in areas characterized by excessive iodine content in the diet, as demonstrated in some areas of Japan where seaweed is largely consumed. Deficiencies of selenium (present in glutathione peroxidase and deiodinases), iron (present in TPO), and vitamin A (relevant for suppression of the TSHb gene) can worsen iodine deficiency.

Familiarity, female gender, and genetic predisposition are among the endogenous pathogenetic factors. Undisclosed genetic defects of thyroid hormone synthesis may be responsible for the common finding of familiarity of goiter.

2.5 PATHOPHYSIOLOGY, PATHOLOGY, AND NATURAL COURSE

The variable incidence of goiter in areas with similar levels of iodine deficiency, the observation that only a portion of people living in iodine-deficient areas are affected by goiter, and the presence of goiter in iodine-sufficient areas, particularly in its familial form, demonstrate that variably associated exogenous and endogenous factors contribute to its development. Iodine deficiency is well known to represent the main cause of goiter, as shown by in vivo experiments in animal models. Iodine per se has been shown to be in vitro an inhibitor of thyroid growth, probably through iodine compounds. The main mechanism, however, is that a decrease of iodine intake leads to impaired production of thyroid iodinated hormones T_4 and T_3 and consequently to a rise of TSH.

Although this step is not recognizable in most patients who seek medical attention for an enlargement of the thyroid gland and are euthyroid, subjects living in areas with severe and long-standing iodine deficiency may also have mild hypothyroidism. When iodine intake is insufficient, TSH induces higher NIS expression with increased thyroid iodine uptake and a preferential synthesis of T_3, thus allowing a normal content of intrathyroidal iodine. However, in long-standing and severe iodine deficiency, these mechanisms are not sufficient and thyroid cell proliferation ensues, associated with an increased probability of gene mutations.

These modifications induce the development of goiter, as shown by epidemiological and experimental studies. This process has been defined as a maladaptation to iodine deficiency and has been clearly shown in experimental animals that develop goiter and eventually hypothyroidism when fed iodine-deficient diets[18] or treated with drugs inhibiting iodine uptake and organification. TSH is the main growth factor for thyroid follicular cells as clearly demonstrated by in vivo and in vitro experiments. In vitro experiments on cultured cell lines show that TSH-stimulated growth of follicular cells is strictly linked to the cAMP–adenylate cyclase cascade. This is the main physiological pathway through which TSH regulates both thyroid hormone synthesis and follicular cell replication. However, other cell pathways stimulate thyroid cell growth, both in physiological and pathological conditions, as reported below.

These pathophysiological mechanisms are responsible for the pathological features of nodular goiter. In its initial evolution the goitrogenous process is characterized by small follicules, poor of colloid and with tall cells (parenchymatous or microfollicular goiter) and later by follicules with abundant colloid and flat cells (colloid goiter). As a consequence of the breaks of adjacent follicules, pseudocysts (colloid-cystic goiter) develop. Later, thyroid nodules grow (multinodular goiter). As a consequence of necrotic and scarring events, true cysts develop (cystic goiter) while vascular transformation induces intracystic hemorrhages (hemorrhagic cysts).

Pivotal experiments in rats have been useful for defining the natural evolution of goiter[18] and have underlined that during the goitrogenesis process the development of functioning and non-functioning nodules may be the consequence of stimulation during stress conditions. Animals fed with iodine-deficient diets developed thyroid nodules that appeared very different in size, colloid content, and ability to trap iodine. The thyroid follicles of these rats were shown by isotope imaging studies to be functionally heterogeneous in their iodine uptake and organification ability. Furthermore, follicular cell clones differ in their replicative capacities and abilities to produce thyroid hormones. More recent data may have at least in part clarified these pivotal observations. Many studies confirmed that 60 to 70% of thyroid nodules are of monoclonal origin, starting from a somatic mutation.[19] The clonal development of follicles with high replicative capacity will induce the onset of non-functioning (cold) or hyperfunctioning (hot) nodules, in which the uptake and thyroid hormone synthesis are independent from TSH stimulation.

2.5.1 FUNCTIONING THYROID NODULES

In recent years, the molecular mechanisms involved in the development of thyroid functional autonomy and hyperfunctioning thyroid nodules have been partially identified. The TSH-R or $G_{s\alpha}$ protein undergoes somatic point mutation that induces a permanent and TSH-independent activation of the adenylate–cyclase pathway. This mechanism has been demonstrated in thyroid toxic adenoma and also in hyperfunctioning nodules of multinodular goiter, adenomas (encapsulated microfollicular) and hyperplastic (non-capsulated micro- and macrofollicular) nodules. These mutations induce mutagenesis and activate function, resulting in hyperplastic and hyperfunctioning nodules.

The prevalence of TSH-R mutations and of $G_{s\alpha}$ in toxic adenomas (hot nodules) ranges in various reports (from 8 to 80% for both proteins),[19] probably as a consequence of higher prevalence in iodine-deficient areas. In patients with multiple toxic adenomatous nodules within a goiter, different somatic mutations have been identified in different nodules. There is no exact correlation between the phenotype and the genotype, probably due to the effects of extracellular growth factor on intracellular factors downstream of the TSH-R. The increase of size and function of hot nodules initially induces a slight enhancement of thyroid hormone production characterized by serum thyroid hormones within normal limits and suppressed TSH (subclinical hyperthyroidism). With the further increase of thyroid hormone production, subclinical hyperthyroidism progresses to overt in which an increased level of thyroid hormone is associated with low TSH.

Thus, in a long-standing multinodular goiter, the functional properties of the goiter may also progress from euthyroidism to a state of subclinical and then overt hyperthyroidism (Figure 2.1). Several epidemiological studies performed in Denmark have

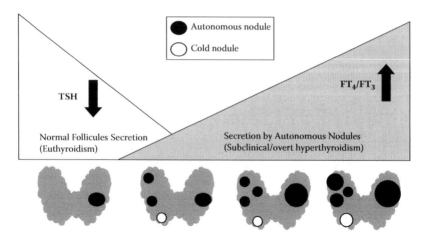

FIGURE 2.1   Development of subclinical and overt hyperthyroidism in long-standing multinodular goiter. (*Source:* Studer, H. and Derwahl, M. 1995. *Endocrinol Rev* 16: 411–426. With permission.)

clearly shown the impact of iodine nutrition on the patterns of thyroid diseases. Iodine deficiency favors the development of nodular goiter and then of toxic multinodular goiter, especially in the elderly. In iodine-sufficient populations, hypothyroidism is more frequent. Comparing the rates of hyperthyroidism and hypothyroidism in an area with low iodine intake (40 to 70 μg/day; Jutland, Denmark) with rates in an area of high iodine intake (400 to 450 μg/day; Iceland), the prevalence of hyperthyroidism was higher in Jutland and that of hypothyroidism was higher in Iceland. The most common causes of hyperthyroidism were multinodular goiter in Jutland and Graves' disease in Iceland.

In other populations living in areas with long-standing mild to moderate iodine deficiencies, the prevalences of multinodular goiter and thyroid hyperfunction are higher while that of hypothyroidism is low.[20,21] The toxic multinodular goiter is more common in the elderly living in areas with mild iodine deficiency and is therefore classified as an IDD.

2.5.2 NON-FUNCTIONING THYROID NODULES

While the pathogenetic mechanisms leading to the growth and development of functioning thyroid nodules have been clarified at least partially, much less is known about the mechanisms underlying the growth of non-functioning thyroid nodules that appear more frequently than functioning nodules. Cold thyroid nodules by definition show reduced uptake on scintiscans as a consequence of failure of iodine transport and/or organification. The nodules are grouped together only because the clinical presentation is very similar, i.e., a neck lump devoid of symptoms. However, they are very heterogeneous and demonstrate several differences in their pathogenesis and pathology.

Table 2.12 depicts a clinical–pathological classification of thyroid nodules that may be cancers, colloid nodules, or adenomas; they may be also pseudonodules that

TABLE 2.12
Clinical–Pathological
Classification of Thyroid Nodules

Benign

Hyperplastic

Adenomas (Nonfunctioning, Hyperfunctioning)

Cystic

Pseudocysts (mixed)

Malignant Nodules

Malignant thyroid tumors

Metastatic tumors

Inflammatory Nodules

Chronic autoimmune (Hashimoto's) thyroiditis

Subacute thyroiditis

Acute thyroiditis

Chronic granulomatous diseases

appear as discrete lesions on palpation but are indeed areas of higher consistency in Hashimoto's thyroiditis or areas of hyperplastic tissue in patients submitted to partial thyroidectomy.

Pathology of nodules that occur in a goiter is inhomogeneous with some nodules showing a macrofollicular pattern and others a macro- and microfollicular pattern; they are often non-capsulated (hyperplastic nodules). Isolated nodules that occur in a gland of normal size are more often capsulated and show a homogeneous micro-follicular pattern with scanty colloid content and high cellularity (adenomatous nodules). Thyroid nodules within a goiter are characterized by a macro- and micro-follicular pattern of growth and are likely to show the same pathogenetic mecha-nisms described for goiter formation in iodine deficiency areas. In the maladaptive process of goiter growth, the generalized activation of thyroid cell replication is associated with a focal increase of thyroid cell proliferation, leading to the develop-ment of thyroid nodules.

As reported above, animal models have shown that iodine deficiency increases thyroid cell activity and proliferation of cell clones that are able to replicate but unable to synthesize thyroid hormones. These events may be associated with a higher mutation rate of genes that may confer a growth advantage (TSH-R and $G_{s\alpha}$ muta-tions). According to this view, some cellular clones with gene mutations providing growth advantage could develop into cold nodules when proliferation only is induced or in functioning nodules when mutations also provide an advantage in hormone synthesis (e.g., TSH-R or G_s).

TABLE 2.13

Growth Factors and Thyroid Nodules

Stimulating Factors	Inhibiting Factors
IGF-1	TGF-β
Epidermal growth factor	IGF binding protein 1
Fibroblast growth factor	
Insulin	

All these factors act on the thyrocytes through a limited number of regulatory pathways. TSH acts through two main cascades: (1) the cyclic adenosine monophosphate (cAMP) pathway that controls expression of NIS, Tg, and TPO, proliferation, and secretion; and (2) the Ca^{++}–inositol 1,4,5 triphosphate (IP_3) cascade that controls H_2O_2 generation, iodide efflux, and secretion. Other physiological factors can activate these two cascades as well.

Other hormones and growth factors have been demonstrated to act on thyrocytes in physiological or pathological conditions (Table 2.13). To exert effects, they require the presence of specific receptors. Insulin, insulin-like growth factor 1 (IGF-1), epidermal growth factor (EGF), and fibroblast growth factor (FGF) have been shown to exert growth-stimulating effects on thyroid cells. TGF-β1 and insulin-like growth factor binding protein 1 (IGFBP-1) show growth-inhibiting activity. IGF-1, EGF, and FGF stimulate proliferation of thyroid follicular cells in vitro and the expression of thyroid growth-stimulating factors is increased in nodular goiters in humans. IGF-1 interacting with insulin receptor on thyroid follicular cells was also shown to stimulate in vitro thyroid cell proliferation. This IGF-1 activity is believed to be the main mechanism of goiter formation in patients with active acromegaly.

The simultaneous overexpression of FGF and FGF receptor in thyrocytes from multinodular goiter may explain their relative TSH independence. TGF-β1 inhibits iodine uptake, iodine organification, and Tg expression and therefore its inactivation in autonomous nodules (caused by the activation of the TSH-R) favors cell proliferation.

Although all these mechanisms and factors may contribute to the development of goiter in individual patients or families, iodine deficiency and TSH stimulation are undoubtedly the main determinants along with the individual genetic settings of genes involved in thyroid hormone synthesis and thyroid follicular cell replication. However, in areas of iodine sufficiency, non-functioning thyroid nodules are isolated lesions in the context of a normal thyroid gland. In this case, the nodules often show a monoclonal, microfollicular pattern of growth and more often are capsulated (adenomatous). It is likely that changes of signalling proteins inducing growth play a role in the development of cold adenomatous nodules. In a minority of patients, mutations in genes involved in development of thyroid cancer (such as BRAF and RAS) have been identified.[19] These data suggest that these nodules represent neoplastic lesions, eventually progressing toward malignancy.

Cold nodules are characterized by a failure in iodide transport or organification. However, NIS gene mutations or other abnormalities leading to reduced functioning of NIS and somatic mutations of the TPO gene inducing an organification defect have not been identified. On the other hand, NIS has been shown to be highly expressed even in these non-functioning adenomas, but with an abnormal intracellular localization rather than location on the apical portions of follicular cells.[22] This would suggest an altered trafficking of NIS with a reduction in its functional properties.

2.6 EPIDEMIOLOGY

Results of epidemiological studies on goiter are largely variable as a consequence of many factors, mainly environment and method of evaluation (palpation or ultrasound). Two studies were conducted in areas where iodine intake was sufficient. In the Whickham survey 15.5% of subjects had goiters, with a female:male ratio of 4.5:1. In the Framingham study, 1% of persons between 30 and 59 years had multinodular goiters revealed by palpation. In an iodine-deficient area, the goiter prevalence was 35% in the age group 12 to 14 years and about 70% in those aged 35 to 75 years.[20] The prevalence of thyroid nodule was much higher when evaluated by ultrasound: Up to 50% of the general population have thyroid nodules, even when thyroid is normal at palpation. Autopsy studies demonstrate the presence of single or multiple nodules in half the population.[23]

Few epidemiological studies have evaluated the clinical evolution of goiter. In the Whickham survey, 20% of women and 5% of men who had goiters in the initial survey showed no evidence of goiter in a follow-up survey. An average growth rate in the multinodular goiter of 5 to 20% was reported in iodine-sufficient areas. Based on the results of the Framingham survey, the estimated lifetime risk for developing a nodule is 5 to 10%. Thyroid nodule size can increase, decrease, or remain stable and thyroid nodules may eventually also disappear over time. Solid nodules more frequently increase while cystic nodules can shrink or disappear.

The rate of progression from euthyroidism to subclinical and overt hyperthyroidism is 10% during a follow-up period of 7 to 12 years. In autonomous nodules, the rate of evolution into toxic nodules is 0 to 6%. Nodule size is crucial; nodules larger than 3 cm present higher risks of developing hyperthyroidism.

2.7 CLINICAL PRESENTATION

2.7.1 SYMPTOMS

The clinical picture of goiter is related to symptoms caused by nodule growth or the development of functional autonomy. Thyroid growth induces cosmetic and pressure symptoms—functional autonomy symptoms of hypersecretion of thyroid hormones (Table 2.14). There is no clear correlation between thyroid size and function and the symptoms cited by patients. Goiter develops insidiously, especially in the elderly. A thyroid gland can easily grow outward but may also grow downward, usually into the anterior mediastinum and less commonly into the posterior mediastinum. Disfigurement is a frequent complaint related to a large goiter (Figure 2.2). Most patients with multinodular goiters have few or no symptoms. Large goitrous masses that are intrathoracic may be discovered incidentally during a chest x-ray and may have caused no symptoms. On the other hand, even small nodular goiters in cervical

TABLE 2.14
Symptoms and Signs of Goiter

Symptoms

Anterior neck mass

Cosmetic

Compression: dyspnea, stridor, cough, dysphagia

Pain, discomfort (intranodular hemorrhage)

Hyperthyroidism

Signs

Obstruction of superior vena cava (Pemberton's sign), no adenopathy

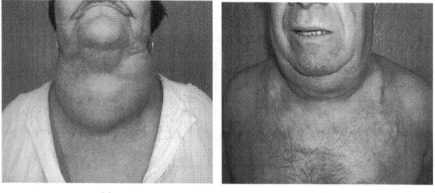

(a)   (b)

FIGURE 2.2   Patient with large non-toxic multinodular goiter (a). Patient with intrathoracic goiter causing vein compression (b).

position at the narrow thoracic inlet may cause tracheal or esophageal compression. Thyroid nodules smaller than 1.5 cm are usually asymptomatic unless intranodular hemorrhage causes pain or discomfort.

The symptoms are related to the compression of the trachea and the esophagus and are more common when a goiter has an intrathoracic extension. Dyspnea, inspiratory stridor, and cough are caused by the tracheal compression common in intrathoracic goiters (Figure 2.2). These symptoms are more apparent in a patient in a recumbent position and during exercise but can be present also at rest. Intranodular haemorrhage may precipitate airway obstruction. Esophageal compression is rarer and usually caused by an intrathoracic goiter. Transient of permanent paralysis of vocal cords can occur due to stretching or compression of laryngeal nerves by a large benign goiter or more commonly by malignant thyroid nodules, resulting in hoarseness and dyspnea, and may require laryngoscope evaluation. Phrenic nerve paralysis and Horner's syndrome due to compression of the sympathetic chain are rare and must raise the suspicion of a malignant thyroid nodule.

2.7.2 PHYSICAL EXAMINATION

The thyroid should be palpated with the patient's head leaning slightly backward. The palpation is aimed to determine thyroid size and the presence of thyroid nodule(s) and neck lymph nodes. A thyroid of normal size can be palpated, but palpation is usually feasible when its size is increased. The possibility of palpating a thyroid nodule depends on the nodule size, localization within the thyroid, neck conformation, and thyroid size. Benign thyroid nodules are usually tender, soft, smooth, and mobile. Malignant nodules may be firm, hard, irregular, and fixed. Intrathoracic extension must be suspected when the lower end of a thyroid is not palpable. Goiters are painful or tender only when recent bleeding has occurred within a nodule.

Compression or thrombosis of the jugular or subclavian veins or the superior vena cava cause facial plethora and dilated neck and upper thoracic veins. They are revealed by the Pemberton sign: When the arms are extended to touch the head, vein distension, facial plethora, cyanosis, and discomfort can be induced as a consequence of the extension of the goiter toward the mediastinum. The presence of enlarged cervical lymph nodes may be the earliest sign of a papillary thyroid carcinoma.

2.8 DIAGNOSIS

The evaluation of goiter includes laboratory investigations, imaging (ultrasound, scintigraphy, neck x-ray, computed tomography, and magnetic resonance) and fine needle cytology (FNC); see Table 2.15. Measurements of thyroid hormones and TSH are required to assess thyroid function. Ultrasound determines thyroid size, the

---

TABLE 2.15
Diagnostic Evaluation of Goiter

Laboratory
TSH
Thyroid hormones
Thyroid autoantibodies (TPOAb, TgAb)
Thyroglobulin, calcitonin

Imaging
Neck ultrasound
Scintigraphy
Radiological (x-ray, CT scan, MR imaging)

Biopsy
Fine needle cytology

---

features of palpable nodules, and the presence of non-palpable nodules. Scintigraphy reveals the functional activities of nodules and FNC shows the benign or malignant nature of the nodules. Radiological studies, in addition, may show compression on the neck or mediastinic organs.

2.8.1 Laboratory Evaluation

TSH is the most sensitive assay for assessing thyroid function. T_4 and T_3 measurements can add useful information. In the presence of endemic goiter, thyroid function is usually normal, although in the past in areas of severe iodine deficiency, findings of slightly elevated levels of serum T_3 and slightly reduced T_4 could be observed. This functional attitude is due to attempts by the thyroid to maintain the euthyroid state by reducing iodine expense. In the same areas, goiter in some individuals can be associated with a slight hypothyroidism. In areas with normal iodine intake or slight to moderate iodine deficiency, the levels of thyroid hormones and TSH are normal with the exception of patients with subclinical hyperthyroidism (functional autonomy).

In patients with non-toxic goiters, the finding of serum antithyroid autoantibodies (TPOAb and TgAb), usually at low titers, is quite common. These autoantibodies may result from focal autoimmune thyroiditis due to the antigenic stimulation induced by the goiter. The classical form of Hashimoto's thyroiditis (autoimmune thyroiditis with goiter) is characterized by high levels of TPOAb and/or TgAb and may be associated with hypothyroidism.[24] The distinction between non-toxic goiter with circulating autoantibodies and Hashimoto's thyroiditis may be only a matter of definition, devoid of any clinical relevance. However, it has been shown that among patients with euthyroidism and goiter, those who show ultrasound patterns peculiar to Hashimoto's thyroiditis (hypoechogenic, inhomogeneous tissue) have massive lymphocytic infiltration of the gland and are prone to develop hypothyroidism.

Serum thyroglobulin (Tg) levels are often elevated in the presence of nodular goiters—those with benign thyroid nodules and those with thyroid carcinoma. Thus, serum Tg is not useful to differentiate malignant from benign thyroid nodules.

Conversely, calcitonin (CT) is a marker of medullary thyroid cancer, a neoplasia with a frequency of about 1 in 200 or 1 in 300 nodules, arising from the parafollicular cells. The normal value of CT as evaluated by modern methods is <10 pg/mL. Measurable CT at low levels is not specific of medullary thyroid carcinoma and can be observed in chronic renal failure, neuroendocrine non-thyroid tumors, and Hashimoto's thyroiditis, during treatment with proton pump inhibitors and in C cell hyperplasia, which is a potentially preneoplastic lesion. When slightly elevated levels of CT are found, stimulation with pentagastrin is recommended: if levels exceed 100 pg/mL, medullary thyroid carcinoma or C cell hyperplasia must be suspected. Although not all authors agree on the routine measurement of CT in the evaluation of a thyroid nodule, it must be underlined that basal or stimulated CT levels are more sensitive than FNC for detecting medullary thyroid carcinoma.

Measurement of urinary iodine (UI), which is necessary to identify iodine deficiency in a population, does not provide useful information for a single patient with goiter.

2.8.2 Imaging

2.8.2.1 Ultrasound (US)

Thyroid US is an easy and low-cost examination. It is very useful for goiter assessment and nodule evaluation, but despite its widespread use, it often detects non-palpable thyroid nodules that are of limited clinical significance but usually require further assessment. US detects five times as many nodules as thyroid palpation; the prevalence of thyroid nodules as evaluated by US ranges from 17 to 67%.[22] As a consequence, the term *thyroid incidentaloma* is now in use.

US provides data about thyroid size, the diffuse or nodular characteristics of a goiter, the number of nodules (unimodular or multinodular goiter), and their sizes and characteristics (solid, cystic, mixed). Thyroid US is much more precise than palpation for defining thyroid size and is useful for the follow-up of patients or in epidemiological studies assessing the presence of goiter in school-age children. Thyroid volume is usually measured by the ellipsoid formula (length × width × depth × π/6). The normal upper limits are 12 mL in adult women and 18 mL in adult males. Thyroid US is also useful to assess whether a goiter is reaching into the mediastinum, locate distinct or coalescent nodules, and determine the presence and echographic patterns of lymph nodes in neck sites (see below).

US is recommended for all patients with thyroid nodules. The features suggesting malignancy of the nodule are hypoechogenicity, microcalcifications, irregular margins, absence of a halo, and a shape more tall than wide (Figures 2.3 through 2.5). However, the sensitivity of ultrasound for diagnosing malignancy of a thyroid nodule is poor because only the coexistence of more than one of these characteristics may be predictive of malignancy.

In a multinodular goiter, only the main nodules and those with suspicious US characteristics must be described in detail. US increases the diagnostic accuracy of thyroid aspiration. It is useful to identify dominant and the suspicious nodules that

Suggestive US Patterns

Benign Nodule	Malignant Nodule
Anechogenic or hyperecogenic	Hypoechogenic
Uniform, thin halo	Absent to thick, irregular halo
Regular margins	Irregular margins
Egg shell calcifications	Microcalcifications
	More tall than wide shape

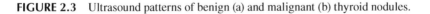

FIGURE 2.3 Ultrasound patterns of benign (a) and malignant (b) thyroid nodules.

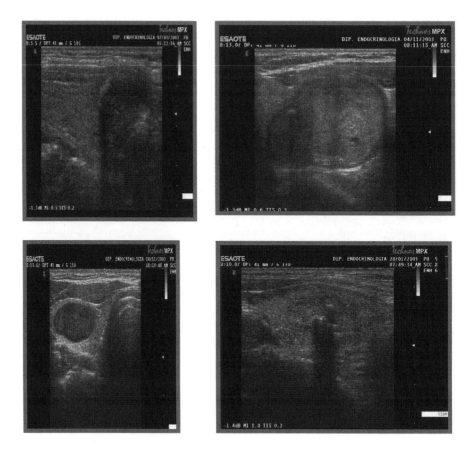

FIGURE 2.4   Ultrasound patterns of benign thyroid nodules.

should undergo aspiration and guide fine needle cytology (FNC). Color flow Doppler ultrasonography enables the study of perinodular and intranodular vascular characteristics (Figure 2.6). In malignant nodules, enhanced intranodular vascular patterns with disorganized distributions can be observed. US elastography is an adjunctive tool to differentiate malignant from benign thyroid nodules: A high elasticity indicating low stiffness is characteristic of benign nodules. A low elasticity indicating high stiffness indicates malignant nodules (Figure 2.7).[25] When a thyroid nodule is detected, the lateral and central neck lymph nodes must be also evaluated by US. Features of metastatic lymph nodes revealed by US include round shape, the loss of hyperechogenic stria corresponding to the hilum, altered echogenicity, and the presence of cystic areas (Figure 2.8).

2.8.2.2   Scintigraphy

Thyroid scans obtained with iodine isotopes (^{131}I or ^{123}I) or more commonly with pertechnate (^{99m}Tc) differentiate the cold (reduced or absent uptake) from the hot (increased uptake) nodules of a nodular goiter (Figure 2.9). Thyroid scintiscans of single or isolated nodules are indicated when TSH is subnormal to exclude a

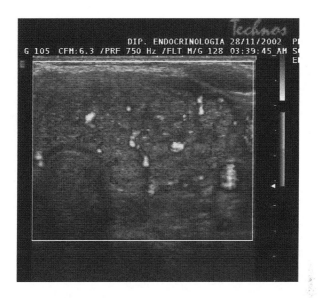

FIGURE 2.5   Ultrasound patterns of papillary thyroid carcinoma.

Thyroid US: Blood Flow

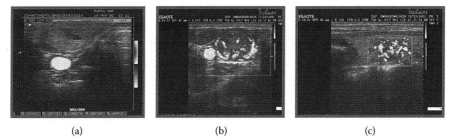

(a)   (b)   (c)

FIGURE 2.6   Color flow Doppler utrasonography of thyroid nodules. (a) Type 1 (absent blood flow). (b) Type 2 (perinodular blood flow). (c) Type 3 (intranodular blood flow).

hyperfunctioning adenoma and in multinodular goiters to identify cold nodules that require FNC and hot nodules that do not. Indeed, because a goiter is only very rarely malignant, a hyperfunctioning nodule does not need evaluation by FNC. TSH suppression by administration of LT$_4$ (levo-thyroxine) allows a better identification of autonomous nodules.

In addition, thyroid scan is required when a follicular nodule is diagnosed by FNC because functioning nodules are mostly benign. Scintigraphy is also useful to confirm the thyroid origin of a mediastinal mass shown by a thorax x-ray or CT scan. Scintigraphy performed with ^{99m}Tc may result in a falsely positive uptake in about 5% of thyroid nodules, whereas iodine isotopes do not create this problem. However, ^{99m}Tc is inexpensive and easier to use than iodine isotopes.

Thyroid US: Elastography

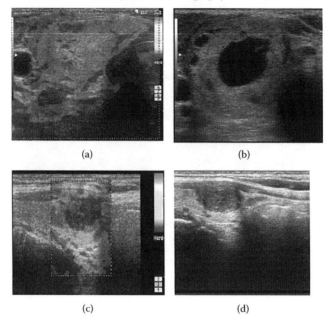

FIGURE 2.7 (a) Elastography and (b) conventional ultrasound of a thyroid nodule with elasticity score 1 (low stiffness). (c) Elastography and (d) conventional ultrasound of a thyroid nodule with elasticity score 5 (high stiffness).

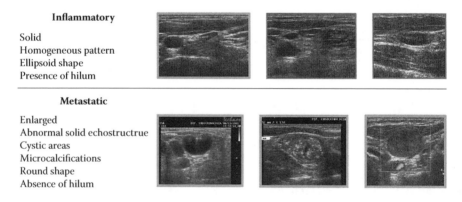

Inflammatory

Solid
Homogeneous pattern
Ellipsoid shape
Presence of hilum

Metastatic

Enlarged
Abnormal solid echostructrue
Cystic areas
Microcalcifications
Round shape
Absence of hilum

FIGURE 2.8 Neck ultrasound of inflammatory and metastatic lymph nodes.

The ^{131}I or ^{123}I uptake (RAIU) is easily performed by administering a tracer dose of radioactive iodine and then measuring the percent of administered radioactivity accumulated in the neck. In iodine-sufficient countries, the upper limit of RAIU 24 hours after administration of the tracer is around 20 to 25% and may exceed 80% in areas with mild to moderate iodine deficiency. However, RAIU has no role in the diagnosis of non-toxic goiter although it represents a mainstay of the differential

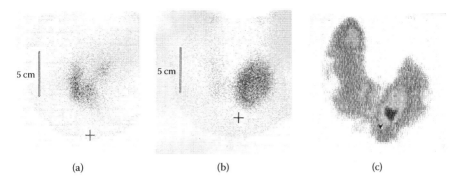

(a)   (b)   (c)

FIGURE 2.9 Thyroid scintiscan of hypofunctioning or cold nodule (a). Functioning or hot nodule (b). Multinodular goiter with hot nodule in left lobe and cold nodule in right lobe (c).

diagnosis of thyrotoxicosis. Indeed, a high RAIU readily identifies true hyperthyroidism (e.g., with thyroid hyperfunction) while a low RAIU indicates a state of thyrotoxicosis caused by either thyroidal destruction (with release of preformed hormone) or an extrathyroidal source of thyroid hormone.[26]

2.8.2.3 Radiological Evaluation

Neck radiological examination with a low penetrance beam and examination of the esophagus with a barium contrast agent enables the identification of tracheal and esophageal compressions and/or deviations (Figure 2.10). Radiological examination can also identify thyroid peripheral and large calcifications typical of benign nodules and small ones that are suspicious for carcinoma.

The pattern of calcifications is, however, not easily assessed. Chest radiography can demonstrate a mediastinal enlargement due to goiter. Computed tomography (CT) or nuclear magnetic resonance (NMR) will enable morphological evaluation of

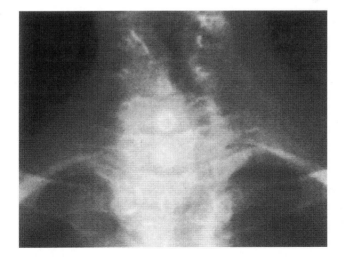

FIGURE 2.10 Neck radiograph showing tracheal deviation and compression by large goiter.

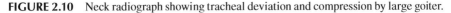

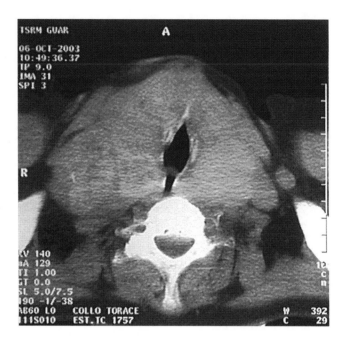

FIGURE 2.11   Computerized tomography scan of neck showing large goiter-inducing tracheal deviation and compression.

the goiter and its relation with the surrounding organs in such patients (Figure 2.11). CT and NMR have no advantage over ultrasound for assessing intrathyroidal structures but are very useful in assessing the extents of substernal goiters. The preference for CT or MR depends on availability and cost.

2.8.3   Fine Needle Cytology (FNC)

Cytological examination using fine needle biopsy can differentiate benign from malignant nodules with high sensitivity and specificity. FNC is easy to perform, well tolerated by patients, and presents no complications. Its accuracy in the diagnosis of non-functioning thyroid nodules is 95%. A plastic syringe with a 21- to 27-gauge needle is used. The needle in inserted perpendicularly to the neck surface, a negative pressure is applied until material appears in the syringe. In mixed nodules, the first aspiration should be followed by a second, on the residual solid component. After removal, the specimen is evacuated onto slides. Air drying is usually used and staining is performed with May-Giemsa-Grünwald or Papanicolaou. The cytological examination results of thyroid fine needle biopsy are classified in five diagnostic categories (Table 2.16):

Thyr 1 (non-diagnostic)—This category should constitute fewer than 15% of total samples; includes specimens defined as "inadequate" due to inappropriate preparation, fixation, or color and "non-representative" specimens containing inadequate numbers of cells. The rate of non-diagnostic cytology depends on operator and

TABLE 2.16
Cytological Categories of
Fine Needle Thyroid Biopsy

Category	Percent
Thyr 1: non-diagnostic	10–15
Thyr 2: negative	50–80
Thyr 3: indeterminate	8–20
Thyr 4: suspicious	2–5
Thyr 5: positive	1–10

cytopathologist experience, nodule characteristics, criteria determining adequacy of samples. The FNC can be repeated after a minimum of 1 month.

Thyr 2 (negative for malignant cells)—This category covers 60 to 75% of cytological examinations and includes colloid-cystic goiter, Hashimoto's thyroiditis, and subacute thyroiditis. The false negative rate is low (about 1%) and repeated FNC during follow-up (suggested particularly when nodule size increases) will further reduce this risk.

Thyr 3 (indeterminate)—This category includes 20% of cytological exams and comprises the follicular and the oxyphilic (or Hürthle) nodules. When a thyroid scan shows a cold nodule, thyroidectomy is advised to establish the diagnosis by histological assessment. At histological examination, about 80% represent benign and 20% represent malignant lesions, mainly the follicular variant of papillary thyroid carcinoma. Some immunocytochemical markers can increase the diagnostic accuracy but at present do not hold a predictive value of certainty. If scintigraphy shows that a solitary indeterminate nodule is hyperfunctioning or TSH is suppressed, the nodule is almost never malignant and surgery can be avoided.

Thyr 4 (suspicious for malignancy)—This category represents a heterogeneous group of lesions that contain too few cells or true cytological atypiae and are insufficient for an unambiguous diagnosis of malignancy. It comprises about 5% of cytological exams.

Thyr 5 (positive for malignant cells)—About 10% of cytological exams fall into this category that includes specimens unequivocally diagnostic for papillary, medullary, anaplastic carcinoma, lymphoma, and metastatic neoplasia. US-guided FNC increases significantly the adequacy of the material aspirated.

All lateral neck lymph nodes with suspicious characteristics must undergo FNC. In addition to cytological evaluation, Tg and CT must be measured in the washing liquid of the needle in order to diagnose a metastatic lymph nodule from a thyroid cancer originating from follicular or parafollicular thyroid cells, respectively.

2.8.4 DIFFERENTIAL DIAGNOSIS

At the anamnestic evaluation and physical examination, it is relevant to ascertain the period of the onset of the goiter. A long-standing goiter whose size has remained unchanged during the years is presumably benign, while a large goiter that develops at puberty is likely dyshormonogenetic. A fast and sudden increase of the size of a goiter, with associated strong pain and local dolorability is typical of an intranodular hemorrhage. In these patients, the differential diagnosis is subacute thyroiditis, characterized by neck pain, fever, slight and transient symptoms of thyrotoxicosis and a previous febrile episode, and an anaplastic tumor of the thyroid (pain is absent), and the neck mass is hard and rapidly growing.

2.9 TREATMENT

Despite iodization programs, nodular goiter still constitutes a major therapeutic challenge: No treatment can be considered ideal. Surgical treatment is advised in patients with compression symptoms if the patients are disturbed by the appearance of goiter (Table 2.17)[23] and in cases where nodules are suspicious for cancer. Clinical observation or medical treatment can be proposed if thyroid enlargement is moderate, the patient is euthyroid, and no symptoms are present. For patients who refuse surgery, the non-surgical treatment options are LT_4 and ^{131}I (Table 2.18). Percutaneous interventional therapy (laser photocoagulation and ethanol injection) has been proposed as an alternative to surgery for benign thyroid nodules.

TABLE 2.17
Common Indications for Surgical Treatment of Multinodular Goiter

Progressive growth of goiter or individual nodular lesions

Suspicion of malignancy at fine needle aspiration

Compression symptoms and signs of trachea, esophagus, recurrent laryngeal nerve, or cervical veins

Unacceptable aesthetic disfigurement

TABLE 2.18
Non-Surgical Treatment of Multinodular Goiter

Treatment	Indication
LT_4	Intended in young- and middle-aged patients to prevent growth and appearances of new nodules, especially in borderline low iodine intake regions
^{131}I	In elderly patients with high surgical risks and cardiopulmonary disease or when surgery is refused
rhTSH + ^{131}I	In patients with large goiters or goiters with low RAIU and cold areas at scintigraphy
Percutaneous ethanol injection	In cystic or prevalently cystic nodules
Laser thermal ablation	Patients with pressure symptoms or cosmetic concerns who decline surgery

2.9.1   IODINE PROPHYLAXIS AND PREVENTION OF GOITER

In many countries, iodine deficiency contributes to a large extent to the high prevalence of diffuse and nodular goiter. This prevalence has been reduced by eliminating iodine deficiency. The most effective method to improve iodine nutrition is through salt iodization, because everyone consumes salt. The addition of iodine is simple and inexpensive and does not change salt taste. However, the iodization of all salt for human and livestock consumption (universal salt iodination or USI) is not commonly achieved.

Iodine is added to kitchen salt at a level of 20 to 40 mg/kg of salt in the form of potassium iodide (KI) or potassium iodate (KIO_3). The fortification with iodine of baker's salt, drinking water, and irrigation water has been used but this method is less practical. When iodization of water is not feasible, iodine can be added to oil. Iodized oil can be administered orally or by intramuscular injection (200 to 400 mg of iodine per year). Iodine can be also given as KI (30 mg monthly) or KIO_3.

In areas where a salt iodization program covering at least 90% of households has been sustained at least 2 years and the median UI indicates iodine sufficiency, there is no need to supplement pregnant and lactating women.[27] In other areas, women should be provided with an intake of at least 150 µg/day of iodine for a long period before conception to restore intrathyroidal stores and ensure a better maternal thyroid function.[28] During pregnancy and lactation, 200 to 250 µg/day should be provided via multivitamin pills containing the correct amount of iodine. Controlled interventions in areas of severe iodine deficiency have shown that iodine supplementation, particularly when given before or early in pregnancy can prevent goiter formation in pregnant women and neurological deficits and also reduce infant mortality.

Iodine supplementation has been clearly shown to prevent the increase in thyroid volume that frequently accompanies pregnancy in women living in iodine-deficient areas. A prospective randomized trial performed to assess the usefulness of iodine supplementation in pregnant women living in a marginally iodine-deficient area showed that 50 µg of iodide per day was a safe and effective measure for preventing thyroid enlargement during pregnancy. A dose of 200 µg per day was even more effective.[29]

After the introduction of iodine prophylaxis, increased incidence of hyperthyroidism was observed. This is due to the development of iodine-induced thyrotoxicosis in subjects with preexisting autonomous multinodular goiter. The condition is transient and correlated to the level of iodine deficiency and the amount of iodine administered. After the initial increase, the incidence of toxic multinodular goiter falls below that observed before the introduction of iodine prophylaxis.

Iodine in pharmacological doses has also been used in the past as a treatment of patients with non-toxic goiter, especially in endemic areas, and has been shown to be effective in reducing goiter size in some individuals. The use of pharmacological doses of iodine as a treatment of multinodular goiter has been abandoned because of its potential for favoring the development of hyperthyroidism that is especially harmful in elderly subjects with nodular goiter and autonomous thyroid function.

2.9.2 Medical Treatment

The only available medical treatment for non-toxic goiter is synthetic LT_4 that reduces TSH secretion and its stimulus of goiter enlargement.[23] In controlled trials, LT_4 therapy was shown to decrease by 15 to 40% thyroid volume measured by ultrasound in non-toxic diffuse goiter. The question of whether LT_4 is an effective treatment for non-toxic nodular goiter has been approached in many studies, most of which focused on its efficacy for reducing the volume of solitary nodules in patients residing in non-endemic areas rather than in patients with multinodular goiters.

The significance of many of these studies is hampered by several limitations including the lack of appropriate methodology (e.g., absence of ultrasonography). In a multicenter, randomized, double-blind, placebo-controlled trial in a European area of borderline iodine sufficiency, patients treated with LT_4 therapy displayed greater reductions in nodule size than controls after 18 months of follow-up.[30] In this study LT_4 treatment was also able to prevent the development of additional nodules. In a long-term study, significant nodular growth was observed in untreated patients followed for 5 years of clinical observation, while LT_4 treatment prevented the appearance of new nodules and increases in the number of nodules and thyroid volume in a control group, clearly indicating that TSH suppression affects the natural history of thyroid nodules.[31]

The degree of serum TSH suppression has been documented in a placebo-controlled, randomized crossover trial that showed that that high level (< 0.1 mU/L) and low level (0.4 to 0.6 mU/L) TSH suppressions were equally effective in reducing thyroid nodule size.[32] A recent guideline does not recommend routine LT_4 therapy, but suggests iodine supplementation or LT_4 in young patients with small nodular goiters and no evidence of thyroid autonomy.[33,34]

It has been recently reported that higher TSH values, even within normal ranges, are associated with a greater risk of thyroid malignancy; the development of thyroid autonomy by reducing TSH levels decreases the frequency of papillary thyroid cancer (PTC) in patients with nodular goiter.[35] In addition, in patients with nodular goiter, treatment with LT_4 is responsible for a reduction of serum TSH and is associated with a decreased frequency of PTC.[36] Further prospective studies are needed to determine whether these observation may have importance in clinical practice.

2.9.2.1 Side Effects

LT_4 treatment may induce subclinical thyrotoxicosis that requires careful monitoring in long-term treatment. Adverse effects involving the cardiovascular system (elevated heart rate and arrhythmias, particularly atrial fibrillation) are potential risk factors for cardiovascular morbidity, especially in elderly patients.[37] TSH suppression induced by LT_4 treatment probably does not affect bone density in men and premenopausal women but may accelerate bone turnover in postmenopausal patients.[37]

2.9.2.2 Main Indications

LT_4 therapy is most likely to be effective in young and middle-aged patients with non-toxic diffuse or multinodular goiters with nodules that are predominantly solid and contain abundant colloid.[23] The degree of the reduction of the size of a goiter is more relevant in recently developed, tender, non-fibrotic goiters and in younger patients. The major goal of LT_4 treatment is to prevent growth and the appearance of new nodular lesions, especially in patients from regions of the world where iodine intake is borderline or low. Pregnancy and lactation stimulate thyroid activity and do not contraindicate the treatment. It is not advisable to start the treatment in patients older than 50 years or maintain it after the age of 55 to 60[23] due to the potential risk of functional autonomy and because elderly subjects and postmenopausal women are more prone to the effects of subclinical hyperthyroidism. Before starting LT_4 treatment, all subjects should have their TSH and thyroid hormones measured to exclude functional autonomy and hyperthyroidism.

LT_4 must be taken in the morning, while fasting, with a starting low dose that must be gradually increased up to the maintaining dose (usually 1.4 to 1.6 μg/kg body weight). Administration of LT_4 at bedtime has recently been proposed.[38]

The aim of the treatment is a TSH level around the lower limit of normal range (0.4 to 0.6 U/L) or partially suppressed (0.1 to 0.4 U/L), while keeping thyroid hormones in the normal range. To check the adequacy of the dose, thyroid hormones and TSH values must be measured not earlier than 3 to 4 months after the start or modification of the LT_4 treatment. A TSH level <0.1 U/L indicates pharmacological thyrotoxicosis.

In multinodular goiter with functional autonomy antithyroid treatment can normalize thyroid function but cannot induce the remission of the disease. Therefore, surgical or ^{131}I treatment is usually advised.

2.9.3 RADIOIODINE THERAPY

Radioiodine has been used for over 60 years to treat clinical and subclinical hyperthyroidism due to Graves' disease or toxic multinodular goiter.[23] The effectiveness of ^{131}I in reducing thyroid size is widely recognized and its use has been extended to symptomatic multinodular goiter. Significant shrinkage results after ^{131}I treatment in patients affected by non-toxic multinodular goiter. Following ^{131}I treatment, an overall decrease of thyroid volume of 34 to 40% after 12 months and 50 to 60% after 2 to 5 years has been reported. Half of the effect is obtained within the first 3 months and a second ^{131}I dose may cause additional thyroid volume reduction. The administered dose of ^{131}I is a determinant of goiter reduction and the outcome of ^{131}I treatment is inversely related to goiter size.

[131]I has been shown to be effective in treatment of large goiters (>100 to 150 ml). A significant volume reduction without any initial clinically significant tracheal compression was observed and the tracheal cross-sectional area improved after 1 year. A transient increase of serum thyroid hormone was observed in a substantial minority of patients during the first 2 weeks after ^{131}I therapy, returning to baseline at 3 weeks. Radiation thyroiditis with tenderness of the neck and slight thyrotoxic symptoms develop in the first 2 weeks after ^{131}I treatment in 4% of patients. Graves-like hyperthyroidism occurs in 5% of patients.

A late effect is the development of hypothyroidism. The long-term risk of extrathyroidal malignancy following ^{131}I therapy for patients with hyperthyroidism has been the object of several studies and is still debated. In a large study series carried out on hyperthyroid patients followed up for a mean of 21 years, ^{131}I treatment was not linked to total cancer death.[39] Although specific long-term studies for ^{131}I treatment for non-toxic multinodular goiter are not available, previous experience supports its safety.

[131]I is the treatment of choice for middle-aged and elderly patients and in the presence of nodules smaller than 4 cm that do not compress the near organs and induce subclinical hyperthyroidism. [131]I can be a valid therapeutic option when thyroidectomy is refused or contraindicated because of old age or the presence of concomitant severe diseases.

2.9.3.1   Radioiodine Treatment with rhTSH Prestimulation

A major hindrance in the use of conventional ^{131}I therapy in non-toxic multinodular goiter is the frequent finding of a low thyroid RAIU and non-functioning (cold) area with thyroid scintigraphy. RhTSH increases thyroid RAIU more than twofold and increases iodine concentrations in areas that were previously cold. Although the use of rhTSH prestimulation for ^{131}I treatment in non-toxic multinodular goiter is off-label, different clinical trials have shown its efficacy. rhTSH enhances ^{131}I uptake, permitting a decrease of radiation in the treatment of multinodular goiter.

In randomized controlled trials, rhTSH has been documented to enhance the goiter volume reduction by 35 to 65% when standard ^{131}I therapy is used.[40] Another approach is to reduce the administered ^{131}I activity with a factor corresponding to the increase in RAIU obtained by rhTSH stimulation. The effect is proportional to the dose of rhTSH administered.[41]

2.9.4   SURGICAL TREATMENT

Surgical treatment is advised for a uninodular or multinodular goiter with mediastinal development or compression or when malignant neoplasia is suspected (Table 2.17). The presence of thyroid nodules per se is not an indication for surgery unless large nodules or compressive symptoms are present and thyroid nodules enlarge during LT_4 treatment.

In cases of large diffuse or multinodular goiters, total or subtotal thyroidectomy is advised. For a single nodule, lobectomy or hemythyroidectomy is advised. When a thyroidectomy is performed by an expert surgeon, complications such as palsy of the recurrent laryngeal nerve and transient or permanent hypoparathyroidism are rare. After thyroidectomy LT_4 treatment is advised to prevent goiter recurrence.

Surgical treatment is mandatory when thyroid cytology is positive or suspicious for thyroid carcinoma and is also indicated in most patients that exhibit indeterminate cytology in which histology is required to exclude the presence of the carcinoma.

2.9.5   ULTRASOUND-GUIDED MINIMALLY INVASIVE PROCEDURES

2.9.5.1   Percutaneous Ethanol Injection

Ultrasound-guided percutaneous ethanol injection is advised for the treatment of cystic or mixed (with a prevalent cystic component) thyroid nodules. It is not recommended for solid thyroid nodules, whether hyperfunctioning or not, or for multinodular goiter.[33,34] This procedure is minimally invasive, does not require local anaesthesia, and is well tolerated by patients. After treatment, a patient may complain of cervical pain that can be easily controlled by analgesics. Subcutaneous or intrathyroid hemorrhage and hoarseness are rare.

2.9.5.2 Thermal Ablation with Radiofrequency

Thermal ablation with radiofrequency (RFA) has been proposed for the debulking of large benign thyroid nodules.[33,34] RFA is based on the percutaneous insertion of large needle electrodes (14- to 18-gauge) or hook needles and is usually performed under conscious sedation. Because of some disadvantages and the absence of prospective randomized trials, RFA is currently not recommended for routine management of benign thyroid nodules.

2.9.5.3 Laser Thermal Ablation

US-guided percutaneous laser thermal ablation (PLA) is a minimally invasive procedure, performed under local anesthesia, and is well tolerated. This technique allows the use of small (21-gauge) and multiple (up to four) needles. In the few patients treated by this technique to date, no permanent dysphonia, cutaneous burning, or damage to the vital structures of the neck has been reported.

The treatment is performed on an outpatient basis, is inexpensive, and takes only 30 minutes. After PLA, the patients may return home; the persistence of cervical pain can be controlled by a 2-day course of orally administered analgesics or corticosteroids. In most patients with thyroid nodules, one to three sessions of PLA or a single treatment with multiple fibers induces a clinically significant decrease in nodule volume and the amelioration of local symptoms. Two randomized trials have confirmed PLA's safety and clinical efficacy.[42]

Because of the novelty of the PLA technique, long-term follow-up studies are lacking. PLA should be performed only by experienced operators and at present is restricted to its use on patients with pressure symptoms or cosmetic concerns who decline surgery or are at surgical risk. However, it is expected that in the future the indications of PLA will be extended in terms of type of nodularity (dominant nodule in multinodular goiter, functioning thyroid nodule) and patient features.

REFERENCES

1. Glinoer, D. 2004. The regulation of thyroid function during normal pregnancy: importance of the iodine nutrition status. *Best Pract Res Clin Endocrinol Metab* 19: 133–152.
2. International Council for Control of Iodine Deficiency Disorders. 2008. UNICEF Report 2008. *IDD Newsl* 30 (4).
3. Vitti, P., Delange, F., Pinchera, A. et al. 2003. Europe is iodine deficient. *Lancet* 361: 9364: 1226.
4. Zimmermann, M.B. and Andersson, M. 2011. Prevalence of iodine deficiency in Europe in 2010. *Ann Endocrinol* 72: 164–166.
5. Vanderpump, M.P., Lazarus, J.H., Smyth, P.P. et al. 2011. Iodine status of UK schoolgirls: a cross-sectional survey. *Lancet* 377: 9782: 2007.

6. Vitti, P. and Aghini-Lombardi, F. 2011. The effect of 15 years voluntary iodine prophylaxis through iodized salt in a small rural community: the Pescopagano experience. *Ann Endocrinol (Paris)* 72: 162–163.
7. World Health Organization, UNICEF, and ICCIDD. 2007. *Assessment of Iodine Deficiency Disorders and Monitoring Their Elimination*, 3rd ed. Geneva.
8. Spitzweg, C. and Morris, J.C. 2010. Genetics and phenomics of hypothyroidism and goiter due to NIS mutations. *Mol Cell Endocrinol* 322: 56–63.
9. Bizhanova, A. and Kopp, P. 2010. Genetics and phenomics of Pendred syndrome. *Mol Cell Endocrinol* 322: 83–90.
10. Ris-Stalpers, C. and Bikker, H. 2010. Genetics and phenomics of hypothyroidism and goiter due to TPO mutations. *Mol Cell Endocrinol* 322: 38–43.
11. Grasberger, H. 2010. Defects of thyroidal hydrogen peroxide generation in congenital hypothyroidism. *Mol Cell Endocrinol* 322: 99–106.
12. Targovnik, H.M., Esperante, S.A., and Rivolta, C.M. 2010. Genetics and phenomics of hypothyroidism and goiter due to thyroglobulin mutations. *Mol Cell Endocrinol* 322: 44–55.
13. Moreno, J.C. and Visser, T.J. 2010. Genetics and phenomics of hypothyroidism and goiter due to iodotyrosine deiodinase (DHEAL1) gene mutations. *Mol Cell Endocrinol* 322: 91–98.
14. Gozu, H.I., Lublinghoff, J., Bircan, R. et al. 2010. Genetics and phenomics of inherited and sporadic non-autoimmune hyperthyroidism. *Mol Cell Endocrinol* 322: 125–134.
15. Bayer, Y., Neumann, S., Meyer, B. et al. 2004. Genome-wide linkage analysis reveals evidence for four new susceptibility loci for familial euthyroid goiter. *J Clin Endocrinol Metab* 89: 4044–4052.
16. Medeiros-Neto, G. and Knobel, M. 2010. Iodine deficiency disorders. In *Endocrinology*, DeGroot, L.J. and Jameson, J.S., Eds. New York: Elsevier, 1650–1667.
17. Leung, A.M., Pearce, E.N., and Braverman, L.E. 2010. Perchlorate, iodine and the thyroid. *Best Pract Res Clin Endocrinol Metab* 24: 133–141.
18. Studer, H., Peter, H.J., and Gerber, H. 1989. Natural heterogeneity of thyroid cells: the basis for understanding thyroid function and nodular goiter growth. *Endocrinol Rev.* 10: 125–135.
19. Krohn, K., Fuhrer, D., Bayer, M. et al. 2005. Molecular pathogenesis of euthyroid and toxic multinodular goiter. *Endocrinol Rev* 26: 504–524.
20. Aghini-Lombardi, F., Antonangeli, L., Martino, E. et al. 1999. The spectrum of thyroid disorders in an iodine-deficient community: the Pescopagano survey. *J Clin Endocrinol Metab* 84: 561–566.
21. Teng, W., Shan, Z., Teng, X. et al. 2006. Effect of iodine intake on thyroid diseases in China. *New Engl J Med* 354: 2783–2793.
22. Dohan, O., la De, V., Paroder, V. et al. 2003. The sodium/iodide symporter (NIS): characterization, regulation, and medical significance. *Endocrinol Rev* 24: 48–77.
23. Hegedus, L., Bonnema, S.J., and Bennedbaek, F.N. 2003. Management of simple nodular goiter: current status and future perspectives. *Endocrinol Rev* 24: 102–132.
24. Latrofa, F. and Pinchera, A. 2008. Autoimmune hypothyroidism. In *Autoimmune Diseases in Endocrinology*, Weetman, A.P., Ed. Totowa, NJ: Humana Press, 136–174.
25. Rago, T., Santini, F., Scutari, M. et al. 2007. Elastography: new developments in ultrasound for predicting malignancy in thyroid nodules. *J Clin Endocrinol Metab* 92: 2917–2922.
26. Latrofa, F., Vitti, P., and Pinchera, A. 2011. Causes and laboratory investigations of thyrotoxicosis. In *Oxford Textbook of Endocrinology and Diabetes,* 2nd ed. Wass, J.A.H. and Shalet, S., Eds. Oxford: Oxford University Press, 468–477.
27. Zimmermann, M.B. 2009. Iodine deficiency. *Endocr Rev* 30: 376–408.

28. Moleti, M., Lo Presti, V., Campolo, M.C. et al. 2008. Iodine prophylaxis using iodized salt and risk of maternal thyroid failure in conditions of mild iodine deficiency. *J Clin Endocrinol Metab* 93: 2616–2621.

29. Antonangeli, L., Maccherini, D., Cavaliere, R. et al. 2002. Comparison of two different doses of iodide in the prevention of gestational goiter in marginal iodine deficiency: a longitudinal study. *Eur J Endocrinol* 147: 29–34.

30. Wemeau, J.L., Caron, P., Schvartz, C. et al. 2002. Effects of thyroid-stimulating hormone suppression with levothyroxine in reducing the volume of solitary thyroid nodules and improving extranodular nonpalpable changes: a randomized, double-blind, placebo-controlled trial by the French Thyroid Research Group. *J Clin Endocrinol Metab* 87: 4928–4934.

31. Papini, E., Petrucci, L., Guglielmi, R. et al. 1998. Long-term changes in nodular goiter: a 5-year prospective randomized trial of levothyroxine suppressive therapy for benign cold thyroid nodules, *J Clin Endocrinol Metab* 83: 780–783.

32. Koc, M., Ersoz, H.O., Akpinar, I., Gogas-Yavuz, D., Deyneli, O., Akalin, S. 2002. Effect of low- and high-dose levothyroxine on thyroid nodule volume: a crossover placebo-controlled trial. *Clin Endocrinol (Oxf)* 57: 621–628.

33. Gharib, H., Papini, E., Paschke, R. et al. 2010. American Association of Clinical Endocrinologists, Associazione Medici Endocrinologi, and European Thyroid Association medical guidelines for clinical practice for the diagnosis and management of thyroid nodules. *J Endocrinol Invest* 33 (5): 1–50.

34. Gharib, H., Papini, E., Paschke, R. et al. 2010. American Association of Clinical Endocrinologists, Associazione Medici Endocrinologi, and European Thyroid Association medical guidelines for clinical practice for the diagnosis and management of thyroid nodules: executive summary of recommendations. *J Endocrinol Invest* 33 (5): 51–56.

35. Fiore, E., Rago, T., Provenzale, M.A. et al. 2009. Lower levels of TSH are associated with a lower risk of papillary thyroid cancer in patients with thyroid nodular disease: thyroid autonomy may play a protective role. *Endocr Rel Cancer* 16: 1251–1260.

36. Fiore, E., Rago, T., Provenzale, M.A. et al. 2010. L-thyroxine-treated patients with nodular goiter have lower serum TSH and lower frequency of papillary thyroid cancer: results of a cross-sectional study on 27,914 patients. *Endocrinol Rel Cancer* 17: 231–239.

37. Biondi, B. and Cooper, D.S. 2008. The clinical significance of subclinical thyroid dysfunction. *Endocrinol Rev* 29: 76–131.

38. Bolk, N., Visser, T.J., Nijman, J. et al. 2010. Effects of evening versus morning levothyroxine intake: a randomized double-blind crossover trial. *Arch Int Med* 170: 1996–2003.

39. Ron, E., Doody, M.M., Becker, D.V. et al. 1998. Cancer mortality following treatment for adult hyperthyroidism. Cooperative Thyrotoxicosis Therapy Follow-Up Study Group. *JAMA* 280: 347–355.

40. Nielsen, V.E., Bonnema, S.J., Boel-Jorgensen, H. et al. 2006. Stimulation with 0.3 mg recombinant human thyrotropin prior to iodine 131 therapy to improve the size reduction of benign nontoxic nodular goiter: a prospective randomized double-blind trial. *Arch Int Med* 166: 1476–1482.

41. Graf, H., Fast, S., Pacini, F. et al. 2011. Modified-release recombinant human TSH (MRrhTSH) augments the effect of ^{131}I therapy in benign multinodular goiter: results from a multicenter international, randomized, placebo-controlled study. *J Clin Endocrinol Metab* 96: 1368–1376.

42. Papini, E., Guglielmi, R., Bizzari, G. et al. 2007. Treatment of benign cold thyroid nodules: a randomized clinical trial of percutaneous laser ablation versus levothyroxine therapy or follow-up. *Thyroid* 17: 229–235.

3 Acute Suppurative, Subacute, and Riedel's Thyroiditis

Serafino Lio

CONTENTS

Key words: acute suppurative thyroiditis; subacute (de Quervain, granulomatous) thyroiditis; Riedel's (invasive fibrous) thyroiditis, transient hyperthyroidism; transient hypothyroidism; permanent hypothyroidism.

3.1   ACUTE THYROIDITIS

3.1.1   DEFINITION

Acute suppurative thyroiditis is a rare infectious disease, affecting children, elders and immunologically impaired adults caused by bacterial, fungal, or parasitic organisms. The thyroid gland presents pyogenic and necrotic inflammation with septic clinical manifestations.

3.1.2   EPIDEMIOLOGY

Suppurative thyroiditis is a rare condition, far less common than other forms of thyroiditis; it has a prevalence in the general population of 0.04%[1] and represents 0.1 to 0.7% of all thyroid disease. Only a few hundred cases are reported in the literature. It is more frequent in children.[2] No gender predilection is present; the female:male ratio is 1:1.

3.1.3   ETIOPATHOGENESIS

The thyroid gland is, in general, resistant to infection. This resistance has been attributed to the protective role of the thyroid capsule that anatomically isolates the gland from the other nearby neck structures and to the rich lymphatic drainage and blood supply. Moreover, the high iodine concentration and hydrogen peroxide present create an unfavorable environment for microorganism growth (Table 3.1).

Infectious thyroiditis most likely occurs in children with congenital anomalies, in patients with preexisting thyroid diseases (remnants of thyroglossal duct, diffuse and multinodular goiter, Hashimoto's thyroiditis, thyroid carcinoma), in frail elders, in immunosuppressed patients, and in patients with human immunodeficiency virus (HIV) infection and acquired immunodeficiency syndrome (AIDS). Thyroid gland involvement can occur also through the bloodstream or lymphatic system or by direct

TABLE 3.1

Predisposing Factors and Sources of Infection in Acute Suppurative Thyroiditis

Factors	Sources
Children with congenital neck anomalies	Blood and lymphatic spread
Preexisting thyroid disease (remnant thyroglossal duct)	Adjacent site (tonsillitis, pharyngitis, otitis, parotitis, mastoiditis, lymphoadenitis)
Simple and multinodular goiters	Direct trauma (thyroid surgery, fine needle aspiration, perforated esophagus)
Hashimoto's thyroiditis	
Carcinoma	Pyriform sinus fistulae (especially left), cysts
Frail elderly	Third and fourth bronchial pouches
Immunosuppressed (AIDS, chemotherapy)	

spread from an adjacent site. Spread of an infection from the skin, urinary tract, and gastrointestinal tract can be also responsible.

Very rarely has suppurative thyroiditis been reported as a complication of thyroid surgery or fine needle aspiration[3] or resulting from perforation of the esophagus by chicken bone ingestion,[4]

In children and adolescents, remnant thyroglossal ducts or fistulas from the pyriform sinus are common sources of bacteria. In adults, a recurrent form of suppurative thyroiditis due to a fourth branchial pouch fistula has been described. From the apex of the pyriform left sinus (in human, the right sinus atrophies early), the formation of a fistula runs anteroinferiorly and ends blindly in the perithyroid tissues or in the thyroid gland. Thus, infections of the retro- and lateral pharyngeal spaces (pharyngitis, tonsillitis, parotitis, mastoiditis, and otitis) and upper respiratory infections with possible fistula abscesses can cause a secondary suppurative infection of the thyroid gland. This mechanism has been described for recurrent suppurative thyroiditis in children (during the first decade of life) but rarely in adulthood.

Virtually any microorganism can infect the thyroid gland. Many aerobic bacteria such as *Streptococcus hemolyticus, pneumoniae,* and *viridians; Staphylococcus aureus* and *epidermidis; Klebsiella; Haemophilus influenzae; Salmonella typhi, parathyphi,* and *brandenburg; Escherichia coli; Pseudomonas aeruginosa; Serratia; Acinobacter* and *Pasteurella* and anaerobic bacteria such as *Eikenella corrodens* and *Fusobacterium mortiferum* have been recognized as causative agents. Infections by *Mycobacterium tuberculosis* associated with disseminated or miliary disease, *Mycobacterium chelo*nei and avian intracellular infections are seldom reported. Fungal agents such as *Candida albicans, Nocardia, Aspergillus, Actinomyces, Coccidioides immitis, Cryptococcus neoformans, Histoplasma capsulatum, Blastomyces dermatidis,* and *Allescheria boydii* cause suppurative thyroiditis, more often in patients treated with glucocorticoid therapy. The infection can be also due to parasitic infections as *Strongyloides stercoralis, Taenia solium, Cysticercus, Echinococcus,* and *Pneumocystis carinii* (in patients with AIDS or malignancies) and is very rarely due to *syphilitic bacteria.* Polymicrobial infection is present in 12 to 30% of cases.

3.1.4 PATHOPHYSIOLOGY

The infection of the thyroid induces the typical signs of inflammatory process designated in Latin as "rubor, calor, tumor, and functio laesa" (blush, heat, swelling, and functional harm). Inflammation is characterized by colliquative necrosis and abscess formation often without thyroid function modifications. In the more aggressive cases, formation of fistulas with propagation to surrounding tissues is observed.

3.1.5 CLINICAL SIGNS AND SYMPTOMS

Most cases arise from pharyngitis, tonsillitis and/or upper respiratory tract infection with symptoms and signs of a suppurative infection. The pain in the anterior neck is the first and predominant symptom (Table 3.2). It is acute and may radiate to the ear or homolateral lower jaw of the side of infection and worsens with neck movements, swallowing, and cough.

A single lobe (more frequently the left in 90%, the right in 6 to 8%, and bilateral in 2% of cases) is usually involved with unilateral or bilateral firm enlargement. Tenderness and local compression resulting in dysphagia and dysphonia are also present. Local observations include erythema, chills, and warmth. Very high fever occurs, often associated with features of typical sepsis. After 1 to 3 days, fluctuation of nodules indicates abscess formation and a fistula may develop. Regional laterocervical lymph nodes may be present. Sometimes homolateral ptosis occurs and involves the sympathetic system. The thyroid function is normal in over two-thirds of patients; a thyrotoxic phase at the beginning of the disease is rarely present.[5]

3.1.6 DIAGNOSIS

Acute anterior neck pain that radiates to the ear or lower jaw, worsened by neck movements, swallowing, and cough is a typical clinical feature at the beginning. In acute and subacute thyroiditis, the local signs are similar but systemic manifestations are more severe, with high fever and chills in the acute form, whereas clinical signs and symptoms of thyrotoxicosis are often present in the subacute cases. In persistence of congenital pyriform sinus fistula, the left lobe of the thyroid is involved and the recurrence of suppurative thyroiditis is frequent (Table 3.2).

TABLE 3.2

Clinical Features of Acute Suppurative Thyroiditis

Epidemiology	Rare (0.04% in general population; 0.1 to 0.7% of all thyroid diseases)
Age and sex	Any age; 1:1 male:female ratio
Signs and symptoms	High fever, neck pain neck radiating to ear or mandible homolaterally and worsened by movement (swallowing or cough); unilateral (left) lobe involvement; fluctuation of abscess and fistula possible; tenderness with local compression (dysphonia, dysphagia); local erythema; lymphadenopathy; ptosis, rare

---

The clinical diagnosis is confirmed by laboratory tests. High C-reactive protein (CRP) and erythrocyte sedimentation rate (ESR) and leukocyte counts are present in acute and subacute types of thyroiditis. In the acute form the thyroid function test (TSH) is normal. The determination of thyroid autoantibodies is indicated only after the recovery from inflammation. Screening for HIV is suggested in immune-depressed patients. Ultrasonography (US) examination of the neck is the mandatory imaging investigation. It shows localized involvement of the thyroid gland with single or multiple hypoechogenic areas confluent at the beginning and anechoic areas in the presence of abscess. Ultrasound examination is helpful to detect spreads to near structures and draining of abscess if present.

Fine needle aspiration (FNA) biopsy is essential, especially in solitary nodules to obtain samples for cytology; the cytology shows the presence of polymorpho-nuclear leukocytes, histiocytes, lymphocytes, and cellular debris. This procedure is contraindicated if *Echinococcus* infection is suspected. Gram and Gomori stains, culture for aerobic and anaerobic bacteria, fungi, and other microorganism and relative antibiotic sensitivity tests are useful. A thyroid scan in a patient with suppurative thyroiditis shows a normal uptake while it is very low in subacute thyroiditis.

Computed tomography (CT) of the neck can be useful in the early phase of acute suppurative thyroiditis to identify pyriform sinus fistula when the clinical course suggests the extension of thyroid abscess. CT can also exclude the possibility of cervical abscess outside the thyroid capsule. A CT scan of the neck shows hypodense areas. Radiography of the neck is useful for detecting soft tissue gas produced by anaerobia bacteria and calcifications often due to the involvement of *Pneumocystis carinii* or *Echinococcus*. An esophagram should be performed to identify the fistulous tract of the left pyriform sinus. Hypopharyngolaryngoscopy may not detect the presence of a fistula (Table 3.3).

In summary, for the diagnosis of acute suppurative thyroiditis it is necessary to perform a careful anamnesis and clinical examination, simple laboratory tests (leukocyte count, ESR-CRP, TSH) and ultrasonography of the neck. If the suspicion of thyroiditis is confirmed with abscess of the thyroid, FNAc is indicated for Gram and Gomori stains; germ culture is necessary for appropriate antimicrobial therapy. In recurrent cases, an esophagram with barium to detect the presence of congenital fistula is indicated and CT is recommended if the results are negative.

Differential diagnosis—For differentiation from subacute thyroiditis, see Section 3.2. In rare cases, medullary carcinoma and anaplastic thyroid cancer may suddenly result from infarction of the tissue and induce tenderness. In these cases FNAc is useful to differentiate thyroid neoplasm by suppurative thyroiditis with determination of calcitonin in FNA washout and/or serum level in case of familial history of medullary carcinoma.

3.1.7 THERAPY

The first line therapy is the immediate empirical oral or in cases of clinical and/or laboratory features of systemic sepsis, intravenous antibiotic therapy to avoid abscess formation although abscesses are now rare (Figure 3.1). If absence is detected

TABLE 3.3
Diagnostic Features of Acute Suppurative Thyroiditis

Laboratory	First level tests with good accuracy:
	Thyroid hormones: normal
	C-reactive protein and erythrocyte sedimentation rate: high
	White blood count: leukocytosis
	Second level:
	HIV
	Thyroid autoantibodies: absent
Imaging	First level tests with good accuracy:
	Ultrasound of single or multiple hypoechogenic areas, anechogenic if abscess present
	Second level:
	RAIU thyroid scan: normal
	CT: hypodense areas, pyriform sinus fistula
	Radiography: gas or calcifications
	Esophagogram with barium: pyriform sinus fistula
Fine needle aspiration	First level tests with good accuracy:
	Cytology: leukocytes, histiocytes, lymphocytes, cellular debris
	Gram and Gomori stains and culture for aerobic and anaerobic bacteria, fungal and other microorganism; antibiotic sensitivity tests

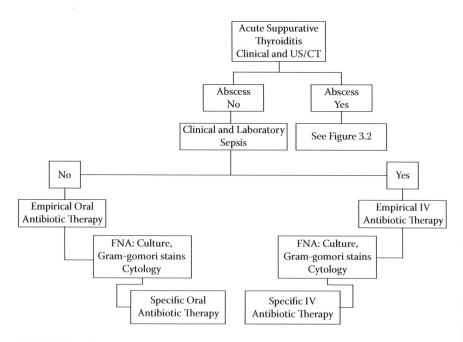

FIGURE 3.1   Management of acute suppurative thyroiditis.

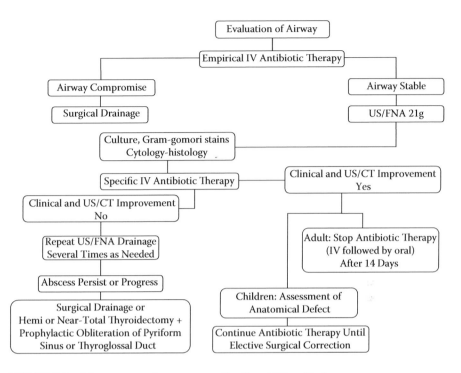

FIGURE 3.2 Management of acute suppurative thyroiditis with abscess.

clinically by fluctuation and by ultrasound or CT, US-FNA or surgical drainage related to airway stability or compromise, respectively, is indicated (Figure 3.2). Intravenous treatment requires hospitalization.

In cases of pyriform sinus and fourth branchial pouch fistula determined by clinical methods and imaging studies, complete resection or endoscopic cauterization of the sinus tract, including the portion of the thyroid where the sinus tract ends, is necessary to prevent recurrent infections. If extensive necrosis develops or a suppurative infection persists despite appropriate antibiotic treatment, thyroidectomy (partial or total) is indicated and the prophylactic obliteration of a pyriform sinus or thyroglossal duct is recommended.[4]

At the beginning of the disease, broad spectrum antimicrobial therapy is administered until culture tests indicate a response. In patients with abscesses who undergo FNAc for Gram and Gomori stains, antibiotic therapy is focused on the early results of the culture and sensitivity tests. Considering the predominance of bacterial etiopathogenesis (65 to 70%), medical history, clinical features and antibiotic allergies, the initial therapy is oral β-lactamase-resistant penicillin (amoxicillin/clavulanic acid 1 g tid). In more severe forms, intravenous amoxicillin/clavulanic acid 2 g tid, piperacillin/tazobactam 4.5 g tid or cephalosporin (adult: ceftriaxone 2 g every 24 h or ceftazidime 1 g tid; child: cefazolin 20 to 50 mg/kg/day bid) are given. Intravenous clindamycin is indicated in patients with allergies or recent exposure to penicillin (adult: 600 to 900 mg tid or qid; child: 10 to 40 mg/kg/day tid). If *Staphylococcus aureus* infection is suspected, intravenous vancomycin is indicated (1 g every 12 h).

TABLE 3.4
Antibiotic and Antifungal Therapy of Acute Suppurative Thyroiditis

Antibiotic	Dosage
β-lactamase-resistant penicillin	
Amoxicillin–clavulanic acid	Tablet, 1 g tid; intravenous, 2 g tid
Piperacillin–tazobactam	Intravenous, 4.5 g tid
Cephalosporin	
Ceftriaxone	Intravenous, 2 g every 24 h
Ceftazidime	Intravenous, 1 g tid
Cefazolin	Intravenous, 1 g tid (adult); 20 to 50 mg/kg/day bid. (child)
Clindamycin	Intravenous, 600 to 900 mg tid or qid (adult); 10 to 40 mg/kg/day tid (child)
Vancomycin	Intravenous, 1 g every 12 h
Trimethoprim–sulfamethoxazole	Intravenous, 100 mg/kg–20 mg/kg every 6 to 8 h for 2 weeks followed by 160 mg–800 mg tablet every 12 h
Fluconazole	Tablet, 100 mg daily

In immunocompromised patients, a combination of β-lactamase-resistant penicillin plus vancomycin is indicated.[4] When culture test results are available, specific antibiotic therapy aimed at the causative agent is administered and should continue at least 14 days. For *Pneumocistis carinii* infections in AIDS patients, therapy consists of intravenous trimethoprim–sulfamethoxazole (100 mg/kg–20 mg/kg every 6 to 8 h) for 2-weeks followed by oral sulfamethoxazole–trimethoprim (160 mg–800 mg every 12 h). In rare cases of fungal infection (about 15%), 100 mg oral fluconazole has been administered. Tuberculosis requires special treatment (Table 3.4).

3.1.8 CLINICAL COURSE

If appropriate therapy is delayed, a thyroid infection can extend to nearby sites and organs (trachea, esophagus, anterior mediastinum) with airway compromise, systemic sepsis, involvement of the sympathetic system and recurrent nerves, and thrombosis of the internal jugular vein (in anaerobic infections). About 50% of patients with congenital anomalies have three or more episodes of suppurative diagnosis before the right diagnosis is made.

3.1.9 PROGNOSIS

The course and prognosis for patients with bacterial thyroiditis are generally excellent (Table 3.5). No significant differences have been reported in the survival course after recovery from disease among patients treated with antibiotics and/or drainage. Recovery is usually complete without thyroid function abnormality; rare cases of permanent hypothyroidism from destruction of thyroid cells are reported. In cases of systemic extension, the disease may be fatal in untreated patients. The mortality rate of suppurative thyroiditis is 8.6%. Death is due to pneumonia, tracheal

TABLE 3.5
Course and Prognosis of Acute Suppurative Thyroiditis

Prognosis	Excellent if treated
Permanent hypothyroidism	Rare
Mortality	8.6% in untreated patients
Causes of death	Pneumonia, tracheal obstruction or perforation, concurrent sepsis, rupture of abscess, mediastinitis, pericarditis, following tracheotomy or incision of abscess

TABLE 3.6
Follow-Up of Acute Suppurative Thyroiditis

Months	Clinical Examination	ESR, CRP, Leukocyte Count	TSH	Ultrasound
1	+	+	+	+
3	+	+	+	+
6	+	–	+	–
12	+	–	+	+

obstruction or perforation, concurrent sepsis, rupture of a thyroid abscess, or mediastinitis and pericarditis related to infection of intrathoracic thyroid tissue. In other cases, death follows tracheotomy or incision and drainage of a thyroid abscess.

3.1.10 FOLLOW-UP

At the beginning of disease an early (after 1 or 2 days) recurrent clinical examination is necessary to control any abscess formation of the thyroid gland that occurs. Subsequently, clinical, ultrasonographic, and laboratory (leukocyte count, CRP, ESR, TSH) controls after 1 and 3 months are indicated; ultrasonography can be eliminated from the testing regimen after 12 months if no local complications occur (Table 3.6).

REFERENCES

1. Berger, S.A., Zonszein, J., Villamena, P. et al. 1983. Infectious disease of the thyroid gland. *Reviews of Infectious Diseases* 5: 108–122.
2. Al-Dajani, N. and Wootton, S.H. 2007. Cervical lymphadenitis, suppurative parotitis, thyroiditis, and infected cystes. *Infectious Disease Clinics of North America* 21: 523–541.
3. Nishihara, E., Miyauchi, F., Matsuzuka, F. et al. 2005. Acute suppurative thyroiditis after fine-needle aspiration causing thyrotoxicosis. *Thyroid* 15: 1183–1187.
4. Paes, J.E., Burman, K.D., Cohen J., et al. 2010. Acute bacterial suppurative thyroiditis: a clinical review and expert opinion. *Thyroid* 20: 247–255.
5. Sicilia, V. and Mezitis, S. 2006. A case of acute suppurative thyroiditis complicated by thyrotoxicosis. *Journal of Endocrinological Investigation* 29: 997–1000.

3.2   SUBACUTE THYROIDITIS

3.2.1   DEFINITION

Subacute thyroiditis (SAT), also called de Quervain's or granulomatous thyroiditis, is the most common cause of pain and tenderness of the thyroid gland, presumably caused by a viral infection. SAT is a transient and self-limiting inflammatory disease characterized by a multiphasic course—an initial thyrotoxic phase followed by hypothyroidism, generally transient, and finally by recovery.

3.2.2   EPIDEMIOLOGY

SAT is the most common cause of pain and tenderness of the thyroid gland, representing up to 5% of all thyroid diseases. Recent data from the Rochester Epidemiology Project in Olmsted County, Minnesota reported an SAT incidence of 12.1 per 100,000/year (female:male ratio of 4 or 5:1). SAT is less common than Graves' disease and Hashimoto's thyroiditis. The incidence is higher in females (19.1 per 100,000) than in males (4.4 per 100,000), in young adulthood (24 per 100,000/year for ages 30 to 40 years) and in middle age (35 per 100,000/year for ages 40 to 50), declining with increasing age.[1] Moreover, SAT is extremely rare during the first decade of life and during pregnancy. A seasonal and geographical distribution has been suggested with high prevalence during summer and early autumn[2] not confirmed in other studies.[3,4] SAT often follows viral epidemics.

3.2.3   ETIOPATHOGENESIS

Viral infection or a postviral inflammatory condition is commonly considered a cause of subacute thyroiditis although the virus cause is not always demonstrable. Most patients have histories of recent upper respiratory infections, sore throats characterized by a prodromic phase suggesting a viral infection. Reports have associated SAT with infections due to mumps, measles, influenza, adenovirus, Epstein-Barr virus, cytomegalovirus, herpesvirus, enterovirus (echovirus, coxsackieviruses A and B), rubella, and *Chlamydia psittaci*. Recently subacute thyroiditis has been observed after administration of the H1N1 vaccine; direct evidence in the thyroid tissue of foamy virus and mumps in humans is only occasionally reported.

An association between subacute thyroiditis and human leukocyte antigen (HLA) has been reported. In particular, the presence of the HLA-B35 haplotype in the familial occurrence and recurrence of the disease is reported. In Japanese patients, HLA-B67 is associated with a greater risk of developing a hypothyroid phase, thus confirming a genetic vulnerability in patients with SAT. The direct involvement of autoimmunity in the etiopathogenesis of the disease has not been confirmed.

The occasional and transient presence of antithyroglobulin (TgAb), antiperoxidase (TPOAb), and antiTSH receptor (TRAb) is probably related to damage of the thyroid follicles with release of sequestered antigens. This induces an immune response by B cells with autoantibody production and T cell reactivity with granuloma formation

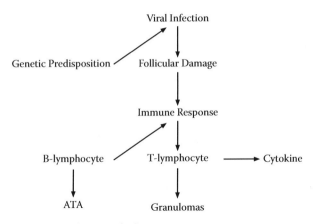

FIGURE 3.3 Pathogenesis of subacute thyroiditis.

(Figure 3.3). The presence of a predisposing HLA haplotype probably induces the capacity of a virus to trigger a cytotoxic T cell response against the thyroid tissue and the development of transitory autoimmune thyroid response. The immune surveillance is subsequently restored with the subsequent suppression of autoantibody synthesis.

SAT has been described in patients treated with interferon-α (IFN-α) alone or in combination with ribavirin, PEG-IFN-α2a, interleukin-2, tumor necrosis factor-α (TNF-α), and etarnecept. It has been associated with acute febrile neutrophilic dermatosis (Sweet's syndrome), giant cell arteritis, and appeared after bone marrow transplantation and gastric bypass and with paraneoplastic manifestations of renal cell and lung carcinoma.

3.2.4 PATHOPHYSIOLOGY

SAT is a destructive thyroiditis manifesting as a typical multiphase disease. The inflammation causes the destruction of follicular epithelium that induces the release in the blood of thyroid hormones, thyroglobulin, and iodinated compounds in variable amounts, with early suppression of TSH secretion.

Cell destruction and TSH suppression induce the depletion of hormone storage and transitory impairment of new thyroid hormone synthesis and secretion that results in hypothyroidism, often subclinical, 2 to 3 months after the onset of the disease. As the inflammation subsides, thyroid cells recover, new follicles are formed, and thyroid hormone synthesis and secretion restart with the reconstitution of storage, thus resulting in euthyroidism. In a minority of cases, the follicular damage develops into fibrosis that may result in permanent hypothyroidism (Figure 3.4). Some authors also suggest that the subtle abnormalities in iodine organification and subsequent impairment of thyroid hormone synthesis may persist years after SAT.[5]

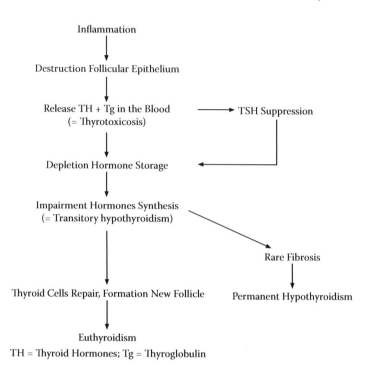

Inflammation

↓

Destruction Follicular Epithelium

↓

Release TH + Tg in the Blood ⟶ TSH Suppression
(= Thyrotoxicosis)

↓

Depletion Hormone Storage ⟵

↓

Impairment Hormones Synthesis
(= Transitory hypothyroidism)

Rare Fibrosis

↓   ↓

Thyroid Cells Repair, Formation New Follicle   Permanent Hypothyroidism

↓

Euthyroidism
TH = Thyroid Hormones; Tg = Thyroglobulin

FIGURE 3.4   Physiopathology of subacute thyroiditis.

3.2.5 CLINICAL SIGNS AND SYMPTOMS

SAT is characterized by three functional phases: hyperthyroidism, hypothyroidism, and finally euthyroidism. The clinical onset is characterized by systemic symptoms including fatigue, myalgia, malaise, anorexia, and often fever accompanied by signs and symptoms resembling an upper respiratory tract infection. The predominant features are pain and tenderness of the anterior upper neck. The pain appears suddenly, frequently bilateral, migrant, often radiating to the homolateral jaw, ear, and throat; coughing and swallowing worsen the pain. Local skin manifestation is less evident than in suppurative thyroiditis.

The thyroid is mildly to moderately enlarged, painful and tender to palpation with involvement of one or both lobes, firm to hard in consistency. Palpation is often difficult and causes unbearable pain. The right lobe is affected more often than the left; solitary painless nodules are rarely reported. The involvement of the thyroid gland is often unilateral at the beginning and migrates to the other side days or weeks later. The severity of pain differentiates SAT from an intranodular hemorrhage that manifests as a unilateral nodule.

At the beginning, the clinical features of hyperthyroidism are present in about 50% of patients and include palpitations, heat intolerance, tremors, hyperreflexia, sweating, diarrhea, nervousness, and moderate weight loss (Table 3.7). This phase, lasting 3 to 6 weeks, is followed, based on progress of the destructive process, by a euthyroid or subclinical hypothyroid phase (30 to 50% of patients) that is often asymptomatic or may be accompanied by fatigue, hyporeflexia, mild cold intolerance,

TABLE 3.7

Clinical Features of Subacute Thyroiditis

Age	30 to 50 years; very rare in children and during pregnancy
Sex	Female:male ratio = 4 or 5:1
History	Sometimes previous upper respiratory tract infection; seasonal distribution suggested
Symptoms	Pain and tenderness of anterior upper neck, sudden, may be monolateral but commonly bilateral, migrant, often radiating to homolateral jaw, throat, ears, aggravated by coughing and swallowing; clinical thyrotoxicosis
Signs	Painful goiter with involvement of one or both lobes that are firm to hard in consistency; palpation is often difficult because it causes severe pain

and constipation. The hypothyroid phase lasts from weeks to 3 to 6 months, rarely continuing for 12 months. Complete recovery is the common course. Permanent hypothyroidism has been reported in 5 to 15% of cases.[3,6]

3.2.6 Diagnosis

At onset, in addition to clinical findings (typically neck pain, fever, malaise, and mild hyperthyroidism), confirmatory tests are needed. Laboratory tests in the initial phase as in suppurative thyroiditis reveal a generalized systemic illness with elevation of erythrocyte sedimentation rate (ESR), C-reactive protein (CRP), and white and red blood cell counts (mild increase of leukocyte count and mild anemia). Liver function abnormalities have been observed with elevation of transaminases and more frequently elevation of alkaline phosphatise and α_2-globulin. The thyroid cell damage caused by inflammation related to SAT may induce a non-specific rise of interleukin-6, a pleiotropic cytokine.

The thyroid function in more than half of cases revealed mild thyrotoxicosis with elevation of thyroid hormones (FT_3 and FT_4) and thyroglobulin (Tg) serum levels, low TSH but absence of antithyroid autoantibodies (ATA: antithyroglobulin and antiperoxidase). After 3 to 6 weeks, the thyroid function returns to normal with normalization of ESR, CRP, and liver function (leukocyte count is related to choice of therapy, see Section 3.2.7). Subclinical hypothyroidism can be observed 2 to 3 months after the hyperthyroid phase. In this phase, the mild positivity of ATA is likely related to release of sequestered antigens that induce immune responses by autoantibodies and T cell reactivity and not a real autoimmune process.

In the recovery phase, thyroid hormones and TSH serum levels return to normal but permanent hypothyroidism is reported in about 5 to 15% of patients arising from fibrosis of the thyroid tissue and not to autoimmune response. Elevated Tg serum levels may persist until recovery. In some patients, the associated positivity of TRAb has been reported in the transitory hypothyroidism phase and is associated with the development of permanent hypothyroidism.

Thyroid ultrasonography (US) plays a supporting role in the noninvasive diagnosis and follow-up of SAT. During the initial phase, US shows mild and inhomogeneous gland enlargement and diffuse or focal hypoechoic to anechoic areas with unclear contours, corresponding to extension of inflammation but not related to early thyroid function impairment. The vascularization in this phase under color Doppler sonography (CDS) appears normal to low. During the recovery phase, US may reveal isoechogeneity or sometimes dyshomogeneity with pseudonodular areas of tissue with slightly increased vascularization that becomes normal at the end of follow-up. It has been suggested that the extension of hypoechoic areas may considered a possible marker for development of thyroid dysfunction.[7] Recently, ultrasound elastography (USE) has shown markedly decreased elasticity of affected areas.[8]

Thyroid scintigraphy with ^{99m}Tc performed to differentiate SAT from true hyperthyroidism in the acute phase shows a markedly reduced or absent visualization of the gland. Radioactive iodine uptake (RAIU) is typically very low (less than 1%) along with low urine iodine values in the initial phase of the disease, whereas the low RAIU due to excess exogenous iodine exposure is characterized by an elevation of urine iodine.

In a minority of cases, fine needle aspiration cytology (FNAc) is indicated. FNAc is unlikely to be proposed in the initial phases of SAT and it may show atypical follicular cells of unclear significance. FNAc reveals plump transformed follicular cells, multinuclear cells and epithelioid granulomas, lymphocytes, and macrophages; often are present follicular cells with intravacuolar granules and polymorphonuclear cells. FNAc is indicated for differential diagnosis from atypical presentation of thyroid carcinoma; if suspicion of carcinoma is low, FNAc can be postponed until resolution of SAT symptoms.

In summary, diagnosis of SAT is fundamentally clinical and is confirmed by laboratory (ESR, CRP, leukocyte counts, α_2-globulin, thyroid hormones) and imaging findings (US, thyroid scintigraphy, radioactive iodine uptake); cytological confirmation is rarely needed (Table 3.8).

Differential diagnosis—SAT, particularly in children, must be differentiated from acute suppurative thyroiditis (more obvious local skin manifestations, more elevated fever, marked leukocytosis, euthyroidism, normal RAIU, mixed area on US, FNAc with neutrophils, culture positive for microorganisms; Table 3.9 and Table 3.10) and from hemorrhagic pseudocyst (more sudden, unilateral, less painful thyroid nodule; no fever, ESR and CRP normal, euthyroidism, US shows anechoic mixed area).

Occasionally autoimmune thyroid diseases (Graves's hyperthyroidism, Hashimoto's thyroiditis) present neck pain and tenderness. All of the above diseases are less severe than SAT with normal ESR-CRP and in SAT, the alteration of thyroid hormone serum levels is more evident. US also shows hypoechoic images in Graves' disease and in Hashimoto's thyroiditis but RAIU is high. In particular, in a painful variant of Hashimoto's thyroiditis, the hyperthyroid early phase with near absent RAIU and elevated ESR and CRP elevated is similar to SAT. However, in Graves' disease and Hashimoto's thyroiditis, the upper respiratory tract infection and systemic symptoms are absent; the thyroid autoantibodies are clearly elevated and anti-inflammatory therapy has no influence on clinical course. In these cases, FNAc is useful and in rare cases, surgical therapy and histological examination are indicated as well and permanent hypothyroidism is frequent. In some cases, unilateral SAT can mimic or be associated with thyroid cancer or lymphoma and FNAc is required (Table 3.11).

TABLE 3.8
Diagnostic Features of Subacute Thyroiditis

Laboratory   First level tests with good accuracy
   ESR and CRP: elevated
   White blood count: high
   Red blood count: mild anemia
   α_2-globulin: elevated
   Thyroid hormones and ATAs
     Early phase
       thyrotoxicosis
     Intermediate phase
       transient subclinical hypothyroidism
       euthyroidism
     Late phase
       euthyroidism
       rare permanent hypothyroidism
   Second level tests
     Liver function (transaminase, alkaline phosphatase): elevated
     ATA: possible mild positivity

Imaging   First level tests with good accuracy
   Ultrasonography: diffuse or focal hypoechoic to anechoic areas
   Scintigraphy/RAIU: reduced (<5%) or absent visualization of gland
   Second level tests
     CDS: normal-low vascularity
     USE: marked decreased elasticity affected area

Note: ATA = antithyroid autoantibodies. CDS = color Doppler sonography. USE = ultrasound sonoelastography.

TABLE 3.9
Differential Clinical Features of Acute Suppurative and Subacute Thyroiditis

	Acute Suppurative	**Subacute**
Epidemiology	0.1 to 0.7%	5%
Age (years)	Any age (pyriform sinus fistula in children)	30 to 50
Sex: F:M ratio	1:1	4 or 5:1
Agent	Bacterial, fungal, parasitic	Viral
Predisposition	Pyriform sinus fistula (children); preexisting thyroid disease	HLA Bw35, B67
Prodrome	Upper respiratory illness	Viral illness
Goiter	Painful, unilateral, left	Painful, migraine
Systemic symptoms	Yes	Yes
Local erythema	Yes	No

TABLE 3.10

Differential Diagnostic Features of Acute Suppurative and Subacute Thyroiditis

	Acute Suppurative	Subacute
ESR-CRP	High	High
Transaminases + alkaline phosphatase	Normal	High
Thyroid function	Euthyroidism	Early thyrotoxicosis (50%) Transient hypothyroidism (30 to 50%) Late euthyroidism (85 to 95%)
Ultrasound	Hypoechogenic and anechogenic areas	Hypoechogenic areas
RAIU	Normal	Very low (5%)
FNAc	Purulent, microorganisms, polymorphonuclear leukocytes	Multinuclear cells, granulomas
Therapy	Medical Surgical (abscess drainage) until hemi-near total thyroidectomy; prophylactic or therapeutic obliteration of pyriform sinus or thyroglossal duct	Medical
Recurrence	If pyriform sinus fistula (children)	Early: 20%; late: 2%
Permanent hypothyroidism	Rare	5 to 15 %

TABLE 3.11

Differential Diagnosis of Subacute Thyroiditis

Acute suppurative thyroiditis	Children; recurrence; more evident local skin manifestations; more elevated fever; marked leukocytosis; generally euthyroidism; normal RAIU; mixed area on US; FNAc with neutrophils and culture positive for microorganisms
Hemorrhagic pseudocyst	More sudden, unilateral, less painful thyroid nodule; no fever; ESR and CRP normal; euthyroidism; US shows anechoic and mixed areas
Painful Hashimoto's thyroiditis	No previous upper respiratory tract infection; hyperthyroidism; ATA elevated; response anti-inflammatory therapy less affect clinical course; FNAc useful; surgical therapy sometimes indicated; permanent hypothyroidism frequent
Thyroid neoplasm	Often unilateral; FNAc (carcinoma); also biopsy needed if lymphoma is suspected

3.2.7 THERAPY

SAT is a self-limited disease and does not require hospitalization. The treatment is usually oral administration of drugs and should be directed to relieving the neck pain and thyroid dysfunction.

For painful goiters, acetylsalicylic acid (0.5 to 1 g every 8 to 12 h) or nonsteroidal anti-inflammatory drugs (NSAIDs) such as ibuprofen (400 to 600 mg every 8 to 12 h) are indicated and produce similar effects. If pain is not relieved within 72 h, cortico-steroids are indicated to achieve rapid effects in more severe forms of the disease.[9] The common initial dose of prednisone or an equivalent is 40 to 60 mg in one or two doses or 10 mg qid. The response should be prompt. If tenderness and painful goiter do not respond within 72 h, the diagnosis of SAT should be reconsidered.

Therapy for the neck pain should be continued for 1 to 2 weeks at the initial dosage and tapered slowly with the halving of dose after that and withdrawal after 6 to 8 weeks of therapy. The early recurrence of symptoms is observed in about 20% of patients when the dosage is reduced and in such cases it is necessary to restart and prolong the weeks of therapy.[3] With the anti-inflammatory therapy, a gastric protector (e.g., inhibitor of protonic pump) is indicated. In a laboratory follow-up, it is useful to remember that leukocyte counts are higher in patients treated with corticosteroids. In pregnant women with severe SAT, prednisolone (20 mg orally at the beginning and gradual reduction of dose) is indicated.[10]

At the beginning of SAT, therapy is not required for the mild and short-lived symptoms of hyperthyroidism. Antithyroid therapy with thionamides is not indicated because the thyroid hormone serum level excess results from the release of preexisting hormones by follicular damage and not from their overproduction. If symptomatic, thyrotoxicosis can be treated with β-blockade therapy. Propranolol (20 to 40 mg bid) or atenolol (25 to 50 mg in single dose) can be administered; the former has the advantage of inhibiting the conversion of T_4 to T_3 and the latter is better tolerated. The therapy can usually be withdrawn in 2 to 6 weeks. In patients who cannot tolerate β-blockers, verapamil (80 to 160 mg bid) can be used. Specific therapy is required to treat anxiety if present.

The subsequent phase is often characterized by transient and subclinical hypo-thyroidism and generally does not require treatment. In rare cases of hypothyroid symptoms, L-thyroxine at a substitutive dose (25 to 100 µg daily to keep TSH in the normal range) may be used for about 6 months. TSH should be monitored periodi-cally during use and after withdrawal. The transient substitutive therapy is beneficial when indicated and may help prevent future recurrences; in fact elevated TSH may aggravate or precipitate SAT. In rare cases of permanent hypothyroidism, usually in patients treated with corticosteroids.[3] L-thyroxine supplementation and monitoring of serum TSH levels are necessary. See Section 3.2.9 and Table 3.12.

Antibiotic therapy is not indicated; thyroidectomy is indicated only if the coexistence of thyroid neoplasm is suspected.

3.2.8 CLINICAL COURSE

SAT is a self-limited disease with three-four phases of the clinical course. The initial phase, characterized by mild thyrotoxicosis (about 50% of cases) and painful goiter, lasts 3 to 6 weeks or occasionally longer. The transient euthyroid phase, often not identified, follows and mild subclinical hypothyroidism in 30 to 50% of patients lasts for weeks or even several months. Finally, the recovery phase follows after 6 to 12 months, with return to normal function and often to normal morphology. Permanent hypothyroidism occurs in 5 to 15% of cases (Figure 3.5).

TABLE 3.12
Therapy of Subacute Thyroiditis

Drug	Oral Dose
Anti-inflammatory	
Aspirin	0.5 to 1 g every 8 to 12 h bid
Ibuprofen	400 to 600 mg every 8 to 12 h bid
Prednisone	40 to 60 mg bid or single dose; or 10 mg qid
Antiarrhythmic	
Propranolol	20 to 40 mg bid
Atenolol	25 to 50 mg in single dose
Verapamil	80 to 160 mg bid
Substitutive	
L-thyroxine	25 to 100 μg in single dose

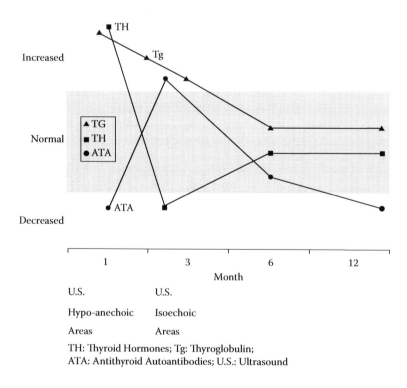

TH: Thyroid Hormones; Tg: Thyroglobulin;
ATA: Antithyroid Autoantibodies; U.S.: Ultrasound

FIGURE 3.5   Clinical course of subacute thyroiditis.

3.2.9 PROGNOSIS

During the first weeks, often due to low initial dosage or excessive rapid reduction of NSAIDs or steroid therapy, exacerbations of painful goiter occur in 20% of cases. Late recurrences after prolonged periods of latency (even many years after the first episode) occur in about 2% of patients.[11] No particular clinical and/or laboratory features are reported to predict early or late recurrence. Early relapse occurs in about 10% of cases treated with corticosteroids.[3,12] Moreover, these drugs are utilized in more severe cases with more extensive inflammation; more diffuse involvement of thyroid tissue explains the relation.[12]

Recovery from SAT is usually complete in 85 to 95% of cases within 6 to 12 months and in rare cases within 18 months. An incidence of 5 to 15% of permanent hypothyroidism is reported and is related to the occurrence of the transient phase of subclinical hypothyroidism[7] or the positivity of TRAb.[13] Permanent hypothyroidism is related to the degree of postinflammation fibrosis even if some authors reported associations in some patients with the above-mentioned transitory positivity of TRAb. Because of the possibilities of permanent hypothyroidism or recurrence of SAT, follow-up for years is mandatory (Table 3.13). In endemic areas, residual goiter is described; moreover, in the follow-up of SAT, isolated cases of the occurrence or relapse of Graves' disease and Riedel's thyroiditis in patients with histories of SAT have been reported.

3.2.10 FOLLOW-UP

Between 3 and 6 months after onset of SAT, it is necessary to control thyroid hormones, ATA, and index of inflammation. After 12 months, US control is useful. Furthermore, annual or biennial control of thyroid hormones is suggested (Table 3.14).

TABLE 3.13
Clinical Course and Prognosis of Subacute Thyroiditis

Clinical course	Thyrotoxic phase: 50 to 60% of cases
	Transitory hypothyroidism: 30 to 50% of cases
	Complete recovery in 85 to 95% of cases
	Permanent hypothyroidism in 5 to 15% of cases
Prognosis	Early recurrence in 10% of cases
	Late recurrence in 2% of cases
	Permanent hypothyroidism in 5 to 15% of cases

TABLE 3.14
Follow-Up of Subacute Thyroiditis

Months	Thyroid Hormones	Antithyroid Antibodies	Ultrasound
3	+	+	−
6	+	−	−
12	+	+	+

REFERENCES

1. Golden, H.S., Robinson, K.A., Saldanha, I. et al. 2009. Prevalence and incidence of endocrine and metabolic disorders in the United States: a comprehensive review. *Journal of Clinical Endocrinology & Metabolism* 94: 1853–1878.
2. Nishihara, E., Ohye, H., Amino, N. et al. 2008. Clinical characteristic of 852 patients with subacute thyroiditis before treatment. *Internal Medicine* 47: 725–729.
3. Fatourechi, V., Aniszewski, J.P., Fatourechi, G.Z. et al. 2003. Clinical features and outcome of subacute thyroiditis in an incidence cohort: Olmsted County, Minnesota study. *Journal of Clinical Endocrinology & Metabolism* 88: 2100–2105.
4. Benbassat, C.A., Olchovsky, D., Tsevetov, G. et al, 2007. Subacute thyroiditis: clinical characteristics and treatment outcome in 56 consecutive patients diagnosed between 1999 and 2005. *Journal of Endocrinological Investigation* 30: 631–635.
5. Roti, E., Minelli, R., Gardini, E. et al. 1990. Iodine-induced hypothyroidism in euthyroid subjects with a previous episode of subacute thyroiditis. *Journal of Clinical Endocrinology & Metabolism* 70: 1581–1585.
6. Lio, S., Pontecorvi, A., Caruso, M. et al. 1984. Transitory and permanent hypothyroidism in the course of subacute thyroiditis. *Acta Endocrinologica (Cph)* 106: 67–70.
7. Nishihara, E., Nietzsche, A., Ohye, H. et al. 2009. Extent of hypoechogenic area in the thyroid is related with thyroid dysfunction after subacute thyroiditis. *Journal of Endocrinological Investigation* 32: 33–36.
8. Ruchala, M., Szczepanek, E., and Sowinski, J. 2011. Sonoelastography in de Quervain thyroiditis. *Journal of Clinical Endocrinology & Metabolism* 96: 289–290.
9. Bahn, R.S., Burch, H.B., Cooper, D.S. et al. 2011. Hyperthyroidism and other causes of thyrotoxicosis: management guidelines of the American Thyroid Association and American Association of Clinical Endocrinologists. *Thyroid* 21 (6): 593–646.
10. Hiraiwa, T., Kubota, S., Imagawa, A. et al. 2006. Two cases of subacute thyroiditis presenting in pregnancy. *Journal of Endocrinological Investigation* 29: 924–927.
11. Iitaka, M., Momotani, N., Ishii, J. et al. 1996. Incidence of subacute thyroiditis recurrence after a prolonged latency: 24-year survey. *Journal of Clinical Endocrinology & Metabolism* 81: 466–469.
12. Mizukoshy, T., Noguchi, S., Murakami, T. et al. 2001. Evaluation of recurrence in 36 subacute thyroiditis patients managed with prednisolone. *Internal Medicine* 40: 292–295.
13. Iitaka, M., Momotani, N., Hisaoka, T. et al. 1998. TSH receptor antibodies-associated thyroid dysfunction following subacute thyroiditis. *Clinical Endocrinology* 48: 445–453.

3.3 RIEDEL'S THYROIDITIS

3.3.1 DEFINITION

Riedel's or invasive fibrous thyroiditis is a very rare chronic inflammatory disease often extended beyond the capsule into surrounding tissues and associated with multifocal fibrosclerosis. The etiology is unknown but likely to be autoimmune.

3.3.2 EPIDEMIOLOGY

Riedel's thyroiditis is extremely rare. In the experience of the Mayo Clinic between 1920 and 1984, the surgical frequency of Riedel's thyroiditis was 0.06% (37 cases among 57,000 thyroidectomies). The overall prevalence in outpatients was 1.06 in

100,000.[1] It occurs mainly in adults (30 to 50 years of age) and the elderly; women are more often affected than men (female:male ratio = 4:1).[2]

3.3.3 ETIOPATHOGENESIS

The etiopathogenesis of Riedel's thyroiditis is unclear. Whether the disease is a primary autoimmune process, a variant of Hashimoto's thyroiditis, or a primary fibrotic disease remains controversial. It is still considered an idiopathic syndrome. An autoimmune mechanism is suggested by the presence of antithyroid autoantibodies (45 to 67% of cases) with a mixed polyclonal population of B and T cells, occasional coexistence with autoimmune disorders (Hashimoto's thyroiditis, Graves' disease, Addison's disease, pernicious anemia, type 1 diabetes mellitus) and favorable response to glucocorticoid therapy.

The immune reaction may represent a response to antigens released from destroyed thyroid tissue; the association with other autoimmune diseases may be coincidental; the response to glucocorticoid therapy may be due to reduced production of cytokines with fibrogenic activity. The infiltration of mononuclear cells and eosinophils, particularly in the early phase, suggests an immunomediated process; the marked tissue eosinophilia called autoallergy may be important in the genesis of fibrosis. The stimulus for the fibrosis is unknown.

A few authors propose a genetic basis and in case of mediastinal involvement, fungal infection (*Histoplasma, Aspergillus*) must be considered. Also a vessel involvement has been theorized. In fact, Riedel's first description of this thyroiditis suggested the presence of endoarteritis, i.e., vasculitis. Recently an occlusive phlebitis has been reported and postulated as a diagnostic pathological feature of Riedel's thyroiditis and related to possible formation of sterile abscess of the thyroid. A few cases of Riedel's thyroiditis during Epstein-Barr virus infection and in patients with histories of SAT have been reported.

3.3.4 PATHOPHYSIOLOGY

Riedel's thyroiditis is characterized by progressive fibrosis with complete destruction of the involved parts of thyroid gland. The fibrogenesis may be related to abundant eosinophil infiltration and to the inhibition of action of transforming growth factor-β (TGF-β), a potent growth inhibitor of immature fibroblasts and epithelial cells.

The possible encasement of blood vessels may be associated with occlusive phlebitis and thrombosis. The fibrosis of thyroid tissue extends through the capsule into the extrathyroidal soft tissue of the neck, resulting in hypothyroidism in 30 to 40% of cases. Tracheal and esophageal compression, fibrous parotitis, occlusive vasculitis, superior vena cava syndrome and cerebral venous sinus thrombosis, hypoparathyroidism, recurrent laryngeal nerve injury, and Horner's syndrome have been related to fibrotic infiltration of the cervical sympathetic trunk.

This form of thyroiditis (34% of reported cases) may be associated with multifocal extracervical fibrosclerositis involving the orbit, mediastinum, lung, myocardium, hepatobiliary duct, and retroperitoneal tissue. Patients with Riedel's thyroiditis often have histories of tobacco use. The exact mechanism is unclear but it is possible that tobacco use, as in Graves' ophthalmopathy, increases immune processes and activates fibroblasts.[3]

3.3.5 CLINICAL SIGNS AND SYMPTOMS

The clinical appearance is characterized by a painless slow enlargement of the thyroid gland and a preexisting goiter,[4] initially unilateral and later involving the controlateral lobe. The interval between the early appearance of the disease and the diagnosis is about 4 to 10 months. A patient may remain stable over years; the disease progresses very slowly. The clinical manifestations are related to local involvement of near neck structures. Dyspnea, dysphagia for solids and liquids, dysphonia, and stridor all relate to a progressive increase of firm thyroid volume with local obstructive phenomena.

The thyroid mass is fixed, often rock-hard, and painless. Neck discomfort or pain may be present. Sometimes the severity of local symptomatology is disproportionate in relation to the size of the mass. The gland feels ligneous on palpation and fixed to surrounding structures. The clinical distinction from malignancy is very difficult. Fever is absent. The clinical differential diagnosis of Riedel's thyroiditis includes differentiated and undifferentiated thyroid carcinoma, lymphoma, and Hashimoto's thyroiditis.

In these diseases, the extent of the fibrosis is not so relevant and often cervical lymphadenopathy is present. Where thyroid involvement is part of a systemic fibrosing process, clinical characteristics referable to other areas may be present. In particular, vagal involvement may induce bradycardia and sometimes syncope. Occasionally extension to the cervical sympathetic trunk may induce Horner's syndrome (ptosis, meiosis of the eye).[5] The presence of palpable cervical lymphadenopathy is rare. If the fibrotic process progresses with significant reduction of thyroid hormone synthesis, the clinical signs and symptoms of hypothyroidism appear. Also the involvement of the parathyroid results in clinical features of hypoparathyroidism (Table 3.15).

3.3.6 DIAGNOSIS

Clinical diagnosis of Riedel's thyroiditis is difficult. It is clinically suspected in middle-aged patients by the presence of a ligneous, non-painful goiter upon palpation of the thyroid gland. Initially, the goiter is unilateral, with local compression; the size of the mass and clinical symptoms are disproportionate. This inflammatory thyroid

---

TABLE 3.15

Clinical Features of Riedel's Thyroiditis

Age	30 to 50 years or elderly
Sex	Female:male ratio = 4:1
Signs and symptoms	Painless, slow, unilateral, then bilateral enlargement; fixed, ligneous, often on preexisting goiter; neck discomfort, compression symptoms (dyspnea, dysphonia, dysphagia); one third: extracervical manifestation

disease does not show characteristic biochemical findings. CRP, ESR, and white blood cells may be normal or elevated.

The thyroid function is normal in most patients; in some cases, hypothyroidism (30%) and hyperthyroidism (4%) have been reported. The thyroid hormone serum levels are in concordance with the clinical symptoms and with radioactive iodine uptake.

Typically, thyrotoxicosis is associated with lack of radioactive iodine uptake present in euthyroid patients; uptake is low in hypothyroid patients. On thyroid scan, Riedel's may appear similar to other forms of chronic thyroiditis and may reveal heterogeneous patterns with decreased uptake in affected areas of the gland. Antithyroid autoantibodies are often present in 40 to 70% of patients at lower serum levels (Table 3.16).

US of the neck will show hypoechoic and heterogeneous areas, sometimes pseudonodular and extended unilaterally or bilaterally in relation to the progression of the fibrosis. In color Doppler sonography (CDS) imaging, the absence of vascular flows in the areas involved is a consequence of the fibrotic involution of glandular parenchyma. Ultrasound elastography (USE) shows heterogeneity in the stiffness values of the thyroid parenchyma.[6] The exact extension of the disease is detected by computed tomography (CT) or magnetic resonance (MR) imaging. In CT, the thyroid appears hypodense with slight contrast medium enhancement. In MR, the gland is hypointense on both T1- and T2-weighted images. Both imaging techniques are important to show the encasement and/or compression of vascular structures, trachea, and esophagus. Fluorine-18 fluorodeoxiglucose positronic emission tomography (FDG PET) can show sites of multifocal fibrosclerosis with intense hypermetabolic mass and the activity can predict the response to corticosteroid therapy.[7]

TABLE 3.16
Diagnostic Features of Riedel's Thyroiditis

Laboratory	Normal thyroid function (hypothyroidism 30%, hyperthyroidism 4%); low levels of thyroid autoantibodies (40 to 70%); ESR and CRP: not significant
Imaging	First level tests with good accuracy
	Ultrasound: hypoechoic, dyshomogeneous
	Chest x-ray and abdominal ultrasound for extracervical involvement
	CT: hypodense, slight enhancement; for extension examination
	Second level tests
	CDS: absence of vascular flow
	USE: heterogeneity in stiffness values
	Scan: heterogeneous pattern with decreased uptake in affected areas
	MR: hypointense T1-T2; for extension examination
	FDG-PET: increased uptake in involved areas; decreased activity after successful corticosteroid therapy
Pathology	First level tests with good accuracy
	Histology (mandatory for diagnosis): fibroinflammatory cells: occlusive; vasculitis; normal parenchyma alternated with complete destruction of thyroid tissue
	FNAc often useless

Chest x-rays and abdominal US are also useful and more economical for detecting possible sites of multifocal extracervical fibrosclerosis. Fine needle aspiration cytology (FNAc) is often nonspecific. The smear is often scanty or acellular (THY 1) for the presence of fibrotic tissue. Hence, for a main differential diagnosis with malignancy, an open biopsy or thyroidectomy is required.[8] The histological features are the extension, in absence of encapsulation, of the fibroinflammatory process to the near structures of the neck including the carotid sheaths, jugular vein, trachea, esophagus, strap muscles, nerves, and parathyroid. Relatively normal functional parenchyma may alternate with complete destruction of thyroid tissue. The evidence of occlusive phlebitis with intimal proliferation, medial destruction, adventitial inflammation and frequent consequent thrombosis is observed. Furthermore, a reaction to a marker of connective tissue (vimentin and actin) at the periphery of the lesion has been reported.[9]

Lymphocytes (predominantly T cells) a similar ratio of CD4 to CD8, and plasma cells almost exclusively concentrated on the border between the fibrotic mass and the normal tissue are seen. Eosinophils may be present as well. The disease is neither associated with follicular epithelial and Hürthle cells as in chronic lymphocytic thyroiditis nor with granulomatous inflammation. In 25 to 50% of cases, a central adenoma may be detected in the preserved thyroid parenchyma. An anecdotal association between Riedel's thyroiditis and acute suppurative thyroiditis as well as subacute thyroiditis, Hashimoto's thyroiditis, Graves' disease, follicular carcinoma, and anaplastic carcinoma has been noted.

In summary, Riedel's thyroiditis is an underdiagnosed but important clinical condition. Differential diagnosis to distinguish it from Hashimoto's thyroiditis and thyroid carcinoma is difficult and usually requires histological examination by open biopsy[10] (Table 3.16).

3.3.7 THERAPY

Untreated Riedel's thyroiditis is usually slowly progressive and self-limiting through stabilization or spontaneous regression (Table 3.17). Because differential diagnosis, particularly with cancer, is often possible only with histology, a surgical approach is required. A wedge resection of the thyroidal isthmus or minimally invasive surgery such as isthmectomy or hemithyroidectomy is initially preferred. This approach allows histological diagnosis and relieves compression on the trachea and/or esophagus.

Generally an extensive resection of the thyroid should not be attempted because the fibrotic involvement of the neck structure with no plane of cleavage increases the risk of damage to the structure. In fact, surgery may be complicated by transient or permanent vocal cord paralysis and severe hypoparathyroidism as well as the emergency need for intraoperative tracheostomy.[3] Because no therapy option has been reported as the best in prospective randomized trials, corticosteroids have been indicated (Table 3.18). A dramatic improvement of compression symptoms is observed with systemic administration of high doses of corticosteroids. The efficacy of drug therapy is greater when given in the initial phase of the disease and less effective in the end stage when fibrogenesis is almost complete.

TABLE 3.17
Therapy, Clinical Course, Prognosis and Follow-Up of Riedel's Thyroiditis

Therapy	*Surgical*
	Wedge resection of isthmus or minimally invasive procedure for differential diagnosis and relief of compression
	Medical
	Prednisone
	Tamoxifen
	Mycophenolate mofetil
	L-thyroxine
Clinical course	Slowly progressive, often self-limiting
Prognosis	*Recurrence:* 16% of cases
	Mortality: 4 to 10% of cases related to extrathyroid and/or extracervical involvement
	Hypothyroidism: rare
Follow-up	*Euthyroidism:* annual control of thyroid function
	Hypothyroidism: control as in hypothyroidism

TABLE 3.18
Medical Therapy of Riedel's Thyroiditis

Therapy	Oral Dose
Prednisone	1 mg/kg bid, reducing 20% of total dose every 2 weeks over 10-week period for 4 to 6 months
Tamoxifen	10 to 20 mg bid (if and until tolerated)
Mycophenolate mofetil	1 g bid (until surgical resection)
L-thyroxine	50 to 150 µg/day related also to cardiovascular disease until TSH normalization
Calcium carbonate	1,000 to 1,500 mg/day (associated to corticosteroid therapy)
Calcitriol	0.5 µg/day (associated to corticosteroid therapy)

When the glucocorticoids are interrupted, relapses of invasive fibrous thyroiditis and unrecognized multifocal extracervical fibrosis are frequent. The initial dose of oral prednisone is 1 mg/kg bid, reduced by 20% of total dose every 2 weeks. The therapy is administered for about 10 weeks but a maintenance dose of 10 mg/daily for 2 more weeks is advised. Some authors suggest maintenance therapy for 4 to 6 months. With corticosteroid therapy, it is necessary to pump protonic inhibitors for gastric protection and administer calcium carbonate (1,000 to 1,500 mg/daily) and calcitriol (0.5 µg/daily) to prevent osteoporosis.

The pharmacotherapy of Riedel's thyroiditis also includes tamoxifen with or without prednisone. Tamoxifen, an antiestrogen drug, inhibits connective tissue proliferation by the stimulating TGF-β, a growth inhibitor of both immature fibroblasts and epithelial cells. This drug produces both subjective and objective improvements with a decrease of goiter size and in some cases complete resolution of the disease. The oral dose is 20 mg once or twice daily; often the dose must be reduced to 10 mg bid because of side effects such as hot flashes, menstrual irregularity, and increased endometrial cancer risk in women and decreased libido in men.

Tamoxifen therapy can be used in patients who do not respond to corticosteroids or those who relapse after withdrawal; moreover the combination of prednisone and tamoxifen is also effective. A recent proposal is the association of tamoxifen- and prednisone-resistant Riedel's thyroiditis with oral mycophenolate mofetil, an immunomodulatory agent recently used with prednisone for other idiopathic fibrotic diseases. This association resulted in decreased size of the mass and a subsequent successful subtotal thyroidectomy has been very recently reported.[11]

If hypothyroidism appears, L-thyroxine is administered indefinitely at a substitutive dose level. In fact, the sustained elevation of TSH serum levels may contribute to a more rapid progression of the disease. Data explaining the natural history of Riedel's thyroiditis are minimal. L-thyroxine therapy is empirically suggested also in euthyroid patients to reduce the thyroid size (Tables 3.17 and 3.18). In rare cases of hypoparathyroidism, supplemental therapy with calcium carbonate and vitamin D is mandatory.

3.3.8 CLINICAL COURSE

Riedel's thyroiditis is generally considered a slowly progressive disease, often self-limiting. Spontaneous remission and stabilization are possible but few data are available. Recurrence is observed in 16% of cases.

3.3.9 PROGNOSIS

Prognosis is poor and ominous and relates more to extrathyroid and/or extracervical involvement with impairment of vital functions rather than the thyroiditis. The mortality ranges from 4 to 10%. The occurrences of hypothyroidism and hypoparathyroidism are rare (Table 3.17).

3.3.10 FOLLOW-UP

In patients with spontaneous or postsurgical hypothyroidism, the functional control is the same as the one for hypothyroidism. In cases of Riedel's thyroiditis in the euthyroid phase, the suggestion is annual or biennial control of thyroid function (FT_4 and TSH) and determination of serum calcium levels in well-stabilized patients (Table 3.17). In patients showing extrathyroid and/or extracervical progression of the disease, the diagnostic methodology detailed in Section 3.3.6 is mandatory.

REFERENCES

1. Hay, H.D. 1985. Thyroiditis: a clinical update. *Mayo Clinic Proceedings* 60: 836–843.
2. Lu, L., Gu, F., Dai, W.X. et al. 2010. Clinical and pathological features of Riedel's thyroiditis. *Chinese Medical Science Journal* 25: 129–134.

3. Fatourechi, M.M., Hay, I.D., McIver, B. et al. 2011. Invasive fibrous thyroiditis (Riedel thyroiditis): the Mayo Clinic experience, 1976–2008. *Thyroid* 21 (7): 1–8.
4. Annaert, M., Thijs, M., Sciot, R. et al. 2007. Riedel's thyroiditis occurring in a multinodular goiter, mimicking thyroid cancer. *Journal of Clinical Endocrinology & Metabolism* 92: 2005–2006.
5. Yasmeen, T., Khan, S., Patel, S.G. et al. 2002. Riedel's thyroiditis: report of a case complicated by spontaneous hypoparathyroidism, recurrent laryngeal nerve injury, and Horner's syndrome. *Journal of Clinical Endocrinology & Metabolism* 87: 3543–3547.
6. Siman, R., Monpeyssen, H., Desarnaud, S. et al. 2011. Ultrasound, elastography, and fluorodeoxyglucose positron emission tomography/computed tomography imaging in Riedel's thyroiditis: report of two cases. *Thyroid* 21 (7): 1–6.
7. Kotilainen, P., Airas. L., Kojo, T. et al. 2004. Positron emission tomography as an aid in the diagnosis and follow-up of Riedel's thyroiditis. *European Journal of Internal Medicine* 15: 186–189.
8. Harigopal, M., Sahoo S., Recant, W.M. et al. 2004. Fine-needle aspiration of Riedel's disease: report of a case and review of the literature. *Diagnostic Cytopathology* 30: 193–197.
9. Papi, C., Corrado, S., Carapezzi, C. et al. 2003. Riedel's thyroiditis and fibrous variant of Hashimoto thyroiditis: a clinicopathology and immunohistochemical study. *Journal of Endocrinological Investigation* 26: 444–449.
10. Shahi, N., Abdelhamid, M.F., Jindall, M. et al. 2010. Riedel's thyroiditis masquerading as anaplastic thyroid carcinoma: a case report. *Journal of Medical Case Reporting* 4: 15–18.
11. Levy, J.M., Hasney, C.P., Friedlander, P.L. et al. 2010. Combined mycophenolate mofetil and prednisone therapy in tamoxifen- and prednisone-resistant Riedel's thyroiditis. *Thyroid* 20 (1): 105–107.

4 Chronic Autoimmune Thyroiditis

Stefano Mariotti

CONTENTS

Key words: antithyroglobulin autoantibodies, antithyroid peroxidase autoantibodies, antithyrotropin receptor autoantibodies, autoimmune diseases, autoimmunity, hypothyroidism, immune system, immune tolerance, polyglandular autoimmune syndromes, thyroiditis, thyroid autoantibodies, thyroid ultrasound, fine needle aspiration cytology; thyroid cancer, L-thyroxine.

4.1   DEFINITION

First described in 1912 by Hakaru Hashimoto as "struma lymphomatosa," this disease has been also called Hashimoto's thyroiditis, chronic thyroiditis, lymphocytic thyroiditis, lymphadenoid goiter, and more recently chronic autoimmune thyroiditis (CAT), after its recognition as the original paradigm for organ-specific autoimmune diseases. CAT includes several variants (Table 4.1) sharing different proportions of common pathological features including diffuse lymphocytic infiltration, fibrosis, atrophy, and oncocytic changes of follicular cells.

The classical variant is represented by a painless, diffuse enlargement of the thyroid gland, often associated with different degrees of hypothyroidism and occurring almost exclusively in young to middle-aged women. The atrophic variant is associated with

TABLE 4.1
Variants of Chronic Autoimmune Thyroiditis (CAT)[a]

Variant	Main Pathological Features	Main Clinical Features
Focal	Scattered, diffuse lymphocytic infiltration	Euthyroidism or subclinical hypothyroidism; detectable serum ATA
Classical (goitrous)	Goiter, diffuse lymphocytic infiltration with germinal centers, fibrosis	Entire spectrum of thyroid dysfunction (most frequently mild to severe hypothyroidism)
Juvenile	Lymphocytic infiltration without other pathological changes	Euthyroidism or subclinical hypothyroidism
Fibrous	Fibrosis and massive destruction of follicular cells	Severe hypothyroidism; may mimic aggressive thyroid cancer or Riedel's thyroiditis

[a] Silent thyroiditis and postpartum thyroiditis represent transient subacute destructive phases of chronic autoimmune thyroiditis and are described in detail in Chapter 5.

the most severe thyroid failure (once called idiopathic myxedema). The asymptomatic forms (mostly frequently the focal variant) can now be detected by antithyroid auto-antibody (ATA) tests, thyroid ultrasound, and fine needle aspiration cytology, CAT is now one of the most common thyroid disorders,[1,2] at least in iodine-sufficient areas.[3]

4.2   INCIDENCE AND PREVALENCE

The presence of several variants, most of them asymptomatic, and the occurrence of hyperthyroid syndromes overlapping with Graves' disease make accurate calculation of CAT incidence extremely difficult. The incidence of symptomatic CAT has been estimated in epidemiological studies at 0.3 to 1.5 cases per 1,000 population per year, with a female:male ratio ranging 8 to 15:1.[1] CAT may be observed at all ages and even in children, but the classic variant is predominant in women aged 30 to 50 years. Atrophic thyroiditis is more frequent in subjects aged around 60 to 65 years. Pathological studies (see Section 4.4) clearly show that the prevalence of CAT is higher than that reported in clinical series, but the prevalence in surgical series can be altered by selection bias.[1]

The current general availability of ATA and ultrasound studies probably explains the apparent increase in the frequency of CAT, which is now easily and often serendipitously detected in asymptomatic patients. Although the presence of serum ATA is not always indicative of CAT, there is a strong correlation in the general population between ATA and thyroid local lymphocytic infiltration[4] on one hand and with thyroid hypoechoic pattern[5] and/or a slight increase in serum thyrotropin (TSH) concentration[6] on the other. Thus, it is conceivable that most subjects who show no signs of apparent thyroid disease except for detectable ATA have mild cases of focal CAT. The prevalence of CAT is also variable in different geographic areas. It is more common in regions with high iodine intake and in genetically susceptible populations.[3]

A rough estimation of the CAT prevalence in women is 10% for asymptomatic cases and 2% for those with clinical symptoms; a prevalence about one-tenth lower can be estimated in men.[7]

4.3 ETIOLOGY AND PATHOGENESIS

CAT represents a typical organ-specific autoimmune disease that fulfills the classical criteria proposed by Milgrom and Witebsky and modified by Rose[8] (Table 4.2). These include lymphocytic infiltration of the target organ, the identification of several well characterized thyroid autoantigens and related autoantibodies, the presence of thyroid-specific cellular immunity, and the association with other autoimmune diseases and several spontaneous or induced animal models of CAT. An important concept is that CAT is not the only consequence of thyroid autoimmunity, which is responsible also for Basedow-Graves' disease as shown in Figure 4.1. Autoimmune thyroid diseases (AITDs) encompass the entire spectrum of thyroid function ranging from severe hypothyroidism (atrophic variant of CAT or primary myxedema) to the hyperthyroidism of Basedow-Graves' disease.

The ultimate cause of thyroid autoimmunity remains elusive and may result from a combination of undetermined genetic and endogenous or exogenous environmental factors (Figure 4.2) that lead to the loss of immunological tolerance.[9,10] As exemplified in Figure 4.3, this phenomenon implies failure of the mechanisms that prevent the emergence of T cells to react with thyroid autoantigens (central tolerance, mainly in the fetal thymus) and control the activity of the normal immune response (peripheral tolerance from regulatory cells such as CD4+ and CD25+ T lymphocytes and T-reg cells).

Several exogenous and endogenous environmental factors (Figure 4.2) combine with a complex genetic background to produce full expression of CAT and other AITDs.[11] The best documented examples of environmental factors are high iodine intake, cytokine administration (interleukin-2, interferons, and other "biological" treatments employed in wide spectrum of neoplastic, viral and immunological diseases), stressful events, and estrogens.

TABLE 4.2
Milgrom and Witebsky's Criteria for Organ-Specific Autoimmune Disease

Classical	Revised
Lymphocyte infiltration of target organ	Direct evidence from transfer of disease with autoantibodies or T lymphocytes
Circulating autoantibodies and/or cellular immunity to target organ	Indirect evidence from reproduction of disease in experimental animal models
Identification of organ-specific antigens	Circumstantial evidence from clinical studies
Induction of humoral and cellular immune response in animals immunized with autologous antigens	
Strict association with other autoimmune diseases	

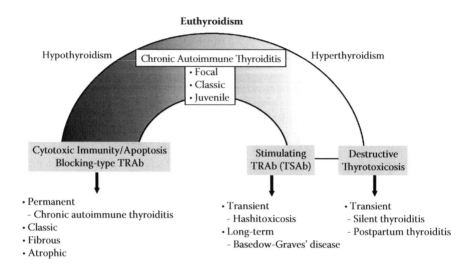

FIGURE 4.1   Spectrum of autoimmune thyroid diseases.

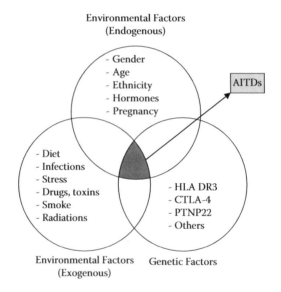

FIGURE 4.2   Genetic and exogenous or endogenous environmental factors involved in the pathogenesis of autoimmune thyroid diseases (AITDs).

An overwhelming mass of experimental and clinical data indicate that CAT is genetically controlled.[12] This concept stems from the observation of the high familiar clustering of CAT and other AITDs with a concordance in monozygous twins about 10 times higher than that of dizygous twins. The main genes involved in susceptibility to thyroid autoimmunity are listed in Table 4.3. The roles of the major human histocompatibility complex (MHC) genes (called human leukocyte antigens

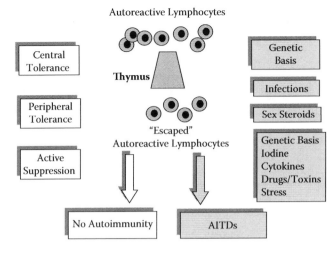

FIGURE 4.3   Sequence of events potentially involved in loss of immunological tolerance in autoimmune thyroid diseases (AITDs).

TABLE 4.3

Main Genes Involved in Genetic Predisposition to Autoimmune Thyroid Diseases

Genes	Alleles
HLA	DR-3 (DRB1*03)
	DQ-2 (DQB1*02)
CTLA-4	ATn106
	49 A/G
	60 C/T
CD 40	5'-UTR C/T
PTPN22	R620W
Tg	Several SNPs
TSHR	Several SNPs

Note: HLA = human leukocyte antigen; CTLA-4 = cytotoxic T lymphocyte-associated antigen 4; CD40 = membrane receptor molecule member of tumor necrosis factor (TNF) superfamily mainly expressed by B lymphocytes monocytes, dendritic cells (in nervous system), endothelial cells (in blood vessels), and epithelial cells; PTPN22 = protein tyrosine phosphatase, non-receptor type 22; Tg = thyroglobulin; TSHR = thyrotropin receptor.

or HLAs) are well known. HLA genes encode highly polymorphic cell surface proteins deeply involved in antigen presentation to the immune system (Figure 4.4). The peculiar HLA haplotype HLA DR3(DRB1*03)/DQB1*0201 is associated with increased susceptibility to AITDs and other organ-specific autoimmune diseases, possibly linked to a specific polymorphism of the amino acid in position 74 (arginine favoring and glutamine preventing thyroid autoimmunity). Other non-HLA genes involved in thyroid autoimmunity include CTLA-4, CD40, the thyrosine phosphatase PTPN22 (all molecules involved in controlling immune responses; Figure 4.4), and thyroid autoantigens as thyroglobulin (Tg) and TSH receptor (TSH-R).[12]

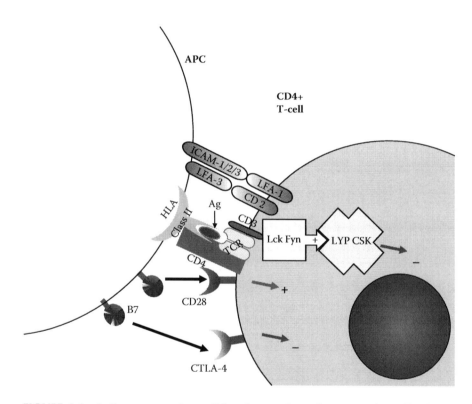

FIGURE 4.4   Antigen presentation to T lymphocytes by antigen-presenting cells (APCs). For its specific recognition, the antigenic epitope must interact with T cell receptors (TCRs) in strict association with class I HLA (for suppressor/cytotoxic T lymphocytes) or class II HLA proteins (for helper T lymphocytes as depicted). Activation of T lymphocytes needs also the interaction of other costimulatory (ICAM-1, 2, 3/LFA-1) and regulatory (B-7/CTLA-4; B-7/CD28) molecules. The interaction B-7/CTLA-4 suppresses immune response through regulatory T lymphocytes while binding of CD-28 to B-7 exerts stimulatory activity. Lymphoid protein phosphatase (LYP) encoded by the *PTPN22* gene represents an additional factor inhibiting T lymphocyte activation. Antigen binding to TCR leads to the activation of specific kinases (Lck and Fym) and the formation of a complex of LYP and the CSK kinase with consequent inhibition of lymphocyte activation.

The initial phase of thyroid autoimmunity involves recruitment of thyroid-specific T lymphocytes through locally produced chemokines (particularly the IFN-γ-induced chemokines CXCL9 e CXCL10 and other chemokines of the CX family: CXCR3, CCR5 and CCL4) that favor the passage of mononuclear cells from peripheral blood into the thyroid gland.[13] Thyroid-specific T lymphocytes subsequently undergo clonal expansion, cytokine production, and further recruitment of mononuclear cells that will constitute the final thyroid infiltrate.[9,10]

As summarized in Figure 4.5, thyroid autoimmunity exerts its pathologic effects via different immune mechanisms involving production of complement (C′)-fixing autoantibodies, immune complex formation, cell-mediated cytotoxic mechanisms including antibody-dependent cellular cytotoxicity (ADCC), natural killer (NK) and specific T-cell cytotoxicity, and local cytokines (IL-2, IFN-γ, and TNF-α, produced by a specific subset of T helper [TH] cells of the TH₁ subtype that predominate in thyroid infiltrates).[9,10] With the exception of stimulating autoantibodies to TSH-R that are directly responsible for hyperthyroidism in Basedow-Graves' disease, all of the above mechanisms along with blocking autoantibodies to TSH-R promote destruction and apoptosis of thyroid cells, providing the basis for different degrees of hypothyroidism, the predominant functional alteration of CAT.

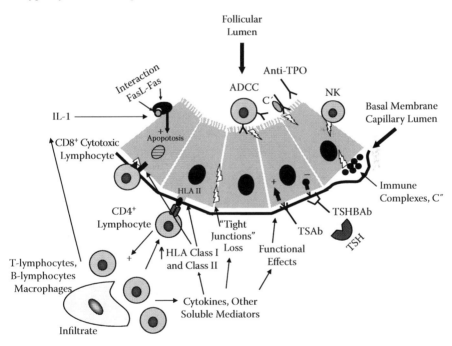

FIGURE 4.5   Effector immune mechanisms involved in thyroid damage in thyroid autoimmunity. ACDD = antibody-dependent cellular cytotoxicity. Anti-TPO = antithyroid peroxidase antibodies. C′ = complement. Fas = main receptor involved in chain of events leading to thyroid cell apoptosis. FasL = Fas ligand. NKs = natural killer cells. TSAbs = stimulating antibodies to TSH receptor. TSHBAbs = blocking antibodies to TSH receptor.

4.4 PATHOLOGY

Although lymphocytic infiltration of the thyroid gland is the pathological hallmark of CAT, several subtypes of CAT encompass the spectrum of AITDs.[14] In the classical variant of CAT, the thyroid shows diffuse infiltration of lymphocytes and plasma cells that may aggregate with macrophages to form lymphoid follicles with germinal centers (Figure 4.6c). The normal architecture of the gland is disrupted, some follicular cells may show oxyphilic changes in the cytoplasm (Askenazy or Hürthle cells), and a variable degree of fibrosis is present in most cases.

In the atrophic variant, the gland is markedly reduced in size due to atrophy of the follicular epithelium that is fully replaced by fibrous tissue and residual lymphocytic infiltration. The juvenile variant is characterized by lymphoid infiltration in the absence of other pathological changes. In rare cases (fibrous variant), extensive fibrosis associated with lymphocytic infiltration is the predominant feature and differentiation from Riedel's thyroiditis may be difficult. Focal CAT (generally detected

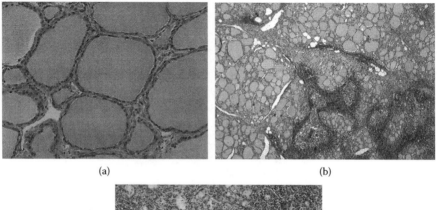

(a)   (b)

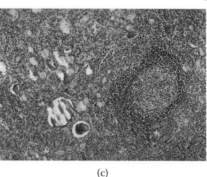

(c)

FIGURE 4.6   Histologic appearance of normal thyroid (a) as compared with focal (b) and classic (c) variants of CAT. Classic variant shows typical pathological changes represented by diffuse lymphocytic infiltration leading to lymphoid follicle formation with germinal centers and extensive damage of thyroid follicles with Hürthle cell metaplasia. Focal variant shows scattered lymphocytic infiltrates with substantially conserved thyroid follicular structure. Stain: hematoxylin and eosin. Magnification: a = 250×; b = 40×; c = 250×. (Source: Images kindly provided by Dr. M.L. Lai, Department of Cytopathology, University of Cagliari, Cagliari, Italy.)

at autopsy or in surgical samples of glands removed because of other diseases, especially in elderly women) is characterized by scattered foci of lymphocytic infiltration (Figure 4.6b) and is asymptomatic, although frequently associated with detectable serum ATA.[15] Accordingly, this condition may also be called *asymptomatic (or mild) atrophic thyroiditis* and represents the most common variant of CAT.

4.5 CLINICAL FEATURES

Most cases of CAT are represented by asymptomatic young or middle-aged women. The diagnosis is made by detection of positive thyroid autoantibodies and/or slightly increased circulating TSH concentration and/or a hypoechoic pattern on thyroid ultrasound. A small to moderate non-tender diffuse goiter (Figure 4.7) of somewhat rubbery consistence on palpation is often the hallmark of the disease. One or more prevalent nodules may be felt on physical examination or more often detected by thyroid ultrasound (see Section 4.6.3).

The nodules may be direct expressions of the disease (as hyperplastic nodules resulting from chronic TSH stimulation or pseudonodules consisting of areas of intense lymphocytic infiltration and/or fibrosis). They may also result from associated benign or malignant thyroid neoplasias, as discussed in detail later. Based on hardness, irregular shape, and tendency for adjacent soft tissue infiltration, the fibrous variant may mimic aggressive thyroid tumors (anaplastic carcinomas, lymphomas) or Riedel's thyroiditis.[16] Thyroid enlargement in CAT is generally not associated with significant local symptoms, with the exception of a feeling of tightness in the neck—a rather frequent complaint. CAT may very rarely present with thyroid pain and tenderness, often accompanied by fever and general malaise, in the absence of any evidence of local invasion: this clinical picture may be very difficult to differentiate from subacute thyroiditis.[17]

Most cases of CAT are associated with euthyroidism or subtle to mild primary hypothyroidism. Overt hypothyroidism (often represented by frank myxedema) is

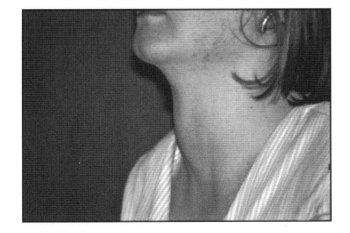

FIGURE 4.7   CAT of 27-year-old woman presenting with diffuse euthyroid goiter.

typical of the atrophic and fibrous variants, but may be observed also in the classical form. For a complete description of the clinical picture of primary hypothyroidism, the reader is referred to Chapter 10. In a minority of cases, CAT may present with transient hyperthyroidism due to the destructive thyrotoxicosis typical of sporadic or postpartum painless (silent) thyroiditis (see Chapter 5 for a complete descriptions of these conditions) or to thyroid hyperfunction with detectable stimulating anti-TSH-R antibodies (TRAb) in syndromes overlapping with Graves' disease. The latter condition is also called (especially in Japanese literature) Hashitoxicosis, although the term has been also used to describe the thyrotoxic phase of silent thyroiditis.[7]

The association of CAT with differentiated thyroid tumors and particularly papillary thyroid carcinoma (PTC) is always possible and known for a long time on the basis of retrospective surgical studies.[18] While these reports may have been affected by selection bias, further support for this association has been provided by recent studies on unselected thyroid nodules submitted to fine needle aspiration cytology (FNAC).[19] Increased TSH[20] and possibly autoimmune inflammation are the most probable factors involved in this association, whose definition deserves further investigation.

A rare and life-threatening complication of CAT is thyroid lymphoma developing from lymphocytic infiltration of the gland and representing a variant of the so-called maltomas (lymphomas arising from, mucosa-associated lymphoid tissues [MALTs] such as palatine tonsils, stomach, and salivary glands).[21] Lymphoma should be suspected in the presence of sudden, rapid developing asymmetric enlargement of a gland affected by CAT, often associated with pain, tenderness, hoarseness, and enlargement of regional lymph nodes. Primary thyroid lymphomas are of B cell origin and prolonged stimulation of intrathyroidal B lymphocytes is presumably responsible for the emergence of malignant clones.[21] The incidence of lymphoma in CAT is very low, but this condition should be considered during long-term follow-up, since primary thyroid lymphoma arises exclusively from thyroid glands affected by CAT.

Association with other autoimmune diseases is a well-established feature of CAT and one of the most convincing clinical criteria supporting its autoimmune pathogenesis.[22] When compared to a control population, a higher prevalence (5 to 30%) of CAT or AITD has been reported in Addison's disease, pernicious anemia, autoimmune gastritis, celiac disease, alopecia areata, type 1 diabetes mellitus, primary biliary cirrhosis, myasthenia gravis, thrombocytopenic purpura, autoimmune hemolytic anemia, vitiligo, Sjøgren's disease, and systemic lupus erythematosus. However, due to the very low prevalence of other autoimmune diseases, the proportion of AITD patients showing each single associated disease remains low and not easily detected unless specifically investigated.[22,23]

AITDs are also frequently found in patients with autoimmune Addison's disease and/or type 1 diabetes mellitus as a part of the autoimmune polyglandular syndrome (APS) type 2. In contrast, AITDs are infrequent features of the much rarer APS type 1 (autoimmune Addison's disease, idiopathic hypoparathyroidism, and cutaneous mucocandidiasis) caused by mutation of the autoimmune-related (aire) gene. All these associations are much more frequently observed at the serological rather than at the clinical level (see Section 4.6.2).

4.6 DIAGNOSIS

4.6.1 CLINICAL DIAGNOSIS

Since most cases of CAT are nearly asymptomatic, a clue to diagnosis is often provided by laboratory tests (positive ATAs, increased serum TSH, and typical hypoechoic pattern on thyroid ultrasound), generally performed in the course of general screening or targeted high risk case finding procedures in subjects with familial histories of thyroid autoimmunity. Less frequently, local signs and symptoms and/or overt thyroid dysfunction dominate the clinical picture. The rare cases of CAT associated with painful thyroid must be differentiated from subacute (De Quervain's) thyroiditis. This differential diagnosis is difficult based only on a clinical ground. Generally, painful CAT is less responsive to glucocorticoid therapy and more frequently relapses for longer periods.

4.6.2 LABORATORY TESTS

The presence of detectable serum ATAs is an important clue to the diagnosis of CAT although ATAs may be undetectable in some cases (mostly juvenile variant or atrophic CAT treated with long-term thyroid hormone substitution therapy). ATAs, the corresponding autoantigens, and the techniques presently employed for antibody detection are listed in Table 4.4. ATAs are not specific for CAT, but, if they are present at medium to high titers, they are generally indicative of AITD.[24] Low titer ATAs are detected in a substantial minority of apparently normal subjects (especially in women aged over 55 years) and in patients with other non-autoimmune thyroid diseases. Thus, ATA testing should always be interpreted in the specific clinical context and compared to other diagnostic procedures before a diagnosis of CAT can be made.

Anti-TPO antibody (TPOAb), formerly known as an antithyroid microsomal antibody, is the antibody test that most frequently shows abnormal results in CAT and other AITDs (Figure 4.8).[25] Most (90 to 95%) sera with positive anti-Tg antibodies (TgAbs) are also positive for TPOAbs, while TgAbs are not detected in about 30 to 50% of TPOAb-positive sera.[25] Testing for TPOAb is therefore the first choice in the diagnostic evaluation of suspect thyroid autoimmunity, although TgAbs, despite lower general sensitivity for AITDs, is more specific for CAT.[24]

ATA titer is an important diagnostic parameter because high levels of serum antibodies are almost exclusively found in full-blown AITDs.[25] However, the precise evaluation of ATA titer is still a difficult task. Although levels exceeding 1,000 international units (IU)/mL are generally observed only in AITDs, current immunometric assays still show marked differences between normal, borderline, and pathological ranges, and no true standardization of the IU has been achieved.[24] Moreover, the effect of long-term treatment with thyroid hormone may reduce ATA titers to the point of disappearance, especially in primary myxedema, due to the atrophic variant of CAT.[9] Assay of TRAb is not generally required for the diagnosis of CAT except in thyrotoxic patients where destructive thyrotoxicosis (painless thyroiditis) must

TABLE 4.4

Thyroid Autoantigen–Autoantibody Systems Employed for Laboratory Diagnosis of AITDs

Autoantigen	Molecular Weight	Amino Acid Sequence	Main Function	Detection Methods
Thyroglobulin (Tg)	640 kD	Determined	Prothyroid hormone	Methods employed in clinical practice: passive agglutination, RIA, ELISA, other immunometric techniques Other methods: precipitation, immunofluorescence, Western blotting
Thyroid peroxidase (TPO)	101 to 107 kD	Determined	Iodide oxidation and coupling of iodothyrosine residues	Methods employed in clinical practice: passive agglutination, RIA, ELISA, other immunometric techniques Other methods: C′ fixation, immunofluorescence, cytotoxicity
TSH receptor	Extracellular (α) subunit: 53 kD; transmembrane and cytoplasmic (β) subunit: 30 to 42 kD	Determined	Transduction of TSH message	Methods employed in clinical practice: radioligand and other competitive receptor assays (TRAb) Functional assays (research only): stimulation (TSAb) and TSH-blocking (TBAb) assays

be distinguished from autoimmune hyperthyroidism in conditions with overlapping features of both CAT and Basedow-Graves' disease.[24] Blocking-type TRAbs may be present in sera of hypothyroid CAT patients, especially in the atrophic variant, but these antibodies do not need to be assayed in clinical practice with the possible exception during pregnancy to identify women at risk of fetal and/or neonatal hypothyroidism due to placental transmission of maternal antibodies.[26]

In selected cases (e.g., a suspicious clinical picture and/or a CAT patient with a personal or family history of multiple autoimmunity), the assay of other non-thyroidal

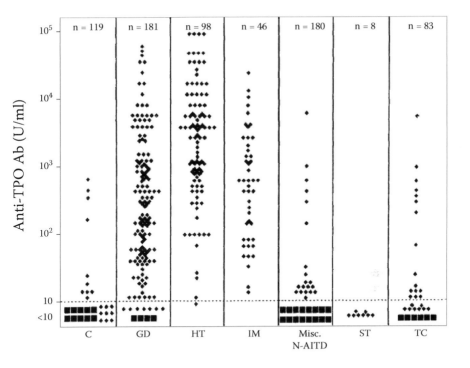

FIGURE 4.8 Antithyroid peroxidase antibodies (Anti-TPO Abs) determined by RIA in 119 normal controls (C) and 596 patients with different thyroid diseases [Graves' disease (GD), classic CAT (Hashimoto's thyroiditis: HT), atrophic CAT (idiopathic myxedema: IM), miscellaneous non-autoimmune thyroid diseases (Misc-N-AITD), subacute thyroiditis (ST), and thyroid carcinoma (TC)]. Values above the dotted line (>10 U/mL) were considered positive. Larger symbols indicate 10 sera. (*Source:* Mariotti, S. et al. 1990. *J Clin Endocrinol Metab* 71: 661–669. With permission from Endocrine Society.)

autoantibodies may allow the identification of mild or preclinical forms of associated autoimmune diseases.[22,23] Presently, due to the low prevalence of clinically autoimmune disease in CAT, routine autoantibody screening is not recommended except perhaps gastric parietal cell antibodies (markers of autoimmune atrophic gastritis) and transglutaminase antibodies (markers of celiac disease).[23]

The laboratory evaluation of thyroid function does not differ from the procedure described in the chapters dealing with hypothyroidism and hyperthyroidism. It is worthwhile to remember that most cases of CAT are associated with TSH at the upper limit of the normal range (2.5 to 4.0 mU/L) or slightly increased (4.0 to 10 mU/L), with normal free thyroxine (FT$_4$) and free triiodothyronine (FT$_3$) concentrations.

Other common laboratory abnormalities may include increased gamma-globulin fraction (in patients with very high ATA titers) and mild elevation of erythrocyte sedimentation rate (ESR) and C-reactive protein (CRP) in forms associated with painful thyroid, in contrast with subacute thyroiditis, where both ESR and CRP are extremely increased.

4.6.3 THYROID IMAGING

Thyroid scintiscan has no role in the diagnosis of euthyroid and hypothyroid CAT although it may be helpful when combined with 24-hour radioiodine uptake tests in hyperthyroid patients to identify destructive thyrotoxicosis. Thyroid ultrasound in combination with color Doppler sonography (CDS) is presently the single best test for diagnosing CAT.[27]

Imaging will show a diffusely hypoechoic pattern of the thyroid gland due to lymphocytic infiltration, which in some cases may assume a typical "honeycomb" appearance due to interstitial fibrosis (Figure 4.9). Evaluation of thyroid blood flow by CDS allows differentiation of euthyroid or mild hypothyroid CAT from Basedow-Graves' disease (where thyroid is also hypoechoic, but blood flow is markedly increased). Increased thyroid blood flow may be observed in hypothyroid CAT due to increased TSH stimulation. Thyroid ultrasound is valuable for diagnosing nodular lesions often found in glands affected by CAT and may be caused by very different pathological conditions.[28] In some cases, these lesions are not strictly thyroid nodules and represent foci of intense mononuclear cell infiltration with germinal centers (pseudonodules); see Figure 4.9.

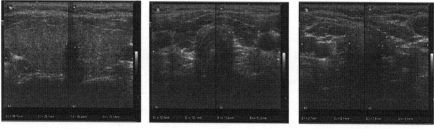

(a)   (b)   (c)

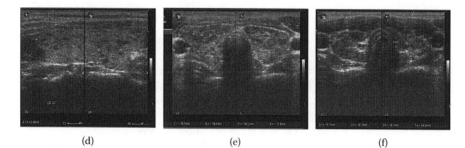

(d)   (e)   (f)

FIGURE 4.9 Thyroid ultrasound features observed in different forms of CAT. (a) Diffuse thyroid enlargement with mild hypoechogenicity; (b) reduced thyroid volume with marked hypoechogenicity; (c) typical appearance of atrophic variant of CAT with marked thyroid atrophy and hypoechogenicity; (d) thyroid showing multiple small hypoechoic areas; (e) gland with hypoechoic areas and hyperechoic striae (honeycomb appearance); (f) markedly hypoechoic gland with pseudonodular pattern.

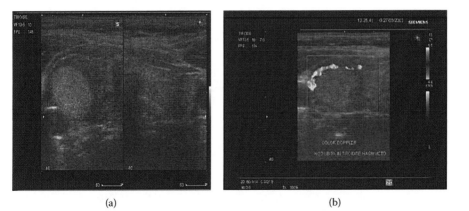

(a)   (b)

(c)   (d)

FIGURE 4.10 Echographic appearance of CAT associated with thyroid nodules. (a) Hyperechoic nodule of right lobe with benign appearance surrounded by hypoechoic slightly enlarged gland (transverse scan); (b) same nodule showing perinodular vascularization assessed by color Doppler sonography (CDS, longitudinal scan); (c) hypoechoic nodule of left lobe suspicious for malignancy (microcalcifications, irregular borders, transverse scan); (d) same nodule evaluated by CDS showing intranodular signal (longitudinal scan).

True thyroid nodules arising from follicular cells are often present in CAT and range from hyperplastic lesions to benign or malignant tumors (Figure 4.10). Although ultrasound may be sufficient to exclude thyroid malignancy, in most cases of nodular CAT, ultrasound-guided fine needle aspiration cytology (FNAc) is required for a reliable diagnosis.

4.6.4 FINE NEEDLE ASPIRATION CYTOLOGY (FNAC)

The typical cytological picture of CAT[29] shows autoimmune infiltrate (lymphocytes and plasma cells) with scattered follicular cells (some of which may present oxyphilic changes) and scarce colloid (Figure 4.11a and b). FNAc is generally not required in CAT cases without nodular lesions, while it is the best tool to differentiate benign from malignant associated thyroid nodules (Figure 4.11d and e).

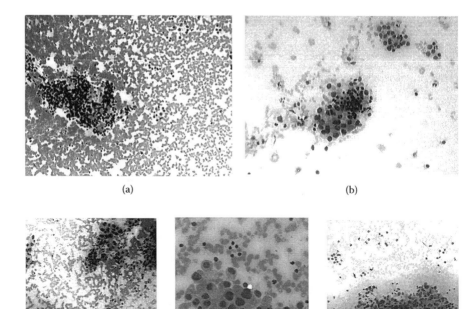

(a)   (b)

(c)   (d)   (e)

FIGURE 4.11   (a) and (b): Cytological appearance of material obtained by fine needle aspiration from nodular and pseudonodular areas of CAT not suggestive of associated neoplastic lesions. (a) Mixture of epithelial cells in background of typical lymphocytes (100× magnification); (b) cluster of Hürthle cells suggestive of oxyphilic metaplasia in background of lymphocytes and plasma cells (250× magnification); (c) through (e): cytological appearance of material obtained by fine needle aspiration from nodular CAT suggestive of associated neoplasia; (c) thyroid cell with microfollicular pattern with atypias (indeterminate; 100× magnification); (d) and (e): cytological features indicative of papillary thyroid carcinoma associated to CAT showing typical nuclear abnormalities (D = 400×) and papillary structures (E =100×). (Source: Images kindly provided by Dr. M.L. Lai, Department of Cytopathology, University of Cagliari, Cagliari, Italy.)

Cytological evaluation of CAT-associated thyroid nodules requires specific expertise because non-specific cytological alterations of follicular cells sometimes mimicking suspicious nodules (Figure 4.11c) are frequently observed.[30] In the presence of thyroid lymphomas, a differential diagnosis with an active thyroid lymphocytic infiltration on one hand and with small cell, poorly differentiated carcinoma on the other may be very difficult on cytological ground. In these cases, the reverse transcription polymerase chain reaction (RT-PCR) for detecting the monoclonality of immunoglobulin heavy chain mRNA may be useful for the correct identification of lymphoma.[7]

4.7 THERAPY

Most patients with CAT do not require treatment. Since the disorder is asymptomatic and goiter small or absent, thyroid function may remain stably normal for a long time. In euthyroid or mildly hypothyroid patients with significant thyroid enlargements and/or associated but not suspicious nodules, thyroid hormone therapy (preferentially L-thyroxine or LT_4) is indicated at doses able to maintain serum TSH in the lower portion of the normal range.

In young patients, partially or fully suppressive (<0.1 mU/L) TSH may be employed with periodical thyroid ultrasonography to control thyroid volume and the numbers, dimensions, and ultrasound characteristics of associated nodules that may show rapid and impressive improvement, especially in children and adolescents, with reduction of thyroid volume (more evident in hypothyroid, but significant also in euthyroid children)[31] even with non-TSH suppressive LT_4 doses.[32] In contrast, TSH suppression (even unintentional) must be avoided in older patients, especially in postmenopausal woman and in men over 60 years of age due to the high risk of bone and cardiac complications and the low chance of shrinking the gland or nodules by irreversible fibrotic changes.

In overt hypothyroidism, full replacement therapy with appropriate doses of LT_4 to maintain stable serum TSH (0.5 to 2.0 mU/L) are required (see Chapter 10). Treatment with LT_4 is indefinitely required in most patients, but up to 20% of initially overt hypothyroid individuals may later recover normal thyroid function. From a practical view, interruption of LT_4 is rarely indicated, because restoration of normal thyroid function is often of only short duration. In rare cases, CAT presenting with overt hypothyroidism may progress to transient or persistent thyrotoxicosis due to painless thyroiditis or evolution to Basedow-Graves' disease. These cases, particularly common in the postpartum period (see Chapter 5), should be promptly identified and the LT_4 immediately withdrawn.

Although the question remains unsettled, a widely spread opinion (shared by the present writer) is that most patients with established diagnoses of CAT and subclinical hypothyroidism (increased serum TSH, normal FT_4) should be treated by LT_4 even in the absence of goiter and nodules because the progression to overt thyroid failure is frequent, particularly in the presence of high titers of circulating ATAs. Elderly patients (75 to 80 years) may represent remarkable exceptions due to high cardiovascular risk and possible protective effects of mild hypothyroidism in the oldest old population (see Chapter 29). Although a fall of serum ATA titers has been reported during long-term LT4 therapy in hypothyroid patients with CAT,[9] no clear evidence indicates that thyroid hormones may halt the disease progression.

Glucocorticoids have no role in CAT therapy, with the possible exception of treating aggressive forms of the fibrous variant[16] and some cases associated with subacute symptoms (pain, hoarseness, dysphagia, severe destructive thyrotoxicosis).[17] Supplementation with selenium (Se) has recently been reported to reduce serum ATA titer and the frequency of postpartum thyroiditis[33] considered to be a consequence of exacerbation of thyroid autoimmunity (see Chapter 5). The action of Se (a fundamental constituent of a large number of key enzymes controlling several metabolic pathways) is believed to be related to its antioxidant properties that lead to reduction of free radicals.[33]

A recent report of the positive effects of Se supplementation (100 mg bid as selenium selenite) on mild forms of thyroid orbitopathy in patients with Basedow-Graves' disease[34] (see Chapter 26) provides further support for the effectiveness of Se as a possible down regulator of the thyroid autoimmune response. Further studies are needed to clarify whether and to what extent Se may be considered an effective treatment of CAT.

Surgery should be employed in the presence of suspicious nodules or large, irregular goiters with compressive local symptoms. Thyroidectomy may be indicated for exceptionally painful variants of CAT (persistent pain not resolving after a course of LT_4 and/or steroids or non-steroidal anti-inflammatory drug administration).

4.8 PROGNOSIS

The most frequent complication of CAT is the development of overt thyroid dysfunction. In patients with CAT and subclinical hypothyroidism, about 5% per year will progress to overt thyroid failure,[1] but age, gender, ATA titer, and absolute serum TSH concentration may affect the progression rate.[2] As stated earlier, the course of CAT may present transient thyrotoxic phases due to destructive thyrotoxicosis (see Chapter 5), but in rare cases the disease may progress to full-blown hyperthyroid Basedow-Graves' disease with active orbitopathy.

In rare cases of fibrous variants of CAT, severe dyspnea and/or dysphagia may mimic aggressive thyroid tumors, but these symptoms always recede after surgical or even medical (corticosteroid) therapy. The association of papillary thyroid carcinoma (PTC) with CAT has been discussed earlier. Independently of this association, CAT may affect the prognosis of PTC, although present data are conflicting. PTCs detected in the background of CAT are often multicentric and in more advanced stages, but lower rates of recurrence and/or metastases have been described in differentiated thyroid tumors associated to thyroid autoimmunity.

The only potentially lethal condition directly arising from CAT is primary thyroid B cell lymphoma. However, primary thyroid lymphomas are observed only in patients with long-standing CAT. The absolute probability of this event is low, estimated below 0.1%.

4.9 FOLLOW-UP

Most patients with CAT need periodical evaluation of thyroid function (TSH and FT_4 measurement) and morphology (color Doppler ultrasonography) before or after institution of long-term substitution therapy with LT_4. In such cases, the criteria for follow-up planning are the same as those discussed for primary hypothyroidism (see Chapter 10). It should be noted that goitrous CAT may present with overt thyroid failure, then progress toward thyrotoxic or hyperthyroid phases including the evolution into a condition indistinguishable from Basedow-Graves' disease. Thus, frequent control of serum TSH should be planned if this condition is suspected.

Even more difficult is to predict the evolution of euthyroid CAT, generally characterized only by positive circulating ATAs that may also herald the appearance of hyperthyroid Basedow-Graves' disease. The odds ratio (OR) for subsequent clinical thyroid dysfunction conferred by positive serum ATAs in otherwise euthyroid subjects were calculated only recently.[35] According to this study, detectable ATAs were associated with a markedly increased OR (about 10 to 80 for TgAb and 10 to 20 for TPOAb) to develop hypothyroid CAT at any time before the diagnosis during a 7-year period.

Euthyroid ATA-positive subjects face increased risk of Basedow-Graves' disease, although the odds significantly increased approaching diagnosis, reaching values similar to those found for CAT only about 6 months to 2 years before the diagnosis. This finding confirms the lack of specificity of TgAb and TPOAb for prediction of Basedow-Graves' disease and the faster progression of autoimmune hyperthyroidism when compared to thyroid failure. Assay of TRAbs, although highly specific for Basedow-Graves' disease is devoid of predictive value since these stimulating antibodies often become detectable simultaneously with the development of clinical hyperthyroidism.

REFERENCES

1. Dayan, C.M. and Daniels, G.H. 1996. Chronic autoimmune thyroiditis. *New Engl J Med* 335: 99–107.
2. Pearce, E.N., Farwell, A.P., and Braverman, L.E. 2003. Thyroiditis. *New Engl J Med* 348: 2646–2655.
3. Laurberg, P., Cerqueira, C., Ovesen, L. et al. 2010. Iodine intake as a determinant of thyroid disorders in populations. *Best Pract Res Clin Endocrinol Metab* 24: 13–27.
4. Arai, T., Kurashima, C., Utsuyama, M. et al. 2000. Measurement of anti-thyroglobulin and anti-thyroid peroxidase antibodies using highly sensitive radioimmunoassay: an effective method for detecting asymptomatic focal lymphocytic thyroiditis in the elderly. *Endocrinol J* 47: 575–582.
5. Vitti, P. and Rago, T. 2003. Thyroid ultrasound as a predicator of thyroid disease. *J Endocrinol Invest* 26: 686–689.
6. Hollowell, J.G., Staehling, N.W., Flanders, W.D. et al. 2002. Serum TSH, T_4, and thyroid antibodies in the United States population (1988 to 1994): National Health and Nutrition Examination Survey (NHANES III). *J Clin Endocrinol Metab* 87: 489–499.
7. Akamizu, T., Amino, N., and De Groot, L. 2008. Hashimoto's thyroiditis. In *Thyroid Disease Manager,* L. De Groot, Ed. http://www.thyroidmanager.org/Chapter8/8-frame.htm
8. Rose, N.R. and Bona, C. 1993. Defining criteria for autoimmune diseases (Witebsky's postulates revisited). *Immunol Today* 14: 426–430.
9. Mariotti, S. and Pinna, G. 2003. Autoimmune thyroid disease. In *Contemporary Endocrinology: Diseases of the Thyroid*, Braverman, L.E., Ed. Totowa, NJ: Humana Press, 107–160.
10. Weetman, A. P. 2004. Cellular immune responses in autoimmune thyroid disease. *Clin Endocrinol (Oxf)* 61: 405–413.
11. Prummel, M.F., Strieder, T., and Wiersinga, W.M. 2004. The environment and autoimmune thyroid diseases. *Eur J Endocrinol* 150: 605–618.
12. Tomer, Y. 2010. Genetic susceptibility to autoimmune thyroid disease: past, present, and future. *Thyroid* 20: 715–725.
13. Rotondi, M., Chiovato, L., Romagnani, S. et al. 2007. Role of chemokines in endocrine autoimmune diseases. *Endocrinol Rev* 28: 492–520.
14. LiVolsi, V.A. 1994. The pathology of autoimmune thyroid disease: a review. *Thyroid* 4: 333–339.

15. Arain, A., Abou-Khalil, B., and Moses, H. 2001. Hashimoto's encephalopathy: documentation of mesial temporal seizure origin by ictal EEG. *Seizure* 10: 438–441.
16. Heufelder, A.E. and Hay, I.D. 1994. Evidence for autoimmune mechanisms in the evolution of invasive fibrous thyroiditis (Riedel's struma). *Clin Invest* 72: 788–793.
17. Kon, Y.C. and DeGroot, L.J. 2003. Painful Hashimoto's thyroiditis as an indication for thyroidectomy: clinical characteristics and outcome in seven patients. *J Clin Endocrinol Metab* 88: 2667–2672.
18. Okayasu, I., Fujiwara, M., Hara, Y. et al. 1995. Association of chronic lymphocytic thyroiditis and thyroid papillary carcinoma: a study of surgical cases among Japanese, and white and African Americans. *Cancer* 76: 2312–2318.
19. Boi, F., Lai, M. L., Marziani, B. et al. 2005. High prevalence of suspicious cytology in thyroid nodules associated with positive thyroid autoantibodies. *Eur J Endocrinol* 153: 637–642.
20. Boelaert, K. 2009. The association between serum TSH concentration and thyroid cancer. *Endocrinol Relat Cancer* 16: 1065–1072.
21. Graff-Baker, A., Sosa, J.A., and Roman, S.A. 2010. Primary thyroid lymphoma: a review of recent developments in diagnosis and histology-driven treatment. *Curr Opin Oncol* 22: 17–22.
22. Weetman, A.P. 2011. Diseases associated with thyroid autoimmunity: explanations for the expanding spectrum. *Clin Endocrinol (Oxf)* 74: 411–418.
23. Weetman, A.P. 2005. Non-thyroid autoantibodies in autoimmune thyroid disease. *Best Pract Res Clin Endocrinol Metab* 19: 17–32.
24. Baloch, Z., Carayon, P., Conte-Devolx, B. et al. 2003. Laboratory medicine practice guidelines: laboratory support for the diagnosis and monitoring of thyroid disease. *Thyroid* 13: 3–126.
25. Mariotti, S., Caturegli, P., Piccolo, P. et al. 1990. Antithyroid peroxidase autoantibodies in thyroid diseases. *J Clin Endocrinol Metab* 71: 661–669.
26. Stagnaro-Green, A., Abalovich, M., Alexander, E. et al. 2011. Guidelines of the American Thyroid Association for the diagnosis and management of thyroid disease during pregnancy and postpartum. *Thyroid* 21: 1081–1125.
27. Vitti, P., Rago, T., Barbesino, G. et al. 1999. Thyroiditis: clinical aspects and diagnostic imaging. *Rays* 24: 301–314.
28. Tonacchera, M., Pinchera, A., and Vitti, P. 2010. Assessment of nodular goitre. *Best Pract Res Clin Endocrinol Metab* 24: 51–61.
29. Baloch, Z.W. and LiVolsi, V.A. 2008. Fine-needle aspiration of the thyroid: today and tomorrow. *Best Pract Res Clin Endocrinol Metab* 22: 929–939.
30. MacDonald, L. and Yazdi, H.M. 1999. Fine needle aspiration biopsy of Hashimoto's thyroiditis: sources of diagnostic error. *Acta Cytol* 43: 400–406.
31. Svensson, J., Ericsson, U.B., Nilsson, P. et al. 2006. Levothyroxine treatment reduces thyroid size in children and adolescents with chronic autoimmune thyroiditis. *J Clin Endocrinol Metab* 91: 1729–1734.
32. Karges, B., Muche, R., Knerr, I. et al. 2007. Levothyroxine in euthyroid autoimmune thyroiditis and type 1 diabetes: a randomized, controlled trial. *J Clin Endocrinol Metab* 92: 1647–1652.
33. Duntas, L.H. 2010. Selenium and the thyroid: a close-knit connection. *J Clin Endocrinol Metab* 95: 5180–5188.
34. Marcocci, C., Kahaly, G.J., Krassas, G.E. et al. 2011. Selenium and the course of mild Graves' orbitopathy. *New Engl J Med* 364: 1920–1931.
35. Hutfless, S., Matos, P., Talor, M.V. et al. 2011. Significance of prediagnostic thyroid antibodies in women with autoimmune thyroid disease. *J Clin Endocrinol Metab* 96: E1466–E1471.

5 Postpartum and Silent Thyroiditis

Stefano Mariotti

CONTENTS

Key words: antithyroglobulin autoantibodies, antithyroid peroxidase auto-antibodies, autoimmune diseases, autoimmunity, hypothyroidism, immune system, immune tolerance, painless thyroiditis, postpartum depression, postpartum thyroiditis, pregnancy, thyroiditis, thyroid autoantibodies, thyroid ultrasound, L-thyroxine.

5.1   DEFINITIONS

Silent thyroiditis (ST) and postpartum thyroiditis (PPT) are two strictly related conditions characterized by transient thyroid dysfunction (typically thyrotoxicosis, hypothyroidism, and final recovery of normal thyroid function). ST and PPT are clinically and pathologically indistinguishable. ST is also known as sporadic (silent) thyroiditis when it occurs outside the postpartum period.

These conditions were identified in the late 1970s[1,2] and along with subacute granulomatous (de Quervains's) thyroiditis represent typical examples of thyroid dysfunctions resulting from rapidly progressing thyroid injury leading to a massive release of thyroid hormone-rich thyroglobulin into the circulation with consequent thyrotoxicosis (also called destructive thyrotoxicosis).

Unlike subacute thyroiditis, ST and PPT are not associated with thyroid pain and tenderness, fever and/or malaise. Their typical presentation is characterized by the sudden appearance of (mostly mild) thyrotoxic symptoms, sometimes accompanied by thyroid enlargement. Many other names have been used in the past to describe sporadic atypical forms of thyroiditis associated with destructive thyrotoxicosis, for example, painless subacute thyroiditis, painless thyroiditis with transient hyperthyroidism, hyperthyroiditis, occult subacute thyroiditis, atypical thyroiditis, spontaneous resolving lymphocytic thyroiditis, and transient thyrotoxicosis with lymphocytic thyroiditis. At present *silent thyroiditis* and *painless thyroiditis* are the most universally accepted and used terms.[3,4]

As indicated by its name, PPT is a form of painless thyroiditis that occurs postpartum. Symptoms suggestive of both hyperthyroidism and hypothyroidism occurring shortly after delivery have been reported since the 1940s, but the complete description of this syndrome (encompassing several types of thyroid dysfunctions) and the recognition of its autoimmune etiology were not reported until the late 1970s.[5]

5.2   INCIDENCE AND PREVALENCE

5.2.1   Sporadic Silent Thyroiditis (ST)

The incidence of sporadic ST is still poorly recognized. According to studies conducted in the United States and Canada during the 1980s, ST accounted for an unexpectedly high proportion (5 to 23%) of consecutively referred thyrotoxic patients. This finding was not confirmed in similar reports from Europe and South America and a possible explanation was that several North American cases were subsequently found to arise from ingestion of ground beef contaminated with thyroid tissue ("hamburger thyrotoxicosis").[6] Since then, the incidence of ST appears to be declining in spite of the recognition of several forms of drug-induced destructive thyrotoxicosis (see Section 5.3 below) associated with a clinical picture of ST. Presently, sporadic ST is believed to account for about 1% of all cases of thyrotoxicosis.[3]

5.2.2   Postpartum Thyroiditis (PPT)

PPT is a very common condition whose incidence is reported in 2 to 17% of pregnancies. Several differences including genetic and environmental factors, diagnostic criteria, and study designs may be responsible for the wide variability. Independent of such potential bias factors, the incidence of PPT is probably between 5 and 10%[3,6] and represents an average of 7.5% in unselected pregnant women.[7]

A strong predictor of a PPT is a previous PPT episode; up to 70% of women have chances to develop recurrences after subsequent pregnancies.[7] This phenomenon is the consequence of the autoimmune pathogenesis of PPT, as will be discussed in detail below. Associated thyroid autoimmunity is also the most probable explanation of the increased occurrence of PTT (10 to 25%) in women with type 1 diabetes mellitus (T1D), corresponding to a prevalence three to four times higher than that reported in non-diabetic women.[7] PPT occurs also after miscarriage, but its frequency is not known.[7]

5.3 ETIOLOGY AND PATHOGENESIS

5.3.1 SPORADIC ST

Although a few cases of true painless subacute thyroiditis have been reported,[8] pathological, serological, and clinical data support the notion that most cases of ST are represented by subacute exacerbation of chronic (Hashimoto's) autoimmune thyroiditis (CAT; see Chapter 4) often triggered by exogenous factors.

The most direct evidence supporting the autoimmune nature of ST is represented by biopsy specimens showing consistently diffuse lymphocytic infiltration in the absence of granulomatous lesions (Figure 5.1). Phenotypical characterization of intrathyroid T lymphocytes is similar to that found in typical CAT. Patients with ST often have personal or family histories of autoimmune thyroid diseases and show increased frequency of HLA haplotypes associated with thyroid autoimmunity (DR3 and DR5).[6]

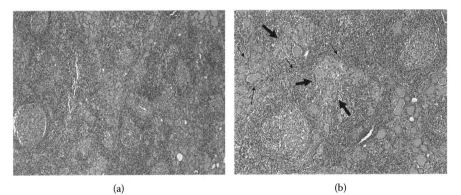

(a)   (b)

FIGURE 5.1   Histologic appearance of thyroid gland taken at autopsy from a 39-year-old man who died from Kaposi's sarcoma. The patient developed during his last 6 months a clinical picture of "silent thyroiditis" (transient thyrotoxicosis with low radioiodine uptake, followed by overt hypothyroidism and subsequent partial recovery of thyroid function. (a) Low magnification (20×) field: diffuse lymphocytic infiltration with lymphoid follicles and germinal center formation, extensive destruction of thyroid follicles within lymphocytic infiltrates; oncocytic metaplasia of thyroid cells (Hürthle cells) and interstitial fibrosis. (b) Higher magnification (40×) field: Hürthle cells (thick arrow) and fibrosis (thin arrow) are better visualized. (*Source:* Johns Hopkins Department of Pathology. With permission.)

Detectable serum antithyroid autoantibodies (ATAs), mostly represented by thyroid peroxidase antibodies (TPOAbs), are found in about 50% of women with PPT. Antibody titers are lower than in typical Hashimoto's thyroiditis.[3] In addition, although most women undergo complete restoration of normal thyroid function, in some cases the remission may be only partial and several patients show persistent and/or increased serum ATAs, thyroid enlargement, and progression to permanent overt hypothyroidism—a clinical picture very similar to that observed in the course of classical CAT. In general, high titers of TPOAbs herald subsequent development of persistent and irreversible hypothyroidism since these antibodies reflect the activity of underlying autoimmune reaction, as best exemplified in PPT (see below).

Occasionally, the appearance of both stimulating and blocking TSH receptor antibodies (TRAbs) has been described after a course of ST (or PPT). While blocking TRAbs may contribute to the development of transient stable thyroid failure, in rare instances the appearance of stimulating TRAbs may favor the progression to typical hyperthyroid Basedow-Graves' disease.

Most cases of ST are therefore considered variants of CAT, characterized by early and atypical presentation due to sudden destructive exacerbation of the chronic autoimmune process. Although several endogenous and exogenous factors (including infections, other hormones, and drugs and other chemical substances) may be implicated, attention has recently focused on iodine and drugs that may act indirectly as positive modulators of the autoimmune response and also exert direct toxic effects on thyroid follicular cells.

In several cases, both mechanisms may be involved; thus, drug-induced thyroiditis[3] has been proposed to indicate courses of ST observed during or shortly after the use of specific drugs. It should be noted that drug-induced ST must be distinguished from the more frequent alteration of thyroid function that may be associated with the administration of several medications.[3,9]

Examples of drug-induced ST are amiodarone-induced destructive thyrotoxicosis (also called type II amiodarone-induced thyrotoxicosis), lithium-induced thyrotoxicosis, thyroid dysfunction observed after administration of interferon-α, interleukin (IL)-2, or other biologic drugs, and during chemotherapy of advanced tumors with multiple kinase inhibitors. For further details on the effects of drugs on thyroid function, see Chapter 30.

The clinical picture of drug-induced ST may include the typical sequence of a thyrotoxic phase followed by hypothyroidism and then recovery or may present directly with hypothyroidism. It is not always easy to differentiate the immune-modulating effects of a drug and its direct toxic effects on thyroid epithelial cells. A typical example is represented by amiodarone.[10] The excess iodine contained in this drug may be responsible for exacerbation of thyroid autoimmunity leading to acceleration of the course of underlying CAT with a rapid appearance of persistent overt hypothyroidism. In other cases, excess iodine may trigger hypothyroidism by exacerbating thyroid autoimmunity in glands with underlying preclinical Basedow-Graves' disease or by other non-immunogenic mechanisms such as the so-called Jod-Basedow effect in partially autonomous glands.

The effects of interferon-γ, IL-2, and other cytokines are other examples of potential dual mechanisms.[9,11] While preexisting thyroid autoimmunity is an established risk factor for patients exposed to these drugs (particularly hepatitis C patients treated with interferon-α), direct toxic effects of cytokines on thyroid follicular cells have been demonstrated, suggesting that episodes of ST may occur in treated patients independently of thyroid autoimmunity. Other rare but possible causes of ST are traumas such as external palpation during physical examination and previous neck surgery such as parathyroid surgery with thyroid gland manipulation to isolate and remove a hyperfunctioning parathyroid gland.[6]

5.3.2   Postpartum Thyroiditis (PPT)

PPT is an autoimmune disorder due to exacerbation of cellular and humoral immune responses observed during the first months after delivery in women with underlying thyroid autoimmunity.

As in ST, evidence supporting the autoimmune nature of PPT derived from pathological data (thyroid biopsies showing lymphocytic infiltration similar to CAT), immunogenetic studies revealing association with the HLA haplotypes characteristic of thyroid and other organ-specific autoimmunity (DR-3, DR-4, and DR-5), and strict association with ATA (TPOAb) titer. In particular, women with detectable TPOAb at the beginning of pregnancy have up to 50% probability to develop PPT, as compared to 0.5% of ATA-negative women.[12]

The basis of postpartum exacerbation of thyroid autoimmunity is the "immunological rebound" following the immunosuppression of pregnancy needed to prevent rejection of the fetus that may be considered a type of allograft. For a detailed discussion of this complex issue, the reader is referred to a recent extensive review.[13] Briefly, the T helper cell cytokine profile during pregnancy displays a Th2 pattern, while in the postpartum period the cytokine profile switches to Th1, favoring the activation of cytotoxic immunological effector mechanisms. This scenario was derived from studies providing phenotype and functional characterization of both peripheral and intrathyroidal mononuclear cells, combined with serological studies involving serial determination of serum ATA during pregnancy and postpartum (Figures 5.2 and 5.3).

Regarding serum ATAs, ATA-positive women before or shortly after conception display progressive decreases of the antibody titer until delivery, in keeping with the relative immunosuppression of pregnancy. In the postpartum period, increases in ATA titer are consistently observed, particularly in women developing clinical pictures of PPT.[14] As in ST, the increase in ATA titer is not directly responsible for thyroid damage, but indirectly reflects the general activation of the immune system and cellular-, cytokine-, and complement-mediated cytotoxic mechanisms (see Chapter 4). Interestingly, a direct correlation between indices of complement activation and disease activity has been documented clearly only in PPT.[6]

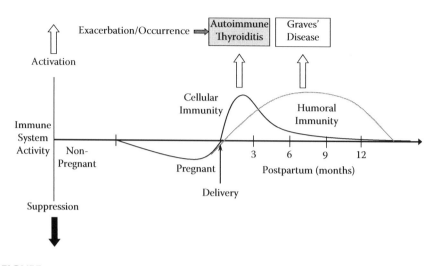

FIGURE 5.2 Various types of postpartum thyroid dysfunctions (for details, see text). (*Source:* Redrawn from Amino, N. et al. 1996. *J Endocrinol Invest* 19: 59–70. With permission of Editrice Kurtis S.r.l. Milan, Italy.)

5.4 PATHOLOGY

Due to the benign and transient natures of both ST and PPT, complete pathological studies are lacking, and most available data rely on a few cases of patients submitted to open thyroid biopsy or more frequently to fine needle aspiration cytology (FNAc). In both ST and PPT, the most consistent finding is focal or diffuse lymphocytic infiltration (Figure 5.1). Unlike classical CAT, lymphocytic germinal centers, Hürthle cell metaplasia, and fibrosis are rarely found but the two conditions cannot be clearly distinguished on histological data alone.[6]

As in subacute thyroiditis, during the thyrotoxic phase different degrees of thyroid follicle disruption with intrafollicular macrophages and rare, scattered multinucleated cells occur. During the hypothyroid and early recovery phases, regenerating small thyroid follicles containing scarce colloid may be observed along with persisting lymphocytic infiltration that may in some cases subside after 6 to 12 months.[6]

5.5 CLINICAL FEATURES

5.5.1 Silent Thyroiditis

The clinical picture of ST usually includes signs and symptoms of mild thyrotoxicosis, with nervousness, tachycardia, and fatigue as the most frequent complaints. In about 10% of cases, the disease may be fully asymptomatic and diagnosis is made serendipitously on the basis of abnormal thyroid function tests. Although ST may on occasion progress into hyperthyroid Graves' disease, orbitopathy, pretibial myxedema, and thyroid acropathy are not observed.[2,6] A mild, generally symmetrical

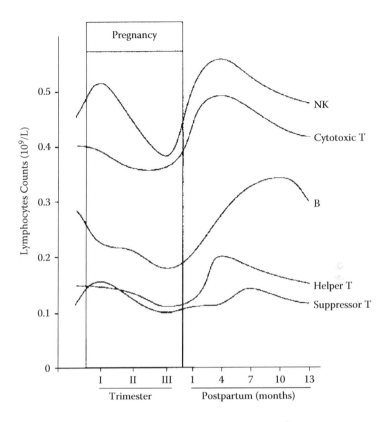

FIGURE 5.3 Changes in lymphocyte counts during pregnancy and postpartum period in normal subjects. (Source: Amino, N. et al. 1996. *J Endocrinol Invest* 19: 59–70. With permission of Editrice Kurtis S.r.l. Milan, Italy.)

enlargement of the thyroid gland is found in more than 50% of cases, but ST may occur in uninodular or multinodular glands and even in ectopic thyroid tissue. Fever and general symptoms and mild thyroid pain and tenderness are generally absent, but may be occasionally reported.[2,6]

The typical course of ST observed in 60 to 70% of cases is represented by a transient thyrotoxic phase lasting 1 to 5 weeks followed by recovery of thyroid function (Figure 5.4). In about one-third of cases, hyperthyroidism is followed by a longer (4 to 16 weeks) hypothyroid phase before normalization of thyroid function. Diagnosis is mostly made during the thyrotoxic phase.

5.5.2 POSTPARTUM THYROIDITIS

PPT encompasses a complex spectrum of thyroid dysfunction (also called postpartum thyroid dysfunction or PPTD; Figure 5.5).[7,14] The typical sequence of PPTD caused by PPT is transient thyrotoxicosis presenting shortly (average 14 weeks) after delivery followed after 4 or 5 weeks by transient hypothyroidism. Many cases appear

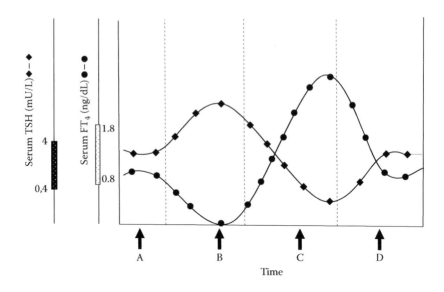

FIGURE 5.4 Sequential serum thyroid free thyroxine (FT$_4$) and thyrotropin (TSH) concentrations during a typical course of silent thyroiditis (ST). A: euthyroid state preceding episode of ST. B: thyrotoxic phase. C: hypothyroid phase. D: recovery of normal thyroid function.

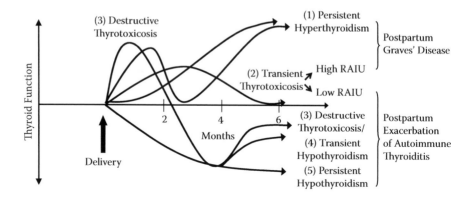

FIGURE 5.5 Various types of postpartum thyroid dysfunctions (for details, see text). (*Source:* Redrawn from Amino, N. et al. 1996. *J Endocrinol Invest* 19: 59–70. With permission of Editrice Kurtis S.r.l. Milan, Italy.)

to lack thyrotoxic phases because the thyrotoxicosis may escape detection due to its short duration and mild severity. Non-specific symptoms are fatigue and irritability. In contrast, hypothyroid symptoms are often profound (marked fatigue, diffuse aches and pain, dry skin, memory defects and cold intolerance), may appear before the onset of overt laboratory abnormalities, and persist after apparent normalization of circulating TSH and thyroid hormone concentrations.

According to an extensive review of 371 episodes described in 13 prevalence studies carried out before 2002, PPTD presented as thyrotoxicosis alone in 32%,

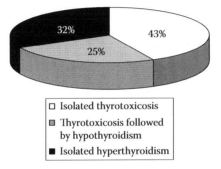

FIGURE 5.6 Clinical presentation of postpartum thyroiditis in 371 episodes of postpartum thyroid dysfunction reported in prevalence studies published before 2002. (Figure drawn from data reported by Stagnaro-Green, A. 2002. *J Clin Endocrinol Metab* 87: 4042–4047.)

hypothyroidism alone in 43%, and the typical biphasic sequence (thyrotoxicosis–hypothyroidism) in 25% of cases (Figure 5.6).[15] Hypothyroidism is generally followed by restoration of normal thyroid function, although persistent mild subclinical or overt thyroid failure may be observed. The probability of developing persistent thyroid failure is higher in patients developing multiple episodes of PPT in subsequent pregnancies.

Hyperthyroidism may occur in the postpartum period also as a relapse of hyperthyroid Basedow-Graves' disease, on occasion after a course of destructive thyrotoxicosis.[7,14] If exophthalmos, other signs of orbitopathy, or other extrathyroidal manifestation of Basedow-Graves' disease are not present, this condition may be difficult to differentiate only on clinical grounds (see Section 5.6). It should be pointed out, however, that in postpartum hyperthyroidism the prevalence of PPT is about 20 times higher than the prevalence of Basedow-Graves' disease.[7]

Women with PPT frequently complain of depressive symptoms. An association between PPT and postpartum depression has been envisaged, although the precise relationship has not been clarified.[7,16] The sequential changes of thyroid function and the specific events of the postpartum period may obviously play an important role in psychiatric symptoms. Postpartum depressive symptoms have been also more frequently reported in euthyroid thyroid antibody-positive women than in antibody-negative women,[17] suggesting that immune system activation may negatively affect mood, but this hypothesis remain to be proven.[18]

5.6 DIAGNOSIS

5.6.1 CLINICAL DIAGNOSIS

A diagnosis of sporadic ST only on clinical grounds is almost impossible. As discussed earlier, thyroid function tests and/or thyroid ultrasound required to examine mild thyrotoxic symptoms or the detection goiter by physical examination generally represent the first clues to the diagnosis. PPT is expected in about 50% of euthyroid women with positive serum ATA. Clinical detection of the corresponding PPTD should be easy in women with known preexisting thyroid autoimmunity. In women without previous histories of thyroid disease or dysfunction, the clinical diagnosis of the thyrotoxic phase is difficult and thyrotoxicosis is often recognized retrospectively at the time of the diagnosis of the hypothyroid phase whose symptoms are generally important, but may be confused with postpartum depression.

5.6.2 LABORATORY TESTS

The interpretation of laboratory tests in ST and in PPT requires the understanding of the rapid sequential variations of the thyroid function characteristics of both conditions.

During the thyrotoxic phase of ST, both total (TT_3, TT_4) and free (FT_4, FT_3) serum thyroid hormone concentrations are increased and serum TSH is suppressed (<0.1 mU/L) as in any other form of thyrotoxicosis. The T_4-to-T_3 ratio is higher than that observed in Basedow-Graves' disease, reflecting the lack of thyroid stimulation, but calculation of this ratio has little practical diagnostic value.

Serum thyroglobulin (Tg) is markedly increased (up to or greater than 400 to 500 ng/ml) as a consequence of colloid leakage into the circulation through follicles damaged by the inflammatory process. The finding of increased circulating Tg is useful to differentiate from thyrotoxicosis with low radioiodine uptake caused by excessive exogenous thyroid hormone intake, especially in patients with Münchausen syndrome (thyrotoxicosis factitia).[19] Iodine urinary excretion is increased two- to fivefold due to iodide leakage from a damaged thyroid. In some cases, this finding requires a differential diagnosis with different forms of iodine-induced thyrotoxicosis, although in those diseases urinary iodine excretion is higher, often exceeding 1000 µg/24 hours.

ATAs are frequently detected in sera of patients with ST and indeed this finding contributed substantially to clarifying the autoimmune pathogenesis of this condition. On average, both the frequency and the titers of ATAs are lower than those commonly observed in CAT. Anti-Tg antibodies (TgAbs) are present in about one-fourth and TPOAbs in two-thirds of cases during the thyrotoxic phase of ST. TRAbs are not found in typical ST, but may became detectable at progressively increasing titers in rare patients showing the appearance of typical Basedow-Graves' disease after a course of ST. Circulating ATAs reach the highest levels during the hypothyroid phase, followed by a progressive decrease.

Acute-phase proteins are increased in ST, accounting for a high erythrocyte sedimentation rate (ESR) and C-reactive protein (CRP) levels.[6] This increase is less marked than that commonly found in typical, painful, subacute thyroiditis. Several serum cytokines (IL-6 and IL-12) are also increased in a consistent proportion (about 50%) of patients with ST, but rarely represent a clinically useful assay, with the possible exception of IL-6, which has been proposed in the diagnostic work-up of amiodarone-induced thyrotoxicosis to identify the destructive (type II) variant of this condition.[10]

Laboratory diagnosis of the thyrotoxic phase of PPT is based on the presence of low serum TSH associated with increased serum FT_3 and FT_4 on at least two consecutive occasions[6] since no abnormality in thyroid function is expected in the postpartum period. The hypothyroid phase of PPT may be identified by a borderline increase of serum TSH (>3 or 4 mU/L) associated with low (<6 to 7 pg/ml) FT_4, or definitively increased serum TSH (>10 mU/L) on two or more occasions. TPOAbs and/or TgAbs are positive in most (>90%) of women with PPT and their titers increase progressively 6 to 12 months postpartum. Differences in timing, assay method, sensitivity, and ethnic background may explain the minority of women with clinical and hormonal features of PPT and undetectable circulating TPOAbs and TgAbs.

TRAbs are typically detected in postpartum hyperthyroidism due to Basedow-Graves' disease, but occasionally this antibody is transiently found also in PPT.[7] Positive TPOAbs at different times during pregnancy are highly predictive of PPT and assay of TPOAbs has been proposed at different times before and after delivery.[20] However, current guidelines do not support universal screening. A case-finding attitude is advised in subjects at risk for thyroid autoimmunity.[21] This is mainly due to the low positive predictive value for PPT of a positive TPOAb test (only about 50% of TPOAb-positive women actually develop PPTD); moreover, PPT is a mild self-resolving condition for which no effective prevention strategy is available.

5.6.3 Thyroid Imaging

Twenty-four hour radioiodine (^{131}I or ^{123}I) uptake is typically very low or absent during all the thyrotoxic and first weeks of the recovery phases of both ST and PPT. In spite of the benefits of ultrasound diagnosis (see below), the simple uptake test remains essential for the correct identification of ST and other forms of destructive thyrotoxicosis; 24-hour radioiodine uptake testing is contraindicated in lactating women with PPT.

Thyroid ultrasonography reveals diffuse hypoechogenicity similar to that observed in CAT and different degrees of thyroid enlargement in both ST and PPT. In pregnant women with positive ATAs, thyroid hypoechogenicity is also predictive of later development of PPT, although the clinical value of this finding is modest because many ATA-positive pregnant women with hypoechoic thyroids remain euthyroid during the postpartum period.[7] Color and power Doppler evaluations show reduced thyroid blood flow in both ST and PPT, in keeping with the destructive nature of these conditions. This test is particularly helpful in clinical settings in which radioactive tests must be avoided.

5.6.4 Fine Needle Aspiration Cytology (FNAc)

The findings observed in FNAc obtained from glands affected by ST and PPT are described in Section 5.4 (Pathology). However, unless distinct nodules are clearly detected by thyroid ultrasound, FNAc is rarely needed in the diagnostic evaluation of these conditions. In cases of associated nodules, FNAc should be employed according to the criteria discussed for CAT (Chapter 4).

5.7 THERAPY

The destructive nature of thyrotoxicosis caused by ST and PPT represents a clear contraindication to the use of thionamide antithyroid drugs. In most cases, the thyrotoxic phases of both conditions are mild and transient and do not need pharmacological treatment. Rather, patients should be reassured and the transient nature of the disturbance explained. The possibility of a subsequent transient hypothyroid phase with possible evolution to permanent thyroid failure should be explained to patients, particularly in PPT (where the hypothyroid phase is more severe and symptomatic).

Serum TSH should be therefore measured after 4 to 6 weeks and then every 2 months until 9 to 12 months pass after delivery.[7] In more symptomatic cases, short-term administration of beta-blockers (10 to 20 mg propranolol qid, titrated on symptom severity) may be envisaged in both conditions. In the few cases (generally ST) with disabling thyrotoxicosis, anti-inflammatory drugs may be proposed as for subacute thyroiditis. Prednisone and other synthetic glucocorticoids reduce serum thyroid hormone concentrations by reducing inflammatory activity and the consequent thyroid destruction, but may also inhibit peripheral T4 conversion to T3. Glucocorticoids have been used in ST on an empirical basis[22] and optimal doses have been not established. A starting dose corresponding to 30 to 60 mg prednisone/day followed by progressive tapering by 7.5 to 15 mg/week for a total period of therapy of 4 to 6 weeks is considered adequate.[6] In exceptional cases of severe ST with recurring thyrotoxic phases, thyroidectomy or radioiodine (^{131}I) administration (when thyroid uptake has recovered) has been proposed.[6]

Most patients with ST have mild and transient hypothyroidism and do not require treatment. In some cases, administration of LT$_4$ is needed to control hypothyroid symptoms. Care should be exercised to not suppress serum TSH, since the stimulating effect of this hormone is needed to accelerate the recovery of normal thyroid function.[6] LT$_4$ may then be progressively tapered until full withdrawal in order to assess final thyroid status. Since a minority of patients develop permanent thyroid failure, no further attempt to withdraw LT$_4$ is advised if hypothyroidism is still present after 6 months.

Unlike ST, most cases of hypothyroidism due PPT are symptomatic and require treatment, often started with a fixed daily dose of LT$_4$ (100 μg), followed by individual tailoring of the dose to maintain serum TSH between 0.5 and 2.0 mU/L (see Chapter 10). In more symptomatic cases, replacement with a submaximal dose of T$_3$ (60 to 80 mg/day in 3 to 4 administrations) has been proposed to relieve symptoms more quickly and allow easier detection of spontaneous recovery by increasing serum T$_4$.[4]

Since the course of the hypothyroid phase in PPT is difficult to predict and up to 30% of affected women develop persistent thyroid failure, a practical useful protocol is to treat with thyroid hormone for at least 1 year, then stop and reevaluate thyroid function.[6] As an alternative, based on the high recurrence rate of PPT and the negative impact of even mild or subclinical hypothyroidism on subsequent pregnancies, LT$_4$ therapy should be offered until completion of the family[7] to maintain a euthyroid state while a woman is attempting pregnancy, pregnant, or breast feeding.[21]

5.8 PROGNOSIS

The most important consequence of ST and PPT is the development of permanent thyroid dysfunction. Permanent hypothyroidism is rather rare in ST (observed in about 5% of affected patients). Persistent high titers of circulating ATAs are predictive of permanent thyroid failure, while recovery of stable euthyroidism is consistently observed in about one-half of patients in whom ATAs progressively decrease until disappearance.[6]

Although most women with PPT recover normal thyroid function by the end of the first postpartum year, recent studies suggest that up to 50% may develop late permanent hypothyroidism.[23] Factors associated with an increased risk of developing permanent hypothyroidism are multiparity, hypoechogenicity on ultrasound, severity of initial hypothyroidism, TPOAb titer, maternal age, and a history of miscarriage.[21]

5.9 FOLLOW-UP

For patients recovering from the euthyroid state, the follow-up is similar to that described for CAT (see Chapter 4), taking into account that previous episodes of ST and PPT (especially if repeated) are associated with a high risk (>50%) of developing permanent thyroid failure. For hypothyroid patients who do not recover normal thyroid function, the follow-up is the same as for autoimmune primary hypothyroidism (described in Chapter 10).

REFERENCES

1. Amino, N., Miyai, K., Yamamoto, T. et al. 1977. Transient recurrence of hyperthyroidism after delivery in Graves' disease. *J Clin Endocrinol Metab* 44: 130–136.
2. Woolf, P.D. 1980. Transient painless thyroiditis with hyperthyroidism: a variant of lymphocytic thyroiditis? *Endocrinol Rev* 1: 411–420.
3. Pearce, E.N., Farwell, A.P., and Braverman, L.E. 2003. Thyroiditis. *New Engl J Med* 348: 2646–2655.
4. Akamizu, T., Amino, N., and DeGroot, L. 2008. Hashimoto's thyroiditis. In *Thyroid Disease Manager,* DeGroot, L.J., Ed. http://www.thyroidmanager.org/Chapter8/8-frame.htm.
5. Smallridge, R.C. 1999. Postpartum thyroid diseases through the ages: a historical view. *Thyroid* 9: 671–673.
6. Lazarus, J.H. 2005. Sporadic and postpartum thyroiditis. In *Werner & Ingbar's The Thyroid" A Fundamental and Clinical Text,* Braverman, L. and Utiger, R., Eds. Philadelphia: Lippincott Williams & Wilkins, 524–535.
7. Stagnaro-Green, A. 2004. Postpartum thyroiditis. *Best Pract Res Clin Endocrinol Metab* 18: 303–316.
8. Daniels, G.H. 2001. Atypical subacute thyroiditis: preliminary observations. *Thyroid* 11: 691–695.
9. Prummel, M.F., Strieder, T., and Wiersinga, W.M. 2004. The environment and autoimmune thyroid diseases. *Eur J Endocrinol* 150: 605–618.
10. Martino, E., Bartalena, L., Bogazzi, F. et al. 2001. The effects of amiodarone on the thyroid. *Endocrinol Rev* 22: 240–254.
11. Tomer, Y. and Menconi, F. 2009. Interferon-induced thyroiditis. *Best Pract Res Clin Endocrinol Metab* 23: 703–712.
12. Stagnaro-Green, A. and Glinoer, D. 2004. Thyroid autoimmunity and the risk of miscarriage. *Best Pract Res Clin Endocrinol Metab* 18: 167–181.
13. Weetman, A.P. 2010. Immunity, thyroid function and pregnancy: molecular mechanisms. *Nat Rev Endocrinol* 6: 311–318.

14. Amino, N., Tada, H., and Hidaka, Y. 1996. Autoimmune thyroid disease and pregnancy. *J Endocrinol Invest* 19: 59–70.

15. Stagnaro-Green, A. 2002. Clinical review 152: Postpartum thyroiditis. *J Clin Endocrinol Metab* 87: 4042–4047.

16. Lucas, A., Pizarro, E., Granada, M.L. et al. 2001. Postpartum thyroid dysfunction and postpartum depression: are they two linked disorders? *Clin Endocrinol (Oxf)* 55: 809–814.

17. Kuijpens, J.L., Vader, H.L., Drexhage, H.A. et al. 2001. Thyroid peroxidase antibodies during gestation are a marker for subsequent depression postpartum. *Eur J Endocrinol* 145: 579–584.

18. Mariotti, S., Carta, M., and Piga, M. 2007. Thyroid autoimmunity and mood disorders. In *The Thyroid and Autoimmunity*, Wiersinga, W. et al., Eds. Stuttgart: Georg Thieme, 153–161.

19. Mariotti, S., Martino, E., Cupini, C. et al. 1982. Low serum thyroglobulin as a clue to the diagnosis of thyrotoxicosis factitia. *New Engl J Med* 307: 410–412.

20. Amino, N., Tada, H., Hidaka, Y. et al. 1999. Therapeutic controversy. Screening for postpartum thyroiditis. Screening for postpartum thyroid dysfunction in the general population Is beneficial. *J Clin Endocrinol Metab* 84: 1813–1816.

21. Stagnaro-Green, A., Abalovich, M., Alexander, E. et al. 2011. Guidelines of the American Thyroid Association for the diagnosis and management of thyroid disease during pregnancy and postpartum. *Thyroid* 21: 1081–1125.

22. Nikolai, T.F., Coombs, G.J., McKenzie, A.K. et al. 1982. Treatment of lymphocytic thyroiditis with spontaneously resolving hyperthyroidism (silent thyroiditis). *Arch Intern Med* 142: 2281–2283.

23. Stagnaro-Green, A., Schwartz, A., Gismondi, R. et al. 2011. High rate of persistent hypothyroidism in a large-scale prospective study of postpartum thyroiditis in southern Italy. *J Clin Endocrinol Metab* 96: 652–657.

6 Single Thyroid Nodule

Rossella Elisei and Eleonora Molinaro

CONTENTS

Key words: thyroid nodule, neck ultrasound, fine needle aspiration, calcitonin, thyroid cancer.

6.1 DEFINITION

A single nodule on a thyroid is a swelling clearly distinct from the surrounding thyroid parenchyma caused by a hemorrhagic or colloid fluid collection (cyst) or an abnormal proliferation of cells (solid nodule). It can be visible and palpable on neck inspection, not visible but palpable, or not visible or palpable. This latter case is better defined as an incidentaloma[1] since it is usually discovered unexpectedly and will be discussed in a separate chapter.

Thyroid nodules smaller than 3 to 4 cm are usually asymptomatic. Larger nodules can cause some difficulties in swallowing or a bothersome cough or create more serious problems such as dysphagia and dyspnea. Functioning nodules represent only 5 to 15% of all thyroid nodules. Non-functioning nodules and cysts do not affect thyroid function but they may be associated with other thyroid disorders such as Hashimoto's thyroiditis or Graves' disease that frequently affect thyroid function by leading to hypothyroidism and hyperthyroidism, respectively.

6.2 PREVALENCE

The prevalence of thyroid nodules depends highly on the screening method and the population evaluated. However, we know that it positively correlates with population age and palpable nodules are present in about 10% of middle-aged people. This prevalence is much greater, up to 50%, when the same age population is screened with neck ultrasound.

As with many other thyroid diseases, thyroid nodules are rare in children and are five times more frequent in females than in males. As shown in Table 6.1, other factors can greatly influence thyroid nodule prevalence. In countries where iodine deficiency has been corrected by prophylaxis, thyroid nodules are clinically detectable in 4 to 7% of the general adult population. Prevalence is much greater in countries affected by moderate or severe iodine deficiency where nodules are usually in the context of a goiter and usually multiple. Epidemiological studies on large populations before and after iodine fortification reported that even small changes in iodine intake significantly influenced goiter prevalence, nodule incidence, and thyroid dysfunction.[2]

Another environmental factor influencing the prevalence of thyroid nodules is exposure to both external and internal ionizing radiation, especially during childhood. Several studies performed in populations exposed to external radiation therapy for head and neck diseases and studies on survivors of atomic bomb explosions or exposed to radioactive fallout from nuclear accidents clearly demonstrated a greater prevalence of thyroid nodules than that found in the general population.[3] A linear dose–response curve between thyroid nodule prevalence and radiation dose shows no evidence of a threshold at low doses. The risk reaches a plateau and possibly tapers off at high doses.

TABLE 6.1

Risk Factors for Thyroid Nodules

Advanced age (rare in children)

Female sex (female:male ratio = 5:1)

Iodine-deficient area (frequently associated with goiter and other nodules)

External or internal ionizing radiation exposure (linear response with absorbed dose)

TABLE 6.2
Clinical and Pathological Classification of Thyroid Nodules

Pseudonodules

Inflammatory: lymphocytic or subacute thyroiditis

Hyperplastic: compensatory after lobectomy or in hemiagenesia

Benign Nodules

Functioning: Hot nodule on scintigraphy; solid or mixed at ultrasound, usually accompanied by clinical or subclinical hyperthyroidism[a]

Non-functioning: Cold nodule on scintigraphy; liquid, solid, or mixed on ultrasound, with no alteration of thyroid function[b]

Malignant Nodules

Non-functioning: Cold nodules on scintigraphy; solid or mixed at ultrasound, usually with no functional alterations

[a] Hot nodules have been found malignant only in anecdotal cases.

[b] Non-functioning and liquid nodules are usually pure cysts and very rarely malignant.

6.3 CLINICAL AND PATHOLOGICAL CLASSIFICATION OF THYROID NODULES

As shown in Table 6.2, thyroid nodules are of several types and three major categories can be distinguished: (1) pseudonodules; (2) benign nodules; and (3) malignant nodules.

6.3.1 PSEUDONODULES

Pseudonodules are mainly observed in lymphocytic (Hashimoto's) thyroiditis and result from lymphocytic infiltration. They can be observed also in subacute thyroiditis as granulomas related to the inflammation of the gland. Both the ultrasound readings and cytological features will be of diagnostic value to distinguish pseudonodules from classical nodules. A thyroid nodule can be also mimicked by the hyperplasia of the remaining lobe after contralateral lobectomy or in cases of congenital hemiagenesis. A neck ultrasound will aid diagnosis (Figure 6.1a) in this situation.

6.3.2 BENIGN NODULES

Benign nodules can be further distinguished in functioning and non-functioning thyroid nodules. Functioning nodules that represents 5 to 15% of all thyroid nodules can concentrate iodine. They are thus defined as hot nodules on scintigraphy (Figure 6.2a) and they produce and secrete thyroid hormones. For that reason, they are also defined toxic based on the presence of clinical or subclinical hyperthyroidism. The possibility that they are malignant is so rare that there is no indication to perform fine needle aspiration for diagnostic purposes.

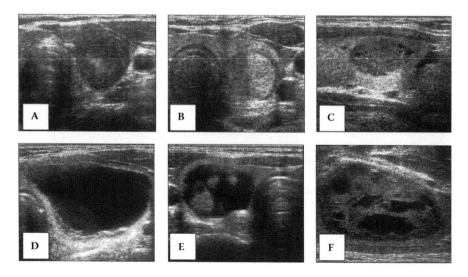

FIGURE 6.1 Echographic patterns of thyroid nodules. (A) Pseudo nodule of Hashimoto's thyroiditis (no FNAc). (B) Solid nodule with no suspicion of malignancy (FNAc if size exceeds 1 cm). (C) Solid nodule with microcalcifications and irregular border, suspicious of malignancy (FNAc if size exceeds 1 cm). (D) Pure cystic nodule (FNA only for evacuation of liquid). (E) Cystic nodule with solid component that must be submitted to FNAc. (F) Mixed nodule (FNAc if size exceeds 1 cm).

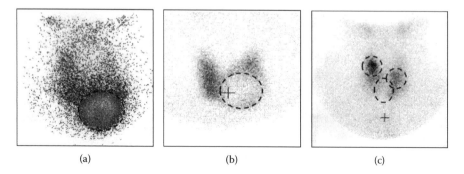

FIGURE 6.2 $^{I}123$ Scintigraphy of hot nodule (a), cold nodule (b), and hot and cold multinodular goiter (c).

The pathogenesis of toxic adenomas is strictly correlated to the presence of activating somatic mutations of the thyrotropin-stimulating hormone (TSH) receptor (60 to 70% of cases); in a minority of cases (15 to 20%), the cause is the Gsα protein[4] involved in the intracellular signalling pathway of the TSH receptor (Figure 6.3; Table 6.3).

Non-functioning thyroid nodules are cold on scintigraphy (Figure 6.2b) and do not release thyroid hormones. Thus, they do not affect thyroid gland function. They account for more than 80% of thyroid nodules and their ultrasound patterns classify them into three types: solid (50 to 60%; Figure 6.1B and C), cystic (10 to 20%; Figure 6.1D), and mixed (20 to 40%; Figure 6.1E and F).

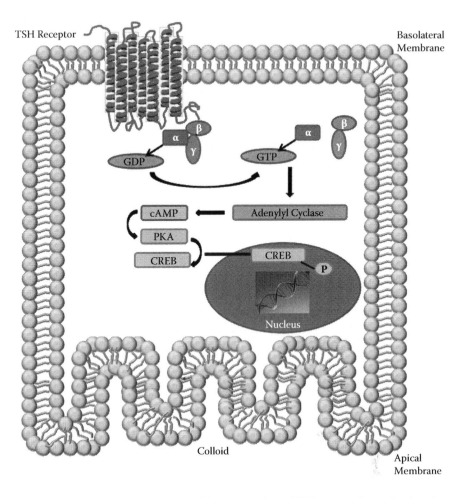

FIGURE 6.3 Thyroid follicular cell with transmembrane TSH receptor located at basolateral level and cAMP pathway involving Gsα protein. Activating point mutations of either the TSH receptor or Gsα protein are involved in the pathogenesis of hyperfunctioning adenomas and toxic adenomas.

Purely cystic nodules may be hemorrhagic or colloidal based on whether they contain blood or colloid, respectively. They are almost invariably benign although 10% of cold nodules that are solid or mixed can be malignant. However, aspiration of cyst fluid for cytologic analysis almost always indicates complex cysts exceeding 2 cm in diameter without suspicious features. Fine needle aspiration (FNA) of pure cysts is not necessary unless it is for therapeutic reasons.

Single solid nodules, especially when developed in a normal thyroid, are follicular adenomas (FAs) revealed by histology. Nodules in the context of a multinodular goiter are more frequently represented by hyperplastic nodules. FAs are characterized grossly and microscopically by a complete capsule and clear follicular cell differentiation (Figure 6.4). Their sizes are highly variable and larger tumors are

TABLE 6.3
Genetic Alterations in Thyroid Nodules

Nodule Classification	Form	Genetic Alteration
Benign	Cysts	Nd
	Functioning adenoma	Activating mutations of TSH receptor
		Gsα activating mutations
	Follicular adenoma	Ras activating mutations, mainly N-Ras
		PAX-8/PPARγ translocations
		Other chromosomal alterations
Malignant	Papillary carcinoma	RET/PTC rearrangement
		TRK rearrangement
		BRAF V600E
	Follicular carcinoma	Ras activating mutations, mainly N-Ras
		PAX-8/PPARγ translocations
		Other chromosomal alterations
	Medullary carcinoma	RET activating mutations (75% of sporadic cases and 25% of familial cases)
		Ras mutations
	Other	P53 inactivating mutations, PTEN inactivating mutations, etc.

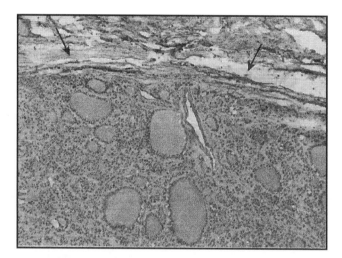

FIGURE 6.4 Histology of typical follicular adenoma with microfollicular pattern and complete capsule as shown by the two arrows. Only histology can distinguish follicular adenomas from follicular carcinomas on the basis of the absence or presence of invasion of the capsule, respectively.

characterized by necrosis, internal hemorrhages, edema, fibrosis, and calcification. According to follicle size, we can distinguish microfollicular, normofollicular, and macrofollicular tumors.

Sometimes the follicles are few and the pattern is solid or trabecular. A frequent cytological variant is the oxyphilic, oncocytic, or Hürthle cell adenoma composed mainly of large cells with granular and eosinophilic cytoplasm. The cells are characteristically rich in mitochondrias and pleomorphic in their nuclei. FAs and follicular carcinomas (FCs) show the same cytological pattern and cannot be distinguished before surgical treatment. Capsular invasion that may be revealed only by histology is the unique feature that can distinguish FAs from FCs. Some genetic somatic alterations have been discovered in FAs (Table 6.3).

About 40% of FAs show somatic activating point mutations of one of the three *RAS* genes (H-RAS, K-RAS, and N-RAS). They encode a 21-kD protein (p21) involved in signal transduction from cell membrane receptors to growth factors to nuclei. The activating mutations determine a constitutive activation of this signalling cascade called the MAP kinase pathway and induce uncontrolled proliferation. Since these mutations are frequently found in FCs, the question whether FAs with RAS mutations are more prone to become malignant is still under investigation. What we know at present is that a RAS mutation may cause genomic instability that increases the possibility for other mutations to occur.

Another genetic alteration reported in 10 to 15% of FAs is the PAXγ-PPARγ translocation. PAX8 is a thyroid transcription factor involved in thyroid ontogenesis and in the regulation of several thyroid-specific genes among which are thyroglobulin (Tg) and thyroperoxidase (TPO) genes. PPARγ (peroxisome proliferator-activated receptor gamma) is a transcription factor belonging to the hormone nuclear receptor family that plays a role in the regulation of lipid metabolism, inflammatory processes, cellular differentiation, and tumorigenesis.

The fusion protein obtained after the translocation t(2;3)(q13;p25) shows a dominant negative effect that inhibits the cellular differentiation and growth suppression commonly induced by PPARγ agonists. As for RAS mutations, whether the presence of a PAX8-PPARγ translocation in a FA makes it more prone to become a FC is still unknown because, also in this case, a high prevalence (50 to 60%) of PAX8-PPARγ translocation is present in FCs. Finally, a loss of heterozygosity (LOH) or polyploidy of chromosome 7 are frequently found associated with FAs (68 and 52.4%, respectively) and with FCs (100 and 66%, respectively).

6.3.3 MALIGNANT NODULES

With the exception of cases showing clinical evidence of metastatic disease, the clinical presentation of thyroid cancer is a nodule, usually asymptomatic, more frequently solid or even mixed based on neck ultrasound, and rarely completely fluid. Malignant nodules are rarely hot on scintigraphy with radioiodine (^{123}I or ^{131}I) although a nodule may be falsely hot if investigated with ^{99m}Tc. A malignant nodule can be a papillary, follicular, or medullary thyroid cancer. More rarely it can be an anaplastic thyroid tumor or a secondary lesion from another malignancy.

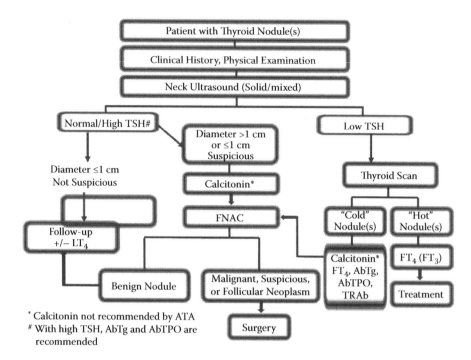

FIGURE 6.5 Suggested algorithm for work-up of patient with thyroid nodule. The algorithm is very consistent with that proposed by the ETA guidelines and by the AME/AACE guidelines and exhibits some differences with algorithm proposed in ATA guidelines.

Malignant nodules account only for 5 to 6% of all thyroid nodules. Whenever possible, they must be distinguished from benign nodules to determine which patients must be treated with thyroidectomy and which patients can be followed and/or treated with medical therapy. A specific diagnostic work-up should be always performed in a patient with a thyroid nodule to clarify the nature of the nodule (Figure 6.5). According to the histological pattern, they can be distinguished as differentiated (papillary and follicular from follicular cells and medullary from C cells) and undifferentiated (anaplastic, lymphoma, sarcoma, etc.). Each nodule seems to have specific hallmarks that will be helpful to better characterize it for decisions about treatment.

6.4 DIAGNOSIS

The clinical importance of thyroid nodule evaluation is primarily related to the need to exclude thyroid cancer, which is present in 5 to 6% of thyroid nodules. Thus, the initial evaluation of all patients with thyroid nodules should include a history, physical examination, and measurement of serum thyroid stimulating hormone (TSH). Ultrasound is also recommended for all patients to confirm the presence of other nodularities, assess sonographic features, and reveal possible lymphadenopathy.

Fine needle aspiration cytology (FNAc) is the most accurate method for evaluating the benign or malignant nature of a thyroid nodule and identifying patients who require surgical resection.[5] Surgery can be avoided only for toxic adenomas and pure cysts. In the latter case, the indication may be to evacuate the liquid content. If a nodule is complex or posterior, ultrasound guidance is strongly recommended to avoid non-diagnostic or incorrect cytology results.

Over the past decade, the routine use of thyroid scintigraphy became less common. The technique is reserved for cases in which it is important to determine functional status of nodules and for patients with multiple thyroid nodules (Figure 6.2c). Scintigraphy is used to reveal nodules that are hypofunctional and therefore may require FNAc.

In recent years, several guidelines give direction on how to handle patients with thyroid nodules. Although the guidelines are very consistent, they exhibit a few disagreements, the most important of which are the measurement of serum calcitonin (CT) and the indications for submitting very small nodules to FNAc. Figure 6.5 summarizes our recommended workup for thyroid nodules that is very consistent with the European Thyroid Association guidelines.[6]

6.4.1 History and Physical Examination

Patient history and physical examination are two important steps to find or exclude risk factors indicating that a nodule could be malignant (Table 6.4). A history of rapid growth of a neck mass, childhood head and neck irradiation, total body irradiation for bone marrow transplantation, family history of thyroid cancer, or thyroid cancer syndromes (e.g., multiple endocrine neoplasia 2, family polyposis, or Cowden's syndrome) are all risk factors for malignancy that must be considered when evaluating a patient.

A fixed hard mass, obstructive symptoms, cervical lymphadenopathy, or vocal cord paralysis suggest the possibility of cancer. Conversely, a soft and elastic consistency of a nodule is more commonly detected when the nodule is a cyst.

6.4.2 Biochemical Diagnosis

Thyroid function should be assessed in all patients with nodules by measuring TSH and free tetraiodothyronine (FT_4). Not all authors agree on the necessity of also measuring free triiodothyronine (FT_3). In this regard, it is useful to consider that toxic adenomas commonly show a relatively higher increase of FT_3 than FT_4 and this may be relevant in older patients. According to the functional activity of a nodule, different workups may be performed (Figure 6.5):

- If serum TSH concentration is low, indicating overt or subclinical hyperthyroidism, the possibility that the nodule is hyperfunctioning is increased and thyroid scintigraphy should be performed as the next step. If the nodule is hot, FNAc is not recommended.
- If serum TSH concentration is normal or elevated and the nodule meets criteria for sampling (i.e., exceeds 1 cm in size or shows suspicious echographic features if smaller than 1 cm), FNAc is indicated. In addition, patients with high serum TSH concentrations require evaluation for hypothyroidism and the measurement of thyroid antibodies is also indicated.

TABLE 6.4
Epidemiological and Clinical Risk Factors Indicating Possible Nodule Malignancy

Examination	Risk Factor
Anamnestic	Rapid growth
	Head and neck radiation exposure
	Total body radiation for bone marrow transplantation
	Family history of thyroid cancer or thyroid cancer syndromes (multiple endocrine neoplasia 2, family polyposis, Cowden's syndrome)
Signs	Fixed hard mass
	Obstructive symptoms
	Cervical lymphadenopathy
	Vocal cord paralysis
Symptoms	Dysphagia
	Dyspnea
	Cough
Biochemical	Calcitonin
Neck scintigraphy	Cold nodule
Neck ultrasound	Solid pattern
	Hypoechogenicity
	Microcalcifications
	Absence of peripheral halo
	Irregular borders
Neck ultrasound + color Doppler	Intranodular blood flow

6.4.3 OTHER LABORATORY TESTS

Routine measurement of serum antithyroid peroxidase (TPO) and antithyroglobulin (Tg) antibodies is not necessary and should be performed only when TSH is elevated or suppressed to better clarify the nature of the thyroid disease. However, the presence of a high titer of TPO antibodies does not negate the need for FNAc of a thyroid nodule in a patient with Hashimoto's thyroiditis. Thyroiditis and thyroid cancer coexist with sufficient frequency, especially after head and neck irradiaton. Thus, a well-defined solid nodule, even with high serum antibody concentration, requires further evaluation, specifically FNAc.

As far as the measurement of circulating Tg is concerned, recall that levels can be elevated in many thyroid diseases. An elevated level does not help discriminate benign from malignant thyroid nodules. Thus, there is a general recommendation to *not* measure serum Tg levels as part of the evaluation of a patient with a thyroid nodule.[6-8] Although the technique has been widely studied,[9] the routine measurement of serum calcitonin (CT) in patients with nodular thyroid disease is still controversial.

In most studies, pentagastrin stimulation tests were performed to confirm C cell hyperplasia in patients with elevated basal calcitonin levels. As an example, in one report of 10,864 patients screened after 1991, 44 (0.4%) had elevated CT confirmed by elevated pentagastrin-stimulated CT testing and all had medullary cancer. Fifty-nine percent of these patients were in complete remission compared with only 2.7% of patients diagnosed with medullary cancer prior to the use of routine screening. This suggests a benefit of early diagnosis.[10] In contrast, in a study of 10,158 patients with thyroid nodules, 5% had elevated basal CT, but only 20% of these patients had elevated values after pentagastrin stimulation, and only 31% of them had medullary cancer.[11]

Despite these differences, all these studies demonstrated that serum CT was more accurate than FNAc because many of the cancers were very small and difficult to puncture or select for FNAc because of the presence of other, more relevant nodules. However, controversy continues concerning the routine use of serum CT measurements because of the high false positive rate (59% or higher) in some studies and the uncertain importance of small tumors.[12] In the United States, pentagastrin is not available and therefore cannot be used to confirm C cell hyperplasia in patients with elevated serum CT levels. Although calcium stimulation of CT may be an alternative to pentagastrin, few data[13] are available.

The American Thyroid Association guidelines noted these uncertainties and have not taken a position for or against screening. The European Thyroid Association guidelines recommend CT measurement in patients with thyroid nodules.[6,7]

Although our own suggestion is to measure serum CT in all patients with thyroid nodules, to those who are not still convinced suggest measuring it at least in patients with nodules who have been already demonstrated to require surgical treatment. The presurgical diagnosis of medullary thyroid cancer will be relevant in planning the extension of the surgical treatment.

6.4.4 THYROID ULTRASONOGRAPHY

Thyroid ultrasound should be performed in all patients with suspected thyroid nodules or nodular goiters found on physical examination. Thyroid ultrasonography can answer questions about both size and ultrasound features of nodules. It also provides information about thyroid gland volume (goiter versus normal volume), nodule structure (solid, cystic, or mixed), grade of echogenicity (hypo or hyper), completeness of halo, and presence of microcalcifications (Figure 6.2).

Thyroid ultrasound can also provide information about the presence of other nodules. It can identify posteriorly located nodules or predominantly cystic nodules and also help distinguish pseudo nodules in Hashimoto's thyroiditis and TSH-induced hyperplasia of follicular tissue. Whenever a malignancy is suspected (Table 6.4), thyroid ultrasound should be expanded to explore the lateral regions of the neck to find or exclude the presence of lymphadenopathies whose echographic patterns are very suggestive (Figure 6.6).

Several ultrasonographic findings are suspicious for thyroid cancer (Table 6.4). The predictive value of these characteristics varies widely, and we do not rely on thyroid ultrasound to diagnose cancer or to select patients for surgery. However, ultrasound findings can be used to select nodules for FNAc.

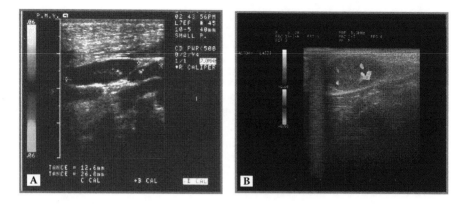

FIGURE 6.6   Ultrasound features of inflammatory (A) and metastatic (B) neck nodes. Metastatic nodes are usually round (AP/LL > 0.7), solidly hypoechoic with microcalcifications, and the halo is not more recognizable. Cystic nodes are invariably metastases of papillary thyroid cancer.

It is worth noting that there are no differences in the neck ultrasound features of papillary, follicular, or medullary thyroid cancers and the diagnosis can be done only by FNAc. In recent years, elastosonography (Figure 6.7), a powerful diagnostic technique that assesses nodule hardness as an indicator of malignancy, has demonstrated great potential as a new tool for diagnosing thyroid cancer, especially in nodules with indeterminate cytology.[14]

6.4.5 Thyroid Scintigraphy

Thyroid scintigraphy is used to determine the functional status of a nodule. A low serum TSH, indicating overt or subclinical hyperthyroidism, increases the possibility that a thyroid nodule is hyperfunctioning. Thus, thyroid scintigraphy should be performed in patients with low serum TSH concentrations. If a nodule is confirmed to be hot, FNAc is not recommended. However, in some cases, the nodule is cold and the rest of the gland is hyperfunctioning because of a concomitant autoimmune thyrotoxicosis. In these cases, the benign or malignant nature of the nodule must be defined by FNAc. Sometimes, several hot and cold nodules are present simultaneously and thyroid scintigraphy is helpful for selecting cold nodules for FNAc (Figure 6.2c).

Scintigraphy utilizes one of the radioisotopes of iodine (preferably ^{123}I) or [99m]Tc (pertechnetate technetium). These radioisotopes are handled differently by thyroid follicular cells. Normal thyroid follicular cells take up both technetium and radioiodine, but only radioiodine is organified and stored (as Tg) in the lumens of thyroid follicles.

Most benign and virtually all malignant thyroid nodules concentrate both radioisotopes less avidly than adjacent normal thyroid tissue. However, 5% of thyroid cancers concentrate pertechnetate, but not radioiodine.[15] These nodules may appear hot or indeterminate (warm) on pertechnetate scans and cold on radioiodine scans. Although most are benign nodules, a few are thyroid cancers. As a result, patients

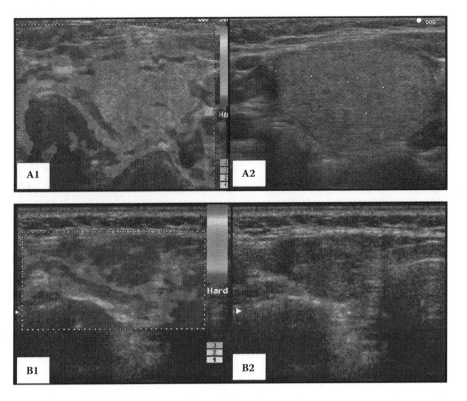

FIGURE 6.7   Elastosonography of benign thyroid nodule (A1) and malignant thyroid nodule (B1). The difference in color expresses their highly different consistencies. A2 and B2 represent the corresponding conventional ultrasound that should always be added to elastosonography.

with nodules that are functioning on pertechnetate imaging should undergo radioiodine imaging to confirm that they are actually functioning.

6.4.6   FINE NEEDLE ASPIRATION CYTOLOGY (FNAc)

FNAc is the procedure of choice for evaluating the benign or malignant nature of thyroid nodules and selecting those that are candidates for surgery.[5] FNAc has resulted in improved diagnostic accuracy, a higher malignancy yield at the time of surgery, and significant cost reductions.[5]

FNA is a simple and safe procedure in which cells for cytologic examination are obtained from a nodule. Commonly a 25-gauge needle is used to puncture the nodule. There is no need for local anesthesia. With experience, adequate samples can be obtained in 90 to 97% of aspirations of solid nodules. Ultrasound-guided FNA is usually preferred, especially for nodules that are technically difficult to aspirate using palpation methods alone, for example, predominantly cystic or posteriorly located nodules. In patients with large nodules (>4 cm), ultrasound-guided FNA directed at several areas within a nodule may reduce the risk of a false negative biopsy.

Increasing evidence indicates that the presence of suspicious ultrasound features is more predictive of malignancy than nodule size alone.[16,17] A decision analysis of thyroid nodule cytology criteria for nodules measuring 1.0 to 1.5 cm favors the approach of selecting nodules with suspicious ultrasonographic characteristics for FNAc over the approach of performing FNAc of all nodules >1 cm.[5,18] Based on this evidence, both the European Thyroid Association and American Thyroid Association guidelines indicate that nodules smaller than 1 cm should be submitted to FNAc only when the ultrasonographic pattern is strongly suggestive.

We usually perform FNAc in solid nodules, both palpable and nonpalpable, measuring more than 1 cm. This recommendation is based on observational studies that show similar rates of cancer in nonpalpable nodules larger than 1 cm and palpable nodules of similar size.[17] Purely cystic nodules (no mural components) do not require diagnostic FNAc but aspiration of the fluid may be part of a therapeutic strategy.

At present, the major concern is the high prevalence of subcentimetric nodules and the real need to submit all of them to FNAc. Evidence indicates the lower the diameter, the higher the prevalence of "non-diagnostic" FNAc that may generate a lot of anxiety and concern for patients. Thus, it is conceivable to submit to FNAc only small nodules with echographical features suggesting malignancy while the others can be kept under surveillance. In patients showing high risk factors for thyroid cancer (Table 6.4), the ATA guidelines recommend ultrasound-guided FNAc also for nodules between 5 and 10 mm.[6] We know of no data to support such an approach, and we prefer to biopsy subcentimetric nodules in both high and low risk patients only if they show suspicious features at neck ultrasound, independently of nodule diameter.

As shown in Table 6.5, five categories of cytological classifications[19] are now widely recognized. Unfortunately, the indeterminate (THY3) and inadequate (THY1) categories pose a relevant issue regarding the need to submit patients to surgical treatments. The terminology used by different cytopathologists to describe follicular thyroid nodules is highly variable. It is essential that physicians interpreting reports be familiar with the terminology used by the specific cytopathologist.

In the last 5 to 10 years, achievements have been made and efforts continue to find molecular features that can differentiate FAs from FCs. Data remain controversial and many researchers are trying to find markers to discriminate these two pathologies without the need for surgery.[20,21]

TABLE 6.5
Categories of Cytological Results

FNAc Category	Identification Code
Non-diagnostic	THY1
Benign	THY2
Indeterminate	THY3
Suspicious for malignancy	THY4
Malignant	THY5

6.4.7 THYROID NODULE DIAGNOSIS DURING PREGNANCY AND CHILDHOOD

Thyroid radionuclide scanning is contraindicated during pregnancy. Otherwise, a pregnant woman found to have a thyroid nodule should be evaluated in the same way as if she were not pregnant. Thus, FNAc of the nodule should be done (as it would for most nonpregnant patients). The therapeutic strategy depends on cytology and is discussed in detail in the guidelines for the management of thyroid disease during pregnancy.

Although rare, thyroid nodules may be detected in children. The workup for this age group is the same as described above. If necessary, thyroid scintigraphy with ^{99m}Tc or ^{123}I may be performed at any time during infancy and childhood. FNAc is recommended because the prevalence of thyroid cancer in childhood nodules is higher than in adults and surgical treatment should not be postponed.

6.5 TREATMENT

The optimal therapy for patients with thyroid nodules varies with the lesions found and whether or not they are functioning. As shown in Table 6.5, five major categories of results may be obtained from FNAc and each requires different subsequent management.

6.5.1 NONDIAGNOSTIC (THY1)

A non-diagnostic cytology is usually due to an inadequate sample that can be related to several conditions such as the nature (cystic) and/or the size (< 1 cm) of a nodule, severe blood contamination, or even the inexperience of the operator. A significant lower prevalence of inadequate samples is obtained when FNAc is performed under ultrasound guidance in both solid and cystic nodules.

It is worth noting that the absence of malignant cells in an inadequate sample should not be interpreted as a negative cytology. Thus, for patients with non-diagnostic FNAc results, the recommendation is to repeat the procedure. If repeated aspiration is still non-diagnostic, surgical excision could be considered, especially for large solid nodules. An additional attempt to obtain adequate cytological material with additional ultrasound-guided FNAc is also reasonable for smaller solid nodules. For nodules that are partially cystic, monitoring is an alternative option as well.

6.5.2 BENIGN NODULE (THY2)

Most benign thyroid nodules tend to grow slowly. It has been demonstrated that after one year of observation fewer than 20% of nodules had grown and they needed 3 years to grow more than 50% of the original volume. Patients with benign nodules are usually followed without surgery but opinions concerning the efficacy of LT_4 therapy for these patients are controversial. Long-term growth of benign nodules appears to be prevalently endogenous and less influenced by exogenous factors including LT_4 therapy.

Whether LT_4 therapy is effective in controlling the sizes of thyroid nodules and safe, particularly if suppression of TSH is long term and performed in a middle-aged population remains unknown. Several parameters should be reviewed when considering the administration of LT_4 therapy: (1) the size and rate of growth of the nodule; (2) thyroid volume; (3) patient age; and (4) absence of functional autonomy. According to prospective studies specifically addressing this issue, only young patients with small or medium goiters and growing nodules are good candidates for LT_4 suppressive therapy.

Recently it has been demonstrated that serum TSH is an independent risk factor for predicting malignancy in a thyroid nodule. In a study of 1,500 patients presenting to a thyroid practice, the malignancy prevalences were 2.8, 3.7, 8.3, 12.3, and 29.7% for patients with serum TSH concentrations below 0.4 mU/L, 0.4 to 0.9 mU/L, 1.0 to 1.7 mU/L, 1.8 to 5.5 mU/L, and 5.5 mU/l, respectively.[22] A similar study demonstrated that when cancer was diagnosed, a higher TSH was associated with a more advanced stage of cancer.[23] A real benefit of LT_4 suppressive therapy in reducing the risk of cancer development is still a matter of discussion.

The follow-up of thyroid nodules (those treated with LT_4 and those not treated) is performed with periodic thyroid ultrasound controls, initially at 6 to 12 months, then at increasing intervals over time. Cystic degeneration and hemorrhage are the most common causes of rapid growth and can be easily detected by ultrasonography. Benign nodules larger than 3.5 to 4 cm should be considered for surgical treatment, especially if accompanied by symptoms and/or signs of tracheal and/or esophagous compression.

Thyroid nodules that are stable in size and reveal unchanged ultrasound features do not need to be resubmitted to FNAc because detection of malignancy in routine repeated FNAc is uncommon; it varies from 0.4 to 1.4% based on different series. Malignancy is such a rare event in benign thyroid nodules that grow over time (1.4%) that a possible false negative result from a previous benign cytology cannot be completely excluded since this can happen in 1 to 5% of aspirated cases and up to 12 or 13% in nodules larger than 4 cm.

From a practical view, a reassessment is warranted when growth is substantial, for example, a >50% change in volume, a 20% increase in at least two diameters, significant change in the structure of a nodule, or new symptoms attributed to a nodule.

Recent research suggests that nonsurgical therapy such as radiofrequency thermal ablation (RTA) and percutaneous laser ablation (PLA) may play a role in treating symptomatic patients.[24] Although very promising, the follow-up of treated patients is still too short to draw conclusions. One study with the longest follow-up of patients treated with RTA (2 years) showed a 75% decrease of nodule size. Compressive symptoms improved in all patients and completely disappeared in 88% of them.

The treatment was well tolerated by all patients. No patient needed hospitalization after RTA and no major complications were observed. According to these data, RTA is an effective and simple procedure for achieving lasting shrinkage of thyroid nodules and controlling compressive symptoms. It is particularly attractive for elderly people for whom surgery and radioiodine therapy are often contraindicated or ineffective.[25]

The PLA study with the longest follow-up (3 years) showed shrinkage of about 50% of the initial volume in a wide size range of benign cold thyroid nodules, with improvements in local symptoms and signs. Side effects and failures were few although not negligible and the authors concluded that long-term controlled studies are needed to establish the eligibility of patients for routine PLA.[26] In our opinion, these types of alternative treatments should be performed only in experienced medical centers at present.

6.5.3 FOLLICULAR NEOPLASM (THY3)

In patients with cytology suggesting follicular neoplasms, we typically perform thyroid scintigraphy, particularly if the TSH is at the lower end of normal range (Figure 6.5). Patients with hyperfunctioning (autonomous) nodules are followed with 6- to 12-month controls. For hyperthyroid patients, radioiodine therapy or surgery is advised. About 15 to 25% of microfollicular or cellular adenomas prove to be cancers, depending on the cytological pattern.[5] The presence of nuclear atypia seems to be an important predictive factor for malignancy. However, there is no consensus as to which nodules should be excised to exclude follicular cancer and studies have been performed to try to identify prognostic clinical or echographic features.

We demonstrated that only the presence of cell atypia at cytology and spot microcalcifications at thyroid ultrasound were significantly associated with malignancy.[27] However, in these patients, other clinical parameters and thyroid ultrasound patterns can be used to select those facing higher risks of malignancy. One approach is to follow patients who have nodules that are less than 50% macrofollicular or have similar proportions of macro- and microfollicles and resubmit them to FNAc after a 3- to 6-month interval before deciding whether to continue to monitor or recommend thyroidectomy. Conversely, most patients with nonautonomous pure microfollicular adenomas should undergo surgery with pathological evaluation for capsular and/or vascular invasion.

Although still not introduced in routine clinical practice, the elastosonography appears to have great practical value in distinguishing benign from malignant nodules (Figure 6.7). In particular, the elastosonography of small microfollicular nodules showed high specificity and sensitivity. If these results will be confirmed in other series, thyroid elastosonography could be a powerful instrument to at least partially resolve this distinction dilemma.[28]

The use of genetic biomarkers is very promising for enhancing the ability to distinguish benign from malignant nodules, especially in cases with indeterminate and/or inadequate cytology but it is still too early for clinical application. Certain proteins that can be detected by immunoistochemistry, particularly HBME-1 and galectin-3, have levels of expression that correlate with the nature of a nodule. However, technical problems surround the amount of tissue needed because cytological smears seem to be insufficient and the interpretation of the stains that is obviously subjective.

Genetic mutations involved in thyroid tumorigenesis (Table 6.3) can be sought in cytological material. Nucleic acids can be extracted with success both directly from a smear by scraping the cells from a slide[29] and from cells remaining in a needle used for FNAc.[20,21] Technically, all candidate oncogenes can be analyzed. The main limitation of this technique at present is that more than 30% of thyroid malignancies are still orphans of oncogenes.

TABLE 6.6

Sensitivity and Specificity of Echographic Patterns
in Predicting Malignancy of Thyroid Nodules

Echographic Pattern	Sensitivity %	Specificity %
Hypoechoic solid pattern	66.6	48.6
Microcalcification	54.0	75.6
Absence of peripheral halo[a]	66.6	77.0
Absence of peripheral halo + hypoechoic solid pattern	66.0	82.4
Absence of peripheral halo + microcalcification	26.6	93.2
Hypoechoic solid pattern + microcalcification	30	79.7
Absence of peripheral halo + hypoechoic solid pattern + intranodular blood flow	43.3	91.8
Absence of peripheral halo + microcalcification + intranodular blood flow	16.6	97.2
Hypoechoic solid pattern + microcalcification + intranodular blood flow	20	89.1

[a] Absence of peripheral halo includes presence of irregular borders.

From a practical view, cases positive for one of the known mutations are candidates for surgery because of a very high probability of thyroid cancer (100% in BRAF-positive cases, 85% in RAS-positive cases, 80% in RET/PTC-positive cases, etc.). The presence of a mutation can be of clinical utility in making the decision to perform a total thyroidectomy instead of a lobectomy. However, nodules without known oncogenic mutations (the majority in the group of those with indeterminate cytology) still have a 30% probability of malignancy and must be treated with surgery.

While the exact indication for a routine mutation analysis is still under investigation, other strategies have been recently applied to nucleic acids extracted from cytological material based on the differential levels of mRNA expression of some candidate genes. Several combinations of genes have been explored but their specificity and sensitivity in discriminating benign from malignant tumors were not sufficient to lead to their introduction into clinical practice. However, studies show that combinations of many genes may greatly improve both the sensitivity and the specificity of the technique.[30] However, because of the complexity of the technique, genes should be engineered as microchips to be applied for clinical purposes. Although these systems are still under evaluation, they seem sufficiently promising to warrant an international clinical trial dedicated to indeterminate thyroid nodules in the next few years.

6.5.4 SUSPICIOUS FOR MALIGNANCY (THY4)

This category includes lesions with some features suggestive of but not definitive for papillary thyroid cancer (PTC). Typically, nodules in this category have a 50 to 75% risk of malignancy. Such patients should be referred for surgery as should those with malignant cytologies.

6.5.5 MALIGNANT (THY5)

The malignant category includes papillary cancer, medullary cancer, thyroid lymphoma, anaplastic cancer, and cancer metastatic to the thyroid. Patients with cytologies diagnostic of malignancy should be referred for surgery. The extent of surgery is related to histological type and extension of local disease. This issue is covered in Chapters 7 and 8.

6.5.6 OTHER NODULE CATEGORIES

6.5.6.1 Autonomous Nodules

The optimal therapy of patients with autonomous nodules is controversial. If a nodule causes hyperthyroidism, a patient should be treated preferably with radioiodine, especially if the biggest diameter is smaller than 3.0 to 3.5 cm. Large nodules would likely require greater ^{131}I activities and multiple treatments. For these reasons, it may be better for them to undergo surgery, possibly after a period of antithyroid drug therapy.

Patients with subclinical hyperthyroidism (low serum TSH and normal serum free T_4 values) present an intriguing problem. Subclinical hyperthyroidism is associated with increased risk of atrial fibrillation in patients over 60 to 65 years of age; it is also associated with decreases in bone mineral density in postmenopausal women. These subjects should be treated according to the above suggestions. Conversely, younger asymptomatic patients can be followed up with 6 to 12 months of controls and treated when local or general symptoms due to enlargement of a nodule or hyperthyroidism, respectively, appear. The main risk is that these patients will drop out of the follow-up protocol, then return when they are clinically hyperthyroid.

In the past, other treatments were proposed for resolving autonomous nodules. Among several, the most apparently promising was the treatment by ultrasound-guided injection of ethanol. However, the rate of success was low and this treatment is currently limited to pure liquid nodules (cysts).

6.5.6.2 Cystic Thyroid Nodules

Cystic nodules represent difficult management issues. Many patients with small cystic nodules of non-diagnostic cytology can be followed with the assumption that the nodules are benign. In some patients, however, recurrent bleeding or cyst reformation may cause discomfort, anxiety, or rarely obstructive symptoms, mandating excision of the nodule. LT_4 therapy was not beneficial in a small randomized study of patients with cystic nodules.

Pure cystic thyroid nodules, especially colloidal cysts, can be successfully treated by ultrasound-guided injection of ethanol or sclerosing agents. A small atrophic nodule will replace the cyst and require only clinical, biochemical, and echographic controls for 12 to 18 months. Repeating FNAc in atrophic nodules secondary to ethanol injection is not recommended.

6.6 CONCLUSIONS

Single nodule is a very common thyroid disease especially in subjects over 50 years of age. Fortunately, only 5% of single nodules are malignant and they can be identified by FNAc. At present, the real challenge in the management of thyroid single nodules is the subgroup of patients who have nodules of indeterminate cytology that represent about 15% of all nodules: they can be malignant in 20 to 30% of cases but at present no diagnostic tools can distinguish benign from malignant cases preoperatively. A distinctive molecular profile could be a very good option to resolve this problem but we are still far from finding it.

REFERENCES

1. Pinchera, A. 2007. Thyroid incidentalomas. *Horm Res* 68 (5): 199–201.
2. Laurberg, P., Cerqueira, C., Ovesen, L. et al. 2010. Iodine intake as a determinant of thyroid disorders in populations. *Best Pract Res Clin Endocrinol Metab* 24: 13–27.
3. Imaizumi, M., Usa, T., Tominaga, T. et al. 2006. Radiation dose–response relationships for thyroid nodules and autoimmune thyroid diseases in Hiroshima and Nagasaki atomic bomb survivors 55–58 years after radiation exposure. *JAMA* 295: 1011–1022.
4. Tonacchera, M., Perri, A., De Marco, G. et al. 2003. TSH receptor and Gs(α) genetic analysis in children with Down's syndrome and subclinical hypothyroidism. *J Endocrinol Invest* 26: 997–1000.
5. Baloch, Z.W., LiVolsi, V.A., Asa, S.L. et al. 2008. Diagnostic terminology and morphologic criteria for cytologic diagnosis of thyroid lesions: a synopsis of the National Cancer Institute Thyroid Fine-Needle Aspiration State of the Science Conference. *Diagn Cytopathol* 36: 425–437.
6. Cooper, D.S., Doherty, G.M., Haugen, B.R. et al. 2009. Revised American Thyroid Association management guidelines for patients with thyroid nodules and differentiated thyroid cancer. *Thyroid* 19: 1167–1214.
7. Pacini, F., Schlumberger, M., Dralle, H. et al. 2006. European consensus for the management of patients with differentiated thyroid carcinoma of the follicular epithelium. *Eur J Endocrinol* 154: 787–803.
8. Paschke, R., Hegedus, L., Alexander, E. et al. 2011. Thyroid nodule guidelines: agreement, disagreement and need for future research. *Nat Rev Endocrinol* 7: 354–361.
9. Elisei, R. 2008. Routine serum calcitonin measurement in the evaluation of thyroid nodules. *Best Pract Res Clin Endocrinol Metab* 22: 941–953.
10. Elisei, R., Bottici, V., Luchetti, F. et al. 2004. Impact of routine measurement of serum calcitonin on the diagnosis and outcome of medullary thyroid cancer: experience in 10,864 patients with nodular thyroid disorders. *J Clin Endocrinol Metab* 89: 163–168.
11. Costante, G., Meringolo, D., Durante, C. et al. 2007. Predictive value of serum calcitonin levels for preoperative diagnosis of medullary thyroid carcinoma in a cohort of 5817 consecutive patients with thyroid nodules. *J Clin Endocrinol Metab* 92: 450–455.

12. Valle, L.A. and Kloos, R.T. 2011. The prevalence of occult medullary thyroid carcinoma at autopsy. *J Clin Endocrinol Metab* 96: E109–E113.

13. Doyle, P., Duren, C., Nerlich, K. et al. 2009. Potency and tolerance of calcitonin stimulation with high-dose calcium versus pentagastrin in normal adults. *J Clin Endocrinol Metab* 94: 2970–2974.

14. Rago, T. and Vitti, P. 2008. Role of thyroid ultrasound in the diagnostic evaluation of thyroid nodules. *Best Pract Res* 22: 913–928.

15. Reschini, E., Ferrari, C., Castellani, M. et al. 2006. The trapping-only nodules of the thyroid gland: prevalence study. *Thyroid* 16: 757–762.

16. Leenhardt, L., Hejblum, G., Franc, B. et al. 1999. Indications and limits of ultrasound-guided cytology in the management of nonpalpable thyroid nodules. *J Clin Endocrinol Metab* 84: 24–28.

17. Papini, E., Guglielmi, R., Bianchini, A. et al. 2002. Risk of malignancy in nonpalpable thyroid nodules: predictive value of ultrasound and color-Doppler features. *J Clin Endocrinol Metab* 87: 1941–1946.

18. McCartney, C.R. and Stukenborg, G.J. 2008. Decision analysis of discordant thyroid nodule biopsy guideline criteria. *J Clin Endocrinol Metab* 93: 3037–3044.

19. Watkinson, J.C., 2004. The British Thyroid Association guidelines for the management of thyroid cancer in adults. *Nucl Med Commun* 25: 897–900.

20. Cantara, S., Capezzone, M., Marchisotta, S. et al. 2010. Impact of proto-oncogene mutation detection in cytological specimens from thyroid nodules improves the diagnostic accuracy of cytology. *J Clin Endocrinol Metab* 95: 1365–1369.

21. Nikiforov, Y.E., Steward, D.L., Robinson-Smith, T.M. et al. 2009. Molecular testing for mutations in improving the fine-needle aspiration diagnosis of thyroid nodules. *J Clin Endocrinol Metab* 94: 2092–2098.

22. Boelaert, K., Horacek, J., Holder, R.L. et al. 2006. Serum thyrotropin concentration as a novel predictor of malignancy in thyroid nodules investigated by fine-needle aspiration. *J Clin Endocrinol Metab* 91: 4295–4301.

23. Haymart, M.R., Repplinger, D.J., Leverson, G.E., et al. 2008. Higher serum thyroid stimulating hormone level in thyroid nodule patients is associated with greater risks of differentiated thyroid cancer and advanced tumor stage. *J Clin Endocrinol Metab* 93: 809–814.

24. Hegedus, L. 2009. Therapy: a new nonsurgical therapy option for benign thyroid nodules? *Nat Rev Endocrinol* 5: 476–478.

25. Spiezia, S., Garberoglio, R., Milone, F. et al. 2009. Thyroid nodules and related symptoms are stably controlled two years after radiofrequency thermal ablation. *Thyroid* 19: 219–225.

26. Valcavi, R., Riganti, F., Bertani, A. et al. 2010. Percutaneous laser ablation of cold benign thyroid nodules: a 3-year follow-up study in 122 patients. *Thyroid* 20: 1253–1261.

27. Rago, T., Di Coscio, G., Ugolini, C. et al. 2007. Clinical features of thyroid autoimmunity are associated with thyroiditis on histology and are not predictive of malignancy in 570 patients with indeterminate nodules on cytology who had a thyroidectomy. *Clin Endocrinol (Oxf)* 67: 363–369.

28. Rago, T., Scutari, M., Santini, F. et al. 2010. Real-time elastosonography: useful tool for refining the presurgical diagnosis in thyroid nodules with indeterminate or nondiagnostic cytology. *J Clin Endocrinol Metab* 95: 5274–5280.

29. Marchetti, I., Lessi, F., Mazzanti, C.M. et al. 2009. A morpho-molecular diagnosis of papillary thyroid carcinoma: BRAF V600E detection as an important tool in preoperative evaluation of fine-needle aspirates. *Thyroid* 19: 837–842.

30. Li, H., Robinson, K.A., Anton, B. et al. 2011. Cost effectiveness of a novel molecular test for cytologically indeterminate thyroid nodules. *J Clin Endocrinol Metab*

7 Differentiated (Papillary and Follicular) and Anaplastic Thyroid Carcinoma

Furio Pacini and Maria Grazia Castagna

CONTENTS

Key words: thyroglobulin, rhTSH, ^{131}I whole body scan, radioiodine therapy.

7.1 DIFFERENTIATED (PAPILLARY AND FOLLICULAR) THYROID CARCINOMA

7.1.1 DEFINITIONS

Follicular thyroid epithelium can give rise to differentiated and undifferentiated carcinomas. Differentiated thyroid carcinoma (DTC) includes the papillary and follicular histotypes and their variants that account for more than 80% of all thyroid cancers. Undifferentiated (or anaplastic) thyroid cancer is still derived from the follicular epithelium but is characterized by the almost complete loss of thyroid differentiation. Frequently, it can arise on the background of preexisting papillary or follicular carcinoma. The undifferentiated type accounts for about 5% of thyroid carcinomas.

7.1.2 EPIDEMIOLOGY

7.1.2.1 Incidence of Thyroid Cancer

Thyroid cancer represents fewer than 1% of all human tumors but is the most common endocrine malignancy. The annual incidence of thyroid cancer varies considerably by geographic area, age, and sex. Worldwide incidence rates vary widely due to ethnic or environmental factors (such as spontaneous background radiation) or dietary habits, but different standards of medical expertise and health care may also play a role in the efficiency of cancer detection. A recent review reported an overall incidence of all types of thyroid cancers in the United States of 7.7 per 100,000 person-years (11.3 per 100,000 woman-years and 4.1 per 100,000 man-years).[1] The incidence was significantly higher in whites than blacks (7.16 per 100,000 and 4.25 per 100,000 person-years, respectively).[2] High rates were observed in certain geographic areas such as Hawaii (11.9 per 100,000 women and 4.5 per 100,000 men).[3]

From 1998 through 2002, the highest rates of age-adjusted thyroid cancer incidence were found in the U.S. and Israel for males (3.5 per 100,000 for both countries) and for females (10.0 per 100,000 and 12.1 per 100,000, respectively). The lowest rates were in Uganda (0.5 per 100,000 in males and 1.5 per 100,000 in females). Considerable variation in thyroid cancer incidence was present within every continent with the exception of Africa where incidence rates were generally low[4] (Table 7.1).

Thyroid cancer is very rare in children under age 15 (0.5 per 100,000 person-years) and represents 1.5 to 3% of all childhood cancers. The annual incidence of thyroid cancer increases with age, peaking at 22 per 100,000 person-years by the fifth to the seventh decade.[2] Female gender is definitely a risk factor for thyroid cancer, with most population studies showing a clearly increased risk in women, yet it seems that the disease may be more aggressive in men.

Despite considerable variation in cancer incidence worldwide, reports of increasing incidence have come from all over the globe during recent decades.[5-8] This phenomenon is mainly due to an increase in micropapillary (<2 cm) histotype. No

TABLE 7.1
Age-Standardized Incidence Rates per 100,000 (World) for Various Countries (1998–2002)

Country	Males (Rate)	Females (Rate)
Europe		
Denmark	1.2	2.9
Norway	1.6	4.2
Sweden	1.3	3.3
Finland	2.2	7.0
France	2.3	5.8
Switzerland	2.0	6.5
United Kingdom	0.9	2.3
Italy	2.9	7.1
Spain	1.4	4.0
Oceania		
New Zealand	1.3	5.1
Australia	2.5	8.1
Americas		
U.S. SEER white	3.5	10.0
Canada	2.1	5.6
Colombia	2.2	9.4
U.S. SEER black	1.6	5.2
Asia		
China	2.2	7.2
Japan	1.3	3.2
Singapore	2	6.6
Israel	3.5	12.1
Africa		
Algeria	1.4	3.6
Egypt	1.1	2.6
Tunisia	1.3	3.1
Uganda	0.5	1.5
Zimbabwe	1.0	3.1

Source: Adapted from Kilfoy, B.A. et al. 2009. *Cancer Causes Control* 20: 525–531.

significant change in the incidence of the less common histological categories (follicular, medullary, and anaplastic cancers) was noted. The increase is attributable to better detection of small papillary carcinomas as a result of improved diagnostic accuracy (neck ultrasound and fine needle aspiration cytology).

It is a common experience in thyroid cancer referral centers that nearly 60 to 80% of thyroid carcinomas detected now are micropapillary thyroid carcinomas (smaller than 1 cm in size) that carry an excellent long-term prognosis.[7] However, more recently, an increased incidence for all sizes of thyroid tumor has been reported in the U.S. Although from 1997 through 2005 the annual percentage change (APC) for primary tumors <1.0 cm was 9.9 in men and 8.6 in women, a significant increase was also observed for tumors >4 cm among men (APC 3.7) and women (APC 5.7).[9] These data suggest that increased diagnostic scrutiny is not the only explanation.

7.1.2.2 Thyroid Cancer Incidence by Histotype

Papillary thyroid carcinoma affects women more often than men, and in 2006 was predicted to represent 3% of all cancers in women, 1% in men and 1.4% in children, thus becoming one of the top seven new cancer cases. The U.S. incidence of papillary thyroid cancer is 5.7 per 100,000 person-years, with a rate of 8.8 per 100,000 woman-years and 2.7 per 100,000 man-years.[1] Follicular cancer occurs more often than papillary cancer in older patients (>40 years of age). In the United States, the incidence of follicular thyroid cancer is 0.82 per 100,000 person-years (1.06 per 100,000 woman-years and 0.59 per 100,000 man-years). The incidence of follicular cancer did not vary substantially by race or ethnicity.[1] The incidence of anaplastic thyroid cancer in the United States is 0.21 per 100,000 person-years without substantial differences of race, ethnicity, and sex.

Regarding prevalence, on January 1, 2008, there were approximately 458,403 thyroid cancer patients in the United States (100,952 men and 357,451 women). This includes all patients alive on January 1, 2008 who had been diagnosed with thyroid cancer, patients with active disease, and those who were cured.[2]

7.1.2.3 Mortality

Despite increasing incidence, the mortality from thyroid cancer has been declining over the last three decades. In the European Union from 1992 to 2002, thyroid cancer mortality declined in both men and women (−23 and −28%, respectively).[9] How much of the decline in mortality is due to early diagnosis or to improved treatment of the disease is unclear. The age-adjusted death rate was 0.5 per 100,000 per year. Approximately 0.1% died under age 20; 0.9% between ages 20 and 34; 2.3% between ages 35 and 44; 8.1% between ages 45 and 54; 17.5% between ages 55 and 64; 24.1% between ages 65 and 74; 30.3% between ages 75 and 84; and 16.8% in patients older than 85 years.[2]

7.1.3 ETIOLOGY AND PATHOGENESIS

Thyroid oncogenesis is characterized by a series of genetic events associated with hypothetical environmental factors. While genetic factors have been well defined in recent decades, the role of environmental factors is still controversial.

TABLE 7.2

Environmental Factors in Thyroid Cancer

Environmental Factor	Evidence
Thyroid radiation	Solid
Dietary iodine	Controversial
TSH	Solid
Estrogens	Controversial

7.1.4 ENVIRONMENTAL FACTORS

Table 7.2 lists the environmental factors involved in thyroid cancer.

7.1,4.1 Thyroid Radiation

The only established environmental risk factor for thyroid carcinoma is exposure to ionizing radiation. The risk, particularly of papillary carcinoma, is greater in subjects of younger age at exposure. This is supported by epidemiological studies in atomic bomb survivors and in children exposed to the radiation fallout after the explosion at the Chernobyl nuclear power plant in 1986. Before the explosion, the incidence of thyroid cancer in Belarus (the most contaminated region) children was very low (0.5 to 1.0 per 1,000,000 children). Following the explosion, a dramatic (80-fold) increase in the incidence of malignant thyroid tumors (mostly papillary) was observed in exposed subjects who were children at the time of the accident.[10,11]

Previous studies in patients subjected to external radiation on their heads and necks as therapy for several benign or malignant diseases already demonstrated a causative role of radiation in the development of thyroid cancer. After radiotherapy to the head and neck for thymic enlargement, tonsillitis, acne, and adenitis, the risk of developing thyroid cancer in subsequent years is around 3%. A linear relationship exists between radiation doses up to 1,800 rads and the occurrence of thyroid nodules and cancer. Also in cases of external radiation, studies demonstrated that the younger the age at the time of exposure the higher the risk and doses ranging from 0.10 to 60 Gy can induce thyroid tumors.[12] Most nodules tend to occur within 10 to 20 years after exposure, but the risk may persist for 40 or more years.

7.1.4.2 Dietary Iodine

Dietary iodine intake is among the possible environmental factors contributing to thyroid diseases in general and thyroid cancer in particular. Low dietary iodine intake can result in increased serum TSH, a thyroid cancer permissive factor in susceptible individuals. Although there continues to be disagreement on whether iodine intake determines the prevalence of DTC, strong evidence indicates that different levels of iodine intake influence the form of presentation, with follicular thyroid carcinoma predominating in areas of deficient iodine intake.

7.1.4.3   TSH and Thyroid Cancer

Thyroid-stimulating hormone (TSH) is the main regulator of thyroid function and is involved in the secretion of thyroid hormones, maintenance of thyroid-specific gene expression (differentiation), and thyroid cell proliferation. TSH is a mitogen, and several in vivo and in vitro studies demonstrated that high TSH levels are associated with stimulation of thyroid cancer cell growth, while TSH suppression is associated with growth inhibition. Recently, it has been reported that in patients with nodular thyroid diseases, the risk of thyroid malignancy increases with serum TSH concentrations, and that even within normal ranges, higher TSH values are associated with a higher frequency and more advanced stages of thyroid cancer.[13]

7.1.4.4   Gender and Thyroid Cancer

Several hypotheses have been proposed to explain the gender disparities observed in the incidence of thyroid cancer, including differential screening, gender-specific behavioral differences, biological sex differences, and variations in tumor biology. The female predominance of thyroid cancer and its peak incidence occurring at reproductive ages suggests that female sex hormones may be involved in the development of thyroid cancer. Despite numerous experimental studies suggesting that sex hormones and their receptors may play a role in tumorigenesis and tumor progression., clinical evidence of their impact on thyroid cancer development remains inconclusive.

7.1.5   GENETIC ALTERATIONS

In recent years, the genetic alterations responsible for thyroid cancer have been extensively studied and partially defined. Mutations in genes coding for elements of the mitogen-activated protein kinase (MAPK) pathway are often responsible for transformation of thyroid follicular cells. The most frequent genetic alterations are represented by somatic activating mutations of proto-oncogenes including BRAF and RAS or rearrangements of RET and TRK or inactivating mutations of tumor suppressor genes such as p53 and PPARγ.[14] Figure 7.1 illustrates the genetic alterations responsible for neoplastic transformation in relation to different histotypes.

Mutations of the BRAF gene are the most frequent alterations of papillary carcinoma, with a prevalence of nearly 50%. The most frequent mutation is V600E, which results in constitutive activation of BRAF protein kinase leading to phosphorylation and activation of the MEK-MAP kinase cascade. The BRAF mutation is more common in the classical variant of papillary carcinoma and is somehow associated with more aggressive tumor behavior.[14] In the case of RET and TRK proto-oncogenes, the genetic alteration is represented by rearrangement of these genes with various ubiquitous genes (rearranged RET/PTC and TRK) along with the formation of a chimeric oncogene by the tyrosine kinase portion of RET or TRK and a ubiquitous gene promoter.

The rearrangement leads to constitutive activation of the RET or TRK domain, resulting in activation of the MAP-kinase. RET/PTC rearrangement is the most frequent alteration found in radiation-induced tumors.[14] Point mutations of the RAS

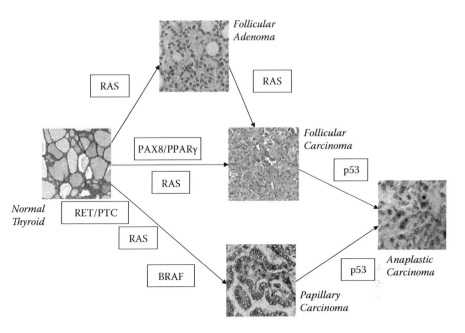

FIGURE 7.1   Genetic alterations responsible for neoplastic transformation in relation to different histotypes.

oncogene have been described for all three variants of the gene (N, H, K). Mutations affect codon 12, 13, or 61. Unlike BRAF and RET/PTC which are papillary carcinoma-specific, RAS mutations are found in a small proportion of papillary carcinomas, follicular adenomas, and follicular carcinomas. RAS mutations represent the major cause of aberrant activation of the phosphatidylinositol-3 kinase (PI3K)/ Akt pathway.[14] The PAX8-PPARγ oncogene results from a chromosomal rearrangement that fuses the thyroid-specific transcription factor PAX8 to the widely distributed nuclear transcription factor PPARγ. The PAX8-PPARγ rearrangement is found in 35 to 45% of follicular carcinomas, 4 to 33% of follicular adenomas, and rarely in oncocytic carcinomas.[14]

Aberrant activation (PIK3CA amplification and RAS mutations) of the phosphatidylinositol-3 kinase (PI3K)/AKT pathway plays a fundamental role in thyroid tumorigenesis, particularly in follicular thyroid cancer (FTC) and aggressive thyroid cancers such as anaplastic thyroid cancer (ATC), and less frequently in papillary thyroid cancer. Epigenetic silencing of the PTEN gene, a negative regulator of the PI3K/AKT pathway, also occurs in thyroid tumors, but its relationship with genetic alterations in this pathway is unclear.[14] Both papillary and follicular thyroid carcinomas may progress to an undifferentiated phenotype by inactivating mutations of p53 proto-oncogene that deprive cells of a major thyroid tumor suppressor gene.[14]

Familial predisposition (in absence of recognized predisposing conditions such as Cowden's syndrome, Werner syndrome, Carney complex, familial adenomatous polyposis) is reported in 3 to 10% of DTC cases. It is well established that the risk of developing the same tumor in first-degree relatives of DTC patients is significantly higher than in the general population. No specific genetic alterations have been demonstrated in the blood of familial non-medullary thyroid carcinoma (FNMTC) patients, apart from susceptibility loci found in a few pedigrees.

Recent studies reported that patients with FNMTC display the features of "anticipation phenomenon"—the tendency for family members of the second generation to develop clinical disease at an earlier age and with more aggressiveness than found in parents in the first generation. This phenomenon, has been correlated with inheritable alteration of the telomere–telomerase complex (short telomeres).[15]

7.1.6 PRESENTATION AND DIAGNOSIS

Thyroid cancer presents as a thyroid nodule detected by palpation or more frequently by fortuitous discovery during neck ultrasonography (US). While thyroid nodules are frequent (4 to 50% of the population, depending on diagnostic procedure and patient age), thyroid cancer is rare (~5% of all thyroid nodules). Thyroid US is a widespread technique used as a first-level diagnostic procedure for detecting and characterizing nodular thyroid disease. US features associated with malignancy are hypoechogenicity, microcalcifications, absence of peripheral halo, irregular borders, solid aspect, and intranodular blood flow and shape (more tall than wide).

All these patterns taken individually are poorly predictive of malignancy but, when multiple patterns suggestive of malignancy are simultaneously present, the specificity of US increases.[16] However, despite the overall utility of US, the "gold standard" for the differential diagnosis of thyroid nodules is still fine needle aspiration cytology (FNAc). According to available guidelines,[17,18] FNAc should be performed on any thyroid nodule larger than 1 cm and in those smaller than 1 cm if the clinical picture (history of head and neck radiation, family history of thyroid cancer, suspicious features at palpation, presence of cervical adenopathy) or ultrasonographic study indicates suspicion of malignancy. The results of FNAc are very sensitive for the differential diagnosis of benign and malignant nodules but the technique has limitations related to inadequate samples and follicular neoplasia. FNAc should be repeated if samples are inadequate. In cases of follicular neoplasia with normal TSH and cold appearance on thyroid scan, surgery should be considered.[17,18]

Among various methods proposed to increase the diagnostic accuracy of FNAc, mutation status of the tumor (presence or absence of oncogene mutations) is gaining increasing attention after reports demonstrated that the integration of traditional cytology and mutation analysis significantly increased sensitivity and specificity.[19] See Table 7.3.

Thyroid function tests and thyroglobulin (Tg) measurement are of little help for diagnosing thyroid cancer. However, measurement of serum calcitonin is a reliable tool for the diagnosis of the few cases of medullary thyroid cancer (5 to 7% of all thyroid cancers), and has higher sensitivity compared to FNAc. For this reason, routine measurement of serum calcitonin should be an integral part of the diagnostic evaluations of thyroid nodules.[20] In cases of undifferentiated thyroid carcinoma, the diagnosis is usually easy based on typical clinical aspects: large, hard mass invading the neck and causing compressive symptoms (dyspnea, cough, vocal cord paralysis, dysphagia, and hoarseness).

TABLE 7.3
Diagnostic Accuracy of Thyroid Ultrasound, FNAc, and Molecular Testing in Differential Diagnosis of Benign and Malignant Thyroid Nodules

Test	Sensitivity (%)	Specificity (%)	PPV (%)	NPV (%)
Thyroid ultrasound				
Microcalcifications	72	72	11	98
Hypoechoicity	81	47	7.0	98
Increased intranodular flow	62	50	5.6	96
Irregular margins	53	81	12	97
FNAc	43–98	72–100	89–98	99
Molecular analysis	79.8	100	100	89.9
FNAc and molecular analysis	90.5	98.7	97.4	94.9

Note: PPV = positive predictive value. NPV = negative predictive value.

7.1.7 Treatment of Differentiated Thyroid Carcinoma

Table 7.4 details DTC treatments.

7.1.7.1 Surgery

The initial first-line treatment for DTC is total or near-total thyroidectomy when the diagnosis is made before surgery. Less extensive surgical procedures may be accepted in cases of unifocal DTC diagnosed at final histology after surgery performed for benign thyroid disorders if a tumor is small, intrathyroidal, and of favorable histological type (classical papillary or follicular variant of papillary or minimally invasive follicular).

The initial treatment of DTC should always be preceded by careful exploration of the neck by ultrasound to assess the status of lymph node chains. The benefit of prophylactic central node dissection in the absence of evidence of nodal disease is controversial. No evidence shows that in papillary thyroid carcinoma it may improve recurrence or mortality. It allows accurate staging of the disease that may guide subsequent treatment and follow-up.[17,18]

TABLE 7.4
Treatment of Differentiated Thyroid Cancer

Total thyroidectomy	When diagnosis is presurgical
Lobectomy	May be allowed in case of incidental finding at histology for surgery performed to treat other thyroid disease
Radioiodine remnant ablation	See Table 7.6 for indication
Levo-thyroxine (LT$_4$) therapy	Suppressive therapy after thyroidectomy and in patients with residual metastatic disease; replacement therapy when disease-free status is documented

Compartment-oriented microdissection of lymph nodes should be performed in cases of preoperatively suspected and/or intraoperatively proven lymph node metastases. Prophylactic lymph node dissection is not indicated in follicular thyroid cancer. In expert hands, surgical complications such as laryngeal nerve palsy and hypoparathyroidism, are extremely rare (below 2%).[17,18]

7.1.7.2 Prognosis, Staging, and Risk Assessment

Both papillary and follicular differentiated thyroid cancers usually have good prognoses; overall mortality is below 10%. Such favorable prognoses result from the biological properties of most thyroid carcinomas and the effectiveness of primary therapy. In recent years, increased emphasis is placed on using individual estimates of risk to guide postablative remnant ablation and follow-up in DTC patients. Several risk stratification systems have been published and the most popular is the AJCC/UICC system. All of them were developed to predict the risk of death but not of recurrence.

Because they are based on clinical pathologic factors available soon after diagnosis and initial surgical therapy, they do not change over time. To overcome this limitation, the American Thyroid Association (ATA) in recently published guidelines[18] classified the risk of recurrence as low, intermediate, or high based on tumor-related parameters (pTNM and histological variant) integrated with other clinical features including results of a postablative radioiodine whole body scan (WBS) and serum Tg measurement.

Low risk—Patients display no local or distant metastases. All macroscopic tumor has been resected; no tumor invasion of locoregional tissues or structures has occurred and no aggressive histology or vascular invasion is noted. If a patient received ^{131}I, no ^{131}I uptake was noted outside the thyroid bed on postablative WBS.

Intermediate risk—Patients show microscopic invasion of tumor into the perithyroidal soft tissues at initial surgery, cervical lymph node metastases, ^{131}I uptake outside the thyroid bed on posttherapeutic WBS, or tumors with aggressive histology or vascular invasion.

High risk—Patients with macroscopic tumor invasion, incomplete tumor resection, distant metastases, and possibly thyroglobulinemia out of proportion to what is seen on the postablative scan.

This system for estimating risks of recurrence and disease-specific death is used to guide subsequent follow-up. See Table 7.5. Similar recommendation are given in the ETA guidelines.[17]

Although the risk stratifications proposed by the ATA and the ETA are good starting points for initial decision making, they are less accurate in predicting long-term outcomes in DTC patients. Recent reports developed the concept of ongoing risk stratification that incorporates the results of initial treatment (surgery and radioiodine ablation). Such risk stratifications are obtained 8 to 12 months after initial treatment or later.[21]

7.1.7.3 Postsurgical Thyroid Remnant Ablation

Surgery is usually followed by the administration of ^{131}I to ablate any remnant thyroid tissue and potential microscopic residual tumors. The impact of ablation on

TABLE 7.5

Risk Stratification Based on ATA Guidelines

Low Risk	Intermediate Risk	High Risk
No local or distant metastases	Microscopic invasion of tumor	Macroscopic tumor invasion
All macroscopic tumor resected	into perithyroidal soft tissues at	Incomplete tumor resection
No tumor invasion of	initial surgery	Distant metastases
locoregional tissues or structures	Cervical lymph node metastases	Thyroglobulinemia out of
No aggressive histology or	[131]I uptake outside thyroid bed on	proportion to what is seen
vascular invasion	posttherapeutic WBS	on postablative scan
If ^{131}I given, no ^{131}I uptake	Tumor with aggressive histology	
outside thyroid bed on	or vascular invasion	
posttherapeutic WBS		

Source: Cooper, D.S., Doherty, G.M., Haugen, B.R. et al. 2009. *Thyroid* 19: 1167–1214. With permission.

recurrence and mortality rate is controversial, but in most series it seems to reduce the risk of regional recurrence and facilitates long-term surveillance based on serum Tg measurement and diagnostic WBS. In addition, the high activity level of ^{131}I allows highly sensitive posttherapeutic WBS. According to several guidelines,[17,18] the recommendations for remnant ablation are modulated on the basis of risk factors. Radioiodine ablation is definitely indicated in high-risk patients but not in low-risk patients. In patients at intermediate risk, radioiodine remnant ablation may be indicated but the decision must be individualized.[17,18] See Table 7.6.

Effective thyroid ablation requires adequate stimulation by TSH that may be achieved by thyroid hormone withdrawal (THW) or exogenous recombinant human TSH (rhTSH) administration. The recombinant procedure is considered the method

TABLE 7.6

Indications for Remnant Ablative Therapy (RAI)

RAI Recommended	RAI Not Recommended
All patients with:	Patients with unifocal cancer <1 cm without other
• Known distant metastases	higher risk features[a]
• Gross extrathyroidal extension of tumor	Patients with multifocal cancer when all foci are
regardless of tumor size	<1 cm in absence of other higher risk features[a]
• Primary tumor size >2 cm even in absence of	
other higher risk features[a]	
Selected patients with 1- to 2-cm cancers confined	
to thyroid with documented lymph node	
metastases or other higher risk features*	

[a] Higher risk features include histological subtypes (tall cell, columnar, insular, solid variant, and poorly differentiated thyroid carcinomas, follicular and Hürthle cell cancers), intrathyroidal vascular invasion, gross or microscopic multifocal disease.

of choice based on several reports[22,23] demonstrating equal efficacy compared to THW even using low-activity [131]I (1110 to 1,850 MBq).[22,23]

7.1.7.4 Levo-Thyroxine (LT₄) Therapy

Thyroid hormone suppression therapy is an important part of the treatment of thyroid cancer. Immediately after surgery, thyroid hormone therapy is initiated with the dual aim to replace the hormone and suppress the potential growth stimulus of TSH on tumor cells (TSH suppressive therapy). The drug of choice is LT₄ and the suppressive dose varies according to the age and body mass index. TSH suppressive treatment is of benefit for high-risk thyroid cancer patients by decreasing progression of metastatic disease, thus reducing cancer-related mortality. No significant benefits are demonstrated in patients who achieved complete remission. These patients may be shifted from suppressive to replacement LT₄ therapy.

7.1.8 FOLLOW-UP

7.1.8.1 Short Term

The aim of follow-up is the early discovery and treatment of persistent or recurrent locoregional or distant disease. Most local recurrences develop and are detected in the first 5 years after diagnosis. However, in a minority of cases, local or distant recurrence may develop late during follow-up, even 20 years after initial treatment.

Two to three months after initial treatment, thyroid function tests (FT₃, FT₄, TSH) should be performed to check the adequacy of LT₄ suppressive therapy. At 6 to 12 months, follow-up should ascertain whether a patient is free of disease. This follow-up is based on physical examination, neck ultrasound, basal and rhTSH stimulated serum Tg measurement (in Tg antibody-negative patients) with or without diagnostic radioiodine WBS.[17,18] See Table 7.7.

At present most patients (nearly 80%) fall into the low-risk category and will disclose normal neck ultrasound and undetectable (<1.0 ng/ml) basal and stimulated serum Tg. Diagnostic WBS does not add clinical information in this setting and may be omitted. These patients may be considered in complete remission; their rate of subsequent recurrence is very low (<1.0% at 10 years).[17,18]

7.1.8.2 Long Term

The subsequent follow-up of patients considered free of disease at the time of first follow-up will consist of annual physical examination, basal serum Tg measurement on replacement LT₄ therapy, and neck ultrasound. No other biochemical or morphological tests are indicated unless some new suspicion arises during evaluation (Table 7.7). The question of whether a second rhTSH stimulated Tg test should be performed in disease-free patients is a matter of debate.

A recent study[24] reported that this procedure has little clinical utility in patients who had no biochemical (undetectable serum Tg) or clinical (imaging) evidence of disease at the time of first control after initial therapy (Table 7.8). Recently, new methods for serum Tg measurement with a functional sensitivity below 0.1 ng/mL became available. Using these systems, some authors reported much higher sensitivity of the

TABLE 7.7
Short- and Long-Term Follow-Up of Patients with Differentiated Thyroid Carcinoma

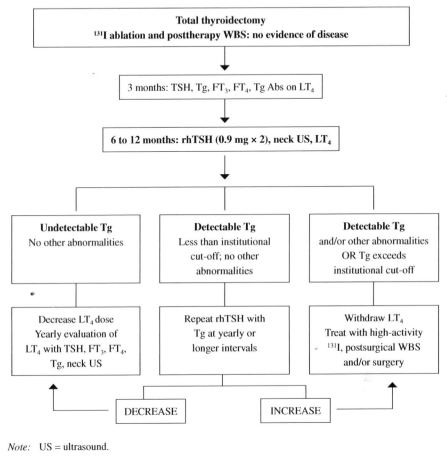

Note: US = ultrasound.

assays. In their experience, an undetectable basal serum Tg (<0.1 ng/ml) using ultrasensitive assays should give the same information of a stimulated Tg value and thus the authors recommended that rhTSH-Tg testing should be abandoned. However, this approach has been questioned.[25,26]

Patients with evidence of persistent disease or increases of detectable levels of serum Tg over time require imaging techniques to assess localization of disease and appropriate treatment including therapeutic doses of [131]I. Included in this category are the 5 to 10% of DTC patients who presented with local or distant metastases at diagnosis and an additional 5 to 10% who develop recurrent disease during follow-up.

During the evaluation of metastatic patients, [18]FDG-PET scanning is gaining more attention as a diagnostic and prognostic tool. In general, the sensitivity of

TABLE 7.8
Prevalence of Recurrence in Patients Free of Disease at First Control after Initial Therapy Based on Stimulated Serum Tg Measurement, Neck Ultrasound, and Diagnostic WBS

Number of Patients	Stimulus	Follow-Up (Years)	Recurrence Rate (%)	References
315	Hypothyroidism	12	0.6	Pacini et al. 2002, *JCEM*
256	Hypothyroidism	5.0	0.9	Cailleux et al. 2000, *JCEM*
68	rhTSH	3.3	1.4	Kloos & Mazzaferri 2005, *JCEM*
68	rhTSH	3.0	1.5	Castagna et al. 2008, *JCEM*
89	rhTSH	3.0	1.1	Crocetti et al. 2008, *Thyroid*

[18]FDG-PET is not superior to the sensitivities of traditional techniques such as CT and MR. Thus, the main indication for [18]FDG-PET is in metastatic patients who lost radioiodine uptake. ^{131}I-WBS negative and [18]FDG-PET positive patients indicate more aggressive and less differentiated disease and carry a worse prognosis with respect to ^{131}I-WBS positive and [18]FDG-PET negative patients.

7.1.8.3 Treatment of Metastatic Disease

Clinically evident lymph node metastases are present in approximately one-third of patients with papillary thyroid carcinoma at presentation. Microscopic metastases are present in one-half. The most common site of lymph node involvement is the central compartment (level 6). The jugular lymph node chains (levels 2 through 4) are the next most common sites of cervical node involvement. Lymph node metastases may also develop in the posterior triangle of the neck (level 5). Approximately 5 to 10% of patients develop distant metastases. Distant spread of papillary carcinoma typically affects the lungs and bone. Unlike papillary carcinoma, cervical metastases from follicular carcinomas are uncommon. However, the rate of distant metastasis is significantly increased (approximately 20%). Lung and bone are the most common sites.

Treatment of locoregional disease is based on surgery when possible. Radioiodine therapy may be an option in cases of small lesions not amenable to surgery. External beam radiotherapy may be indicated when complete surgical excision is not possible or when a tumor shows no significant radioiodine uptake.[17]

Distant metastases are more successfully cured if they take up radioiodine, are of small size, and located in the lungs (not visible on x-rays). Lung macronodules may benefit from radioiodine therapy but the definitive cure rate is very low.[27] Bone metastases have the worst prognosis even when aggressively treated by a combination of radioiodine therapy and external beam radiotherapy.[17] Brain metastases are relatively rare and usually carry poor prognosis. Surgical resection and external beam radiotherapy represent the only therapeutic options.

In cases of diffuse and progressive metastatic disease, systemic therapy should be considered. Chemotherapy is used less frequently due to lack of effective results and should be replaced by enrollment of patients in experimental clinical trials of tyrosine kinase inhibitors (TKIs). Molecules that block kinase activity at distal steps in the MAP kinase pathway are logical candidate drugs for thyroid cancer. TKIs tested against differentiated thyroid cancer in clinical trials include motesanib diphosphate, axitinib, gefitinib, sorafenib, and sunitinib. None of these is specific for one oncogene protein but they target several TK receptors and pro-angiogenic growth factor receptors. The results of Phase II and III clinical trials conducted to date are promising, with partial responses ranging from 14 to 32% and stable disease responses of 50 to 67%.[28] The preliminary results of these trials are promising and indicate that target therapy may become the first-line treatment of metastatic refractory thyroid cancer patients in the near future.

7.2 ANAPLASTIC THYROID CANCER (ATC)

7.2.1 DEFINITION

ATC is fortunately very rare, but is the most aggressive thyroid malignancy.

7.2.2 EPIDEMIOLOGY

ATC affects more women than men, but the female-to-male ratio is about 2 to 3:1, lower than the ratios of papillary and follicular histotypes. It arises from the follicular cells of the thyroid gland but does not retain any of the biological features (iodine uptake and Tg synthesis) of the original cells. The peak incidence is in the sixth and seventh decades (mean age at diagnosis = 55 to 65 years).[1] In most cases, ATC develops from a preexisting well-differentiated thyroid tumor that undergoes additional mutational events, mainly p53 mutation.[29]

7.2.3 DIAGNOSIS

The diagnosis is usually easy, based on typical clinical aspects: large, hard mass invading the neck and causing compressive symptoms (dyspnea, cough, vocal cord paralysis, dysphagia, and hoarseness). About 30% of patients have vocal cord paralysis and cervical metastases are palpable on examination in 40% of patients. Almost 50% of patients present distant metastases, mostly in the lungs but also in bones, liver, and brain. Due to its aggressive behavior, the latest manual of the American Joint Committee on Cancer Staging classifies all ATCs as T4 and stage IV tumors regardless of their size and overall tumor burden. The mean overall survival is less than 6 months despite treatment.

7.2.4 TREATMENT

Treatment of ATC has not been standardized and unfortunately no efficient treatment exists. Surgery, chemotherapy, and radiotherapy, alone or in combination, do not improve survival. The most common single cytotoxic agent used is doxorubicin alone or in combination with cisplatin. The results have been disappointing. Adding bleomycin and other agents does not enhance the efficacy of this combination. Recently, paclitaxel has been used in clinical trial and shown some improvement in response but not in survival. Novel treatment strategies including targeted therapy, suppressor gene therapy, and drugs that can induce cell cycle arrest are under experimental trials.[29]

REFERENCES

1. Aschebrook-Kilfoy, B., Ward, M.H., Sabra, M.M. et al. 2011. Thyroid cancer incidence patterns in the United States by histologic type, 1992–2006. *Thyroid* 21: 125–134.
2. Howlader, N., Noone, A.M., Krapcho, M. et al., Eds. 2011. *SEER Cancer Statistics Review, 1975–2008*. Bethesda, MD: National Cancer Institute. Based on November 2010 SEER data submission posted to SEER website. http://seer.cancer.gov/csr/1975_2008/
3. Goodman, M.T., Oshizawa, Y., and Olonel, L.N. 1988. Descriptive epidemiology of thyroid cancer in Hawaii. *Cancer* 61: 1272–1281.
4. Kilfoy, B.A., Zheng, T., Holford, T.R. et al. 2009. International patterns and trends in thyroid cancer incidence, 1973–2002. *Cancer Causes Control* 20: 525–531.
5. Davies, L. and Welch, H.G. 2006. Increasing incidence of thyroid cancer in the United States, 1973–2002. *JAMA* 10: 295: 2164–2167.
6. Reynolds, R.M., Weir, J., Stockton, D.L. et al. 2005. Changing trends in incidence and mortality of thyroid cancer in Scotland. *Clin Endocrinol*, 62: 156–162.
7. Leenhardt, L., Bernier, M.O., Boin-Pineau, M.H. et al. 2004. Advances in diagnostic practices affect thyroid cancer incidence in France. *Eur J Endocrinol* 150: 133–139.
8. Hughes, D.T., Haymart, M.R., Miller, B.S. et al. 2011. The most commonly occurring papillary thyroid cancer in the United States is now a microcarcinoma in a patient older than 45 years. *Thyroid* 21: 231–236.
9. Bosetti, C., Bertuccio, P., Levi, F. et al. 2008. Cancer mortality in the European Union, 1970–2003, with a joinpoint analysis. *Ann Oncol* 19: 631–640.
10. Pacini, F., Vorontsova, T., Demidchik, E.P. et al. 1997. Post-Chernobyl thyroid carcinoma in Belarus children and adolescents: comparison with naturally occurring thyroid carcinoma in Italy and France. *J Clin Endocrinol Metab* 82: 3563–3569.
11. Jacob, P., Bogdanova, T.I., Buglova, E. et al. 2006. Thyroid cancer among Ukrainians and Belarusians who were children or adolescents at the time of the Chernobyl accident. *J Radiol Prot* 26: 51–67.
12. Sarne, D. and Schneider, A.B. 1996. External radiation and thyroid neoplasia. *Endocrinol Metab Clin North Am* 25: 181–196.
13. Boelaert, K., Horacek, J., Holder, R.L. et al. 2006. Serum thyrotropin concentration as a novel predictor of malignancy in thyroid nodules investigated by fine-needle aspiration. *J. Clin Endocrinol Metab* 91: 4295–4301.
14. Nikiforov, Y.E. and Nikiforova, M.N. 2011. Molecular genetics and diagnosis of thyroid cancer. *Nat Rev Endocrinol*, August 30 [Epub ahead of print].
15. Capezzone, M., Cantara, S., Marchisotta, S. et al. 2008. Short telomeres, telomerase reverse transcriptase gene amplification, and increased telomerase activity in the blood of familial papillary thyroid cancer patients. *J Clin Endocrinol Metab* 93: 3950–3957.
16. Rago, T. and Vitti, P. 2008. Role of thyroid ultrasound in the diagnostic evaluation of thyroid nodules. *Best Pract Res Clin Endocrinol Metab* 226: 913–928.
17. Pacini, F., Schlumberger, M., Dralle, H. et al. 2006. European Thyroid Cancer Taskforce: European consensus for the management of patients with differentiated thyroid carcinoma of the follicular epithelium. *Eur J Endocrinol* 154: 787–803.

18. Cooper, D.S., Doherty, G.M., Haugen, B.R. et al. 2009. Revised American Thyroid Association management guidelines for patients with thyroid nodules and differentiated thyroid cancer. *Thyroid* 19: 1167–1214.
19. Cantara, S., Capezzone, M., Marchisotta, S. et al. 2010. Impact of proto-oncogene mutation detection in cytological specimens from thyroid nodules improves the diagnostic accuracy of cytology. *J Clin Endocrinol Metab* 95: 1365–1369.
20. Elisei, R., Bottici, V., Luchetti, F. et al. 2004. Impact of routine measurement of serum calcitonin on the diagnosis and outcome of medullary thyroid cancer: experience in 10,864 patients with nodular thyroid disorders. *J Clin Endocrinol Metab* 89: 163–168.
21. Castagna, M.G., Maino, F., Cipri, C. et al. 2011. Delayed risk stratification, to include the response to initial treatment (surgery and radioiodine ablation), has better outcome predictivity in differentiated thyroid cancer patients. *Eur J Endocrinol* 165: 441–446.
22. Schroeder, P.R., Haugen, B.R., Pacini, F. et al. 2006. Radioiodine ablation of thyroid remnants after preparation with recombinant human thyrotropin in differentiated thyroid carcinoma: results of an international, randomized, controlled study. *J Clin Endocrinol Metab* 91: 878–884.
23. Pilli, T., Brianzoni, E., Capoccetti, F. et al. 2007. A comparison of 1850 (50 mCi) and 3700 MBq (100 mCi) 131-iodine administered doses for recombinant thyrotropin-stimulated postoperative thyroid remnant ablation in differentiated thyroid cancer. *J Clin Endocrinol Metab* 92: 3542–3546.
24. Castagna, M.G., Brilli, L., Pilli, T. et al. 2008. Limited value of repeat recombinant human thyrotropin (rhTSH)-stimulated thyroglobulin testing in differentiated thyroid carcinoma patients with previous negative rhTSH-stimulated thyroglobulin and undetectable basal serum thyroglobulin levels. *J Clin Endocrinol Metab* 93: 76–81.
25. Schlumberger, M., Hitzel, A., Toubert, M.E. et al. 2007. Comparison of seven serum thyroglobulin assays in the follow-up of papillary and follicular thyroid cancer patients. *J Clin Endocrinol Metab* 92: 2487–2495.
26. Castagna, M.G., Tala, J., Jury, H.P. et al. 2011. The use of ultrasensitive thyroglobulin assays reduces but not abolishes the need for TSH stimulation in patients with differentiated thyroid carcinoma. *J Endocrinol Invest,* March 7 [Epub ahead of print].
27. Durante, C., Haddy, N., Baudin, E. et al. 2006. Long-term outcome of 444 patients with distant metastases from papillary and follicular thyroid carcinoma: benefits and limits of radioiodine therapy. *J Clin Endocrinol Metab* 91: 2892–2899.
28. Brilli, L. and Pacini, F. 2011. Targeted therapy in refractory thyroid cancer: current achievements and limitations. *Future Oncol* 7: 657–668.
29. Smallridge, R.C., Marlow, L.A., and Copland, J.A. 2009. Anaplastic thyroid cancer: molecular pathogenesis and emerging therapies. *Endocr Relat Cancer* 16: 17–44.

8 Medullary Thyroid Cancer and Multiple Endocrine Neoplasia Type 2 (MEN2)

Furio Pacini

CONTENTS

Key words: Medullary thyroid cancer, RET, calcitonin, MEN2.

8.1   DEFINITION

Medullary thyroid carcinoma (MTC) is a tumor of the parafollicular C cells of the thyroid. Normal C cells are located in the basal layers of thyroid follicles, account for about 1% of thyroid cells, and are typically associated with the production and secretion of calcitonin (CT), a calcium lowering hormone, whose secretion is retained also by the neoplastic C cells of MTC at higher rates compared to normal C cells.

TABLE 8.1
Classification and Features of Medullary
Thyroid Carcinoma (MTC)

Sporadic (mostly unifocal)

Hereditary:

Multiple endocrine neoplasia type 2A (MEN 2A) features:
MTC (multifocal)
C cell hyperplasia
Pheochromocytoma
Parathyroid adenoma
Cutaneous lichen amyloidosis

Multiple endocrine neoplasia type 2B (MEN 2B) features:
MTC (multifocal)
Pheochromocytoma
Mucosal neurinoma
Marfanoid habitus
Corneal nerve hypertrophy
Congenital megacolon

FMTC
Isolated familiar medullary carcinoma

8.2   EPIDEMIOLOGY

MTC accounts for fewer than 10% of all thyroid carcinomas. Although mainly sporadic (70 to 80% of all medullary carcinomas), an autosomal dominant hereditary form (20 to 30%) known as multiple endocrine neoplasia (MEN) syndrome type 2 is present in 20 to 30% of patients.[1] The sporadic form shows a peak incidence during the fifth and sixth decades of life, whereas the hereditary form peaks during the second and third decades. MEN2 is characterized by MTC in combination with pheochromocytoma and hyperparathyroidism (MEN2A) or MTC with pheochromocytoma, multiple mucosal neuromas, and marfanoid habitus (MEN2B). When familial MTC recurs in the absence of other neoplasias, it is defined as isolated familial MTC (FMTC). Table 8.1 details the classifications.

8.3   PATHOLOGY AND HORMONE SECRETION

Macroscopically, MTC presents as a firm nodule indistinguishable from other thyroid carcinomas. At histological examination, classic MTC consists of sheets of spindle-shaped, round, or polygonal cells separated by fibrous stroma, forming a nested pattern characteristic of endocrine tumors. The nuclei are usually uniform in shape with rare mitotic figures. Amyloid deposits are seen between tumor cells in 60 to 80%

of tumors. In some instances, particularly cytology studies, MTC may be confused with anaplastic carcinoma, Hürthle cell tumor, or papillary thyroid carcinoma. In all cases, the diagnosis of MTC should be confirmed by positive immunohistochemical staining for CT.

The tumor metastasizes early to central and lateral lymph node compartments. Frequency of lymph node metastases and primary tumor size show clear correlations: 20 to 30% in patients with MTCs smaller than 1 cm in diameter (T1 of TNM classification) and up to 90% in patients with T3 and T4 tumors.[2]

Metastases outside the neck may occur in the liver, lungs, bones, and less frequently in the brain and skin and generally affect multiple organs. In hereditary MTC, the pathology is no different from that of sporadic cases, but multifocal disease and C cell hyperplasia are present.

CT secretion is primarily regulated by extracellular calcium concentrations. Other substances such as gastrin (and pentagastrin), β-adrenergic agonists, growth hormone-releasing hormone, and several gastrointestinal peptides can stimulate CT secretion from C cells. Normal serum CT concentrations are usually below 10 pg/mL.[3] Increased serum CT levels are almost diagnostic of MTC. However, other conditions such as renal insufficiency, autoimmune thyroid disorders, chronic hypocalcemia, hypergastrinemia, and neuroendocrine tumors may also involve CT secretion.

Pentagastrin testing is the most widely used stimulation test for CT secretion.[3] Pentagastrin-stimulated CT remains below 10 pg/mL in 80% of normal subjects, and in the others does not increase above 50 pg/mL. The main clinical interest of pentagastrin stimulation testing is to screen subjects belonging to MTC families and MTC patients who have undetectable postoperative basal serum CT concentrations. Carcinoembryonic antigen (CEA) is also produced by neoplastic C cells. Compared to CT measurement, CEA does not add significant clinical information and does not increase following pentagastrin stimulation.

Paraneoplastic syndromes are reported in patients with metastatic MTC (particularly Cushing's syndrome), and are due to the expression of genes coding for several peptides such as somatostatin, pro-opiomelanocortin, vasoactive intestinal peptide, gastrin-releasing peptide, ACTH-like material, serotonin, and histaminase. These secretory products are probably responsible for the severe diarrhea syndrome associated with metastatic MTC.

8.4 GENETIC ALTERATIONS

Hereditary MTC is autosomal dominant. In 1993, germline gains of function point mutations of the RET proto-oncogene encoding for a tyrosine kinase receptor were demonstrated as causative events in MEN 2A, FMTC, and MEN 2B.[4,5] Germline RET mutations in several exons are found in approximately 98% of MEN 2 patients.[4-6] Mutations affect mainly the cysteine-rich extracellular domains in exons 10 and 11 and also in exons 5, 8, 13, 14, 15, and 16. In MEN 2B, most patients carry a single mutation at codon 918 of exon 16.

Mutations with strong activation of the RET oncogene are associated with more aggressive phenotypes, while mutations providing weaker RET activation result in less aggressive and late onset forms of the disease. Based on these findings, the American Thyroid Association (ATA) recently developed an MTC risk stratification based on genotype.[7] ATA level D mutations carry the highest risks for MTC based on youngest age of onset, highest risk of metastases, and disease-specific mortality. ATA level C mutations carry lower (but still high) risks of aggressive MTC. ATA level B and A mutations carry lower risks for aggressive MTC.

In sporadic MTC, somatic RET mutations at codon 918 (more rarely at codons 618, 634, 768, 804, and 883) have been identified in 25 to 33% of the cases and are associated with less favorable outcomes compared with tumors without RET mutations.[8] Somatic mutations of the RET proto-oncogene have been identified in 10 to 20% of sporadic pheochromocytomas (codons 620, 630, 634, and 918), but not in sporadic parathyroid tumors.

8.5 PRESENTATION AND DIAGNOSIS

8.5.1 Sporadic MTC

The presentation of sporadic MTC is the discovery, often fortuitous, of a neck lump similar to the lump of any other thyroid nodule. Clinical neck lymph node metastases are detected in at least 25% of patients and may be the presenting signs. In a patient with thyroid nodule, the presence of familial history of MTC, pheochromocytoma, or diarrhea syndrome should alert the physician of the possibility of MTC.

Increased serum levels of serum CT are almost diagnostic of MTC (>10 pg/mL). Fine needle aspiration (FNA) cytology with positive immunocytochemical staining for CT and/or CT measurement in the wash-out fluid of FNA[9,10] will confirm the diagnosis. Virtually all patients with clinical MTC have elevated basal circulating CT concentrations. For this reason, routine measurement of serum CT in nodular thyroid disorders has been advocated by authoritative European centers for the detection of MTC.[11,12] Whenever an MTC is suspected, exclusion of familial forms should always be obtained before surgery.

8.5.2 Multiple Endocrine Neoplasia Type 2A

Typical features of MEN 2A are the association of MTC (100% of patients), pheochromocytoma (nearly 59%), and multiple parathyroid adenomas (around 20 to 30%). Interscapular cutaneous lichen amyloidosis has been described in a few MEN 2A families. It is a pruritic and hyperpigmented lesion of the skin occurring early in life even before the onset of the C cell disease. Also Hirschsprung's disease has been observed in a few families.

Presentation of MTC in MEN2A patients depends on whether a patient is the propositus of a new family or the affected member of a family submitted to genetic screening. In the first case, MTC presents as in sporadic MTC, although usually at an earlier age. In the second case, clinical MTC is rarely observed before age 10 and frequency increases with age.[13] However, with genetic testing, the diagnosis should be anticipated and most MTCs should be detected at a very early stage when a tumor is intrathyroidal. At present, genetic testing is recommended before age 5 in all subjects at risk (50% chance) to establish gene carrier status. An affected child has a probability of over 90% of developing an MTC at some point during his life.[7]

The diagnosis of clinically significant adrenal medullary disease invariably follows the diagnosis of C cell disease. Most pheochromocytomas are located in adrenal glands and very few cases have been observed in the retroperitoneal region. Pheochromocytoma is bilateral in 50% of cases, but often after an interval of several years. Clinical symptoms (headache, palpitation, increased sweating, anxiety, and hypertension) fluctuate. Hypertension is rarely present at an early stage. Therefore, pheochromocytoma should be routinely screened by measuring plasma concentration or 24-hour urinary excretion of metanephrine and normetanephrine. If biochemical tests are abnormal, imaging studies (ultrasonography, CT, MRI, or ^{123}I-meta-iodobenzylguanidine scintigraphy) are used to localize the tumor. Follow-up and screening for pheochromocytoma should be repeated at periodical intervals.[7]

Hyperparathyroidism occurs in 20 to 30% of known MEN 2A gene carriers, usually after the third decade of life. It often consists of parathyroid hyperplasia with one or more adenomas in older patients. Measurement of serum ionized calcium and PTH annually is an important part of follow-up in subjects with MEN2A.

8.5.3 Multiple Endocrine Neoplasia Type 2B

MEN2B involves the association of MTC, pheochromocytoma, ganglioneuromatosis, marfanoid features, and skeletal abnormalities.[14] Hyperparathyroidism is never observed in this syndrome. Clinical MTC associated with MEN 2B is the most aggressive form of MTC and occurs early in life, usually before 5 to 10 years of age. It is frequently associated with extension beyond the thyroid capsule, lymph node, and distant metastases at the time of diagnosis.

Pheochromocytomas are identified in about half of the individuals. Mucosal neuromas are typical feature of MEN 2B. They are present in the distal portion of the tongue, in the lips, throughout the intestinal tract, and eventually in the urinary tract. Hypertrophy of corneal nerves is frequent and is evaluated by slit lamp ophthalmic examination. Megacolon and marfanoid habitus are also frequent.

8.5.4 Familial Isolated MTC (FMTC)

A number of families have exhibited hereditary MTC as the only manifestation. MTC presents at a later age and with relatively more favorable prognosis compared to the MEN2-associated MTC. FMTC is defined when a germline RET mutation and MTC are present without other features of MEN2 both in the propositus and in the other affected family members.

8.5.5 Screening of MTC in MEN2 Kindred

The first step in the management of a kindred with MEN 2 is to perform a RET protooncogene analysis on the index case.[6] When a mutation is found, all first-degree relatives are screened for the same mutation to identify gene carriers. Approximately 4 to 10% of patients with apparently sporadic MTC have germline mutations of the RET proto-oncogene and consequently have hereditary forms. Thus, RET proto-oncogene analysis should be performed in patients with apparently sporadic MTC.[8]

8.6 TREATMENT OF MTC AND MEN2

8.6.1 INITIAL TREATMENT OF SPORADIC AND FAMILIAL MTC

All patients with suspicious MTC should undergo accurate staging before surgery. The goal is to define the extent of disease, particularly in the neck area, and identify or rule out hyperparathyroidism and/or pheochromocytoma in cases of hereditary forms. Preoperative biochemical evaluation should include basal serum CT, CEA, and calcium and plasma or urinary metanephrines. Imaging should include neck ultrasound (US) in all patients. Other imaging techniques (chest CT, liver CT or contrast-enhanced MRI, bone scintigraphy) should be performed in patients with documented lymph node metastases or with serum CT exceeding 400 pg/ml.[7]

Several studies have shown that recurrence rates and survival in patients with MTC depend strictly on the radicality of the initial surgical procedure.[15] Multicentric and bilateral MTC is observed in 30% of sporadic cases and in nearly 100% of hereditary cases. Thus, the treatment of choice is always total thyroidectomy and prophylactic central compartment (level VI) neck dissection. The therapeutic option for additional lymph node surgery should be guided by the results of presurgical evaluation.[7]

Patients with positive preoperative imaging in the central and lateral neck compartment should be submitted to central (level VI) and lateral neck compartmental dissection (Levels IIA, III, IV, V).[7] Lymph node metastases in the lateral neck may occur in up to 50% of patients with tumors 1 to 4 cm in diameter and in up to 90% in patients with tumor larger than 4 cm or with T4 tumors.[16] This applies to patients with either sporadic or hereditary MTC.

In the presence of distant metastatic disease or advanced local disease, less aggressive neck surgery may be appropriate to preserve speech, swallowing, and parathyroid function while maintaining locoregional disease control to prevent central neck morbidity.[7] In hereditary cases, the four parathyroid glands should be identified during surgery. If they appear normal, they can be left in place or, when necessary, be implanted in a muscle. In a patient with evidence of hyperparathyroidism, a gland that appears enlarged or any adenoma should be removed. The remaining glands should be transplanted to the non-dominant forearm. If diffuse hyperplasia is found in all three glands, removal of all three with autotransplantation of only a portion of one remaining gland to the non-dominant forearm is performed.[17]

The use of external beam radiation therapy (EBRT) after surgery is controversial. EBRT may be indicated when a surgical report indicates incomplete tumor resection or as an adjuvant treatment to the neck and mediastinum in patients with moderate to high volume disease involving the central and lateral neck compartments.

8.6.2 PROPHYLACTIC THYROIDECTOMY IN MEN 2 GENE CARRIERS

Prophylactic thyroidectomy is indicated in gene carriers of MEN2 or FMTC kindred. The rationale is to prevent the development of MTC that occurs in almost 100% of the patients at different points in life, depending on the aggressiveness of the mutation. The ATA guidelines for MTC state that with mutations belonging to the ATA-C risk level, prophylactic total thyroidectomy should be performed before age 5.[7] With ATA-A and ATA-B mutations, prophylactic thyroidectomy may be delayed beyond the first 5 years provided that basal and pentagastrin-stimulated serum CT levels are normal and cervical US (performed annually starting by age 5) does not show evidence of thyroid nodules or suspicious lymph nodes.[7]

Prophylactic level VI central compartment neck dissection may not be necessary in MEN 2A and FMTC patients who undergo prophylactic thyroidectomy within their first 3 to 5 years of life unless clinical or radiological evidence shows lymph node metastases or thyroid nodules larger than 5 mm (at any age) or serum basal CT exceeds 40 pg/ml in a child older than 6 months.[7]

Patients with MEN 2B (who have the highest ATA-D risk level) should undergo thyroidectomy as soon as possible, within the first year of life. Also in these patients, prophylactic level VI neck dissection may not be necessary unless they show clinical or radiological evidence of lymph node metastases.[7]

All patients with MEN2 and FMTC should undergo annual screening for pheochromocytoma (with plasma or urinary metanephrines and normetanephrines) beginning at age 8 in carriers of the RET mutation associated with MEN 2B and by age 20 in carriers of MEN 2A RET mutations. Patients with FMTC should be screened periodically from the age of 20. Screening for hyperparathyroidism should be performed at the same intervals by measuring serum calcium and PTH.

8.7 POSTSURGICAL MANAGEMENT AND FOLLOW-UP

Replacement doses of L-thyroxine are given postoperatively to maintain serum TSH concentration within the normal range. The postsurgical follow-up is based on measurement of serum CT (and CEA in specific cases). Serum CT levels reflect the absence or presence of persistent or recurrent disease.[18] The first control of serum CT should be performed 2 to 3 months postoperatively (Table 8.2) to allow the presurgical CT concentration to drop according to its biological half-life.[19]

TABLE 8. 2

Follow-Up of Patients Affected by Medullary Thyroid Carcinoma after Surgery

Measure serum calcitonin (CT) after 1 to 3 months

If CT undetectable, pentagastrin test

If CT undetectable on pentagastrin test, no other testing; basal CT annually

If CT detectable (basal or after pentagastrin), search for persistent disease by imaging techniques

---

Undetectable basal and stimulated serum CT levels are very strong predictors of complete remission[20] and the patient does not need to undergo other diagnostic procedures. Serum CT is checked again every 6 months for the first 2 to 3 years after surgery and then annually. The rate of recurrence during long-term follow-up in patients with biochemical remission after initial treatment is less than 3%.[21]

Conversely, if basal serum CT is detectable or becomes detectable after stimulation, a patient is not cured. Note that imaging techniques will not demonstrate disease until basal serum CT approaches levels exceeding 150 pg/mL.[20] In these patients, the disease is usually associated with locoregional nodes and almost never with distant metastases. Imaging should be limited to careful examination of the neck by US. If suspicious lymph nodes are detected, FNA and CT measurement in the wash-out will confirm the diagnosis.

In patients with serum CT evaluation exceeding 150 pg/ml, in addition to neck ultrasound, the evaluation should include the search for distant metastases using the most sensitive techniques (neck and chest CT, liver triphase contrast-enhanced CT or contrast-enhanced MR, liver US, bone scintigraphy, MR of the spine and pelvis, [18]FDG-PET). If all these tests do not reveal sites of metastatic disease, period restaging is indicated at optimal timing based on CT doubling time[22]—a very significant predictor of progressive disease and survival by multivariate analysis.

8.8 TREATMENT OF LOCOREGIONAL RECURRENCES

Whenever feasible, surgery is the treatment of choice for local and regional recurrences. The extent of surgery will be dictated by precise localization of the recurrence determined by complete preoperative workup, type of initial surgical procedures performed, and the nature of the relapse. If initial surgery was complete, resection should be limited to the recurrent tissue; if initial surgery was incomplete, surgery should include completion of initial surgery and resection of the recurrence. In the absence of known distant metastases, EBRT of the neck and mediastinum may be indicated after reintervention, particularly when serum CT remains elevated, which is the general rule.

8.9 MANAGEMENT OF DISTANT METASTASES

Distant metastases are present at the time of diagnosis in nearly half of the patients and represent the main cause of death. They frequently affect multiple organs (such as liver, lungs, and bones) and are multiple within organs. The course of disease is unpredictable, with long survivals even without treatment in a minority of patients and aggressive outcomes in most patients. Reported survivals are 51% at 1 year, 26% at 5 years, and 10% at 10 years.[23]

Management is oriented toward eradication or stabilization of the lesions whenever possible or to the relief of symptoms when therapy fails. Surgery is indicated for a single lesion in any organ, particularly bone, liver, and brain. Bone surgery is also indicated in patients with or at high risk of orthopedic or neurological complications. Unfortunately, even if only one metastasis is seen at imaging, multiple small additional metastases are discovered at surgery.

EBRT is indicated for bone and brain metastases not amenable to surgery, especially when they are painful or present risk of complication. Other procedures such as embolization, chemoembolization in the liver, and injection of cement in bone metastases have been proposed in selected cases.[24]

Systemic chemotherapy with several agents alone or in combination has shown very limited efficacy, achieving only short-term partial responses in no more than 10 to 20% of patients. The use of chemotherapeutic agents is no longer considered first-line therapy in view of the advent of promising new compounds.[7] Several kinase inhibitors are currently undergoing clinical trials for treating advanced MTC. Preliminary results showed partial responses in 6 to 20% of patients and stable disease in 47 to 87% of patients with tolerable and manageable toxicities.[25] In particular, vandetanib (AstraZeneca) has been recently approved by the FDA in the United States for the treatment of metastatic, progressive MTC.[26]

REFERENCES

1. Schlumberger, M. and Pacini, F. 2006. *Thyroid Tumors*. Paris: Edition Nucleon. Chap. 18.
2. Scollo, C., Baudin, E., Travagli, J.P. et al. 2003. Rationale for central and bilateral lymph node dissection in sporadic and hereditary medullary thyroid cancer. *J Clin Endocrinol Metab* 88: 2070–2075.
3. Baloch, Z., Carayon, P., Conte-Devolx, B. et al. 2003. Guidelines Committee, National Academy of Clinical Biochemistry. Laboratory Medicine Practice Guidelines: Calcitonin and RET Proto-Oncogene Measurements. *Thyroid* 13: 68–79.
4. Hofstra, R.M., Landsvater, R.M., Ceccherini, I. et al. 1994. A mutation in the RET proto-oncogene associated with multiple endocrine neoplasia type 2B and sporadic medullary thyroid carcinoma. *Nature* 367: 375–376.
5. Mulligan, L.M., Eng, C., Healey, C.S. et al. 1994. Specific mutations of the RET proto-oncogene are related to disease phenotype in MEN 2A and FMTC. *Nat Genet* 6: 70–74.
6. Eng, C., Clayton, D., Schuffenecker, I. et al. 1996. The relationship between specific RET proto-oncogene mutations and disease phenotype in multiple endocrine neoplasia type 2. *JAMA* 276: 1575–1579.
7. American Thyroid Association Guidelines Task Force. 2009. Medullary Thyroid Cancer Management Guidelines. *Thyroid* 19: 565–612.
8. Elisei, R., Cosci, B., Romei, C. et al. 2008. Prognostic significance of somatic RET oncogene mutations in sporadic medullary thyroid cancer: a 10-year follow-up study. *J Clin Endocrinol Metab* 93: 682–687.
9. Boi, F., Maurelli, I., Pinna, G. et al. 2007. Calcitonin measurement in wash-out fluid from fine needle aspiration of neck masses in patients with primary and metastatic medullary thyroid carcinoma. *J Clin Endocrinol Metab* 92: 2115–2118.
10. Kudo, T., Miyauchi, A., Ito, Y. et al. 2007. Diagnosis of medullary thyroid carcinoma by calcitonin measurement in fine-needle aspiration biopsy specimens. *Thyroid* 17: 635–638.
11. Pacini, F., Fontanelli, M., Fugazzola, L. et al. 1994. Routine measurement of serum calcitonin in nodular thyroid diseases allows the preoperative diagnosis of unsuspected sporadic medullary thyroid carcinoma. *J Clin Endocrinol Metab* 78: 826–829.
12. Elisei, R., Bottici, V., Luchetti, F. et al. 2004. Impact of routine measurement of serum calcitonin on the diagnosis and outcome of medullary thyroid cancer: experience in 10,864 patients with nodular thyroid disorders. *J Clin Endocrinol Metab* 89: 163–168.

13. Gagel, R.F., Jackson, C.E., Block, M.A. et al. 1982. Age-related probability of development of hereditary medullary thyroid carcinoma. *J Pediatr* 101: 941–946.
14. Leboulleux, S., Travagli, J.P., Caillou, B. et al. 2002. Medullary thyroid carcinoma as part of a multiple endocrine neoplasia type 2B syndrome: influence of the stage on the clinical course. *Cancer* 94: 44–50.
15. Gharib, H., McConahey, W.M., Tiegs, R.D. et al. 1992. Medullary thyroid carcinoma: clinicopathologic features and long-term follow-up of 65 patients treated during 1946 through 1970. *Mayo Clin Proc* 67: 934–940.
16. Moley, J.F. and DeBenedetti, M.K. 1999. Patterns of nodal metastases in palpable medullary thyroid carcinoma: recommendations for extent of node dissection. *Ann Surg* 229: 880–887.
17. Wells, S.A. Jr., Farndon, J.R., Dale, J.K. et al. 1980. Long-term evaluation of patients with primary parathyroid hyperplasia managed by total parathyroidectomy and heterotopic autotransplantation. *Ann Surg* 192: 451–458.
18. Stepanas, A.V., Samaan, N.A., Hill, C.S. Jr. et al. 1979. Medullary thyroid carcinoma: importance of serial serum calcitonin measurement. *Cancer* 43: 825–837.
19. Fugazzola, L., Pinchera, A., Luchetti, F. et al. 1994. Disappearance rate of serum calcitonin after total thyroidectomy for medullary thyroid carcinoma. *Int J Biol Markers* 9: 21–24.
20. Machens, A., Schneyer, U., Holzhausen, H.J. et al. 2005. Prospects of remission in medullary thyroid carcinoma according to basal calcitonin level. *J Clin Endocrinol Metab* 90: 2029–2034.
21. Franc, S., Niccoli-Sire, P., Cohen, R. et al. 2001. French Medullary Study Group (GETC). Complete surgical lymph node resection does not prevent authentic recurrences of medullary thyroid carcinoma. *Clin Endocrinol* 55: 403–409.
22. GTE Study Group. 2005. Prognostic impact of serum calcitonin and carcinoembryonic antigen doubling-times in patients with medullary thyroid carcinoma. *J Clin Endocrinol Metab* 90: 6077–6084.
23. Modigliani, E., Cohen, R., Campos, J.M. et al. 1998. Prognostic factors for survival and for biochemical cure in medullary thyroid carcinoma: results in 899 patients. GETC Study Group. *Clin Endocrinol* 48: 265–273.
24. Fromigué, J., De Baere, T., Baudin, E. et al. 2006. Chemoembolization for liver metastases from medullary thyroid carcinoma. *J Clin Endocrinol Metab* 91: 2496–2499.
25. Brilli, L. and Pacini, F. 2011. Targeted therapy in refractory thyroid cancer: current achievements and limitations. *Future Oncol* 7: 657–668.
26. Deshpande, H., Roman, S., Thumar, J. et al. 2011. Vandetanib (ZD6474) in the treatment of medullary thyroid cancer. *Clin Med Insights Oncol* 5: 213–221.

9 Thyroid Incidentaloma

Rossella Elisei and Laura Agate

CONTENTS

Key words: incidentaloma, thyroid nodule, neck ultrasound, fine needle aspiration, microPTC.

9.1 DEFINITION

Incidentaloma is a term commonly used to indicate an asymptomatic tumor (benign or malignant) unexpectedly discovered during imaging procedures performed for other purposes. According to this definition, a thyroid swelling not visible or palpable upon neck inspection is a thyroid incidentaloma.

It is usually serendipitously discovered as an incidental finding during a radiologic procedure, such as carotid ultrasonography (US), neck computed tomography (CT), or positron emission tomography (PET) scanning performed for reasons other than thyroid disease including extensions of gynecological and mammary gland workups, metabolic assessments preceding weight loss programs, routine control for other malignancies, or color Doppler evaluation of the neck to detect carotid vascular disease. In most cases, the nodules are smaller than 1.5 to 2 cm in size but larger asymptomatic non-visible and posteriorly located nodules can belong to this category.[1] Figure 9.1 depicts the various types.

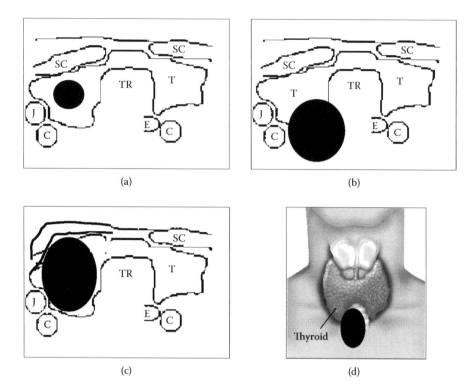

(a)   (b)

(c)   (d)

FIGURE 9.1   Different types of thyroid incidentalomas that are not visible or palpable due to small size or position in the neck. (a) Small subcentimetric nodule in context of thyroid lobe; (b) Larger nodule localized in posterior part of thyroid lobe; (c) Retroclavicular thyroid nodule; (d) Retrosternal jugular thyroid nodule. J = jugular vein. C = carotid artery. E = esophagus. T = thyroid. TR = trachea. SC = sternocleidomastoid muscle.

9.2   PREVALENCE

The prevalence of incidentaloma is very high because of the wide use of neck US and its ability to find very small nodules (2 to 3 mm). Evidence indicates that only 10% of the middle-aged population have palpable thyroid nodules, but more than 50% showed nodules at neck US. This prevalence is very similar to the autoptic prevalence. As for larger nodules, incidentalomas are more frequent in females (up to 45% at 55 years of age) than in males (up to 32% in the same age group).

Incidentaloma prevalence is particularly high in certain risk categories such as subjects treated for malignancies during childhood with external radiation to the head and neck and populations living in iodine-deficient areas. However, studies indicate that 67% of subjects with no known personal or familial history of thyroid disease showed one or more thyroid nodules on neck US. By contrast, only 21% of them had palpable thyroid nodules.

9.3 DETECTION

Thyroid incidentalomas are most commonly found when patients undergo radiographic imaging of the head and neck for other conditions. Thyroid incidentalomas were found in 9.4% of patients who underwent color Doppler evaluation of the carotid circulation without known thyroid disease. Ultrasound of the neck is a relatively economical and very sensitive diagnostic tool that allows high-resolution imaging of the thyroid. It sometimes serves an extension of a workup performed for completely different purposes such as a gynecological examinations or dietetic consultations. Conversely, in many cases, neck US is performed as an adjunct to a physical examination of the thyroid and allows the discovery of non-palpable thyroid nodules (Figure 9.1).

Thyroid incidentalomas may also be detected incidentally during CT or MR imaging of the neck or chest. This is mainly due to the large field of visualization of these imaging procedures whose sensitivity remains much lower (i.e., 1:2) than that of neck US.

Nuclear medicine procedures including Sestamibi scanning and positron emission tomography (PET) can also discover thyroid incidentalomas. Sestamibi is usually performed to study parathyroid glands and is always accompanied by a neck US that can better clarify the features of incidentalomas.

About 2 to 3% of PET or PET and CT scans performed for cancer initial staging or localization of metastatic disease show thyroid incidentalomas. However, in recent years, the resolution power of PET scanning has improved greatly and [18]FDG avid lesions <8 mm in size can be detected. We can predict that with the increasing use of PET/CT, the incidence of thyroid incidentalomas found this way will also increase. It is worth noting that [18]FDG uptake in the thyroid can be focal or diffuse; focal uptake is typical of a thyroid nodule (Figure 9.2a).[2] Diffuse uptake is mainly related to inflammatory thyroid diseases such as thyroiditis (Figure 9.2b).[3]

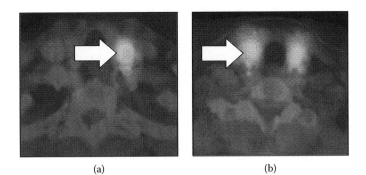

(a) (b)

FIGURE 9.2 Typical examples of [18]FDG thyroid uptake. (a) Focal thyroid uptake usually corresponding to a thyroid nodule; (b) diffuse thyroid uptake usually corresponding to thyroiditis.

9.4 CLINICAL AND PATHOLOGICAL EVALUATION

Incidentalomas present the same risk of malignancy as palpable nodules.[4] Thus, the initial evaluations of all patients with thyroid nodules (discovered by palpation or incidentally noted on a radiologic procedure such as carotid US, neck CT, MR, or PET) includes a history, physical examination, and measurement of serum thyroid stimulating hormone (TSH).

A dedicated thyroid ultrasound is usually recommended for all patients with thyroid incidentalomas, regardless of the type of procedure identified. This US is required to confirm the presence of the nodule, exclude the possibility of a pseudo-nodule other than a real nodule, assess its precise size and sonographic features, and to look for additional nodules and lymphadenopathies. The superiority of US for both physical examinations and in conjunction with other imaging procedures to detect and characterize nodules is well documented. Studies have demonstrated the ability of neck US to reveal additional nodules in about 30% of patients referred to endocrinologists for single incidentalomas.

Thyroid incidentalomas as palpable nodules fall into three classifications: pseudo-nodules, benign nodules, and malignant nodules. The clinical and pathogenic features of these three groups of nodules are the same as those described in Chapter 6. While pseudonodules may be easily identified and distinguished from real nodules by a neck ultrasound expert, the benign or malignant nature of an incidentaloma can be assessed only by fine needle aspiration cytology (FNAc).[5]

9.5 WORKUP

9.5.1 NECK ULTRASOUND

The clinical importance of thyroid nodule evaluation is the need to exclude thyroid cancer that occurs in 5 to 6% of palpable and incidentaloma thyroid nodules.[4] Familial and environmental history will be of particular clinical relevance to identify risk factors for malignancy such as previous exposure to neck radiation or a familial history of papillary thyroid cancer (PTC).

As noted earlier, the imaging modalities that can detect a thyroid incidentaloma cannot distinguish benign from malignant nodules. However, thyroid nodules identified by PET scanning show a greater probability (27 to 47%) of malignancy. The probability that a PET-detected thyroid nodule is a thyroid cancer seems to be greater if the thyroid ^{18}FDG uptake is focal rather than diffuse. A PET-positive incidentaloma must be further studied based on the greater risk of malignancy.[6]

A dedicated thyroid ultrasound is recommended for every patient to adequately confirm the presence of a nodule incidentally found by another imaging technique. It is very important to assess sonographic features of these nodules, particularly the smallest ones, to decide whether FNAc is indicated. Even small, subcentimetric thyroid nodules subjected to neck US can reveal some features that can raise concern that they could be malignant (Figure 9.3). The most important suspicious characteristics include microcalcifications, irregular margins, marked hypoechogenicity,

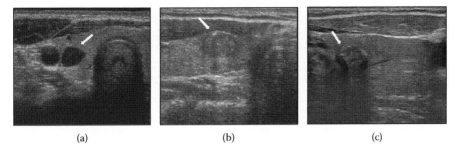

(a)   (b)   (c)

FIGURE 9.3   Different ultrasound patterns of incidentalomas. (a) Hypoanechoic nodule corresponding to small cyst—usually a benign entity. (b) Solid, isoechoic nodule with some intranodular calcifications and complete halo. These features are not strongly suspicious of malignancy but it cannot be excluded. (c) Nodule showing typical echographic features suspicious for malignancy (hypoechogenicity, incomplete halo, and microcalcifications).

TABLE 9.1
Ultrasound Features of Inflammatory and Metastatic Lymph Nodes

Echographic Factor	Inflammatory	Metastatic
Shape	Oval	Round
Echogenicity	Normoechoic	Hypoechoic
Peculiar findings	None	Microcalcifications
Hilus	Present, well defined	No longer visible

incomplete peripheral halo, and intranodular vascular pattern.[7] Nodules with these features are good candidates for FNAc.

Neck ultrasound should also examine the lateral regions to identify abnormal cervical lymph nodes. As reported in Table 9.1, very peculiar features of metastatic lymph nodes[8] can strongly suggest their relationship with a thyroid malignancy. In such cases, even if a thyroid nodule is very small, FNAc of both the nodule and the suspicious lymph node should be performed. Thyroglobulin (Tg) and calcitonin (CT) measurements in the wash-out of the needle used to aspirate the lymph node are also strongly indicated.[9,10]

For larger nodules and also for thyroid incidentalomas, neck US can provide information about thyroid gland volume and structure that may be relevant for defining the therapeutic strategy and timing of follow-up.

9.5.2   FINE NEEDLE ASPIRATION CYTOLOGY (FNAc)

FNAc is the most accurate method for evaluating thyroid nodules and identifying patients who require surgical resection.[5] However, for nodules smaller than 1 cm,

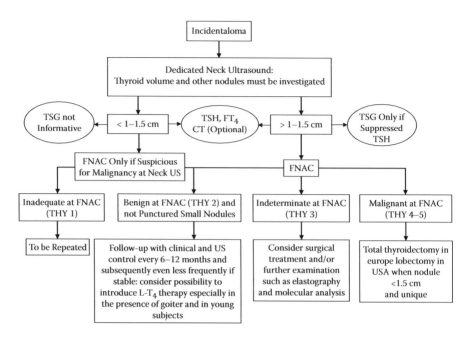

FIGURE 9.4   Algorithm for management of thyroid incidentalomas.

the risk of an inadequate response (i.e., THY1 response, according to the British Thyroid Association classification[11] is very high (36% in nodules smaller than 0.8 cm versus 14% in nodules larger than 1.0 cm). The risk becomes even higher when nodules smaller than 0.5 cm are punctured.[12] Thus, the question of whether all clinically non-palpable thyroid lesions should be assessed by FNAc is still under debate. Furthermore, thyroid incidentalomas are usually small; larger ones are located in positions that make puncture difficult. Thus, ultrasound-guided FNAc is better indicated but this diagnostic approach is not cost effective if performed on all thyroid incidentalomas because only a small proportion of them are microPTCs.

For this reason, thyroid cancer experts agree that FNAc is indicated only for thyroid incidentalomas after US signs suggest malignancy. Incidentalomas with US features suggestive of benignity should be followed with periodic clinical and US evaluation (Figure 9.4).

9.5.3   THYROID SCINTIGRAPHY (TSG)

Over the past decade, the routine use of TSG has become less common and reserved for cases that require determination of nodule functional status. In incidentalomas that are often micronodules, TSG is usually useless because of its inability to distinguish such small areas from the rest of the gland. For large incidentalomas, the indication to perform TSG is the reduced level of TSH as found in palpable nodules (Figure 9.4).

9.5.4 Laboratory Tests

The laboratory tests for examining incidentalomas are the same as those indicated for palpable nodules (Figure 9.4; Chapter 6). Controversial opinions surround the need to measure serum calcitonin (CT) in workups of thyroid incidentalomas. Some authors believe that microMTCs discovered through routine measurement of serum CT may be clinically not relevant.[13]

Recently, it has been demonstrated that microMTCs can be more aggressive than expected because of association with lymph node metastases that are important poor prognostic factors for a definitive cure.[14] However, although several thyroid cancer experts are convinced that routine serum CT measurement in patients with thyroid nodules should be recommended,[15] the American Thyroid Association has published different indications[16,17] from those suggested by European experts.[18,19]

9.6 TREATMENT

The optimal therapy for patients with incidentalomas is based on their functions and benign or malignant nature. However, the significant discrepancy between the high prevalence of thyroid nodules incidentally discovered and the low frequency of clinical relevant thyroid malignancy is in favor of the hypothesis that incidentalomas produce low clinical impacts and justify conservative approaches.[1,20]

All incidentalomas that do not require FNAc or have been documented as benign should be followed with 6 to 12 months of control to monitor their ability to grow and rate of growth. If their growth is very slow, the intervals between the controls can be prolonged. If growth remains stable for 2 to 3 years, a certain stability can be assumed and controls can be performed at 1- to 2-year intervals, then every 3 to 5 years (Figure 9.4).

The unresolved question is what can happen if a small incidentaloma is a microPTC and the diagnosis is missed. It is worth noting that studies of microPTCs demonstrated that the risk of extrathyroidal invasion and/or lymph node metastases was virtually absent if the microPTC was smaller than 0.5 cm[21] and that 70% of microPTCs that were followed up but not submitted to surgical treatment remained stable more than 4 years.[22] The evidence that microPTC usually exhibits non-aggressive biological behavior and follows an indolent course points to a conservative approach for small non-US suspicious incidentalomas based on a wait-and-see strategy.

If an incidentaloma is associated with a goiter, if TSH is relatively high, or if the rate of growth appears significant, it could be useful to introduce levo-thyroxine (LT_4) suppressive therapy to interfere with nodule growth.[23] However, even for larger nodules, some experts disagree with this strategy.[24] Certainly, if a nodule grows to 1 to 2 cm or larger or changes in US patterns are observed and become worrisome, ultrasound-guided FNAc is required.

Also in the case of a thyroid incidentaloma, as well as in the case of nodules of bigger size, the FNAc results fall into five classifications according to the British

Thyroid Association[11] guidelines: inadequate (Thy1), benign (Thy2), indeterminate (Thy3), suspicious for thyroid cancer (Thy4), and thyroid cancer (Thy5). The therapeutic strategy will be based on the same criteria used for larger nodules. However, it is rather uncomfortable to send a surgeon a patient with a Thy3 micronodule that has a 5:1 probability of being benign.

This choice will be easier if the Thy3 response is accompanied by US signs that are highly suspicious of malignancy or (even better) an elastograph strongly indicative of malignancy.[25] See Chapter 8.

These considerations and the evidence that the risk of a Thy1 (inadequate) or Thy3 (indeterminate) cytological diagnosis is far higher in smaller nodules than in larger nodules justify the present practice of restricting FNAc to nodules with clinical, anamnestic, or US features of malignancy. Furthermore, this approach should decrease the burden of repeated inconclusive FNAc procedures and patient concern and anxiety without missing aggressive small microPTCs.

In recent years, several studies have attempted to verify the possibility of molecular diagnosis of thyroid malignancy in FNA material[26,27] by analyzing the most common oncogene mutations involved in thyroid carcinogenesis.[28] A number of controversial opinions have been reported and at present no agreement about the routine application of this approach has been reached. Molecular analysis may be of help in workups of patients with incidentalomas under specific conditions. For example, if long-term follow up confirms that a microPTC with a specific oncogene mutation such as BRAF V600E is apparently more aggressive than others without the mutation or the microPTC harbors less aggressive genetic alterations such as RET/PTC rearrangements,[29] this approach can easily distinguish incidentalomas that must be removed quickly. Concerns about applying this strategy continue, particularly because the prevalence of the BRAF V600E mutation is about 30 to 40% in microPTC,[30] but only 5% of microPTCs exert aggressive biological behaviors.

9.7 CONCLUSIONS

It is expected that the progress and improvement of imaging techniques will further increase the prevalence of incidentalomas. As to incidentaloma management, evidence points to excellent prognoses for most small thyroid malignancies. Patients should be reassured that active surveillance with periodic (wait-and-see) controls will allow early discovery of the few cases with more aggressive behaviors and lead to prompt and successful treatment.

REFERENCES

1. Pinchera, A. 2007. Thyroid incidentalomas. *Horm Res 68 Suppl* 5: 199–201.
2. Zhai, G., Zhang, M., Xu, H. et al. 2010. The role of ^{18}F-fluorodeoxyglucose positron emission tomography/computed tomography whole body imaging in the evaluation of focal thyroid incidentaloma. *J Endocrinol Invest* 33: 151–155.
3. Karantanis, D., Bogsrud, T.V., Wiseman, G.A. et al. 2007. Clinical significance of diffusely increased 18F-FDG uptake in the thyroid gland. *J Nucl Med* 48: 896–901.

4. Papini, E., Guglielmi, R., Bianchini, A. et al. 2002. Risk of malignancy in non-palpable thyroid nodules: predictive value of ultrasound and color Doppler features. *J Clin Endocrinol Metab* 87: 1941–1946.

5. Baloch, Z.W., LiVolsi, V.A., Asa, S.L. et al. 2008. Diagnostic terminology and morphologic criteria for cytologic diagnosis of thyroid lesions: a synopsis of the National Cancer Institute Thyroid Fine-Needle Aspiration State of the Science Conference. *Diagn Cytopathol* 36: 425–437.

6. Shie, P., Cardarelli, R., Sprawls, K. et al. 2009. Systematic review: prevalence of malignant incidental thyroid nodules identified on fluorine-18 fluorodeoxyglucose positron emission tomography. *Nucl Med Commun* 30: 742–748.

7. Rago, T. and Vitti, P. 2008. Role of thyroid ultrasound in the diagnostic evaluation of thyroid nodules. *Best Pract Res Clin Endocrinol Metab* 22: 913–928.

8. Leboulleux, S., Girard, E., Rose, M. et al. 2007. Ultrasound criteria of malignancy for cervical lymph nodes in patients followed up for differentiated thyroid cancer. *J Clin Endocrinol Metab* 92: 3590–3594.

9. Boi, F., Maurelli, I., Pinna, G. et al. 2007. Calcitonin measurement in wash-out fluid from fine needle aspiration of neck masses in patients with primary and metastatic medullary thyroid carcinoma. *J Clin Endocrinol Metab* 92: 2115–2118.

10. Biscolla, R.P. 2007. Cervical lymph node metastases in patients with differentiated thyroid cancer. *Arq Bras Endocrinol Metabol* 51: 813–817.

11. Watkinson, J.C. 2004. The British Thyroid Association guidelines for the management of thyroid cancer in adults. *Nucl Med Commun* 25: 897–900.

12. Leenhardt, L., Hejblum, G., Franc, B. et al. 1999. Indications and limits of ultrasound-guided cytology in the management of nonpalpable thyroid nodules. *J Clin Endocrinol Metab* 84: 24–28.

13. Valle, L.A. and Kloos, R.T. 2011. The prevalence of occult medullary thyroid carcinoma at autopsy. *J Clin Endocrinol Metab* 96: 109–113.

14. Ahmed, S.R. and Ball, D.W. 2011. Clinical review: incidentally discovered medullary thyroid cancer: diagnostic strategies and treatment. *J Clin Endocrinol Metab* 96: 1237–1245.

15. Elisei, R. 2008. Routine serum calcitonin measurement in the evaluation of thyroid nodules. *Best Pract Res Clin Endocrinol Metab* 22: 941–953.

16. Kloos, R.T., Eng, C., Evans, D.B. et al. 2009. Medullary thyroid cancer: management guidelines of the American Thyroid Association. *Thyroid* 19: 565–612.

17. Cooper, D.S., Doherty, G.M., Haugen, B.R. et al. 2009. Revised American Thyroid Association management guidelines for patients with thyroid nodules and differentiated thyroid cancer. *Thyroid* 19: 1167–1214.

18. Paschke, R., Hegedus, L., Alexander, E. et al. 2011. Thyroid nodule guidelines: agreement, disagreement and need for future research. *Nat Rev Endocrinol* 7: 354–361.

19. Pacini, F., Schlumberger, M., Dralle, H. et al. 2006. European consensus for the management of patients with differentiated thyroid carcinoma of the follicular epithelium. *Eur J Endocrinol* 154: 787–803.

20. Gough, J., Scott-Coombes, D., Fausto Palazzo, F. 2008. Thyroid incidentaloma: an evidence-based assessment of management strategy. *World J Surg* 32: 1264–1268.

21. Machens, A., Holzhausen, H.J., Dralle, H. 2005. The prognostic value of primary tumor size in papillary and follicular thyroid carcinoma. *Cancer* 103: 2269–2273.

22. Ito, Y., Uruno, T., Nakano, K. et al. 2003. An observation trial without surgical treatment in patients with papillary microcarcinoma of the thyroid. *Thyroid* 13: 381–387.

23. Papini, E., Petrucci, L., Guglielmi, R. et al. 1998. Long-term changes in nodular goiter: a 5-year prospective randomized trial of levothyroxine suppressive therapy for benign cold thyroid nodules. *J Clin Endocrinol Metab* 83: 780–783.

24. Reverter, J.L., Lucas, A., Salinas, I. et al. 1992. Suppressive therapy with levothyroxine for solitary thyroid nodules. *Clin Endocrinol (Oxf)* 36: 25–28.
25. Rago, T., Scutari, M., Santini, F. et al. 2010. Real-time elastosonography: useful tool for refining the presurgical diagnosis in thyroid nodules with indeterminate or nondiagnostic cytology. *J Clin Endocrinol Metab* 95: 5274–5280.
26. Nikiforov, Y.E., Steward, D.L., Robinson-Smith, T.M. et al. 2009. Molecular testing for mutations in improving the fine-needle aspiration diagnosis of thyroid nodules. *J Clin Endocrinol Metab* 94: 2092–2098.
27. Marchetti, I., Lessi, F., Mazzanti, C.M. et al. 2009. A morpho-molecular diagnosis of papillary thyroid carcinoma: BRAF V600E detection as an important tool in preoperative evaluation of fine-needle aspirates. *Thyroid* 19: 837–842.
28. Cantara, S., Capezzone, M., Marchisotta, S. et al. 2010. Impact of proto-oncogene mutation detection in cytological specimens from thyroid nodules improves the diagnostic accuracy of cytology. *J Clin Endocrinol Metab* 95: 1365–1369.
29. Romei, C., Ciampi, R., Faviana, P. et al. 2008. BRAFV600E mutation, but not RET/PTC rearrangement, is correlated with a lower expression of both thyroperoxidase and sodium iodide symporter genes in papillary thyroid cancer. *Endocr Relat Cancer* 15: 511–520.
30. Ugolini, C., Giannini, R., Lupi, C. et al. 2007. Presence of BRAF V600E in very early stages of papillary thyroid carcinoma. *Thyroid* 17: 381–388.

10 Adult Primary Hypothyroidism

Cesidio Giuliani and Fabrizio Monaco

CONTENTS

Key words: myxedema, permanent hypothyroidism, autoimmune thyroiditis, iatrogenic hypothyroidism, iodine deficiency and excess, thyroid hormone replacement therapy.

10.1 DEFINITION

The term *adult primary hypothyroidism* defines a condition characterized by decreased concentrations of thyroid hormones (T_3 and T_4) in the target tissues due to reduced synthesis and secretion of these hormones by the thyroid gland. The severe form of hypothyroidism, characterized by the accumulation of glycosaminoglycans in the interstitial tissue, is called myxedema. From a clinical view, hypothyroidism can be distinguished as overt and subclinical.

Overt hypothyroidism is characterized by decreases of serum T_3 and T_4 concentrations and elevated serum TSH concentration. Subclinical hypothyroidism is characterized by a slightly elevated serum TSH value with normal values of serum thyroid hormones. Hypothyroidism is also classified as permanent and transient.[1]

The present chapter will focus on the overt and permanent form of primary hypothyroidism since the subclinical and transient forms are discussed elsewhere in this book.

10.2 EPIDEMIOLOGY

Primary hypothyroidism is the most frequent form of hypothyroidism (99%). Its prevalence in the general population is 0.3 to 1% with incidence ranging from 20 to 290 cases/100,000 individuals annually.[2–4] The prevalence of the disease increases with age and reaches 4.5% in the elderly population. The female:male ratio ranges from 4:1 up to 7:1.[2–4]

The Whickham survey, a 20-year follow-up study conducted on a randomly selected sample of the adult population of Great Britain, provided the most extensive information on the epidemiology of thyroid disease.[2] The study has shown that overt hypothyroidism is more common in women than in men (with an incidence of 4.1/1,000 annually in women and 0.6/1,000 annually in men and a prevalence of 1.8/1,000 in women and 0.1/1,000 in men). Furthermore, the risk of developing hypothyroidism increases with age.

The Whickam survey also identified serum thyroid autoantibodies and high serum TSH concentrations as risk factors for developing hypothyroidism. Several cross-sectional studies conducted in Europe, United States, China, and Japan confirmed these findings.[3–5] The variability of hypothyroidism prevalence among the different studies is due to both genetic and environmental factors. Among the latter, iodine intake constitutes an important factor. Several studies have shown an increased frequency of hypothyroidism, both subclinical and overt, in populations with high iodine intakes in comparison with frequency in populations with low intake. The main reason is the increased prevalence of chronic autoimmune thyroiditis associated with high iodine intake.[6]

10.3 ETIOPATHOGENESIS

The causes of adult primary hypothyroidism are reported in Table 10.1. All the reported conditions are responsible for failures of thyroid function due to losses of functional tissue or abnormalities of the biosynthesis of thyroid hormones.

TABLE 10.1

Causes of Adult Primary Hypothyroidism

Autoimmune thyroid diseases

Non-autoimmune thyroiditis

Iatrogenic hypothyroidism (surgery, radiation, drugs)

Severe iodine deficiency

Iodine excess

Infiltrative diseases of thyroid

Adult onset of thyroid congenital diseases

10.3.1 AUTOIMMUNE THYROID DISEASES

Hashimoto's thyroiditis and painless sporadic and painless postpartum thyroiditis are all forms of autoimmune thyroiditis. Hashimoto's thyroiditis or chronic autoimmune thyroiditis is the main cause of adult-acquired hypothyroidism in developed countries.[3] Although most patients with Hashimoto's thyroiditis do not display thyroid dysfunction, hypothyroidism can be the first clinical sign of the disease.

In countries without iodine deficiencies, Hashimoto's thyroiditis is responsible for more than 60% of all the cases of overt hypothyroidism. The risk of developing hypothyroidism in patients with Hashimoto's thyroiditis increases with age. In the Whickam survey, the risk of overt hypothyroidism was 2.1% per year in euthyroid women with positive thyroid autoantibodies and increased to 4.3% per year in the presence of TSH values above 2 mU/L.

The decreased function of the thyroid gland is the result of a diffuse infiltration of the parenchyma by lymphocytes and plasma cells with metaplastic changes and atrophy of the thyroid follicular cells (Figure 10.1). In a later stage, the disease can result in a small gland with extensive fibrosis and atrophic follicles (Figure 10.2). In some cases, hypothyroidism may be a consequence of autoantibodies to the TSH receptor (TSHR) that act as TSH antagonists.

Painless postpartum thyroiditis and painless sporadic (or silent) thyroiditis are usually self-limiting autoimmune diseases characterized by a transient hypothyroidism. However, about 20 to 60% of women affected by postpartum thyroiditis develop permanent hypothyroidism within 5 to 10 years. Silent thyroiditis evolves to permanent hypothyroidism in 5 to 20% of cases.[7,8] Hypothyroidism may develop after several years of remission in patients affected by Graves' disease.

10.3.2 NON-AUTOIMMUNE THYROIDITIS

Rarely, acute thyroiditis may evolve to permanent hypothyroidism as a consequence of parenchymal destruction and fibrosis. Subacute thyroiditis causes a reversible destruction of the thyroid gland with a transient hypothyroidism that usually lasts 1 to 3 months. However, permanent hypothyroidism develops in about 5% of patients. One-third of patients with Riedel's thyroiditis present with primary hypothyroidism as a consequence of the extensive fibrosis involving the entire gland.

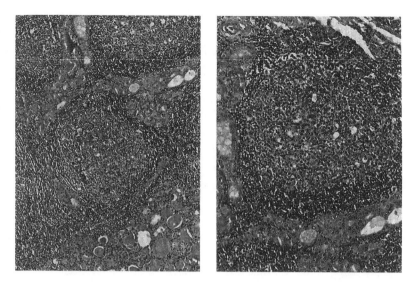

FIGURE 10.1   Hashimoto's thyroiditis. Diffuse infiltration of thyroid parenchyma by lymphocytes and plasma cells, with formation of lymphoid follicles with prominent germinal centers. (*Source:* Lloyd, R.V. et al. *Endocrine Diseases.* Armed Forces Institute of Pathology Atlas of Nontumor Pathology, First Series, Fascicle 1. Washington: American Registry of Pathology. With permission.)

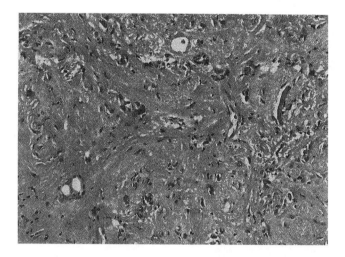

FIGURE 10.2   Hashimoto's thyroiditis. Extensive fibrosis and atrophic follicles. (*Source:* Lloyd, R.V. et al. *Endocrine Diseases.* Armed Forces Institute of Pathology Atlas of Nontumor Pathology, First Series, Fascicle 1. Washington: American Registry of Pathology. With permission.)

10.3.3   Iatrogenic Hypothyroidism

Antithyroid drugs such as methimazole and propylthiouracil may induce hypothyroidism during the treatment of hyperthyroidism especially when high doses are used. The dysfunction recedes after tapering the dose or withdrawing the drug. Permanent primary hypothyroidism is an inevitable effect of total thyroidectomy. In patients who undergo partial thyroidectomies, the risk of developing the disease depends on the extent of surgery and the residual functions of the thyroid remnants.[8,9]

Subtotal thyroidectomy, which leaves approximately 4 to 5 g of tissue, causes hypothyroidism in 15 to 70% of patients, with a cumulative incidence that increases 1 to 2% per year. Thyroid lobectomy causes hypothyroidism, mainly subclinical, in about 22% of patients. The disease is often transient. Permanent hypothyroidism is observed in about 8% of cases. A frequent cause of hypothyroidism is radioiodine treatment for hyperthyroidism.

The incidence of radioiodine-induced hypothyroidism varies according to the cause of hyperthyroidism and the time of follow-up. In a long-term study, the cumulative incidence of hypothyroidism in patients treated for Graves' disease and in those treated for nodular toxic goiter was 24 and 4%, respectively, after 1 year, and increased to 80 to 90% and 24 to 60%, respectively, after 25 years.[10,11] The frequency of hypothyroidism also depends on the cumulative dose of radiation administered. One year after radioiodine treatment, hypothyroidism has been described in fewer than 15% of patients receiving doses below 184 MBq and in 50 to 60% of patients receiving doses above 350 MBq.

Hypothyroidism, mainly subclinical, has been observed also in patients treated for malignancies with ^{131}I-metaiodobenzylguanidine (MIBG) or with monoclonal antibodies radiolabeled with [131]I. Thyroid toxicity is a consequence of free radioiodine. Although the therapeutic protocol defines the administration of a saturated solution of potassium iodide to patients prior and during the treatment with a radiolabeled substance, hypothyroidism is still observed in 21% of patients treated with ^{131}I-MIBG and 25% of patients treated with ^{131}I-rituximab or ^{131}I-tositumomab.[12,13] Primary hypothyroidism may be a consequence of external radiation of the head and neck region for lymphoma or other malignancies. The dysfunction, mainly subclinical, has been described in about 20 to 50% of patients receiving radiation involving the neck, with a peak incidence 2 to 3 years after treatment.[8,14] Several drugs listed in Table 10.2 can lead to overt primary hypothyroidism via different mechanisms. They will be treated in detail in Chapter 30.

10.3.4   Iodine Deficiency

Severe iodine deficiency (iodine intake <25 µg/day) is associated with an increased prevalence of hypothyroidism in the adult population. The most sensitive individuals are persons with slight abnormalities of thyroid hormonogenesis in which the iodine deficiency unmasks the defect. Dietary substances that interfere with thyroid hormonogenesis may aggravate the effect of iodine deficiency. This is particularly

TABLE 10.2

Main Drugs Causing Primary Hypothyroidism

Iodine and compounds containing iodine

Amiodarone

Lithium

Cytokines (interferons, interleukins)

Tyrosine kinase inhibitors (e.g., sunitinib, imatinib, motesanib, sorafenib)

Aminoglutethimide

Resorcinol

Paraaminosalicylic acid

Phenylbutazone

Ethionamide

important in several developing countries where iodine deficiency is associated with a diet rich in foods (such as cassava, lima beans, sweet potatoes) containing cyanogenic glycosides that are metabolized to thiocyanate, an inhibitor of iodide uptake in the thyroid.[15]

10.3.5 IODINE EXCESS

Iodide excess (>500 to 1,000 µg/day) from several sources (food, drugs, radiographic contrast agents, antiseptics) causes hypothyroidism in individuals who fail to escape from the Wolff-Chaikoff effect. This phenomenon is seen mainly in patients who have underlying thyroid anomalies that affect iodide organification. Particularly at risk are patients with autoimmune thyroiditis or patients with a history of previous thyroid disorder such as subacute thyroiditis or treatment with radioiodine or partial thyroidectomy.[5,8] It is important to note that iodine-induced hypothyroidism is often a reversible condition.

10.3.6 INFILTRATIVE THYROID DISEASES

Infiltrative diseases of the thyroid (amyloidosis, cystinosis, sarcoidosis, scleroderma, hemochromatosis, etc.) are rare conditions that cause overt hypothyroidism in up to 50% of affected patients. These conditions are characterized by gland enlargement and infiltration of the parenchyma (Figure 10.3).

10.3.7 ADULT ONSET OF CONGENITAL THYROID DISEASES

Congenital thyroid dysfunctions are usually causes of neonatal hypothyroidism. In some cases, characterized by a partial defect of hormonogenesis, they can develop in adults, especially in the presence of other factors that may interfere with thyroid function (iodine deficiency or excess, drugs, compounds that act as endocrine disruptors).

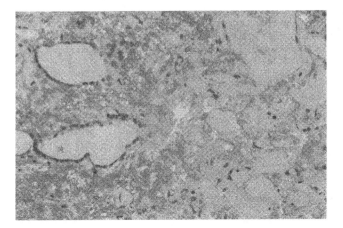

FIGURE 10.3   Amyloidosis of thyroid. Amyloid deposits viewed under polarized light after Congo red staining. (*Source:* Lloyd, R.V. et al. *Endocrine Diseases.* Armed Forces Institute of Pathology Atlas of Nontumor Pathology, First Series, Fascicle 1. Washington: American Registry of Pathology. With permission.)

10.4   PATHOPHYSIOLOGY

Primary hypothyroidism is characterized by decreased production and release of thyroid hormones, 3,5,3'-triodothyronine (T_3) and 3,5,3',5'-tetraiodothyronine or thyroxine (T_4). In an attempt to balance this condition, TSH secretion is increased. The hypothalamus–pituitary–thyroid axis is so sensitive that a significant increase of TSH is the response to very small decreases of thyroid hormones. The increased secretion of TSH stimulates the function of the remnant thyroid gland and may induce its enlargement. Furthermore, the enhanced TSH levels specifically stimulate the production of the active metabolic T_3 hormone in preference over T_4. This effect is the consequence of the induced activity of thyroidal and extrathyroidal type 2 deiodinase. All these changes limit the decrease of circulating T_3, and indicate that the serum T_3 or free T_3 (FT_3) evaluation is less reliable than evaluating T_4 or free T_4 (FT_4) in hypothyroid patients.

10.5   CLINICAL FEATURES

The clinical expression of hypothyroidism varies considerably based on several factors such as the age of the patient, the severity and duration of the disease, and its etiology. Older patients exhibit fewer symptoms and signs than younger patients. Today, most cases of primary hypothyroidism are diagnosed early and characterized by few and non-specific symptoms such as weakness and fatigue, decreased attention span, and sleepiness.

When thyroid failure develops gradually as in Hashimoto's thyroiditis, the typical manifestations of hypothyroidism may take months or years to appear. In cases

Thyroid Diseases

of rapid development of thyroid insufficiency (e.g., after thyroidectomy or radio-iodine treatment), the clinical manifestations appear earlier, after a few weeks, and symptoms like muscle cramps and paresthesia are more frequent.[16] The common symptoms and signs of overt hypothyroidism are listed in Table 10.3. Since this disease can affect virtually all organ systems, we will perform a systematic discussion of the clinical features.

TABLE 10.3
Frequency of Clinical Features in Primary Hypothyroidism

Symptoms and Signs	Frequency (%)
Weakness	90–95
Edema of eyelids	85–90
Sleepiness and lethargy	85–90
Cold intolerance	60–90
Edema of face	60–90
Dry and coarse skin	60–90
Fatigue	60–90
Slow speech	50–90
Thick tongue	60–80
Sparse eyebrows	80
Cold skin	50–80
Hyporeflexia	70
Hair coarseness	70
Weight gain	50–70
Skin pallor	50–70
Dyspnea	50–70
Menstrual disorders	35–80
Slow movement	30–70
Impaired memory	60
Constipation	45–60
Depression	60
Non-pitting edema	55–60
Paresthesia	55
Bradycardia	50
Hair loss	40–50
Anorexia	40–45
Decreasing hearing	30–40
Muscle pain	35
Joint pain	25

TABLE 10.4
Skin Manifestations of Hypothyroidism

Mild peripheral edema
Non-pitting edema
Pallor of skin, in some cases yellowish hue
Dry, thick, coarse, cold skin
Periorbital edema
Coarse, dry, brittle hair
Hair loss (particularly eyebrows and lateral extremities)
Thick, brittle nails

10.5.1 SKIN AND APPENDAGES

Skin changes in hypothyroid patients are summarized in Table 10.4. Thyroid hormone deficiency causes hyperkeratosis with decreased blood flow of the skin and reduction of sebaceous and sweat gland secretions. As a consequence of these changes, the skin appears dry, thick, coarse, pale, and cold. The pallor of the skin is also a consequence of the anemia that is often present in hypothyroidism. In some patients, the skin acquires a yellowish hue due to hypercarotenemia. It may present a mild, pitting, peripheral and periorbital edema, but the characteristic of long-standing hypothyroidism is the non-pitting edema resulting from the accumulation in the dermis and in the connective tissue of glycosaminoglycans (GAGs) such as hyaluronic acid.

This phenomenon may affect all the organ systems. The hydration of GAGs molecules causes a mucinous edema that unlike classic edema does not pit under pressure, and does not change with postural switching. The mucinous edema contributes to the thickness and pallor of the skin. GAGs accumulation is a consequence of the effect of the lack of thyroid hormones on their synthesis and metabolism. Indeed, thyroid hormones inhibit GAGs production and promote their degradation. Hypothyroid patients also show alterations of skin appendages: hair growth may decrease or cease and characteristic is the loss of hair in the lateral extremities of eyebrows. Nails are thick and brittle.

10.5.2 CARDIOVASCULAR SYSTEM

Hypothyroidism induces several hemodynamic alterations, as shown in Table 10.5.[17,18] The main clinical features are bradycardia and the sign of reduced peripheral circulation (cold, pale skin). Dyspnea and exercise intolerance are less frequent and are the signs of cardiac dysfunction. Indeed, echocardiographic studies have shown several characteristic of impaired left ventricular function in hypothyroid patients, particularly the increased ratio PEP/LVET.

TABLE 10.5

Hemodynamic Changes Induced by Hypothyroidism

Cardiac output and stroke volume	↓
Heart rate	↓
Cardiac contractility	↓
Left ventricular preejection time (PEP)	↑
Left ventricular isovolumetric contraction time	↑
Time to peak filling rate	↑
Left ventricular ejection time (LVET)	↓
PEP/LVET	↑
Blood volume	↓
Circulation time	↑
Blood flow in tissues	↓
Systemic vascular resistance	↑

Note: ↑ = increased. ↓ = decreased.

Increased systemic vascular resistance may cause increased diastolic blood pressure in about 20% of patients. A third of patients with overt hypothyroidism exhibit pericardial effusion with a fluid rich in GAGs. This complication is more frequent in long-standing severe forms. Cardiac failure is seen in patients with underlying heart disease, but a very severe hypothyroidism may induce—although rarely—a cardiomyopathy. In this case, histological examination of the heart reveals a mucinous edema of the myocardium (myxedema heart).

Several studies have shown that overt hypothyroidism is a risk factor for atherosclerosis, and coronary atherosclerosis is a frequent finding in hypothyroid patients. Indeed, thyroid hormone deficiency promotes an increase of atherogenic molecules such as low-density lipoprotein (LDL) cholesterol, C-reactive protein, homocysteine, plasminogen activator inhibitor-1, D-dimer.[19] It should be emphasized that since hypothyroidism induces decreased oxygen demand of tissues including the heart, hypothyroid patients may tolerate well the reduction of myocardial blood flow, so that angina is infrequent. Particular care is required in using replacement therapy with LT$_4$ since a sharp increase of tissue oxygen demand may precipitate an ischemic heart stroke.

10.5.3 Respiratory System

A relatively common problem of long-standing hypothyroidism is obstructive sleep apnea that is mainly a consequence of the mucinous infiltration of the tongue and pharynx. In severe cases, pleural effusion and dysfunction of the respiratory muscles along with hypoventilation, atelectasis and dyspnea are present. Rarely, in critical patients, a depression of the ventilatory drive may precipitate a respiratory insufficiency with hypercapnia and hypoxia.

TABLE 10.6
Gastrointestinal Manifestations of Hypothyroidism

Anorexia
Constipation
Paralytic ileus
Weight gain
Malabsorption
Ascitis
Elevation of serum levels of aminotransaminases

10.5.4 Gastrointestinal Tract

The main gastrointestinal manifestations of hypothyroidism are summarized in Table 10.6. Common symptoms are anorexia and constipation. Anorexia reflects the reduced food requirement, whereas constipation is due to decreased peristaltic activity. In older patients, constipation may be severe and unresponsive to laxatives. In severe forms, paralytic ileus may occur.

Weight gain is reported in about two-thirds of patients but it is modest (less than 10% of body weight prior to onset of the disease) and mainly due to the interstitial accumulation of GAGs rather than adipose tissue. Intestinal absorption of food is frequently reduced but only in severe cases does overt malabsorption occur. Liver function is not affected by hypothyroidism, but often an increase of serum aminotransaminases occurs as a consequence of their impaired clearance. Ascitis is a rare complication. About one-third of patients with hypothyroidism of autoimmune etiology show achlorhydria and vitamin B_{12} malabsorption due to autoimmune gastritis.

10.5.5 Nervous System

The nervous system is an important target of thyroid hormones. Numerous neurologic and psychiatric features are present in hypothyroid patients (Table 10.7). Furthermore, the decreased cerebral perfusion contributes to the clinical manifestations.

The most common symptoms are weakness, fatigue, and sleepiness. Often the patients complain of symptoms due to peripheral neuropathy as paresthesia, numbness, and tingling. Less frequently, involvement of the VIII cranial nerve with deafness or vertigo may be noted. All voluntary movements and deep tendon reflexes are slowed. All intellectual functions slacken and cognitive defects (reduced attention span, reduced ability of calculation, memory impairment) are present. Speech is slow and dysarthric. In long-standing hypothyroidism, especially in the elderly, signs of cerebellar dysfunction (ataxia, intention tremor, nystagmus, and dysdiadochokinesia) may be present. Carpal tunnel syndrome is reported in about one-third of the patients as a consequence of the compression of the median nerve by GAGs deposited in the carpal tunnel.

TABLE 10.7
Neurologic and Psychiatric Features
of Hypothyroidism

Neurologic
Weakness, fatigue, slow movement
Sleepiness, lethargy, coma
Paresthesia, numbness, tingling
Reduced deep tendon reflexes
Slow speech, dysarthria
Carpal tunnel syndrome
Cognitive deficits: calculation, memory, attention span
Cerebellar dysfunction: ataxia, nystagmus, tremor
Deafness

Psychiatric
Low emotional level, lack of enthusiasm
Nervousness, irritability
Psychosis: depression, bipolar affective disorders

Relatively common psychiatric disorders are nervousness and irritability. Characteristic of the hypothyroid patient is a low emotional level and lack of enthusiasm. These features contribute to the expressionless face characteristic of overt hypothyroidism. Depression is present in 60% of the patients with hypothyroidism. For this reason, thyroid function tests are included in the diagnostic evaluation of patients presenting with depression. Less frequently, bipolar disorders are observed and occasionally patients may present an overt dementia.

10.5.6 MUSCULOSKELETAL SYSTEM

Up to 80% of hypothyroid patients display symptoms like myalgia, muscle weakness, fatigue, stiffness, and cramps. They are more frequent when hypothyroidism has a rapid onset such as after thyroidectomy or treatment with radioiodine. These symptoms are the consequences of impaired mitochondrial oxidative metabolism caused by the thyroid hormone deficit.

In fewer than 10% of patients, a generalized muscular hypertrophy (hypothyroid myopathy) characterized by severe fatigue and decreased muscle activity have been described. This condition, known as Hoffmann syndrome, presents typical electromyographic abnormalities: polyphasic action potentials, repetition discharge, low-voltage and short-duration motor unit potential. These findings are due to the transition of the muscle fibers from fast type II to slow type I. The muscular hypertrophy is actually a pseudohypertrophy since it is mainly a consequence of muscular infiltration by GAGs.[20]

High serum creatine phosphokinase (CPK), lactate dehydrogenase (LDH), and creatinine are common in hypothyroidism. Joint symptoms are also frequent and include arthralgia, joint stiffness, and occasional synovial effusions. Hypothyroidism does not affect bone density. Although elevated circulating levels of parathormone (PTH) are found frequently, bone turnover is slightly decreased by the presence of a tissue resistance to PTH.

10.5.7 REPRODUCTIVE SYSTEM

In adult premenopausal women, irregular menstrual cycles are frequent. Common symptoms are anovulatory cycles, oligomenorrhea, polymenorrhea, and menorrhagia. Amenorrhea is less frequent. Few studies report the prevalence of infertility in hypothyroid women although the range is high (6% to 70%) and indicates that this condition is frequent.[21] Pregnancy is often associated with abortion, preeclampsia, stillbirth, low birth weight, or premature delivery. In adult men, hypothyroidism is associated with decreased libido and erectile dysfunction. Although past studies have reported normal semen levels, recent studies revealed abnormalities in sperm morphology (pathozoospermia and asthenozoospermia).[21]

10.5.8 ENDOCRINE SYSTEM AND METABOLISM

Hypothyroidism affects the secretion of several hormones (Table 10.8). Primary hypothyroidism is associated with hyperprolactinemia in about one-third of patients resulting from increased secretion of TRH that acts as a stimulator of prolactin (PRL) synthesis and release. Thyroid hormone deficiency causes an enhanced hypothalamic somatostatinergic tone that is responsible for decreased secretion of growth hormone (GH). The GH deficit results in low serum IGF-1, IGF-2, IGFBP-1, and IGFBP-3 concentrations and increased serum IGFBP-2 levels.

In long-standing primary hypothyroidism, the lack of the negative feedback effect of thyroid hormones on TSH secretion may cause thyrotrophic hyperplasia. In rare cases, the hyperplasia may be so bulky as to mimic pituitary macroadenoma including the typical clinical manifestations such as headache, visual field defects, and hypopituitarism. Thyroid hormone replacement will shrink the pituitary mass. In fewer than 10% of patients, inappropriate secretion of vasopressin (AVP) occurs, probably due to the impaired systemic hemodynamic that activates baroreceptor-mediated AVP release.[22]

Adrenal production of cortisol is decreased in hypothyroidism. Since thyroid hormone deficiency causes also decreased cortisol metabolism (due to a reduction of hepatic 11β-hydroxysteroid dehydrogenase type 1 activity), serum cortisol levels and 24-hour urinary excretion of cortisol are normal. In severe, long-standing primary hypothyroidism, ACTH secretion, both basal and after stimulus, and adrenal responsiveness to ACTH may be reduced.

Occasionally adrenal insufficiency may be precipitated by stress or by rapid replacement with thyroid hormones. Adrenal insufficiency due to hypothyroidism should be differentiated from the adrenal primary insufficiency of autoimmune etiology that may be associated with Hashimoto's thyroiditis in the context of a polyglandular autoimmune syndrome. Aldosterone production is decreased, probably due to reduced hepatic synthesis of angiotensinogen and a decrease of plasma renin

TABLE 10.8

Endocrine Changes Induced by Hypothyroidism

PRL	↑
GH, IGF-1, IGF-2, IGFBP-1, IGFBP-3	↓
IGFBP-2	↑
AVP	↑
Cortisol	↔ or ↓
ACTH	↓
Aldosterone	↔ or ↓
Angiotensinogen, renin activity	↓
PTH, 1, 25-(OH)$_2$-vitamin D	↑
FSH, LH	↔
FSH and LH responsiveness to GnRH	↓
SHBG	↓
Estradiol, estrone	↓
Free estradiol	↔
Testosterone, Δ_4-androstenedione	↓
Free testosterone	↔
Progesterone	↔ or ↓
Norepinephrine	↑
Epinephrine	↔ or ↑

Note: ↑ = increased. ↓ = decreased. ↔ = normal.

activity. Plasma aldosterone concentrations are only slightly decreased or even normal due to a reduced metabolism of the hormone.

Serum calcium and phosphate are normal, whereas it is frequent to find increased serum PTH and 1,25-(OH)$_2$-vitamin D concentrations. These findings reflect tissue resistance to the action of PTH and vitamin D. Synthesis and secretion of catecholamines, particularly norepinephrine, are increased, whereas tissue responsiveness is reduced due to the decreased numbers of adrenergic receptors and the impairment of their signaling caused by the thyroid hormone deficiency.

The effects of hypothyroidism on the gonadal function have been described above (see Section 10.5.7). Note that thyroid insufficiency during adolescence may cause sexual immaturity and delayed puberty; occasionally in primary hypothyroidism, the elevated circulating levels of TSH may stimulate the luteinizing hormone (LH) receptor and cause precocious sexual development. The main sexual hormonal changes found in adult hypothyroid patients are consequences of the decreased level of sex hormone-binding globulin (SHBG). Therefore, both total serum testosterone and estradiol are reduced, whereas their unbound fractions remain normal. Usually gonadotropin concentrations are normal, but in premenopausal women the LH ovulatory surge may not happen and secretion of progesterone is inadequate.[21]

TABLE 10.9
Metabolic Changes Induced by Hypothyroidism

Basal metabolic rate	↓
O_2 consumption	↓
Heat production	↓
Energy expenditure	↓
Blood glucose	↔
Plasma insulin	↑
Plasma proteins	↔
Serum total and LDL cholesterol	↑
Serum HDL cholesterol	↔ or ↓
Serum triglycerides	↑
FFA	↓

Note: ↑ = increased. ↓ = decreased. ↔ = normal.

Because of the many metabolic effects of thyroid hormones, several abnormalities of metabolism are described in hypothyroid patients (Table 10.9). Most metabolically active tissues show a decrease of O_2 consumption and heat production, leading to a low basal metabolic rate (35 to 45% below normal), decreased appetite, cold intolerance, and low basal body temperature. The reduced energy expenditure leads to a slight weight gain, although most gain is due to GAGs and water deposition in interstitial tissues. Carbohydrate metabolism is also affected. Glucose intestinal absorption is slow and glucose uptake by tissues is reduced, but blood glucose levels are normal due to decreased liver gluconeogenesis.

The reduced uptake of glucose by the cells is due to a blunted responsiveness of target tissues to insulin as a consequence of impaired expression of the glucose transporter GLUT-4 on the plasma membrane.[23] Plasma insulin levels are usually elevated, mainly due to decreased degradation of the hormone. The latter effect is particularly important in patients with preexisting type 1 diabetes mellitus who develop hypothyroidism because the exogenous insulin half-life increases and therefore its requirement may be reduced.

In hypothyroidism, both the synthesis and the degradation of proteins are decreased, the latter more than the former, producing a positive nitrogen balance. The low protein catabolism explains also the increased pool of albumin in the extravascular space. Blood protein concentrations are normal.

Thyroid insufficiency causes increases of total and LDL cholesterol, associated usually with normal or slightly low concentrations of HDL cholesterol and an increase of LDL:HDL cholesterol ratio. There is also a modest increment of serum triglycerides whereas free fatty acid (FFA) levels are usually reduced. Although animal experimental studies have shown that hypothyroidism is associated with reduced leptin and increased resistin levels, these data are not so clear for humans for whom contradictory results have been found.[8]

Thyroid hormones are necessary for the hepatic conversion of carotene in vitamin A. Hypothyroidism leads to reduced production of this vitamin and an increase of carotene in the bloodstream that causes the yellowish hue of the skin.

Finally, thyroid insufficiency causes a decreased metabolism of several drugs such as digoxin, phenytoin, morphine, and insulin. Therefore, dose adjustments of these drugs are necessary in hypothyroid patients.

10.5.9 RENAL FUNCTION

Decreases of glomerular filtration rate and renal plasma flow are found in adult patients with primary hypothyroidism. These changes are mainly due to the reduction of cardiac output and blood volume. Furthermore, decreased tubular sodium and increased water reabsorption are responsible for the marked fluid retention characteristic of hypothyroidism. Water retention is also due to the increased secretion of AVP. In more than half of the patients, an increase of serum creatinine is present. Hyponatremia is observed in 45% of patients and in 21% of those with normal creatinine levels.[24]

10.5.10 HEMATOPOIETIC SYSTEM

Anemia, usually normochromic and normocytic, is present in at least 30% of hypothyroid patients; in some studies has been described up to 80%. The anemia is caused by the impaired production of erythropoietin. Sometimes the characteristics and pathogenesis of the anemia may be different. In female patients with menorrhagia, the consequent iron deficiency may lead to a hypochromic, microcytic anemia. In patients with associated autoimmune gastritis with deficits of vitamin B_{12}, pernicious anemia (hyperchromic and macrocytic) may occur.

No changes in leukocytes or platelet counts have been described, whereas hemostasis abnormalities are reported and thought to account for the bleeding menstrual disorders. The most frequent anomalies in hemostasis are prolonged bleeding time, decreased platelet adhesiveness, and low concentrations of some clotting factors such as factor VIII and von Willebrand.[25]

10.6 DIAGNOSIS

The clinical suspicion of hypothyroidism, based on the symptoms and signs of the disease (Table 10.3), is confirmed by thyroid hormone assay measuring serum TSH and FT_4 (Table 10.10). The assays of serum TSH and FT_4 are sufficient to establish the diagnosis of overt primary hypothyroidism characterized by serum elevated TSH and low FT_4 values (Figure 10.4). Serum TSH measurement has the highest sensitivity and specificity of all single tests for diagnosing hypothyroidism.[8,16,26] For this reason, it also serves as an initial screening test.

The assessment of FT_4 further increases diagnostic accuracy and allows differentiation of the distinct forms of hypothyroidism (Figure 10.4).[8,16,26] When the hypothalamus–pituitary–thyroid axis is intact, there is an inverse log-linear relationship between FT_4 and TSH. Therefore, a small reduction of FT_4 results in a high

TABLE 10.10
Diagnostic Investigations of Hypothyroidism

Test	Accuracy[a]
I level	
TSH, FT_4	Excellent
Anti-TPO, anti-Tg	Good
Thyroid ultrasound	Good
ECG	Good
II level	
FT_3	Good
24-hour urinary iodine excretion	Poor
Thyroid scintigraphy	Good
TBAb	Good
Chest radiography	Poor
Echocardiography	Poor
Total, LDL, and HDL cholesterol	Poor
Triglycerides	Poor
Iron	Poor
Vitamin B_{12}	Poor
Folic acid	Poor
Gastric parietal cell autoantibodies	Poor

[a] Accuracy is specific for the diagnosis of hypothyroidism and its cause.

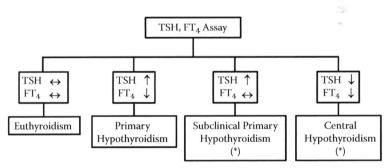

(*) Nonthyroidal illness should be excluded

FIGURE 10.4   Flowchart for biochemical diagnosis of patients with suspected hypothyroidism.

increase of TSH. This relationship makes FT_4 assay highly sensitive for the diagnosis of hypothyroidism. Conversely, FT_3 measurement is less reliable. Indeed, in primary hypothyroidism, the enhanced TSH concentrations stimulate the production of the metabolic active hormone T_3 rather than T_4 as a consequence of induced activity of thyroidal and extrathyroidal type 2 deiodinase.

These processes in patients who still have residual functioning thyroid tissue keep the circulating levels of T_3 within normal range in the initial phase of hypothyroidism. Therefore, the serum FT_3 level tends to be normal for a longer time, and its decrease is an index of the severity of hypothyroidism.

Findings of low FT_4 and high TSH concentrations indicate overt primary hypothyroidism; whereas the association of high TSH with normal FT_4 values suggests a subclinical primary hypothyroidism or nonthyroidal illness (Figure 10.4). When low FT_4 and low or inappropriately normal TSH concentrations are found, central (secondary or tertiary) hypothyroidism is suspected. This panel however can be also observed in non-thyroidal illness or in the transition phase from thyrotoxicosis to hypothyroidism, for instance, in silent thyroiditis.

After a diagnosis of primary hypothyroidism has been established, its cause should be determined. History taking and physical examination are fundamental to differentiate iatrogenic hypothyroidism or forms arising from postpartum and subacute thyroiditis. Detection of thyroid autoantibodies, antithyroperoxidase (anti-TPO), and antithyroglobulin (anti-Tg) allows the diagnosis of the most prevalent form of hypothyroidism, i.e., chronic autoimmune thyroiditis.[8,16,26,27] Indeed, anti-TPO and anti-Tg are found in 90% of patients with Hashimoto's thyroiditis.

Thyroid ultrasound serves as a first-level investigation of primary hypothyroidism (Table 10.10). Indeed, the finding of an atrophic gland or a typical ultrasonographic pattern of autoimmune thyroiditis (hypoechogenic and non-homogeneous) enables the diagnosis of autoimmune thyroiditis in 10% of patients with no detectable thyroid autoantibodies.[16,28] Furthermore, ultrasonography investigates the volumetric characteristic of the gland and eventually reveals thyroid nodules. Ultrasonography is also very useful for the detection of other causes of hypothyroidism such as infiltrative thyroid diseases and congenital hypoplasia. For all these reasons, we prefer to perform thyroid ultrasounds of all patients with hypothyroidism.

Electrocardiogram (ECG) usually reveals only a slow rate and prolonged QT interval but it is useful for finding cardiac complications of hypothyroidism. The observation of T wave changes such as flattening or inversion, anomalies of the ST segment, and low voltage complexes suggest pericardial effusion or ischemic heart disease. The detection of cardiac diseases is extremely important, since it will modify the therapeutic approach for a hypothyroid patient, as will be discussed in the next paragraph.

II level investigations may be useful to get supplemental information about a specific patient. Serum FT_3 measurement will provide more information about the severity of thyroid hormone deficiency. In selected cases, some investigations are needed for a causative diagnosis. When iodine excess is suspected, the detection of high concentrations of 24-hour urinary iodine excretion may confirm the diagnosis. Thyroid scintigraphy, preferentially with ^{131}I (that also allows evaluation of iodine organification) is indicated when ultrasonography is not available. It usually shows a reduced uptake of radioiodine and is also useful to detect congenital thyroid anomalies.

TSH receptor blocking antibodies (TBAbs) are present in about 16% of patients with primary hypothyroidism. TBAbs may be observed in patients with Hashimoto's thyroiditis and in patients previously affected by Graves' disease. This investigation is performed by only a few laboratories because it is based on tissue culture techniques. In cases of cardiac involvement, chest radiography and echocardiography will give more specific information. The measurements of total, LDL and HDL cholesterol and triglycerides often show increased levels that usually return to normal with treatment. When the coexistence of other diseases is suspected, specific investigations may be required. In autoimmune hypothyroidism, a suspicion of atrophic gastritis may be confirmed by measuring serum iron, vitamin B_{12}, and gastric parietal cell autoantibodies. Folic acid determination is useful in cases of megaloblastic anemia.

10.7   THERAPY

Treatment of hypothyroidism is intended to restore and maintain the euthyroid state. Occasionally this can be achieved by removing a causative agent, for instance, discontinuing use of compounds rich in iodine or drugs that interfere with thyroid function. In most cases, thyroid hormone replacement is required. Both T_4 and T_3 thyroid hormones are well absorbed in the gastrointestinal tract and administered orally.

Levothyroxine (LT_4), the first line treatment, is presently the drug of choice, since it has several advantages.[8,16,26,29] The drug has a long half-life (about 7 days); see Table 10.11. Once daily administration is sufficient to achieve adequate replacement. Furthermore, LT_4 is converted to the more metabolically active LT_3 hormone in the extrathyroidal tissues. This process allows tissue production of T_3 on the basis of need. Indeed, in individuals with normal thyroid function, about 87% of circulating T_3 comes from the peripheral tissue conversion of T_4.

LT_3 treatment is not recommended because it has several disadvantages compared to LT_4. LT_3 has a shorter half-life (about one day); see Table 10.11. It must be administered two to three times per day. The short half-life along with decreased binding to plasma proteins causes significant fluctuations of the serum concentrations of the hormone, with peaks above the physiological level. Further, T_3 is four to five times more powerful than T_4 on an equimolecular basis and thus presents more risk of side effects. Hence, LT_3 is a second line drug presently used only for particular conditions of hypothyroidism such as myxedema coma or the management of patients with thyroid cancer to shorten the period of hypothyroidism required for radioiodine treatment in special cases.

TABLE 10.11
Pharmacokinetic Features of Thyroid Hormones

	T_4	T_3
Gastrointestinal absorption	80%	90%
Plasma peak concentration	2–4 hours	1–2 hours
Plasma protein binding	99.97%	99.7%
Plasma free (unbound) hormone	0.03%	0.3%
Plasma half-life	~7 days	~1 day

Some authors recommend replacement therapy with a combination of LT_4 and LT_3. This is based on the observation that about 10% of hypothyroid patients are dissatisfied with LT_4 monotherapy, and under physiological conditions, 13 to 20% of circulating T_3 is produced by the thyroid gland. A combination therapy in which 50 μg of the LT_4 requirement is replaced by 12.5 or 10 μg of LT_3 has been employed, but the studies demonstrated conflicting results about its real advantage compared to monotherapy with LT_4.[8,16,26,29–31] Furthermore, the addition of LT_3 to replacement therapy poses a risk of overtreatment unless doses are carefully controlled. Thus, the current approach is to treat hypothyroidism using LT_4 alone. Combination therapy may eventually be indicated in patients with impaired deiodinase activity although randomized clinical trials are needed to confirm this hypothesis.[32]

The starting dose of LT_4 treatment must be tailored to individual patients on the basis of several factors including age, weight, duration and severity of hypothyroidism, and the presence or absence of other diseases, particularly of the cardiovascular system. We recommend, in adult patients under 65 years old, without coexisting disorders, a starting dose of 25 to 50 μg/day, with incremental increases of 25 to 50 μg every 3 or 4 weeks (Table 10.12). Beneficial effects are seen after 3 to 5 days and patients usually reach the euthyroid state in about 3 months.

In patients over age 65 and those with severe long-standing hypothyroidism or cardiovascular diseases, we recommend starting treatment only after an electrocardiogram (ECG) has been performed. In these patients the replacement dose is reduced. The initial dose will be 12.5 to 25 μg/day, increased by increments of 12.5 to 25 μg every 6 to 8 weeks (Table 10.12). Note that for patients with cardiovascular diseases, particularly ischemic cardiac disease, the replacement must be performed carefully, starting with the lowest dose and slow increments so that determining the maintenance dose will require several months. Indeed, the hypothyroid state induces a decrease of tissue oxygen demand and this has a protective role for the ischemic myocardium. The restoration of the euthyroidism will increase the tissue oxygen demand and may deteriorate cardiac function. Therefore, replacement therapy in patients with coronary artery disease should be started after correction of the heart disease.

The LT_4 maintenance dose in adults is usually 1.2 to 1.7 μg/Kg/day. Pregnant women need doses usually 25 to 50% greater, as do women taking estrogen. Maintenance doses for the elderly are lower—up to 50% less than the dose for a young adult. The best way to establish the appropriate replacement dose is to evaluate serum TSH and FT_4 concentrations. The final goal of maintenance therapy is to obtain TSH values between 0.5 and 2 mUI/L and FT_4 values in the upper third of the normal range.

TABLE 10.12

LT_4 Therapy in Primary Hypothyroidism

Patient	Starting Dose	Incremental Dose	Maintenance Dose
<65 years old	25–50 μg/day	25–50 μg every 3–4 weeks	100–150 μg/day
>65 years old or with cardiovascular diseases	12.5–25 μg/day	12.5–25 μg every 6–8 weeks	50–75 μg/day

TABLE 10.13
Main Drugs Interfering with Thyroid
Hormone Absorption or Metabolism

Drugs Decreasing Thyroid Hormone Absorption

Cholestyramine	Ferrous sulfate
Soy	H_2 antagonist
Calcium carbonate	Protonic pump inhibitor
Sucralfate	Caffeine
Aluminum hydroxide	

Drugs Increasing Thyroid Hormone Metabolism

Rifampin	Statins
Carbamazepine	Sertraline
Phenytoin	Imatinib, sorafenib
Estrogen	

For optimal absorption, LT_4 must be administered in the starvation state; hence, the best time is in the morning upon awakening. Breakfast should be eaten at least 30 minutes after LT_4 ingestion. If a patient takes other drugs, their administration should be delayed 2 to 3 hours. Under optimal conditions, almost 80% of T_4 is absorbed in the gut. A lack of efficacy of the treatment is exceptional. The most common cause of failure is poor compliance by not taking the drug correctly. Other causes are gastrointestinal diseases involving malabsorption or drug interference. Indeed, several drugs may interfere with thyroid hormone absorption and metabolism, as reported in Table 10.13.

In several countries, LT_4 is available in tablets of different dosage (25, 50, 75, 100, 125, 150, 175, and 200 μg). This facilitate the correct titration of a maintenance dose. However, when the appropriate replacement is difficult to achieve, the long half-life of the hormone allows the prescription of different doses on alternate days (e.g., 75 μg one day and 100 μg the next day) or even the withdrawal of a dose for one or two days weekly (e.g., 100 μg daily from Monday to Saturday, no therapy on Sunday). Several countries also recently made available a drop formulation of LT_4; each drop contains 3.57 μg of hormone. This formulation allows easy adjustment of required doses. An inconvenience of the LT_4 solution is that it contains 28.8% ethanol. The product is thus not suitable for children, pregnant women, or patients with liver dysfunction or epilepsy.

LT_4 replacement therapy lacks side effects. They occur only in cases of overdosage with the induction of iatrogenic thyrotoxicosis. Particular caution is required for elderly patients and those with cardiac abnormalities since they may develop atrial fibrillation, ventricular arrhythmia, cardiac ischemia, or heart failure.

If hypothyroidism is associated with adrenal insufficiency, it is important for a patient to take a glucocorticoid replacement before starting LT_4 therapy. Indeed, thyroid hormone administration in patients with adrenal insufficiency may precipitate an adrenal crisis.

LT_4 treatment increases the efficacy of catecholamines, warfarin, and tricyclic antipsychotic agents, whereas it decreases the efficacy of digitalis. Further, in diabetic patients, it increases the requirements for insulin or oral hypoglycemic drugs.

10.8 PROGNOSIS

Patients with overt hypothyroidism face poor quality of life if the disease is not appropriately treated because of the complex organ and tissue involvements of the disease. Severe hypothyroidism is also a life-threatening condition since it may evolve to myxedema coma or serious complications of the cardiovascular system. However, proper treatment allows an excellent prognosis both for the quality of life and for survival.

10.9 FOLLOW-UP

In most patients, we recommend clinical and laboratory evaluations, measuring serum TSH and FT_4 1 or 2 months after the start of the replacement therapy. Thereafter, the clinical and laboratory evaluations are carried out 2 months after every therapeutic adjustment. When the maintenance dose is reached, follow-up will be performed every 6 months for the first year and then annually. If a goiter is present, an annual thyroid ultrasound is recommended. In selected patients (elderly, individuals with severe hypothyroidism or cardiovascular diseases), we recommend an ECG every month for 3 months after the start of therapy; the same procedure is suggested each time a dose adjustment is performed (Table 10.14).

10.10 SCREENING

Screening for adult primary hypothyroidism has been addressed by several studies, but still remains controversial.[16] Although the cost effectiveness of a general population-based screening is unfavorable, case-finding strategies have provided good results. Good targets for such screening are the elderly since overt hypothyroidism has been found in up to 5% of patients (particularly women) admitted to geriatric

TABLE 10.14
Follow-Up of Adult Primary Hypothyroidism

Examination	Schedule	Accuracy
Clinical evaluation	Two months after beginning of therapy or dose adjustment	Excellent
	Every 6 months for first year, then annually when maintenance dose is achieved	
TSH, FT_4	Two months after beginning of therapy or dose adjustment	Excellent
	Every 6 months for first year, then annually when maintenance dose is achieved	
Thyroid ultrasound	Annually in patients with goiter	Excellent
ECG	In selected patients: every month for 3 months from beginning of therapy and every time a dose adjustment is performed	Excellent

TABLE 10.15

Drugs Cited in Chapter 10

Drug	Dosage Forms	Dosage Range
Levothyroxine (LT_4)	Tablets, capsules, solution for intravenous injection,[a] oral solution (drops)[a]	12.5–200 µg/day
Liothyronine (LT_3)	Tablets, solution for intravenous injection[a]	20–120 µg/day
$LT_4 + LT_3$	Tablets	12.5–200 µg/day

[a] Available only in some countries.

units.[8] Screening pregnant women is advantageous based on the poor outcome of a pregnancy if a diagnosis is missed.[33]

The authors of this chapter favor screening by serum TSH measurement of all pregnant women and individuals above 60 years of age who seek medical attention. Further, we suggest screening of individuals with family histories of autoimmune thyroiditis and patients affected by autoimmune diseases.

REFERENCES

1. Monaco, F. 2003. Classification of thyroid diseases: suggestions for a revision. *J Clin Endocrinol Metab* 88: 1428–1432.
2. Vanderpump, M.P.J. 2005. The epidemiology of thyroid diseases. In *Werner & Ingbar's The Thyroid*, Braverman, L.E. and Utiger, R.D., Eds. Philadelphia: Lippincott Williams & Wilkins, 398–406.
3. Kasagi, K., Takahashi, N., Inoue, G. et al. 2009. Thyroid function in Japanese adults as assessed by a general health checkup system in relation with thyroid-related antibodies and other clinical parameters. *Thyroid* 19: 937–944.
4. McGrogan, A., Seaman, H.E., Wright, J.W. et al. 2008. The incidence of autoimmune thyroid disease: a systematic review of the literature. *Clin Endocrinol* 69: 687–696.
5. Laurberg, P., Cerqueira, C., Ovesen, L. et al. 2010. Iodine intake as a determinant of thyroid disorders in population. *Best Pract Res Clin Endocrinol Metab* 24: 13–27.
6. Bürgi, H. 2010. Iodine excess. *Best Pract Res Clin Endocrinol Metab* 24: 107–115.
7. Stagnaro-Green, A., Schwartz, A., Gismondi, R. et al. 2011. High rate of persistent hypothyroidism in a large-scale prospective study of postpartum thyroiditis in Southern Italy. *J Clin Endocrinol Metab* 96: 652–657.
8. Wiersinga, W.M. 2010. Hypothyroidism and mixedema coma. In *Endocrinology, Adult and Pediatric*, Jameson, J.L. and DeGroot, L.J., Eds. Philadelphia: Saunders, Elsevier, 1607–1622.
9. Johner, A., Griffith, O.L., Walker, B. et al. 2011. Detection and management of hypothyroidism following thyroid lobectomy: evaluation of a clinical algorithm. *Ann Surg Oncol* 18: 2548–2554.
10. Metso, S., Jaatinen, P., Huhtala, H. et al. 2004. Long-term follow-up study of radioiodine treatment of hyperthyroidism. *Clin Endocrinol* 61: 641–648.
11. Ross, D.S. 2011. Radioiodine therapy for hyperthyroidism. *New Engl J Med* 364: 542–550.
12. Quach, A., Ji, L., Mishra, V. et al. 2011. Thyroid and hepatic function after high-dose ^{131}I-metaiodobenzylguanidine (^{131}I-MIBG) therapy for neuroblastoma. *Pediatr Blood Cancer* 56: 191–201.

13. Bishton, M.J., Leahy, M.F., Hicks, R.J. et al. 2008. Repeat treatment with iodine-131-rituximab is safe and effective in patients with relapsed indolent B-cell non-Hodgkin's lymphoma who had previously responded to iodine-131-rituximab. *Ann Oncol* 19: 1629–1633.

14. Vogelius, I.R., Bentzen, S.M., Maraldo, M.V. et al. 2011. Risk factors for radiation-induced hypothyroidism: a literature-based meta-analysis. *Cancer.* 117: 5250–5260.

15. Zimmermann, M.B. 2009. Iodine deficiency. *Endocrinol Rev* 30: 376–408.

16. Brent, G.A., Reed-Larsen, P., and Davies, T.F. 2008. Hypothyroidism and thyroiditis. In *Williams Textbook of Endocrinology*, Kronenberg, H.M. et al., Eds. Philadelphia: Saunders, Elsevier, 377–409.

17. Wiersinga, W.M., 2010. The role of thyroid hormone receptor in the heart: evidence from pharmacological approaches. *Heart Fail Rev* 15: 121–124.

18. Biondi, B. and Cooper, D.S. 2008. The clinical significance of subclinical thyroid dysfunction. *Endocrinol Rev* 29: 76–131.

19. Ichiki, T. 2010. Thyroid hormone and atherosclerosis. *Vascul Pharmacol* 52: 151–156.

20. Tuncel, D., Cetinkaya, A., and Gokce, M. 2008. Hoffmann's syndrome: a case report. *Med Princ Pract* 17: 346–348.

21. Krassas, G.E., Poppe, K., and Glinoer, D. 2010. Thyroid function and human reproductive health. *Endocrinol Rev* 31: 702–755.

22. Schrier, R.W. 2008. Vasopressin and aquaporin 2(AQP2) in clinical disorders of water homeostasis. *Semin Nephrol* 28: 289–296.

23. Maratou, E., Hadjidakis, D.J., Kollias, A. et al. 2009. Studies of insulin resistance in patients with clinical and subclinical hypothyroidism. *Eur J Endocrinol* 160: 785–790.

24. Iglesias, P. And Diez, J.J. 2009. Thyroid dysfunction and kidney disease. *Eur J Endocrinol* 160: 503–515.

25. Federici, A.B. 2011. Acquired von Willebrand syndrome associated with hypothyroidism: a mild bleeding disorder to be further investigated. *Semin Thromb Hemost* 37: 35–40.

26. McDermott, M.T. 2009. In the clinic: hypothyroidism. *Ann Intern Med* 151: ITC61.

27. Walsh, J.P., Bremmer, A.P., Feddema, P. et al. 2010. Thyrotropin and thyroid antibodies as predictors of hypothyroidism: a 13-year, longitudinal study of a community-based cohort using current immunoassay techniques. *J Clin Endocrinol Metab* 95: 1095–1104.

28. Carle, A., Pedersen, I.B., Knudsen, N. et al. 2009. Thyroid volume in hypothyroidism due to autoimmune disease follows a unimodal distribution: evidence against primary thyroid atrophy and autoimmune thyroiditis being distinct diseases. *J Clin Endocrinol Metab* 94: 833–839.

29. Todd, C.H. 2009. Management of thyroid disorders in primary care: challenges and controversies. *Postgrad Med J* 85: 655–659.

30. Joffe, R.T., Brimacombe, M., Levitt, A.J. et al. 2007. Treatment of clinical hypothyroidism with thyroxine and triiodothyronine: a literature review and metaanalysis. *Psychosomatics* 48: 379–384.

31. Kansagra, S.M., McCudden, C.R., and Willis M.S. 2010. The challenges and complexities of thyroid hormone replacement. *Lab Med* 41: 338–348.

32. Wiersinga, W.M. 2009. Do we need still more trials on T$_4$ and T$_3$ combination therapy in hypothyroidism? *Eur J Endocrinol* 161: 955–959.

33. Glinoer, D. and Spencer, C.A. 2010. Serum TSH determinations in pregnancy: how, when and why? *Nat Rev Endocrinol* 6: 526–529.

11 Congenital Neonatal Hypothyroidism

Ines Bucci and Cesidio Giuliani

CONTENTS

Key words: congenital hypothyroidism, neonatal hypothyroidism, cretinism, thyroid dysgenesis, thyroid dyshormonogenesis, newborn screening, thyroid hormone replacement therapy.

11.1 DEFINITION

Congenital hypothyroidism (CH) is a condition of thyroid hormone deficiency that is present at birth. CH is one of the most common preventable causes of mental retardation. Without prompt treatment, affected children develop growth failure and neurodevelopmental disabilities.

The term *cretinism* is used to define the condition of severe hypothyroidism with growth and mental retardation related to unrecognized CH. This condition can be considered virtually eliminated since the introduction of the neonatal screening.[1] Cretinism may be endemic or sporadic. Endemic cretinism is present in areas with severe iodine deficiencies and is often associated with goiter. Sporadic cretinism occurs randomly as a consequence of thyroid dysgenesis or dyshormonogenesis.[2] CH is classified into permanent and transient forms. Permanent CH refers to a persistent thyroid hormone deficiency requiring lifelong treatment. Transient CH is a condition of thyroid hormone deficiency present at birth and recovering to normal thyroid function in the first few months or years of life.[2]

11.2 EPIDEMIOLOGY

CH is the most common neonatal endocrine disorder. Before the introduction of newborn screening programs, the incidence of CH as diagnosed on clinical grounds was 1:7,000 to 1:10,000 births. After the onset of screening programs, the incidence increased to 1:3,000 to 1:4,000 births in iodine-sufficient areas, with a 2:1 female:male ratio.[3–5] Primary hypothyroidism is the most frequent form; secondary hypothyroidism incidence has been reported as ~1:50,000.[3,4] With more extensive experience in neonatal screening from regional, state and national programs, wide geographical variation and increased incidence have been reported.

Incidence of CH in Europe is 1:2,709 births and in Italy 1:2.400 births.[6] In the United States, incidence changed from 1:4,094 births in 1987 to 1:2,370 births in 2002.[7] The reasons for the increased incidence are not clear but probably include (1) changes in screening strategy (from primary measurement of T_4 to primary measurement of TSH), (2) changes in testing techniques (from radiochemical-based assay to fluoroimmunoassay or enzyme immunometric assay), (3) lowering the TSH cutoff, (4) increased frequency of preterm and low birth weight newborns, (5) misclassification of transient forms of CH as permanent, and (6) changes in demographic composition.[8,9] Indeed, CH is less frequent in white and black populations in comparison with Hispanics and Asians.[10]

Furthermore, the reduction of the TSH cutoff significantly increased case detection.[11,12] It must be noted that changes in screening practice (strategy, cutoff, assay techniques) do not affect the incidence of the most severe types of CH (such as the forms due to thyroid dysgenesis and thyroid dyshormonogenesis), but allow the identification of additional mild cases mostly with in situ thyroid glands. Note that this form of mild CH may be permanent in up to 78% of cases.[12] In a recent study from Quebec, the reduction of the TSH cutoff increased the incidence of the mild form of CH of unknown etiology, characterized by a normal sized in situ thyroid gland, more than twofold, while the incidence of thyroid dysgenesis or dyshormonogenesis remained stable.[13]

CH is more frequent in twins and multiple births compared to singletons and in newborns from mothers older than 39 years.[7] The incidence of transient forms of CH varies widely, ranging from 10 to 40% in newborns diagnosed with CH.[2] Transient CH is more frequent in areas with low iodine intake. Higher incidences of both permanent and transient CH were reported in preterm infants and in newborns with Down syndrome.[2,12]

11.3 ETIOPATHOGENESIS

The causes of congenital hypothyroidism are reported in Table 11.1. Like acquired hypothyroidism, CH can be classified as primary, central (secondary or tertiary), or peripheral according to etiology. Primary causes include thyroid development defects, impaired thyroid hormone synthesis, and defective TSH binding or signaling.

TABLE 11.1
Causes of Congenital Hypothyroidism

Permanent Hypothyroidism

Primary Hypothyroidism
Thyroid dysgenesis (athyreosis, hemiagenesis, thyroid ectopia, thyroid hypoplasia)
Thyroid dyshormonogenesis
Resistance to TSH binding and signaling

Central Hypothyroidism
Isolated TSH deficiency
TRH deficiency (pituitary stalk interruption or other developmental defects)
Resistance to TRH
Deficiency of transcription factors involved in pituitary development and function

Peripheral Hypothyroidism
Resistance to thyroid hormone
Defects in transmembrane transport

Transient Hypothyroidism
Maternal antithyroid drug therapy
Transplacental transfer of TSH receptor-blocking antibodies
Maternal and neonatal iodine deficiency or excess
Heterozygous inactivating mutations of THOX2 or DUOXA2
Congenital hepatic hemangioma/hemangioendotelioma

Central causes include defects in TSH or TRH synthesis. Peripheral causes are represented by tissue resistance to thyroid hormone action or defects in the transmembrane transport of thyroid hormones. Permanent CH may be due to primary, central or peripheral causes, whereas transient hypothyroidism is almost always due to primary causes except rare conditions of peripheral consumption of thyroid hormones by a hepatic hemangioma or hemangioendothelioma.

11.3.1 PERMANENT PRIMARY HYPOTHYROIDISM

Permanent primary CH is by far the most common form. In iodine-sufficient areas, thyroid dysgenesis accounts for 85% of all cases of primary hypothyroidism. Thyroid dysgenesis is abnormal embryological thyroid gland development ranging from complete absence of a thyroid gland to ectopy and orthotopic hypoplasia. Most patients with thyroid dysgenesis (65%) exhibit defects in normal thyroid migration from the base of the tongue to the neck that result in ectopic and often hypoplastic glands.

The ectopic gland is located along the path of migration from the foramen cecum to the mediastinum.[14] Thyroid ectopy is twice as common in females. The second most common variant of thyroid dysgenesis (35%) is the absence of a functionally active thyroid gland defined as athyreosis or thyroid agenesis. Athyreosis indicates the disappearance of the thyroid due to alterations following the specification of the thyroid anlage. Agenesis is the absence of the gland due to a defective initiation of thyroid morphogenesis.[14]

Developmental defects may affect only one lobe, resulting in hemiagenesis with or without an isthmus. The prevalence of hemiagenesis is about 0.2% in children. It may not cause CH and is generally discovered later in life. The less frequent variant of thyroid dysgenesis (below 5%) is the hypoplasia of an orthotopic thyroid. These small glands may display very low levels of function, exhibiting apparent athyreosis on nuclear medicine imaging.[15]

Although thyroid dysgenesis is sporadic in most cases, several studies support a role of genetic factors in the pathogenesis of this disorder. Indeed, in about 2% of cases, a familial occurrence has been demonstrated. The incidence of asymptomatic developmental anomalies such as hemiagenesis, pyramidal lobe, and thyroglossal duct cyst is higher in first relatives of patients with sporadic thyroid dysgenesis than in control populations.

Thyroid dysgenesis is associated with other congenital anomalies in 5 to 16% of cases. Several defects in genes controlling the embryonic development of the thyroid (TTF-1, TTF-2, PAX-8, and TSH receptor) have been implicated in syndromic and non-syndromic forms of thyroid dysgenesis[15] (Table 11.2). TTF-1, also known as NKX2.1, is a transcription factor that regulates the expression of the thyroglobulin (Tg), thyroperoxidase (TPO), and TSH receptor (TSHR) genes in thyroid follicular cells. It also regulates the transcription of the surfactant protein B gene in epithelial lung cells.[14,15]

TTF-1 gene mutations have been associated with CH (with phenotypes ranging from athyreosis to hypoplasia), respiratory distress, ataxia, and benign chorea.[16] TTF-2, also known as FOXE1, is a transcription factor expressed in the thyroid, in the Rathke's pouch, pharyngeal tissue, and hair follicles during development. Homozygous mutation in TTF-2 gene causes Bamforth-Lazarus syndrome characterized by thyroid dysgenesis with hypothyroidism, choanal atresia, cleft palate or bifid epiglottis, and spiky hair.[15]

PAX-8 is another transcription factor expressed in the thyroid and kidney that has a role in regulating thyroid function and differentiation. Several heterozygous PAX-8 gene mutations have been demonstrated, with variability in phenotypic expression

---

TABLE 11.2
Genes Involved in Thyroid Dysgenesis

Gene	Clinical Manifestations
TTF-1 or NKX2.1	Athyreosis, thyroid hypoplasia, respiratory distress, ataxia, and benign chorea
TTF-2 or FOXE1	Bamforth-Lazarus syndrome: thyroid dysgenesis, cloanal atresia, cleft palate or bifid epiglottis, spiky hair
PAX-8	Ectopic or hypoplastic thyroid, genitourinary malformations
NKX2-5	Athyreosis, thyroid ectopy, cardiac defects
TSHR	Thyroid hypoplasia

ranging from ectopic to orthotopic thyroid gland and from severe hypothyroidism to euthyroidism.[17]

The expression of PAX-8 in the kidney may explain the high incidence of genitourinary malformations in CH and the reported association of thyroid hemiagenesis with ipsilateral renal hemiagenesis.[18] NKX2-5 is a transcription factor related to TTF-1 and expressed in both thyroid and myocardium during development. Mutations in the NKX2-5 gene are associated with thyroid dysgenesis and cardiac anomalies.[15] Homozygous inactivating mutations of the TSHR may cause a hypoplastic thyroid gland with severe hypothyroidism.

From 10 to 15% of all cases of permanent CH are due to defects of thyroid hormonogenesis.

Hereditary defects at virtually all the steps of thyroid hormone synthesis have been described (Table 11.3). With few exceptions, these disorders are transmitted in an autosomal recessive manner and share goiter as a common clinical feature. The most common form of thyroid dyshormonogenesis (46%) is a defect of TPO activity.[19]

TPO is an enzyme located on the apical membranes of thyroid follicular cells. It catalyzes the iodination of thyrosyl residues in Tg and the subsequent iodothyrosine coupling to generate iodothyronines (T_4 and T_3). Mutations of the TPO gene lead to deficient enzyme activity resulting in a total or partial iodide organification defect. The severity of this defect is correlated to the severity of CH. In about 30% of cases, thyroid dyshormonogenesis is due to mutations of the Tg gene. Tg constitutes the matrix for the synthesis of thyroid hormones and serves also for their storage. Tg mutations result in a defect of protein secretion in the follicular lumen or in nonfunctional molecules and cause moderate-to-severe CH with large goiters and low serum Tg concentrations. Less frequently (about 15% of cases), thyroid dyshormonogenesis is caused by mutation of the pendrin (PDS) gene.

Mutations of the PDS gene result in a clinical condition known as Pendred's syndrome characterized by hypothyroidism, goiter, and sensorineural deafness. The PDS protein acts as a chloride and iodide transporter in both the thyroid and the inner ear. In the thyroid, PDS exports iodide across the apical membrane into the colloid space. In Pendred's syndrome, this process is disrupted and although iodide is normally taken up by thyrocytes, it is not efficiently bound to the Tg in the colloid. Mutations of the NIS gene rarely cause CH. NIS protein mediates iodide uptake by thyrocytes

TABLE 11.3
Defects of Thyroid Hormonogenesis

Inactivated Gene	Defect	Inheritance
NIS	Iodide transport defect across basal membrane	Autosomal recessive
TPO	Defective organification of iodide	Autosomal recessive
DUOX2	Defective organification of iodide	Autosomal recessive
PDS	Iodide transport defect across apical membrane	Autosomal recessive
TG	Abnormalities of Tg	Autosomal recessive
DHEAL-1	Defect of iodide recycling	Autosomal recessive and dominant

through the basal membranes. NIS inactivating mutations cause an inability of the thyroid to accumulate iodine. Phenotype may vary with an onset of hypothyroidism and goiter in the neonatal state, infancy, or childhood, depending on the residual NIS activity present.[15]

More recently, mutations of the enzyme dual oxidase 2 (DUOX2) have been described. DUOX2 is located at the apical membranes of thyrocytes and is involved in the H_2O_2 generation that is crucial for TPO activity. Homozygous mutations of the DUOX2 gene result in a complete organification defect with severe CH, whereas heterozygous mutations cause partial defects associated with a mild transient form of CH.[15]

Rarely, thyroid dyshormonogenesis arises from iodothyrosine deiodinase defects. The iodothyrosine deiodinase (DHEAL1) enzyme catalyzes the deiodination of monoiodothyrosine (MIT) and diiodothyrosine (DIT), leading to the formation of free iodide and tyrosine, both of which can be reutilized in thyroid hormone synthesis. Mutations of the DHEAL1 gene impair the intrathyroidal recycling of iodide and induce an excessive urinary loss of iodide as MIT and DIT. As result, iodide deficiency occurs and may cause CH and goiter.

Very rarely, CH is a consequence of thyroid resistance to TSH binding or signaling. The TSH receptor has a role in a later stage of the thyroid development, acting mainly to maintain the differentiated function of the gland. Inactivating mutations of the TSH receptor gene have been described. They are associated to a variable phenotype ranging from asymptomatic hyperthyreotropinemia to a hypoplastic gland with CH. CH may be present in patients with pseudohypoparathyroidism type 1 in which mutations of the Gsα protein cause resistance of the target organs to multiple hormones including TSH. The resistance tends to be mild, and overt clinical hypothyroidism is not always present at birth.

11.3.2 Permanent Central Hypothyroidism

Permanent central CH is almost always a part of congenital hypopituitarism resulting from developmental defects of the hypothalamic and/or pituitary axis such as midline defects. Familial hypopituitarism caused by gene mutations of transcription factors controlling pituitary development (PIT-1, HESX1, LHX3, LHX4, SOX-3) has also been described.

More rarely, congenital tumors of the hypothalamic–pituitary region (such as hamartoma) may cause permanent CH. Generally all these conditions are characterized by a deficiency of all other pituitary hormones. Selective central hypothyroidism is a rare entity resulting from defective TSH synthesis or secretion of a biologically inactive TSH. The defect of TSH production may be caused by a mutation of the β subunit of the TSH gene or by the resistance of thyrotroph cells to TRH signaling (mainly caused by mutations in the TRH receptor).

11.3.3 Permanent Peripheral Hypothyroidism

Peripheral resistance to thyroid hormones caused by mutations in the thyroid hormone receptor β gene can cause hypothyroidism characterized by a slightly or moderately elevated serum TSH and mildly elevated serum FT_4. Another rare cause of peripheral hypothyroidism is a mutation in the gene encoding the thyroid hormone membrane monocarboxylase transporter 8 (MCT8) that facilitates the passage of thyroid hormones through plasma membranes of target cells. The MCT8 defects result in X-linked hypothyroidism associated with mental retardation, hypotonia, weakness, quadriplegia, reduced muscle mass, and delay of developmental milestones.[20]

11.3.4 TRANSIENT HYPOTHYROIDISM

Most transient CH is of the primary type. Moderate iodine deficiency is the most common cause. Also iodine overload resulting from maternal and neonatal exposure to antiseptic preparations may cause transient CH, particularly in preterm infants that are very sensitive to the blocking effect of iodine.[21] Maternal therapy with antithyroid drugs such as propylthiouracil, carbimazole, methimazole, or high-dose iodine can induce a transient CH that usually recedes in 2 to 3 weeks. Maternal TSHR blocking antibodies (TRBAbs) cross the placenta and may persist for 4 to 6 months after birth, impairing newborn thyroid function. A genetic form of transient CH is caused, as noted above, by heterozygous mutations of the DUOAX2 gene. This condition is the first example of a genetic basis for transient CH.

Finally, a very rare form of peripheral transient CH has been described in newborns affected by congenital liver hemangioma or hemangioendothelioma. These tumors produce large quantities of the type 3 iodothyronine deiodinase enzyme that catalyzes the conversion of T_4 in the metabolically inactive reverse T_3 (rT_3). Removal of the tumor or its spontaneous involution restores euthyroidism in these patients.

11.4 PATHOPHYSIOLOGY

Under physiological conditions, the thyroid gland starts development at 3 weeks of gestation. TSH is detectable in fetal serum at 12 weeks of gestation and then gradually rises to a maximum of 6 to 8 mU/L at term. The fetal thyroid gland begins secretion of thyroid hormones at 12 weeks of gestation and the hypothalamus–pituitary–thyroid axis is fully functioning at about 24 to 27 weeks of gestation.[21] Thyroid hormones are necessary for brain development and are specifically involved in the processes of myelination and neuronal connection.

The action of the hormones on the nervous system is not restricted to fetal life; it continues through the first months of postnatal life. Therefore, thyroid hormone deficiency will cause an irreversible cognitive impairment and neurological damage if not promptly treated. During the first half of gestation, thyroid hormone supply to the developing brain is assured by maternal thyroid hormone transfer across the placenta.

Additionally, the fetal brain shows a highly efficient conversion of T_4 to T_3 that guarantees sufficient tissue T_3 concentration despite low serum T_4 concentration. In the hypothyroid fetus, the protective role of maternal T_4 on brain development is demonstrated by the absence of clinical symptoms and signs of hypothyroidism at birth and by a normal or near-normal cognitive outcome if a prompt neonatal treatment with Levothyroxine is started.

The adequacy of placental transfer of thyroid hormones depends on maternal thyroid status and iodine intake. Indeed, hypothyroid newborns from mothers with impaired thyroid function, whether resulting from maternal thyroid disease or severe iodine deficiency, will show signs and symptoms of impaired neurological and cognitive development.

11.5   CLINICAL FEATURES

After the introduction of neonatal screening for CH, affected children are diagnosed before they develop overt clinical signs. Most newborns with CH have no or only subtle symptoms and/or signs at birth, as well as at the time the results of neonatal screening become available (usually with a time lag of 2 weeks). In severe cases, suspicious findings at birth include postmaturity, macrosomia, open posterior fontanel, and jaundice. The clinical presentation of CH according to age is illustrated in Table 11.4.

It is noteworthy that a relationship exists between the severity of the disease reflected by serum thyroid hormone levels and the clinical presentation. More features

TABLE 11.4
Clinical Features of Congenital Hypothyroidism

Age	Symptoms	Signs
Birth to 2 weeks	May be absent	May be absent
	Feeding difficulty	Gestational age >42 weeks
	Sleepiness	Birth weight >4 kg
	Constipation	Large posterior fontanel (>5 mm)
	Periorbital edema	Prolonged jaundice
		Umbilical hernia
		Goiter
		Coarse features
First month	Hoarse cry	Macroglossia
	Feeding difficulty	Dry and cold skin
	Constipation	Peripheral cyanosis and mottling
	Decreased activity	Growth failure
	Lethargy	Bradycardia
		Respiratory distress
		Umbilical hernia
Third month	Feeding difficulty	Macroglossia
	Constipation	Dry, pale, rough skin
	Decreased activity	Puffy face, myxedema
	Lethargy	Hypotonia
	Noisy breathing	Delayed reflexes
	Hoarse cry	Developmental delay
		Umbilical hernia
		Delayed bone maturation

TABLE 11.5

Syndromic Forms of Congenital Hypothyroidism

Syndrome	Characteristics
Pendred's	Hypothyroidism, sensorineural deafness, goiter
Bamford-Lazarus	Hypothyroidism, cleft palate, spiky hair
Ectodermal dysplasia	Hypothyroidism, hypoidrosis, ciliary dyskinesia
Kocher-Debré-Sémélaigne	Hypothyroidism, muscular pseudohypertrophy
Other associations	Hypothyroidism, facial dysmorphism, postaxial polydactyly, severe mental retardation
	Hypothyroidism, benign chorea
	Hypothyroidism, choreoathetosis, neonatal respiratory distress
	Hypothyroidism, obesity, colitis, craniosynostosis, cardiac hypertrophy, developmental delay

are expected in thyroid agenesis and athyreosis compared to thyroid ectopy or milder forms of CH. At the time of diagnosis, the most striking features are prolonged jaundice, lethargy, feeding difficulty, constipation, and wide posterior fontanel.[2,3]

Newborns with thyroid dyshormonogenesis may have visible and palpable goiters. With advancing age and lack of treatment, the symptoms and signs increase up to myxedematous appearance[22] (Table 11.5). Prior to the introduction of the neonatal screening in the 1970s, diagnosis would be delayed for months or even years and an unequivocal complete phenotype could be observed. Typical features were represented by what can be defined as cretinous appearance: large head, puffy face, flat nasal bridge, pseudohypertelorism, open mouth with macroglossia, short stature with delayed bone age, hoarse voice, developmental delay, waddle gait or ataxia, and severe, irreversible, mental retardation (intelligence quotient far under 70). See Figure 11.1. These features can be still observed in developing countries where neonatal screening for CH has not been introduced.

As previously noted, CH may be associated with other congenital malformations. This may occur in the genetic forms of thyroid dysgenesis and dyshormonogenesis (Tables 11.2 and 11.5). Newborns with central congenital hypothyroidism present mild features of hypothyroidism and more striking symptoms of multiple pituitary hormone deficiencies such as hypoglycemia, micropenis, and cryptorchidism. Signs of midline malformation such as cleft lip or palate may also be observed.

11.6 DIAGNOSIS

Diagnosis of CH based only on clinical features is performed in 10% of cases within the first month of life, in 35% within the third month, in 70% within 1 year, and in 100% within 3 to 4 years of life. As previously noted, irreversible neurological damage has already occurred by the time clinical symptoms and signs become evident. The paucity and slow development of clinical features and the importance and efficacy of early treatment to prevent mental and somatic retardation provided the rationale for introducing neonatal screening programs.

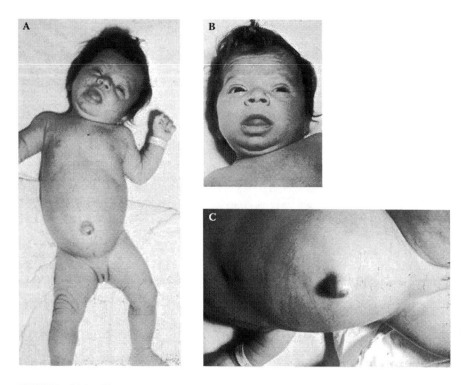

FIGURE 11.1 Three-month-old infant with untreated congenital hypothyroidism. (A) Hypotonic posture; (B) myxedematous face and macroglossia; (C) abdominal distension, umbilical hernia, and skin mottling. (*Source:* Rastogi, M.V. and LaFranchi, S.H. 2010. *Orphanet J Rare Dis* 5: 17–22. With permission.)

Indeed, CH meets the requirements for a mass population screening: (1) the disorder is frequent, (2) early diagnosis only on clinical grounds is difficult, (3) delay or lack of treatment will cause significant severe morbidity, (4) reliable diagnostic tests are available, (5) cost of the diagnosis is compatible with extensive application and is far lower than costs related to lifelong medical care of subjects with neurological and cognitive disabilities, (6) effective therapy is available, and (7) the cost-to-benefit ratio is favorable.

Neonatal CH screening was introduced in Canada in the late 1970s when methods for T$_4$ and TSH assay on blood spots became available.[3] Thereafter, thyroid screening programs were established progressively in the United States, Australia, Japan, and Europe. Screening is now provided to all newborns in developed countries. Neonatal CH screening is part of a wider testing for other congenital conditions such as phenylketonuria (PKU), cystic fibrosis, congenital adrenal hyperplasia, and other inborn errors of metabolism.

CH newborn screening is one of the major achievements in preventive medicine. It is performed using a heel-prick specimen of whole blood spotted onto a filter paper card that is sent to a centralized laboratory for testing. The specimen is collected between 2 and 4 days after birth. Earlier collection will lead to a false positive test due to the physiological postnatal rise of TSH and T_4. In case of a postnatal hospital stay shorter than 24 hours, the specimen must be collected at discharge and a second sample collection is suggested by the fourth day after birth. Preterm neonates and infants with very low birth weights require special attention since they may have delayed increases of TSH after birth and some cases of CH may be missed.[23,24]

These observations support the need for a second screening at 2 to 6 weeks of age in this selected newborn population. The same modification of specimen collection must be applied in acutely ill newborns, in newborns with other congenital malformations (e.g., cardiac defects, genitourinary defects, genetic diseases such as Down syndrome) or treated with drugs interfering with the hypothalamus–pituitary–thyroid axis (e.g., dopamine, steroids, iodine), and monozygotic twins.[25] Some CH screening centers including the authors' also screen newborns from mothers affected by autoimmune thyroid diseases. Some laboratories routinely perform second specimen collections without regard to risk factors in order to avoid missing the diagnosis of some forms of CH characterized by late appearance.

Several neonatal CH screening strategies can be used: (1) initial TSH measurement alone, (2) initial TSH measurement followed by T_4 measurement in samples with elevated TSH, and (3) initial T_4 measurement followed by TSH measurement in samples with low T_4 levels.[2,21,26] At the beginning of screening programs, most laboratories in the United States employed the initial T_4 assay strategy. In Europe and Japan, initial TSH assay was preferred. With the increasing accuracy of TSH assay techniques, a shift from initial T_4 measurement to initial TSH measurement has been registered also in the United States.[26]

Each strategy presents advantages and disadvantage. Generally the most severe cases of primary CH are not missed with any strategy. The initial TSH strategy misses central congenital hypothyroidism and cases with delayed TSH rises can be also missed. However, this approach has the advantage of detecting milder (subclinical) forms of primary CH characterized by normal T_4.

The initial T_4 strategy has the main advantage of detecting central hypothyroidism, but it may miss primary subclinical CH. Both strategies may miss the rare condition in which newborns with CH have delayed TSH increases. For this reason a routine or discretionary second specimen collection can help overcome this problem. The recall rate (percentage of newborn requiring second tests) differs between the screening strategies. The recall rate is higher for initial T_4 than for initial TSH measurements.[26] Simultaneous T_4 and TSH measurements would serve as the best strategy but it is used in only a minority of screening centers.

A critical point in CH newborn screening, whatever strategy is used, is the establishment of a cutoff value of TSH or T_4 that differentiates normal from abnormal results. Both TSH and thyroid hormone levels are higher immediately after birth and decline thereafter, reaching normal infant levels by 2 to 4 weeks of age. Therefore, age-specific normal ranges must be considered in establishing cutoffs[27] (Table 11.6).

Since the introduction of the screening, the increasing sensitivity of TSH assays and changes in measurement techniques led to a progressive reduction of the TSH cutoff from initial serum values of 40 to 50 mU/L (corresponding to 20 to 25 mU/L in whole blood) to serum values of 30 to 20 mU/L (corresponding to 15 to 10 mU/L in

TABLE 11.6

Normal Ranges of Thyroid Function Tests in Infants

Age	TSH mU/L	T$_4$ µg/dL	FT$_4$ ng/dL	FT$_3$ pg/dL
1–4 days	1.0–39.0	14.0–28.0	2.2–5.3	180–760
2–20 weeks	1.7–9.1	7.2–15.7	0.9–2.3	185–770
5–24 months	0.8–8.2	7.2–15.7	0.8–1.8	215–720

whole blood). Instead of predetermined TSH values, most laboratories now develop their own cutoffs by studying the TSH distributions of full-term normal-weight newborns and using an upper (>97th) percentile TSH cutoff. Therefore, TSH cutoffs among different screening programs vary widely. The typical cutoff for serum T$_4$ is between 5 and 13 µg/dL.[8]

Note that neonatal CH screening does not provide a definitive diagnosis of hypothyroidism; confirmatory serum tests are needed (Figure 11.2). Newborns with abnormal screening results should be recalled immediately for examination and venous blood samples should be collected for serum TSH and FT$_4$ measurements. In cases of slight screening test abnormalities, a second blood specimen may be requested before referral. The laboratory results of serum TSH and FT$_4$ measurement should be available within 24 hours and the values obtained should interpreted based on age-normal reference ranges (Table 11.6).

Ideally, the entire procedure from abnormal screening result to serum assay measurement should be completed by 2 weeks of age to allow immediate initiation of therapy when appropriate. Replacement therapy should be started without waiting for serum confirmatory test in cases showing unequivocally abnormal results at screening.

A finding of a normal serum TSH and FT$_4$ values is consistent with a transient elevation of TSH detected at screening. Although such finding does not have clinical implications since no therapy is needed, it is worth noting that this finding was recently considered a risk factors for development of subclinical hypothyroidism later in childhood.[28] A finding of elevated serum TSH and low FT$_4$ values confirms the diagnosis of primary hypothyroidism and initiation of replacement therapy should be immediate.[29]

A finding of elevated serum TSH with normal FT$_4$ value is consistent with subclinical primary hypothyroidism. Since more care is required to ensure an optimal thyroid hormone level for a newborn's developing brain, it is reasonable to start the therapy in all the newborns with a TSH above the age reference range (Table 11.6; Figure 11.2). Since subclinical CH can be transient, an off-therapy trial at age 3 should be performed to establish a definitive diagnosis.[22] A finding of low serum FT$_4$ with a low or inappropriately normal serum TSH concentration is consistent with central hypothyroidism that requires immediate therapy. Alternatively, this biochemical finding can be consistent with neonatal hypothyroxinemia (frequent in premature or acutely ill newborns), a condition that does not require therapy.

Serum thyroid function tests are sufficient to establish a diagnosis of CH. Further laboratory and imaging studies are needed to determine the underlying etiology

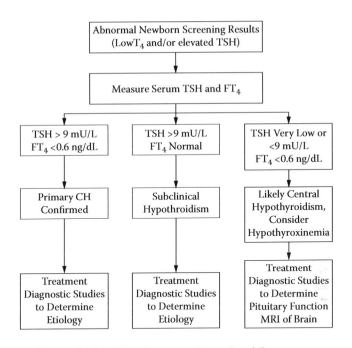

FIGURE 11.2 Diagnostic algorithm of congenital hypothyroidism.

TABLE 11.7
Diagnostic Investigations of Congenital Hypothyroidism

Test	Accuracy
I level	
TSH, FT$_4$	Excellent
Tg	Poor
Thyroid ultrasound	Excellent
Radionuclide uptake and scan	Excellent
II level	
TRBAbs, anti-TPO, anti-Tg	Good
Urinary iodine excretion	Poor
Perchlorate discharge	Good
Genetic analysis	Good

(Table 11.7). Diagnostic studies are chosen on the basis of maternal history (for autoimmune thyroid disease and/or antithyroid drug therapy), family history (relatives with congenital thyroid diseases), and perinatal features (weeks of gestation, perinatal or delivery complications, weight at birth). It is noteworthy to mention that the diagnostic studies should not cause a delay in the initiation of therapy; time consuming or not readily available tests (such as thyroid uptake and scan) should be deferred to the time of re-evaluation (3 years) if they cannot be performed in the first few days of treatment.

Laboratory studies include serum thyroglobulin (Tg), thyroid autoantibodies (TRBAbs, anti-TG and anti-TPO), and urinary iodide determination. Serum Tg levels are low or undetectable in thyroid agenesis, intermediate in thyroid ectopy, and high in dyshormonogenetic goiter, but a certain degree of overlap of these conditions exists. High levels of Tg in newborns with the absence of thyroid radionuclide uptake suggest trapping defects, TSH receptor inactivating mutation, or maternal TRBAbs. TRBAbs measurement is performed if there is a maternal history of autoimmune thyroid disease and/or the mother had a previous child with transient CH. Urinary iodide determination is useful for infants born in areas of endemic iodine deficiency or excess iodine exposure.

Imaging studies include thyroid ultrasound and radionuclide uptake and scan. Ultrasound scanning of the neck is a non-invasive, readily available diagnostic tool that gives useful information about the presence of the thyroid gland in a eutopic location. It is less accurate in demonstrating ectopic glands. Improvements in sensitivity can be obtained using color Doppler ultrasonography.[30] The technique is very accurate in detecting thyroid agenesis/athyreosis (Figure 11.3) and thyroid hemiagenesis (Figure 11.4). The finding of a goiter is consistent with dyshormonogenesis defects.

Radionuclide uptake and scan are the most accurate tests for identifying functioning thyroid tissues and thus distinguishing normal, absent, hypoplastic, or ectopic glands.[31] [123]Iodine yields the most accurate uptake and scan results but is not always readily available. [99]Technetium is used more commonly because it is readily available and less expensive. [131]Iodine should be avoided because it exposes the children to higher doses. The finding of an absent thyroid uptake in conjunction with an empty thyroid bed on ultrasound confirms thyroid agenesis/athyreosis.

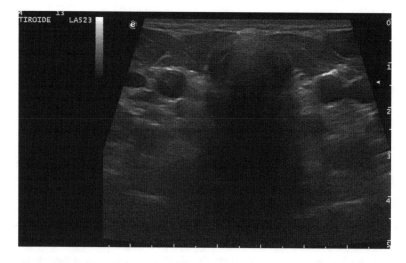

FIGURE 11.3 Thyroid agenesis in 18-year-old woman. Transverse sonogram shows absence of normal thyroid tissue.

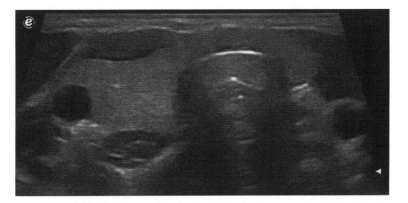

FIGURE 11.4 Thyroid hemiagenesis in 15-year-old girl. Transverse sonogram shows right lobe and isthmus.

If a normal thyroid gland is found at ultrasound, an iodine trapping defect, TSH receptor inactivating mutation, or maternal TRBAbs can be the cause of CH. The finding of an enlarged thyroid gland with increased uptake is suggestive of a dyshormonogenetic defect beyond iodine trapping, such as Tg or iodine organification defects. In the former case the determination of serum Tg levels helps detect Tg defects; iodine organification defects can be diagnosed by a perchlorate discharge test (see Chapter 13). Whenever abnormalities in thyroid location and/or uptake are demonstrated, a permanent form of CH can be established. Conversely, infants with normal thyroid scans and ultrasounds will probably have transient hypothyroidism.

Genetic analyses aimed to identify germline mutations of the genes involved in the pathogenesis of thyroid developmental defects and dyshormonogenesis are currently performed only on a research basis and may be restricted to patients with family histories or suggestive phenotypes. Knee x-rays to determine bone age are used to estimate the severity of CH. Radiography allows the evaluation of the secondary ossification center of the distal femoral epiphysis (whose absence is consistent with hypothyroidism). Alternatively, ultrasonography of the knee has been proposed since it displays good sensitivity and does not involve radiation exposure. In children with diagnoses of central hypothyroidism, additional laboratory and imaging studies are needed to evaluate the hypothalamus–pituitary axis function.

11.7 THERAPY

In all infants with CH, thyroid hormone replacement therapy should be started immediately after the biochemical diagnosis, even before an etiological diagnosis has been achieved. Euthyroidism should be reached as promptly as possible. The goal of therapy is to ensure growth and neurological development as close as possible to genetic potential. The timing of the therapy and the adequacy of the treatment are crucial to a satisfactory developmental outcome. There is an inverse relationship between intelligence quotient (IQ) and the age at which therapy is initiated.[32] Infants treated early may still be subject to impaired development outcomes if euthyroidism is not achieved and maintained by correct dosing.[33]

Levothyroxine (LT_4) is the treatment of choice and no benefits have been shown from the use of triiodothyronine (LT_3). Levothyroxine tablets should be crushed and mixed with water or breast milk, or formula fed and given with a spoon. Interference of levothyroxine absorption by soya milk, fiber, iron, calcium, and sucralfate must be considered. Parents must be given adequate information to ensure correct therapy administration.

The dosage of levothyroxine is crucial for attaining the goals of therapy. There may be a relationship between the etiology of the hypothyroidism, reflected by serum FT_4 levels at diagnosis, and the dose of thyroid hormone required. Higher doses are required in newborns with thyroid agenesis, and lower doses in newborns with thyroid dyshormonogenesis.

Most importantly, in determining a dose regimen, keep in mind that the goal of the therapy is to normalize serum FT_4 levels in 2 weeks and serum TSH levels within a month. Lower scoring on cognitive and behavioral tests is reported in children whose FT_4 serum concentrations are not normalized in 2 weeks.[2]

Several studies have examined different dosage schedules for achieving prompt normalization of thyroid function. The previous starting dose of 6 to 8 µg/kg/day is no longer recommended. Currently the American Academy of Pediatrics and the European Society of Paediatric Endocrinology recommend a levothyroxine dose of 10 to 15 µg/Kg/day[22] (Table 11.8). However, in infants with very low serum FT_4 levels, a higher initial dose (12 to 17 µg/Kg/day) can be used for a few days, then tapered to a lower dose.[22] Thyroid hormone requirements decrease with age, reaching almost half of the neonatal dose at 1 to 3 years of age (Table 11.8). In the first 3 years, replacement therapy should be tailored to obtain a serum FT_4 concentration in the upper half of the age reference range and serum TSH value between 0,5 and 2 mU/L.

As stated above, therapy for CH is warranted even if a diagnosis of permanent hypothyroidism has not been made; it is also warranted in children with transient hypothyroidism. If a diagnosis of permanent hypothyroidism has not been established at the age of 2 to 3 years, a 30-day removal of levothyroxine therapy can be scheduled. If low FT_4 and high TSH serum values result, permanent hypothyroidism is confirmed and therapy is immediately restarted. If serum FT_4 and TSH concentrations

---

TABLE 11.8

Recommended LT$_4$ Doses in Congenital Hypothyroidism

Age of Child	Dose (µg/Kg/day)
0–6 months	10–15
6–12 months	8–10
1–5 years	4–6
5–10 years	3–4
Older than 10 years	2–3

are normal, transient hypothyroidism can be diagnosed and the replacement therapy is no longer needed. However these children need close follow-up because of the risk of thyroid impairment later in childhood, at puberty, and during pregnancy.

11.8 PROGNOSIS

Unrecognized or late treated CH leads to growth failure and severe mental retardation.[34] The prognosis of CH has dramatically improved since the introduction of the newborn screening programs in the late 1970s. Before that, the diagnosis was made after the development of typical clinical features, usually later than 3 months of age in more than 50% of patients. By that time, irreversible brain damage had occurred. The degree of mental retardation, as reflected by IQ testing, was inversely correlated to the age at diagnosis ranging from a mean of 89 (range of 64 to 107) if the diagnosis was made within 3 months, to 54 (range of 25 to 80) if the diagnosis was delayed beyond the sixth month.

After the introduction of the newborn screening, the early recognition and treatment of CH resulted in the attainment of significantly higher IQ levels and normal growth patterns. However, even though overt intellectual disabilities are no longer observed, minor developmental delays, subtle cognitive impairments, and IQ points lower than matched controls have been reported.[35,36] The neurological outcome correlates with severity of hypothyroidism, age at initiation of therapy, levothyroxine starting dose, and maintenance of adequate treatment in the first 3 years.

11.9 FOLLOW-UP

Hypothyroid children require frequent follow to assess growth (weight, length, head circumference), neurodevelopmental milestone attainment, and thyroid functional status. The American Academy of Pediatrics recommend the following schedule for thyroid hormone and TSH assays: (1) 2 and 4 weeks after start of treatment, (2) every 1 to 2 months during the first 6 months of life, (3) every 3 to 4 months between 6 months and 3 years, of age, (4) every 6 to 12 months thereafter, and (5) 4 weeks after any change of dose (Table 11.9).

More frequent follow-up is needed in cases of inadequate treatment or poor compliance. Levothyroxine dose adjustment is required when serum TSH exceeds 10 mU/L or is between 5 and 10 mU/L and is associated with serum FT_4 in the lower half of the age reference range.[37]

TABLE 11.9
Follow-Up of Congenital Hypothyroidism

Clinical evaluation	2 to 4 weeks after start of therapy
Serum TSH and FT_4	Every 1 to 2 months for first 6 months
	Every 3 to 4 months between 6 months and 3 years of age
	Every 6 to 12 months above 3 years of age
	1 month after any change of dose regardless of age

TABLE 11.10
Drugs Cited in Chapter 11

Drug	Dosage Forms	Dose Range
Levothyroxine (LT₄)	Tablets, capsules	25–100 µg/day

REFERENCES

1. Chen, Z.P. and Hetzel, B.S. 2010. Cretinism revised. *Best Pract Res Clin Endocrinol Metab* 24: 39–50.
2. Rastogi, M.V. and LaFranchi, S.H. 2010. Congenital hypothyroidism. *Orphanet J Rare Dis* 5: 17–22.
3. Van Vliet, G. 2005. Hypothyroidism in infants and children: congenital hypothyroidism. In *Werner & Ingbar's The Thyroid*, Braverman, L.E. and Utiger, R.D., Eds. Philadelphia: Lippincott Williams & Wilkins, 1033–1040.
4. Van Tijn, D.A., de Vijlder, J.J., Verbeeten, B. et al. 2005. Neonatal detection of congenital hypothyroidism of central origin. *J Clin Endocrinol Metab* 90: 3350–3359.
5. Olney, R.S., Grosse, S.D., and Vogt, F.R. Jr. 2010. Prevalence of congenital hypothyroidism: current trends and future directions. *Pediatrics* 125: 31–36.
6. Olivieri, A. and Study Group for Congenital Hypothyroidism. 2009. The Italian National Register of infants with congenital hypothyroidism: twenty years of surveillance and study of congenital hypothyroidism. *Riv Ital Pediatr* 35: 2.
7. Harris, K.B. and Pass, K.A. 2007. Increase in congenital hypothyroidism in New York State and in the United States. *Mol Genet Metab* 91: 268–277.
8. Hertzberg, V., Mei, J., and Therrell, B.L. 2010. Effect of laboratory practices on the incidence rate of congenital hypothyroidism. *Pediatrics* 125: S48–S53.
9. Parks, J.S., Lin, M., Grosse, S.D. et al. 2010. The impact of transient hypothyroidism on the increasing rate of congenital hypothyroidism in the United States. *Pediatrics* 125: S54–S63.
10. Hinton, C.F., Harris, K.B., Borgfeld, L. et al. 2010. Trends in incidence rates of congenital hypothyroidism related to select demographic factors: data from the United States, California, Massachusetts, New York, and Texas. *Pediatrics* 125: S37–S47.
11. Mengreli, C., Kanaka-Gantenbein, C., Girginoudis, P. et al. 2010. Screening for congenital hypothyroidism: the significance of threshold limit in false-negative results. *J Clin Endocrinol Metab* 95: 4283–4290.
12. Corbetta, C., Weber, G., Cortinovis, F. et al. 2009. A 7-year experience with low blood TSH cutoff levels for neonatal screening reveals an unsuspected frequency of congenital hypothyroidism (CH). *Clin Endocrinol* 71: 739–745.
13. Deladoey, J., Ruel, J., Giguere, Y. et al. 2011. Is the incidence of congenital hypothyroidism really increasing? A 20-year retrospective population-based study in Québec. *J Clin Endocrinol Metab* 96: 2422–2429.
14. De Felice, M. and Di Lauro, R. 2010. Anatomy and development of the thyroid. In *Endocrinology, Adult and Pediatric*, Jameson, J.L. and DeGroot, L.J., Eds. Philadelphia: Saunders, Elsevier, 1342–1361.
15. Topalogu, A.K. 2006. Athyreosis, dysgenesis and dyshormonogenesis in congenital hypothyroidism. *Pediatr Endocrinol Rev* 3: 498–502.
16. Ferrara, A.M., De Michele, G., Salvatore, E. et al. 2008. A novel NKX2.1 mutation in a family with hypothyroidism and benign hereditary chorea. *Thyroid* 18: 1005–1009.

17. Montanelli, L. and Tonacchera, M. 2010. Genetics and phenomics of hypothyroidism and thyroid dys-and agenesis due to PAX8 and TTF1 mutations. *Mol Cell Endocrinol* 30: 64–71.
18. Kumar, J., Gordillo, R., Kaskel, F.J. et al. 2009. Increased prevalence of renal and urinary tract anomalies in children with congenital hypothyroidism. *J Pediatr* 154: 263–266.
19. Avbelj, M., Tahirovic, H., Debeljak, M. et al. 2007. High prevalence of thyroid peroxidase gene mutations in patients with thyroid dyshormonogenesis. *Eur J Endocrinol* 156: 511–519.
20. Zamproni, I., Grasberger, H., Cortinovis, F. et al. 2008. Biallelic inactivation of the dual oxidase maturation factor 2 (DUOXA2) gene as a novel cause of congenital hypothyroidism. *J Clin Endocrinol Metab* 93: 605–610.
21. Mann, N.P. 2011. Congenital hypothyroidism: what's new? *Paediatr Child Health* 21: 295–300.
22. Rose, S.R., Foley, T., Kaplowitz, P.B. et al. 2006. Update of newborn screening and therapy for congenital hypothyroidism. *Pediatrics* 117: 2290–2303.
23. Woo, H.C., Lizarda, A., Tucker, R. et al. 2011. Congenital hypothyroidism with a delayed thyroid stimulating hormone elevation in very premature infants: incidence and growth and developmental outcome. *J Paediatr* 158: 538–542.
24. LaFranchi, S.H. 2011. Congenital hypothyroidism: delayed detection after birth and monitoring treatment in the first year of life. *J Paediatr* 158: 525–527.
25. Miller, J., Tureck, J., Awad, K. et al. 2009. Newborn screening for preterm, low birth weight, and sick newborns: approved guidelines. *CLSI,* Document 1/LA31-A 29: 1–69.
26. LaFranchi, S.H. 2010. Newborn strategies for congenital hypothyroidism: an update. *J Inherit Metab Dis* 33: 225–233.
27. DeBoer, M.D. and LaFranchi, S.H. 2007. Pediatric thyroid testing issues. *Pediatr Endocrinol Rev* 5: 570–577.
28. Leonardi, D., Polizzotti, N., Carta, A. et al. 2008. Longitudinal study of thyroid function in children with mild hyperthyrotropinemia at neonatal screening for congenital hypothyroidism. *J Clin Endocrinol Metab* 93: 2679–2685.
29. Zung, A., Tenebaum-Takover, Y., Barkan, S. et al. 2010. Neonatal hyperthyrotropinemia: population characteristics, diagnosis, management and outcome after cessation of therapy. *Clin Endocrinol* 72: 264–271.
30. Chang, Y.W., Hong, H.S., and Choi, D.L. 2009. Sonography of the pediatric thyroid: a pictorial essay. *Clin Ultrasound* 37: 149–157.
31. Reed-Larsen, P., Davies, T.F., Schlumberger, M.J. et al. 2008. Thyroid physiology and diagnostic evaluation of patients with thyroid disorders. In *Williams' Textbook of Endocrinology*, Kronenberg, H.M. et al., Eds. Philadelphia: Saunders, Elsevier, 299–332.
32. LaFranchi, S.H. and Austin, J. 2007. How should we be treating children with congenital hypothyroidism? *J Pediatr Endocrinol* 20: 559–578.
33. Bongers-Schokking, J.J. and de Muinck Keizer-Schrama, S.M. 2005. Influence of timing and dose of thyroid hormone replacement on mental psychomotor, and behavioral development in children with congenital hypothyroidism. *J Pediatr* 147: 768–774.
34. Selva, K.A., Harper, A., Downs, A. et al. 2005. Neurodevelopmental outcomes in congenital hypothyroidism: comparison of initial T_4 dose and time to reach target T_4 and TSH. *J Pediatr* 147: 775–780.
35. Leger, J., Ecosse, E., Roussey, M. et al. 2011. Subtle health impairment and socioeducational attainment in young adult patients with congenital hypothyroidism diagnosed by neonatal screening: a longitudinal population-based cohort study. *J Clin Endocrinol Metab* 96: 1771–1782.

36. Van Vliet, G. and Grosse, S.D. 2011. The continuing health burden of congenital hypothyroidism in the era of neonatal screening. *J Clin Endocrinol Metab*, 96: 1671–1673.
37. Balhara, B., Misra, M., and Levitsky, L.L. 2011. Clinical monitoring guidelines for congenital hypothyroidism: laboratory outcome data in the first year of life. *J Pediatr* 158: 532–537.

12 Central Hypothyroidism

Paolo Beck-Peccoz and Luca Persani

CONTENTS

Key words: TSH, TRH, thyroid hormones, isolated congenital hypothyroidism, combined pituitary hormone deficiencies, PROP1, POU1F1/PIT1, nonthyroidal illnesses (NTIs), levothyroxine.

12.1 DEFINITION

Central hypothyroidism (CH) is a condition characterized by defective thyroid hormone synthesis and secretion due to insufficient stimulation by thyrotropin (TSH) of an otherwise normal thyroid gland.[1,2] This disease can be a consequence of disorders affecting either the pituitary gland or the hypothalamus, but most frequently both of them. For this reason, the term *central hypothyroidism* is preferred to *secondary hypothyroidism,* which indicates hypothyroidism of pituitary origin, or *tertiary hypothyroidism,* which defines hypothyroidism of hypothalamic origin.

12.2 EPIDEMIOLOGY

The prevalence of CH in the general population is estimated to range from 1:20,000 to 1:80,000. Data from neonatal screening for hypothyroidism based on combined TSH and T_4 TBG determinations indicate a presence of CH ranging from 1:16,000 to 1:100,000 live newborns.[3] CH can affect patients of all ages and, contrary to ratios found in patients with primary hypothyroidism, the female:male ratio for CH is around 1.0. CH does not reduce life expectancy but the hypothyroid state can severely affect quality of life.[3]

12.3 ETIOPATHOGENESIS

The etiopathogenesis of CH is very heterogeneous and most of the disease mechanisms remain elusive. Depending on the underlying organic or genetic cause, sporadic

TABLE 12.1

Etiology of Central Hypothyroidism (9 Is)

1. INVASIVE LESIONS: pituitary macroadenoma, craniopharyngioma, glioma, meningioma, metastases, empty sella
2. IATROGENIC CAUSES: cranial surgery, radiation, drugs
3. INJURIES: head trauma, breech delivery
4. INFARCTIONS: postpartum necrosis (Sheehan), pituitary apoplexy, vascular accident affecting pituitary or hypothalamus
5. IMMUNOLOGIC DISEASES: lymphocytic hypophysitis
6. INFILTRATIVE LESIONS: sarcoidosis, hemochromatosis, histiocytosis X
7. INFECTIVE DISEASES: tuberculosis, syphilis, mycoses
8. INHERITABLE FORMS: pituitary transcription factor defect (occasionally with childhood onset), TSHβ and TRHR mutations
9. IDIOPATHIC FORMS: unknown causes

and familial forms of CH have been described. Moreover, CH may be isolated or combined with other pituitary hormone deficiencies (CPHD) in both congenital and acquired forms of the disease. Indeed, isolated CH is more frequently due to specific genetic defects, such as TSHβ subunit or TRH receptor gene mutations. The major causes of CH are reported in Table 12.1.

The defect in TSH secretion is mainly quantitative in genetic forms of CH. Serum TSH levels are indeed undetectable in most cases. A typical example is the mutation of the TSHβ gene resulting in the synthesis of truncated TSHβ subunits unable to dimerize with the glycoprotein hormone α subunit (α-GSU). The defect is frequently both quantitative and qualitative in acquired CH. A quantitative defect in the number of functional pituitary thyrotrope cells is probably the pathogenic mechanism accounting for most CH cases. This quantitative defect in TSH-producing cells is frequently associated with a qualitative defect in the secreted TSH isoforms that conserve immunoreactivity but display severe impairment in their biological activity, thus losing the ability to stimulate TSH receptors on thyroid cells.[4,5]

The secretion of bioactive TSH was documented in CH secondary to hypothalamic lesions, pituitary tumors, breech delivery, external head irradiation, and Sheehan's syndrome. It is well documented that glycosylation plays a fundamental role in modulating the expression of TSH bioactivity. Impaired control of TSH synthesis and secretion by TRH and other neuroendocrine or paracrine factors may be associated with alterations of posttranslational processing of the molecule, resulting in the release of TSH forms with altered glycosylation and variable bioactivity.[6] This qualitative defect in TSH secretion provides an explanation for the lack of correlation between circulating thyroid hormone and TSH concentrations in patients with CH.

Defective TRH action due to natural mutations in the TRH receptor (TRHR) gene has been described in only two families. In our experience, the infancy of patients with complete TRH resistance appeared uneventful and the diagnosis in the male proband with homozygous TRHR mutations was reached at the age of 11 years when growth retardation accompanied by fatigue was recorded.[7]

TSHβ defects appear to be relatively frequent causes of inheritable isolated CH.[8] Missense, truncating, and intronic variants have been described. They all cause defective dimerization with the α-GSU, thus preventing the production of entire and bioactive TSH molecules. As a result of this impaired dimerization, a finding of excess circulating α-GSU levels in a patient with isolated CH is indicative of a TSHβ gene defect.

In patients with defects of pituitary transcription factor genes, CH is due to defective differentiation of pituitary structures.[9] Nevertheless, CH may become manifest only during childhood in patients with PROP1 or POU1F1/PIT1 mutations. Pituitary macroadenomas represent the most frequent causes of acquired CH, accounting for more than half the cases. The tumors can be nonfunctioning or may secrete GH, prolactin, ACTH, or gonadotropins. Different degrees of hypopituitarism frequently result from compression of the nontumoral portion of the pituitary. The pituitary stalk and the hypothalamus may be directly affected by suprasellar extension of a tumor. Metastases to the hypothalamic–pituitary region arising from carcinomas of the breast, lung, and occasionally other sites are infrequent and usually reflect advanced disease.

Extrasellar brain tumors can also cause CH by affecting mainly hypothalamic function. In this case, hypopituitarism is usually accompanied by diabetes insipidus. Craniopharyngioma is the most frequent extrasellar brain tumor causing hypopituitarism and CH, especially in children. Meningiomas, gliomas, empty sella, and nontumoral lesions are less frequent CH causes.

Medical interventions for the treatment of sellar and extrasellar tumor masses present additional risks for CH. External radiotherapy for tumors of the head has been described to affect both the hypothalamus and the pituitary, and CH often results from damage of these structures. Overall, the risk of the development of central hypothyroidism is related to total radiation dose higher for intracranial solid tumors treated with higher radiation doses. TSH deficiency also can result from direct radiation of the pituitary by conventional external radiotherapy or γ-knife for pituitary lesions. If not present initially, CH may result from surgical therapy of pituitary tumors. The dimension and extrasellar extension of a pituitary mass along with neurosurgeon expertise are critical factors in this context.

Among the causes of acquired CH, traumatic brain injuries and cardiovascular accidents such as subarachnoid hemorrhages and infarcts represent relevant causes. In all these conditions, the most frequent anterior pituitary defect is growth hormone (GH) deficiency followed by central hypogonadism and CH. Due to the recent development of sophisticated imaging and biochemical assays, increasing numbers of patients have been diagnosed with lymphocytic hypophysitis.[10] The autoimmune process frequently leads to variable CPHDs. Although isolated forms of autoimmune GH or gonadotropin deficiencies have been reported, at present there is no evidence of isolated forms of autoimmune CH.

All the other causes of CPHDs are infrequent and involve either infective or infiltrative granulomatous diseases such as sarcoidosis or histiocytosis. Depending on the extent of pituitary involvement, varying degrees of hypopituitarism can be observed. The neurohypophysis is also affected in most patients, leading to diabetes insipidus.

TABLE 12.2
Factors Affecting TSH Secretion and Causing Transient/Reversible CH

Nonthyroidal Illnesses
Major medical illness (liver or kidney insufficiency, heart failure, carcinoma)
Major surgery and organ transplantation
Severe burns and trauma
Infective diseases
Bipolar disorders
Anorexia nervosa and prolonged fasting
Malnutrition
Aging

Suppressed TSH Secretion after Thyrotoxicosis
Antithyroid drug treatment
Radioactive iodine therapy
Subacute thyroiditis
Newborns from hyperthyroid mothers

Use of Drugs Inhibiting TSH Secretion
Withdrawal of levothyroxine suppressive therapy
Glucocorticoids
Dopaminergic agents
Cocaine
Retinoid X-receptor selective ligands

Transient or reversible forms of CH (Table 12.2) may be noted during nonthyroidal illnesses (NTIs). NTIs can induce down-regulation of hypothalamic TRH synthesis and feedback set points, producing a sort of central hypothyroidism. This mechanism is generally considered protective against unwanted thyroid hormone-mediated metabolic stimulation, but in more severe cases a state of true CH is manifest. Moreover, recovery from a thyrotoxic state may also be followed by a transient form of CH whose prolongation generally depends on the duration and severity of thyrotoxicosis.

Finally, many drugs[11] may affect the mechanisms of neuroendocrine TSH regulation. Cocaine addicts may present with CH and other pituitary deficits. Somatostatin analogs, glucocorticoids, and dopaminergic compounds may acutely induce inhibition of TSH secretion with a consequent reduction of thyroid stimulation. However, activation of the thyroid hormone feedback mechanism is generally effective in maintaining adequate thyroid stimulation over the long term.

Transient central hypothyroidism may be induced in neonates by corticosteroids or dopamine given to the mother during a complicated preterm delivery. Antineoplastic agents acting through the retinoid X nuclear receptor can cause profound TSH inhibition and CH that are reversible upon drug discontinuation. As an example, bexarotene is known to form functional heterodimers with thyroid hormone receptors, thus contributing to the inhibition of TSHβ gene transcription.

12.4 CLINICAL FEATURES AND DIAGNOSTIC PROCEDURES

The clinical and biochemical features of central hypothyroidism are listed in Table 12.3. The hypothyroid state is mild to moderate in most CH patients and although manifestations of CH are similar to those of primary hypothyroidism, they can be masked by signs and symptoms of other pituitary deficits. For this reason, the diagnosis of CH is generally obtained on a biochemical basis either incidentally or in patients under evaluation for hypothalamic or pituitary diseases.

Inheritable forms of CH are generally associated with severe neonatal onset and characterized by typical manifestation of congenital primary hypothyroidism (jaundice, macroglossia, hoarse cry, failure to thrive and retarded growth, umbilical hernia, hypotonia, etc.). If neonates are not treated promptly with LT_4, cretinism may develop. In pituitary transcription factor defects, the presence of CPHDs is suggested by an association with hypoglycemia, adrenal insufficiency, typical craniofacial abnormalities, and severe growth retardation.

The diagnosis of CH cannot be reached solely by TSH determination. A combined evaluation of TSH and FT_4 as a first-level investigation is required for the diagnosis of any form of CH. The hallmark of CH is the finding of serum FT_4 concentrations

---

TABLE 12.3
Features Characteristic of Central Hypothyroidism

Clinical Manifestations

Signs and symptoms of hypothyroidism

Manifestations of concomitant or preexisting hypothalamic/pituitary disease (low radioiodine thyroidal uptake that normalizes after exogenous TSH stimulation; altered imaging of hypothalamic–pituitary region)

Findings Excluding Primary Thyroid Defect

Negative antithyroid autoantibodies

Homogeneous and small or normal thyroid gland on ultrasound

Biochemical Findings

First Level

Low serum FT_4 levels

Low serum FT_3 levels, but only in about 70% of patients

Low or normal TSH concentrations in absence of interference in TSH immunoassay

Low bioactivity of circulating TSH

Second Level

Blunted nocturnal TSH surge, reduced amplitude of circadian TSH oscillation

Variable TSH response to TRH testing

Anti-TPO and anti-Tg antibodies

Imaging Investigations

First Level

TC or MR of hypothalamic–pituitary region

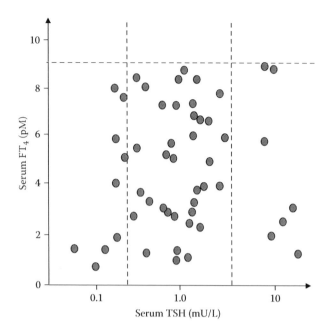

FIGURE 12.1   Serum free T_4 and TSH levels in 52 patients with central hypothyroidism followed at our institution. The lack of correlation is consistent with a qualitative alteration (i.e., altered glycosylation and decreased bioactivity) of circulating TSH molecules.

into the hypothyroid range associated with low or normal TSH levels. Indeed, some CH patients with prevalent hypothalamic defects may show high serum TSH levels, a finding potentially leading to a misdiagnosis of subclinical primary hypothyroidism (Figure 12.1). Measurement of antithyroid autoantibodies, a second level test, may help differentiate CH from primary hypothyroidism. In CH patients, the autoantibodies must be undetectable. A diagnostic workup of CH should also include the exclusion of factors that may interfere in TSH measurement methods by performing appropriate tests of dilution and recovery. Moreover, it should be underlined that FT_4 measurements provide the highest accuracy for the diagnosis of CH. The measurement of FT_3 is highly unreliable; more than 30% of CH patients show normal levels of this hormone. The measurements of different parameters of peripheral thyroid hormone action, such as sex hormone-binding globulin, ferritin, bone markers, serum lipids, and others do not appear diagnostically useful because they lack sufficient sensitivity and specificity to diagnose hypothyroidism. Moreover, patients with CPHDs may have additional pituitary hormone deficiencies that may bias the interpretation of many parameters of peripheral thyroid hormone action.

Following this strategy, only manifest forms of CH, but not the subclinical defects characterized by FT_4 levels still within normal range, can be recognized. It has been reported that the diagnosis of hidden CH in survivors of childhood cancer may be reached by evaluating nocturnal TSH surge. The failure of nocturnal TSH to rise may therefore be useful in the diagnosis of CH patients although the test requires hospitalization. Furthermore, Alexopoulou and coworkers[12] gave a diagnostic value to time-related decreases in circulating T_4 concentrations larger than 20% as compared with the basal T_4 values. This approach would allow the diagnosis and treatment of mild hypothyroid states of central origin, analogous to the subclinical forms of primary hypothyroidism.

TRH testing may be of help in the differential diagnosis of tertiary (hypothalamic) and secondary (pituitary) origin of the central defect since hypothalamic defects are associated with exaggerated, prolonged, or delayed TSH responses. Recent studies indicate that a clear distinction between the two forms of CH may be difficult because both sites are affected in most patients and the distinction is only of limited utility for CH patients. Nevertheless, the presence of abnormal TSH responses to TRH may help confirm suspected CH.

In every patient with CH, a CT scan or MR study of the hypothalamic–pituitary region should be carried out. In the past, radioiodine thyroidal uptake (RAIU) was performed both in basal conditions and after stimulation with bovine TSH (Ambinon® testing), and more recently by recombinant human TSH to document low thyroidal uptake that normalizes after stimulation, thus confirming normal functioning of the thyroid gland. This diagnostic approach is now obsolete.

Finally, patients with nonthyroidal illnesses (NTIs) have values of thyroid function testing that largely overlap values for CH patients, suggesting NTI as a form of CH whose outcome may be amenable to improvement by thyroid hormone treatment. Therefore, the presence of concomitant diseases at the time of blood withdrawal should always be excluded before suspecting true CH (Table 12.3).

12.5 THERAPEUTIC APPROACHES

Treatment of CH is aimed to restore normal serum concentrations of circulating thyroid hormones. Theoretically, this may be achieved in CH patients by TSH or TRH administration, but these treatments were abandoned because of cost and restricted applicability. Today, standard levothyroxine (LT_4) therapy is generally preferred in patients with CH.[13] LT_4 replacement is easily tuned in primary hypothyroidism by evaluating circulating TSH levels. However, this measurement cannot guide LT_4 treatment in CH patients even though a finding of unsuppressed TSH levels during LT_4 treatment strongly indicates undertreatment.[14]

The evaluation of circulating free thyroid hormones plays a major role in monitoring LT_4 treatment in CH. Nonetheless, several recent papers dealing with substitutive LT_4 therapy in CH patients underlined the pitfalls in achieving optimal replacement. Koulouri and collaborators approached the problem by using their department clinical information system to identify all patients with hypothalamic–pituitary lesions and classified their risk of CH as high and low.[15] They then compared FT_4 values in these groups of patients with patients with primary hypothyroidism adequately treated with LT_4, i.e., those with normal levels of circulating TSH during replacement therapy. The authors concluded that CH patients are generally undertreated. Moreover, they suggest that levels of FT_4 around 16 pmol/L (their laboratory reference range was 9 to 25 pmol/L) may represent an appropriate target in treated CH patients. Interestingly, this conclusion is similar to the one we reached, i.e., targeting FT_4 values at the middle of the laboratory range of normal values.[14]

Finally, measurement of FT_3 in addition to FT_4 levels has been suggested. However, most current methods of measuring FT_3 are inaccurate and rarely used in follow-ups of CH patients. The evaluation of clinical and biochemical indices of peripheral thyroid hormone action play limited roles in monitoring LT_4 treatment in CH patients. However, they may be useful in discovering overtreatment.

In patients at risk of CPHDs, concomitant central adrenal insufficiency must always be excluded before starting LT_4 therapy because of the risk of precipitating an adrenal crisis. If adrenal function cannot be assessed before the start of LT_4, prophylactic treatment with steroids is advised and assessment of adrenal function can be postponed. LT_4 treatment should be started at a low daily dosage (25 µg/day), particularly in long-standing hypothyroid states, and then progressively incremented to reach full replacement dose.

Significant differences in LT_4 doses also depend on concomitant treatments for CPHDs. It is well known that recombinant human growth hormone (hGH) treatment interferes with the activity of the hypothalamic–pituitary–thyroid axis and may unmask central hypothyroidism or render LT_4 substitutive therapy insufficient.[16–18] Moreover, estrogens were reported to increase LT_4 requirements also in primary hypothyroidism. Since this is a likely consequence of an increase in thyroxine-binding globulin (TBG) levels, the effect of estrogens and the required adjustment of LT_4 should be transient in order to saturate the increased T_4-binding capacity of plasma proteins.

Finally, treatment strategies are different for CH with neonatal to childhood onset. In fact, normal infants and children have higher circulating free thyroid hormone levels. Therefore, higher LT_4 doses are recommended in CH children and treatment should be started at full-replacement doses (10 to 15 µg/kg of LT_4), particularly in cases with neonatal onset, to protect neurological development.

In conclusion, LT_4 substitutive therapy may be optimal if certain conditions are fulfilled: (1) start therapy only after exclusion of adrenal insufficiency, (2) establish final dose based on age and sex (about 1.4 to 1.7 µg/Kg body weight), (3) maintain levels of circulating FT_4 in the middle range of laboratory reference values, (4) reassess LT_4 dosage whenever additional replacement with other pituitary hormones is necessary, (5) ensure during follow-up that blood for FT_4 measurement is withdrawn before ingestion of daily LT_4 tablets, and (6) suspect undertreatment when TSH levels exceed 0.2 mU/L. In iodine-deficient countries, consider the possible presence of nodular goiter with autonomous thyroid hormone secretion to prevent possible LT_4 overtreatment.

REFERENCES

1. Yamada. M. and Mori, M. 2008. Mechanisms related to the pathophysiology and management of central hypothyroidism. *Nat Clin Pract Endocrinol Metab* 4: 683–694.
2. Lania, A., Persani, L., and Beck-Peccoz, P. 2008. Central hypothyroidism. *Pituitary* 11: 181–186.
3. LaFranchi, S.H. 2010. Newborn screening strategies for congenital hypothyroidism: an update. *J Inherit Metab Dis.* 33 (Suppl 2): S225–S233.

4. Beck-Peccoz, P. and Persani, L. 1994. Variable biological activity of thyroid-stimulating hormone. *Eur J Endocrinol* 131: 331–340.

5. Persani, L., Ferretti, E., Borgato, S. et al. 2000. Circulating TSH bioactivity in sporadic central hypothyroidism. *J Clin Endocrinol Metab* 85: 3631–3635.

6. Szkudlinski, M.W., Fremont, V., Ronin, C. et al. 2002. Thyroid-stimulating hormone and thyroid-stimulating hormone receptor structure-function relationships. *Physiol Rev* 82: 473–502.

7. Bonomi, M., Busnelli, M., Beck-Peccoz, P. et al. 2009. A family with complete resistance to thyrotropin-releasing hormone. *New Engl J Med* 360: 731–734.

8. Bonomi, M., Proverbio, M.C., Weber, G. et al. 2001. Hyperplastic pituitary gland, high serum glycoprotein hormone a-subunit, and variable circulating thyrotropin levels as hallmarks of central hypothyroidism due to mutations of the TSHβ gene. *J Clin Endocrinol Metab* 86: 1600–1604.

9. Pfäffle, R. and Klammt, J. 2011. Pituitary transcription factors in the aetiology of combined pituitary hormone deficiency. *Best Pract Res Clin Endocrinol Metab* 25: 43–60.

10. Caturegli, P., Newschaffer, C., Olivi, A. et al. 2005. Autoimmune hypophysitis. *Endocr Rev* 26: 599–614.

11. Haugen, B.R. 2009. Drugs that suppress TSH or cause central hypothyroidism. *Best Pract Res Clin Endocrinol Metab* 23: 793–800.

12. Alexopoulou, O., Beguin, C., De Nayer, P. et al. 2004. Clinical and hormonal characteristics of central hypothyroidism at diagnosis and during follow-up in adult patients. *Eur J Endocrinol* 150: 1–8.

13. Beck-Peccoz, P. 2011. Treatment of central hypothyroidism. *Clin Endocrinol* 74: 671–672.

14. Ferretti, E., Persani, L., Jaffrain-Rea, M.L. et al. 1999. Evaluation of the adequacy of L-T4 replacement therapy in patients with central hypothyroidism. *J Clin Endocrinol Metab* 84: 924–929.

15. Koulouri, O., Auldin, M.A., Agarwal, R. et al. 2011. Diagnosis and treatment of hypothyroidism in TSH deficiency compared to primary thyroid disease: pituitary patients are at risk of underreplacement with levothyroxine. *Clin Endocrinol (Oxf)* 74: 744–749.

16. Porretti, S., Giavoli, C., Ronchi, C. et al. 2002. Recombinant human GH replacement therapy and thyroid function in a large group of adult GH-deficient patients: when does L-T4 therapy become mandatory? *J Clin Endocrinol Metab* 87: 2042–2045.

17. Agha, A., Walker, D., Perry, L. et al. 2007. Unmasking of central hypothyroidism following growth hormone replacement in adult hypopituitary patients. *Clin Endocrinol (Oxf)* 66: 72–77.

18. Giavoli, C., Porretti, S., Ferrante, E. et al. 2003. Recombinant hGH replacement therapy and the hypothalamus-pituitary-thyroid axis in children with GH deficiency: when should we be concerned about the occurrence of central hypothyroidism? *Clin Endocrinol (Oxf)* 59: 806–810.

13 Congenital Dyshormonogenetic Goiter

Cesidio Giuliani and Ines Bucci

CONTENTS

Key words: congenital hypothyroidism, congenital goiter, Pendred's syndrome, thyroid dyshormonogenesis, LT_4 suppressive therapy.

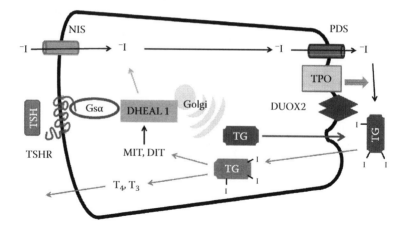

FIGURE 13.1   Schematic drawing of thyrocyte illustrating main steps of thyroid hormonogenesis. See text for explanation.

TABLE 13.1
Defects of Thyroid Hormonogenesis: Molecular Mechanisms

Defect	Molecular Mechanism	Goiter
TSHR or signaling defects	Inactivating mutation of TSHR or Gsα gene	No
Iodide transport defect	Inactivating mutations of NIS gene	Yes
Iodide apical efflux defect	Inactivating mutations of PDS gene	Yes
Defective organification of iodide	Inactivating mutations of TPO or DUOX-2	Yes
Abnormalities of thyroglobulin (Tg)	Mutations of Tg genes	Yes
Defect of iodide recycling	Inactivating mutations of DHEAL-1 gene	Yes

13.1   DEFINITION

Congenital dyshormonogenetic goiter is an inherited form of goiter resulting from
a defect of thyroid hormone biosynthesis. Virtually all the steps but one of thyroid
hormonogenesis may be affected (Figure 13.1 and Table 13.1). The goiter constitutes
the effort of the thyroid gland to overcome the defective hormone biosynthesis and it
can be associated with normal thyroid function or with hypothyroidism. Goiter does
not occur in cases of defects in thyroid-stimulating hormone receptor (TSHR) or its
signaling in which a hypoplastic gland is usually observed.

13.2   EPIDEMIOLOGY

Dyshormonogenetic goiter has a prevalence ranging from 1:30,000 to 1:50,000 in
the general population and constitutes about 10 to 15% of all cases of congenital
hypothyroidism.[1,2] The partial or total inactivation of the thyroid peroxidase (TPO)

gene constitutes the most common defect (46%),[3] followed by mutations of the thyro-globulin (Tg) gene (about 30%).

Mutations of the pendrin (PDS) gene account for about 15% of the defects with an incidence of 7.5 to 10 per 100,000 individuals.[4] The abnormalities of the remaining genes, i.e., TSHR, sodium–iodide symporter (NIS), dual oxidase (DUOX2), dual oxidase maturation factor A2 (DUOXA2), and iodothyrosine deiodinase (DHEAL)-1, are rare and constitute all together fewer than 10% of cases of dyshormonogenetic goiter.

13.3   ETIOPATHOGENESIS

The defects of thyroid hormones biosynthesis are inherited disorders, transmitted in most instances as an autosomal recessive trait (Table 13.2).

13.3.1   DEFECTS IN TSHR OR ITS SIGNALING

Because of the fundamental role of TSH in regulating thyroid hormonogenesis, the inborn errors of TSHR and its signaling are treated in this chapter even if the defects are not associated with goiter. Thyroid resistance to TSH may be due to alterations of the TSHR or the several proteins involved in TSH signal transduction. To date only mutations of the TSHR and the Gsα protein subunit have been described.[5]

The human TSHR gene is located on chromosome 14q31. It encodes a glyco-sylated protein of a 744 amino acid sequence that is a member of the G-protein coupled receptor superfamily. TSHR mediates TSH action on thyrocytes, regulating thyroid cell growth and function. Several TSHR inactivating mutations have been identified. They may cause absent or decreased expression of the receptor on the cell surface or abnormalities of receptor function such as impaired binding of TSH or the inability to translate the message. These loss-of-function mutations are distributed along the receptor sequence without significant hot spots.[6] The defect is inherited in most cases as an autosomal recessive trait, but an autosomal dominant

TABLE 13.2
Gene-Activated Defects of Thyroid Hormonogenesis

Gene Inactivated	Defect	Inheritance
TSHR or Gsα	Regulation of thyroid growth and function	Autosomal recessive and dominant
NIS	Iodide transport defect across basal membrane	Autosomal recessive
PDS	Iodide transport defect across apical membrane	Autosomal recessive
TPO	Defective organification of iodide	Autosomal recessive
DUOX2	Defective organification of iodide	Autosomal dominant
DUOXA2	Defective organification of iodide	Autosomal recessive
Tg	Abnormalities of Tg	Autosomal recessive
DHEAL-1	Defect of iodide recycling	Autosomal dominant with incomplete penetrance

transmission has been described. The latter forms are characterized by a milder clinical expression.[6]

Inactivating mutations of the Gsα protein subunit are responsible for the syndrome known as pseudohypoparathyroidism type 1a, characterized by impaired functions of several hormone receptors associated with this protein. TSHR is one of the receptors involved and a mild form of hypothyroidism is a component of this disorder. The syndrome has an autosomal dominant inheritance with a maternal imprinting.

Others defects causing a thyroid resistance to TSH have also been described. They are transmitted as autosomal dominant traits but the genes involved are not yet identified.[5,6]

13.3.2 IODIDE TRANSPORT DEFECT

The iodide transport defect is due to inactivating mutations of the NIS gene (official gene name: SLC5A.5) located on chromosome 19p12-13.2. The gene encodes for a 13-transmembrane domain glycoprotein of 643 amino acids, localized in the basolateral membranes of thyrocytes. NIS is a member of the sodium–solute symporter family that actively cotransports one iodide ion with two sodium ions across the membranes of thyroid cells. To date, 13 loss-of-function mutations that cause an inability of the thyroid to accumulate iodine have been identified.[7]

Some mutations cause a quantitative defect with absent or decreased expression of the protein on the basolateral membranes; others cause a reduced activity of the protein. The defect is transmitted as an autosomal recessive trait, with affected patients harboring homozygous or compound heterozygous mutations.

13.3.3 IODIDE APICAL EFFLUX DEFECT

Iodide apical efflux defect is caused by inactivating mutations of the PDS gene (official gene name: S.LC26A4). The gene, located on chromosome 7q31, encodes for a protein of 780 amino acids that is a member of the solute carrier family. The protein mediates the exchange across the membrane of chloride with bicarbonate and iodide. In the thyroid, where it is expressed on the apical membrane of the thyrocyte, PDS mediates iodide efflux in the follicular lumen.

PDS is also expressed in the inner ear where it acts as a chloride–bicarbonate exchanger in the endolymphatic ducts and sacs. Inactivating mutations of the PDS gene result in a clinical condition, known as Pendred's syndrome, characterized by hypothyroidism, goiter, and sensorineural deafness. The syndrome is transmitted in an autosomal recessive fashion and more than 150 mutations of the PDS gene have been described.[8]

13.3.4 DEFECTS IN IODIDE ORGANIFICATION

Defects in iodide organification may be due to the mutations of three genes involved in this process: the TPO, the DUOX2, and the DUOX2A genes.

TPO is a 933 amino acid glycoprotein containing a heme group located on the apical membrane of a thyrocyte. The protein exerts enzymatic activity and catalyzes the iodination of the thyrosyl residues of Tg and the subsequent iodothyrosine coupling to generate iodothyronines (T_4 and T_3). Sixty-one inactivating mutations of the TPO gene (mapped on chromosome 2p25) have been reported, most of them found on exons 7, 8, 10 and, 13.[9] Affected individuals carry homozygous or compound heterozygous mutations supporting the autosomal recessive inheritance. TPO inactivating mutations lead to deficient enzyme activity, resulting in a total or partial iodide organification defect.

TPO activity requires the generation of hydrogen peroxide (H_2O_2) as an electron acceptor. Generation of H_2O_2 occurs in the apical membranes of thyrocytes under the control of two enzymes: dual oxidase 1 (DUOX1) and dual oxidase 2 (DUOX2). DUOX1 and DUOX2 are membrane-bound NADPH-dependent glycoproteins with seven transmembrane domains of 1551 and 1548 amino acid sequences, respectively.

The corresponding genes map to chromosome 15q15.3. To date at least 25 different inactivating mutations of the DUOX2 gene have been described, whereas no mutation in the DUOX1 gene has been identified.[10] The defect is transmitted in an autosomal dominant fashion since a single defective allele is sufficient to cause the disease. However, in heterozygous patients, the defect occurs in a milder form with a transient congenital hypothyroidism during the first months of life, when the thyroid hormone requirements are highest.

Recently, two proteins, called DUOX maturation factors (DUOXA1 and DUOXA2) have been identified. The proteins (whose genes are located contiguous to the DUOX1 and 2 genes on chromosome 15q15.3) are crucial for the DUOX1 and DUOX2 maturation process in the Golgi apparatus and for their expression on the plasma membrane. Two different loss-of-function mutations of the DUOXA2 gene have been identified, both inherited as autosomal recessive traits.[11]

13.3.5   Abnormalities of Thyroglobulin (Tg)

Tg is a glycoprotein homodimer of 660 KDa that is secreted into the follicular lumen where it constitutes the scaffold for thyroid hormone synthesis. The Tg monomer is encoded by a single gene that maps on chromosome 8q24.2-3 and is composed of 2749 amino acids. The prevalence of Tg defects is about 1:100,000 live births and to date up to 52 inactivating mutations have been reported, with phenotypes ranging from euthyroidism to severe hypothyroidism.[12] The Tg defects are inherited in an autosomal recessive manner and affected individuals are either homozygous or compound heterozygous for the mutations.

Both quantitative and qualitative abnormalities of Tg have been observed. They include: (1) absent or decreased synthesis of the protein, (2) a defective protein that is normally secreted in the follicular lumen but it has impaired function or only residual functional activity, and (3) a defective intracellular transport of the protein that accumulates in the endoplasmic reticulum and is not secreted in the follicular lumen.

13.3.6   Defect of Iodide Recycling

Rarely, thyroid dyshormonogenesis is due to iodothyrosine deiodinase (DHEAL1) defects. DHEAL1 is a nitroreductase-related enzyme that catalyzes the deiodination of monoiodotyrosine (MIT) and diiodotyrosine (DIT). This reaction leads to the formation of free iodide and tyrosine, both of which can be further reused within the thyroid for hormone synthesis. The DHEAL1 gene maps on chromosome 6p24 and encodes a 293 amino acid sequence protein. Inactivating mutations of the DHEAL1 gene impair the intrathyroidal recycling of iodide and induce excessive urinary loss of iodide as MIT and DIT. As result, iodide deficiency occurs and may cause CH and goiter. The defect is transmitted as an autosomal dominant trait with incomplete penetration.[13]

13.4 PATHOPHYSIOLOGY

Thyroid dyshormonogenesis induces decreased synthesis and secretion of thyroid hormones. In an attempt to balance this condition, increased secretion of TSH stimulates the growth and function of the thyroid gland. With the exception of the defects of TSHR and its signaling, in all the inborn errors of thyroid hormonogenesis, the increased TSH stimulation leads to gland enlargement. Therefore, the goiter is a compensatory mechanism and its size is directly related to the severity of the thyroid defect, ranging from absence (in cases of minimal deficit) to mild or marked enlargement.

The goiter may be present at birth or develop later in life. In general, earlier appearance correlates with a more severe defect. Further, the onset and severity of hypothyroidism also correlate with the extent of the hormonogenesis defect. Hence, thyroid function may vary from a euthyroid state to severe hypothyroidism and cretinism. In several cases, clinical heterogeneity has been observed even in patients harboring the same mutations.

This phenomenon is due to several factors, such as the efficiency of the other steps involved in thyroid hormone biosynthesis or environmental conditions such as iodine intake or goitrogen compounds. Other unknown factors may also be involved. Although these thyroid abnormalities are clinical manifestations of inborn disorders, they may not be present at birth and may occur later in life when the increased requirements for thyroid hormones precipitate the onset of a goiter or hypothyroidism.

The clinical hallmark of Pendred's syndrome is sensorineural deafness. This defect is the consequence of the important role of PDS protein in the inner ear. Indeed PDS is expressed in the endolymphatic duct and sac, where it acts as a chloride–bicarbonate exchanger. Inactivating mutations of the protein cause an alteration of the resorption process of endolymph, leading to structural abnormalities of the cochlea (see below).

13.5 CLINICAL FEATURES

13.5.1 DEFECTS IN TSHR OR ITS SIGNALING

As already noted, these defects are not associated with goiters but rather with hypoplastic glands. TSHR mutations cause a congenital hypothyroidism of different degrees, depending on the extent of thyroid resistance. Milder forms of TSH resistance are associated with a thyroid gland of normal size and subclinical hypothyroidism. In patients with pseudohypoparathyroidism type 1a, hypothyroidism is always mild and the clinical picture is dominated by the other components of the syndrome.

13.5.2 Iodide Transport Defect

Mutations of the NIS gene cause goiter and hypothyroidism. Goiter may appear before, concomitantly with, or after the onset of the hypothyroidism. In most of the patients observed, it occurred during childhood. Frequently the goiter is large and may be diffuse or nodular. Hypothyroidism may be present at birth and may cause cretinism or it may appear later during infancy or childhood. Some patients have only hypothyroidism without goiter.

13.5.3 Iodide Apical Efflux Defect (Pendred's Syndrome)

Mutations of the PDS gene cause Pendred's syndrome, characterized by sensorineural deafness, goiter, and a partial defect in iodide organification. Clinical heterogeneity among patients affected by this syndrome is significant because both thyroid function and goiter presence and size depend on iodine intake. Goiter usually develops during childhood and only rarely is present at birth. Most patients are euthyroid at diagnosis and hypothyroidism is present in conditions of low iodine intake. About half the patients lack thyroid abnormalities and are diagnosed as having familial deafness.[8] The hearing defect arises from abnormalities of the inner ear—an enlarged vestibular aqueduct or the presence of a Mondini cochlea (rudimentary cochlea or single cavity). The hearing loss is severe and prelingual.

13.5.4 Defects in Iodide Organification

Mutations of the TPO gene may cause a total or a partial iodide organification defect, whereas mutations of the DUOX2 and DUOX2A genes cause only partial defect. The total organification defect is clinically characterized by goiter and a permanent congenital hypothyroidism. In cases of partial defect, the patients have goiters associated with euthyroidism or mild hypothyroidism. Transient congenital hypothyroidism has also been observed in these patients.

13.5.5 Abnormalities of Tg

Most patients with Tg mutations have a congenital goiters or goiters that appear shortly after birth. Thyroid function ranges from euthyroidism to severe hypothyroidism, based on the extent of the defect.

13.5.6 Defect of Iodide Recycling

The defect is clinically characterized by goiter and severe hypothyroidism that appear usually during infancy.

13.6 DIAGNOSIS

The presence of a goiter at birth or during childhood with or without hypothyroidism strongly suggests the possibility of a defect of thyroid hormonogenesis. The disorder

---

TABLE 13.3

Diagnostic Investigations of Thyroid Dyshormonogenesis

Test	Accuracy[a]
I Level	
TSH, FT_4	Excellent
Thyroid ultrasound	Excellent
Anti-TPO, anti-Tg	Good
II Level	
Chest radiograph	Good
CT, MR	Good

[a] Accuracy relates to diagnosis of thyroid dyshormonogenesis.

---

is suspected also when familial cases of goiter and/or hypothyroidism are observed, particularly with an early onset in life. A diagnostic evaluation for Pendred's syndrome should be performed in patients with sensorineural deafness, particularly if relatives are also affected by the disease.

First-level investigations for the diagnosis of thyroid dyshormonogenesis are reported in Table 13.3. TSH measurement of a blood specimen collected for the neonatal screening program (see Chapter 11) allows detection of patients with congenital hypothyroidism. The measurements of serum TSH and FT_4 permit confirmation of congenital hypothyroidism or evaluation of thyroid function when these defects are suspected after birth. Serum autoantibodies anti-Tg and anti-TPO are very useful to exclude autoimmune thyroid diseases that may present with goiter and hypothyroidism.

Thyroid ultrasound is a noninvasive, easily available diagnostic tool that allows accurate determination of a goiter and its size. Thyroid ultrasound may also yield information about the presence of a substernal goiter or tracheal compression or deviation. However, these complications are better evaluated with a chest radiograph, a computed tomography (CT) scan, or magnetic resonance (MR) imaging of the neck and thorax.

Further investigations may be performed to confirm the thyroid dyshormonogenesis and identify the type of defect and the gene mutation causing it.

13.6.1 Defects in TSHR or Its Signaling

Diagnostic features of the defect are: (1) a hypoplastic gland revealed by thyroid ultrasound, (2) absent or reduced thyroid radioiodine uptake (RAIU) preferably using ^{123}I, (3) normal serum Tg concentration, and (4) a lack of increase of RAIU, FT_4, and FT_3 serum levels after the administration of human recombinant TSH (rhTSH; Table 13.4). Verification of the diagnosis can be made by genetic analyses showing the mutation.

TABLE 13.4
Diagnosis of TSHR Defects

Test	Finding
I Level	
TSH	Increased
FT_4, FT_3	Decreased
Thyroid ultrasound	Hypoplastic gland
RAIU	Absent or reduced
II Level	
Tg	Normal
RAIU after rhTSH	No change
FT_4, FT_3 after rhTSH	No change
Genetic analyses	Identification of mutation

13.6.2 IODIDE TRANSPORT DEFECT

Diagnostic clues of this defect are the presence of a goiter associated with decreased RAIU (<5% after 24 hours from the administration of radioiodine) that does not increase after administration of rhTSH. The confirmatory test is the ratio between salivary and plasmatic iodine (Table 13.5). Indeed, NIS is normally expressed not only in the thyroid, but also in other tissues such as salivary glands. Hence, under physiological condition 1 hour after the administration of radioiodine, a gradient between salivary and plasmatic concentrations of iodine with a ratio ranging from 25 to 140 occurs. In patients with iodide transport defects, the ratio is below 20 and in most cases is around 1.

TABLE 13.5
Diagnosis of Iodide Transport Defect

Test	Finding
I Level	
TSH	Usually increased
FT_4, FT_3	Usually decreased
Thyroid ultrasound	Goiter in most cases
RAIU	Absent or reduced
Ratio salivary/plasmatic iodine concentrations	<20
II Level	
Tg	Normal or elevated
RAIU after rhTSH	No change
FT_4, FT_3 after rhTSH	No change
Genetic analyses	Identification of NIS mutations

TABLE 13.6

Diagnosis of Iodide Organification Defects

Test	Finding
I Level	
TSH	Usually increased
FT_4, FT_3	Usually decreased
Thyroid ultrasound	Goiter in most cases
Perchlorate discharge test	>10%
CT or MR of inner ear	Morphological abnormalities of cochlea
II Level	
Tg	Normal
Genetic analyses	Identification of gene mutations

13.6.3 IODINE ORGANIFICATION DEFECTS

The diagnostic hallmark of the iodine organification defect is the perchlorate discharge test (Table 13.6). In physiological conditions, more than 90% of radioiodine is bound to the tyrosine residues of Tg within minutes from its entry into thyroid follicular cells. When a defect of the organification process is present, a larger amount of radioiodine is unbound and can be dismissed from the gland.

A perchlorate discharge test is performed administering 500 mg of potassium perchlorate orally 2 hours after oral administration of radioiodine (preferably ^{123}I) and evaluating its effect on RAIU in the next hour. In normal individuals, perchlorate inhibits further radioiodine uptake from the plasma, but since the intrathyroidal radioiodine is almost all bounded to the Tg, the discharge from the gland of free intrathyroidal radioiodine is <10%. Conversely, in patients with organification defects, all the unbound radioiodine will be discharged and this amount exceeds 10%.

Iodine organification defects are distinct in total or partially on the basis of the entity of the radioiodine discharged. In case of a total defect, over 90% of radioiodine is discharged, whereas in partial defects the amount ranges from 90% to 10%. In Pendred's syndrome, a CT or MR of the inner ear will show the morphological abnormalities. Since the organification defects may be caused by mutations of different genes (PDS, TPO, DUOX2, DUOX2A), genetic analyses are needed to identify the gene involved.

13.6.4 ABNORMALITIES OF TG

The diagnosis of this defect is performed by the finding of low or absent basal serum Tg concentrations that do not increase after rhTSH administration (Table 13.7). The patients are usually hypothyroid and show large goiters on thyroid ultrasound along with elevated radioiodine uptake. Genetic analyses may be useful to identify the mutations involved in the defect.

TABLE 13.7
Diagnosis of Tg Defects

Test	Finding
I Level	
TSH	Usually increased
FT_4, FT_3	Usually decreased
Thyroid ultrasound	Goiter in most cases
Basal serum Tg	Decreased or absent
II Level	
Serum Tg after rhTSH test	No change
Radioiodine uptake	Increased
Genetic analyses	Identification of Tg mutations

TABLE 13.8
Diagnosis of Iodothyrosine Deiodinase Defect

Test	Finding
I Level	
TSH	Usually increased
FT_4, FT_3	Usually decreased
Thyroid ultrasound	Goiter in most cases
Plasma and urine MIT and DIT	Increased
II Level	
Radioiodine uptake	Increased with spontaneous discharge
Genetic analyses	Identification of DHEAL1 mutations

13.6.5 DEFECT OF IODIDE RECYCLING

This defect is highly suspected in patients with goiter and hypothyroidism who exhibit high radioiodine uptake followed by a rapid and spontaneous release of the radionuclide. The diagnosis is confirmed by elevated plasma and urine levels of MIT and DIT, evaluated with radioimmunoassay or with high performance liquid chromatography and tandem mass spectrometry (HPLC-MS/MS) that has better diagnostic accuracy (Table 13.8). Genetic analyses may be performed to identify the mutation of the DHEAL1 gene.

13.7 THERAPY

Both euthyroid and hypothyroid dyshormonogenetic goiters are treated with levothyroxine (LT_4) in an attempt to reduce TSH concentrations and therefore decrease the thyroid enlargement. LT_4 is administered at a suppressive dose, i.e., the dose that brings serum TSH values between 0.4 and 1 mU/L. Therapy is personalized on the basis mainly of age, weight, and body composition (lean versus fat mass) as described in Chapters 10 and 11.

In patients with large goiters that cause tracheal and/or esophageal deviation or compression or in cases of goiters show substernal growth, a total or near total thyroidectomy is recommended followed by LT_4 replacement. In patients with iodide recycling defects or mild defects of iodide transport, iodine supplementation (Lugol solution, 10 to 20 drops/day) has been suggested as an alternative approach to LT_4. Fetal large goiter identified by ultrasonography may be treated with intra-amniotic injection of LT_4. Several treatment regimens have been reported in the literature with doses ranging from 5.5 to 33 µg/Kg/injection and number of injections varying from 1 to 6.[14]

13.8 PROGNOSIS

The introduction of newborn screening for congenital hypothyroidism allows early diagnosis and treatment of all patients with hypothyroidism at birth. For patients with thyroid dyshormonogenesis, the best results for the management of both goiter and hypothyroidism are obtained by early LT_4 therapy. Failure to promptly diagnose the disease during infancy and childhood may irreversibly impair growth and mental development and may make a goiter resistant to suppressive hormonal therapy. However, proper treatment allows an excellent prognosis for the quality of life and for survival.

13.9 FOLLOW-UP

As already discussed in Chapter 11, hypothyroid children require frequent follow-up aimed to assess growth (weight, length, head circumference), neurodevelopmental milestone attainment, and thyroid functional status. Table 13.9 reports the recommended follow-up schedule. Thyroid status must be evaluated at follow-up also in patients with diagnosis of euthyroid goiters since hypothyroidism may develop later due to increased thyroid hormone requirements. Table 13.10 details levothyroxine doses.

TABLE 13.9
Follow-Up of Patients with Dyshormonogenetic Goiter

Age	Clinical Evaluation, TSH and FT_4 Assays	Thyroid Ultrasound
Newborns and infants	2 to 4 weeks after starting therapy	Every 3 months
	Every 1 to 2 months for first 6 months	
	Then every 3 to 4 months	
Children and adolescents	Every 6 months	Every 6 months
Adults	Every 12 months	Every 12 months

Note: Clinical evaluation and TSH and FT_4 assays are recommended 1 month after any change of dose regardless of age.

13.10 SCREENING

Screening for dyshormonogenetic goiter is recommended in all cases of goiter and/or hypothyroidism of unidentified etiology that occur at birth or early in life. Furthermore, all the relatives of patients with thyroid dyshormonogenetic defects should be also screened even if they are asymptomatic. Indeed, screening allows identification of heterozygous carrier and affected individuals who are asymptomatic at screening but at risk to develop goiter and hypothyroidism later.

TABLE 13.10
Drug Cited in This Chapter

Drug	Dosage Forms	Dose Range
Levothyroxine (LT$_4$)	Tablets, capsules, solution for intravenous injection,[a] oral solution (drops)[a]	25–200 µg/day

[a] Not available in every country.

REFERENCES

1. Thompson, L. 2005. Dyshormonogenetic goiter of the thyroid gland. *Ear Nose Throat J* 84: 200.
2. Rastogi, M.V. and LaFranchi, S.H. 2010. Congenital hypothyroidism. *Orphanet J Rare Dis* 5: 17–22.
3. Avbelj, M., Tahirovic, H., Debeljak, M. et al. T. 2007. High prevalence of thyroid peroxidase gene mutations in patients with thyroid dyshormonogenesis. *Eur J Endocrinol* 156: 511–519.
4. Bizhanova, A. and Kopp, P. 2010. Genetics and phenomics of Pendred syndrome. *Mol Cell Endocrinol* 322: 83–90.
5. Macchia, P.E. and Fenzi, G.F. 2010. Genetic defects in thyroid hormone synthesis and action. In *Endocrinology, Adult and Pediatric*, Jameson, J.D. and DeGroot, L.J. Philadelphia: Saunders, Elsevier, 1721–1732.
6. Persani, L., Calebiro, D., Cordella, D. et al. 2010. Genetics and phenomics of hypothyroidism due to TSH resistance. *Mol Cell Endocrinol* 322: 72–82.
7. Grasberger, H. and Refetoff, S. 2011. Genetic causes of congenital hypothyroidism due to dyshormonogenesis. *Curr Opin Pediatr* 23: 421–428.
8. Kopp, P., Pesce, L., and Solis, J.C. 2008. Pendred syndrome and iodide transport in the thyroid. *Trends Endocrinol Metab* 19: 260–268.
9. Ris-Stalpers, C. and Bikker H. 2010. Genetics and phenomics of hypothyroidism due to TPO mutations. *Mol Cell Endocrinol* 322: 38–43.
10. Grasberger, H. 2010. Defects of thyroidal hydrogen peroxide generation in congenital hypothyroidism. *Mol Cell Endocrinol* 322: 99–106.
11. Hulur, I., Hermanns, P., Nestoris, C. et al. 2011. A single copy of the recently identified dual oxidase maturation factor (DUOXA) 1 gene produces only mild transient hypothyroidism in a patient with a novel biallelic DUOXA2 mutation and monoallelic DUOXA1 deletion. *J Clin Endocrinol Metab* 96: E841–E845.
12. Targovnik, H.M., Citterio, C.E., and Rivolta, C.M. 2011. Thyroglobulin gene mutations in congenital hypothyroidism. *Horm Res Paediatr* 75: 311–321.
13. Moreno, J.C. and Visser, T.J. 2010. Genetics and phenomics of hypothyroidism and goiter due to iodotyrosine deiodinase (DHEAL1) gene mutations. *Mol Cell Endocrinol* 322: 91–98.
14. Ribault, V., Castanet, M., Bertrand, A.M. et al. 2009. Experience with intraamniotic thyroxine treatment in nonimmune fetal goitrous hypothyroidism in 12 cases. *J Clin Endocrinol Metab* 94: 3731–1739.

14 Syndromes of Reduced Sensitivity to Thyroid Hormones

Paolo Beck-Peccoz, Irene Campi, and Luca Persani

CONTENTS

Key words: TRβ, thyroid response element (TRE), resistance to thyroid hormones, GRTH, PRTH, TSH-oma, glycoprotein hormone α-subunit (α-GSU), SHBG, transporters, MCT8, deiodinases, selenoproteins, SECISBP2.

14.1 DEFINITIONS

Thyroid hormone resistance encompasses a number of syndromes that cause reduced end-organ responsiveness to thyroid hormones (T_4 and T_3). The classical form of thyroid hormone resistance, first described in 1967 by Refetoff and collaborators,[1] is characterized by elevated levels of circulating T_4 and T_3 in the presence of measurable serum TSH concentrations as a consequence of mutations of thyroid hormone beta receptor (TRβ). Recently, other forms of insensitivity due to defects in cell surface transporter (monocarboxylate transporter 8: MCT8) or genetic disorder of thyroid hormone metabolism due to alterations of selenoprotein synthesis involving the deiodinase enzymes have been identified.[2–6]

14.2 THYROID HORMONE ACTION

Biological actions of thyroid hormones (THs) on target tissues depend on a number of variables that include cell surface transporters, intracellular deiodination, and nuclear action via thyroid hormone receptors[7] (Figure 14.1). The effects of TH are essentially intracellular and require transport of iodothyronines across plasma membranes. Different cell surface transporters such as MCT8 mediate TH uptake. The discovery of specific thyroid hormone transporters into cells was one of the most important scientific advances in the field of thyroidology.[8] Moreover, recent data suggest that the complex hormone binding proteins may enter cells, thus providing another pathway for cellular uptake of biologically active hormones.[9] Therefore, the old dogma that thyroid hormones passively cross plasma membranes must be revised and the so-called free hormone hypothesis entirely revisited.

The systemic and local bioavailability of iodothyronine is regulated by three different iodothyronine deiodinases. They are selenocysteine-containing enzymes that remove iodide from thyroxine and its metabolites, thus activating (mainly by mediating the T_4 to T_3 conversion) or inactivating the iodothyronines. Genetic mutations in proteins belonging to the multiprotein complex involved in selenium incorporation, such as the selenocysteine insertion sequence-binding protein 2 (SECIBP2), cause a deficient production of selenoprotein and consequently an abnormal thyroid hormone metabolism.[3,10]

TH effects at nuclear level are mediated by two TH receptors (TRα and TRβ) encoded by separate genes that are differently expressed in the various tissues. TRβ is expressed mainly in the hypothalamus, pituitary, and liver. TRα predominates in the CNS and skeletal and cardiac muscle. A number of cofactor proteins (coactivators and corepressors) are also involved in TH receptor signaling. Thyroid hormone receptors belong to the nuclear receptor superfamily. They act by binding as heterodimers with retinoid X receptor (RXR) or less frequently as homodimers to regulatory DNA sequences defined as thyroid response elements

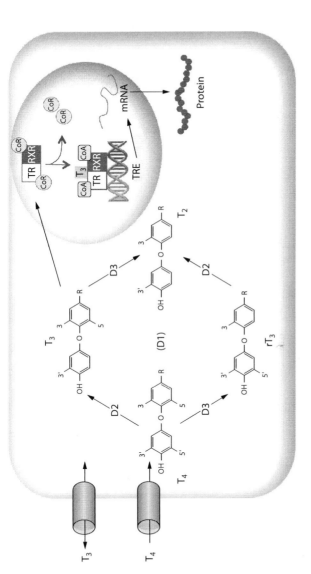

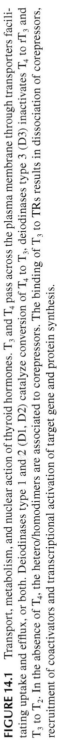

FIGURE 14.1 Transport, metabolism, and nuclear action of thyroid hormones. T_3 and T_4 pass across the plasma membrane through transporters facilitating uptake and efflux, or both. Deiodinases type 1 and 2 (D1, D2) catalyze conversion of T_4 to T_3, deiodinases type 3 (D3) inactivates T_4 to rT_3 and T_3 to T_2. In the absence of T_4, the hetero/homodimers are associated to corepressors. The binding of T_3 to TRs results in dissociation of corepressors, recruitment of coactivators and transcriptional activation of target gene and protein synthesis.

(TREs) in the promoters of target genes. In the absence of T_3, the heterodimers and homodimers are associated to corepressors. Binding of T_3 to TRs results in dissociation of corepressors, recruitment of coactivators, and transcriptional activation (Figure 14.1).

14.3   HIGH T_4 AND T_3 WITH UNSUPPRESSED TSH: DIFFERENTIAL DIAGNOSIS

Several genetic disorders (Table 14.1) and different clinical contexts (Table 14.2) are characterized by the presence of elevated serum T_4 and/or T_3 levels along with measurable TSH. In the first instance, the recognition and exclusion of any assay interferences is critical, hence the use of the direct two-step method or equilibrium dialysis to assay FT_4 and FT_3 is highly recommended.[11]

Familial dysalbuminemic hyperthyroxinemia is an autosomal dominant condition caused by albumin gene mutations that lead to increased affinity of the mutated protein for T_4 or T_3. Consequently, serum total T_4 is raised, whereas free T_4 is normal. However, single-step or analog immunometric assays, unlike the two-step methods or equilibrium dialysis, are susceptible to interference on FT_4 measurement. Interference in TSH measurement may be caused by circulating anti-TSH or heterophilic antibodies. The latter may bind the animal monoclonal antibodies used in a given immunoassay and produce erroneous results. The use of blocking reagents,

---

TABLE 14.1

Genetic Disorders Characterized by Increased Serum Thyroid Hormone Levels and Detectable TSH Concentrations

Disorder	Gene	Free T_4	Free T_3	TSH	Total Reverse T_3	SHBG
Familial dysalbuminemic hyperthyroxinemia (FDH)	*ALB*	N[a]	N[a]	N	↑	N
Resistance to thyroid hormone (RTH)	*TRB*	↑	↑	N or slightly ↑	↑	N
Defect of thyroid hormone transport (Allan-Herndon-Dudley syndrome)	*MCT8*	N or borderline ↓	↑	N or slightly ↑	↓	↑
Defect of thyroid hormone metabolism (SBP2 deficiency)	*SBP2*	↑	N or borderline ↓	N or slightly ↑	↑	N

Note: Interferences leading to spuriously high levels of FT_4 and FT_3 may appear if other methods are used. N = normal. SHBG = sex hormone-binding globulin.

[a] As measured by equilibrium dialysis or direct two-step measurement methods.

TABLE 14.2

Causes of Elevated Serum Thyroid Hormone Levels with Detectable TSH Concentrations in Different Clinical Contexts

Condition	TT_4	TT_3	Free T_4	Free T_3	rT_3	TSH
Raised serum binding proteins	↑	↑	N	N	N	N
Familial dysalbuminemic hyperthyroxinemia	↑	N/↑	N[a]	N[a]	↑	N
Antiiodothyronine autoantibodies	↑	↑	N	N	N	N
Hyperthyroidism in presence of antithyroid-stimulating hormone (TSH) antibodies	↑	↑	↑	↑	N	N
Non-thyroidal illness	↓	↓	N/↓	↓	↑	N/↓
Acute psychiatric disorders	↑	N	↑	N	N	N/↑
Neonatal period	N	N/↑	N/↑	N/↑	N	N
Drugs (e.g., amiodarone)	↑	N	↑	N/↓	↑	N
Thyroxine replacement therapy (including noncompliance)	N	N	↑	N	N	N
TSH-secreting pituitary adenoma	↑	↑	↑	↑	↑	N
Resistance to thyroid hormone	↑	↑	↑	↑	↑	N
Disorder of thyroid hormone transport	N or slightly ↓	↑	N	↑	↓	N or slightly ↑
Disorder of thyroid hormone metabolism	↑	N/↓	↑	N/↓	↑	N/↑

Note: Interferences leading to spuriously high levels of FT_4 and FT_3 may appear if other methods are used. N = normal.

[a] As measured by equilibrium dialysis or direct two-step measurement methods.

the preanalytic removal of immunoglobulins from the serum (e.g., by PEG precipitation), the modification of assay antibodies by removal of the Fc fragment, and using chimeric "humanized" antibodies are well-known methods for avoiding this interference. In practice, a serial serum dilution and recovery test may help identify an incorrect result due to interfering factors.

Finally, acute systemic illnesses, psychiatric disorders, neonatal period, and certain drugs (heparin and amphetamines) have been associated with abnormal TH levels. These potential causes can be easily ruled out by a return to a normal thyroid function following recovery or drug withdrawal. Levothyroxine replacement therapy taken intermittently can be another cause of hyperthyroxinemia with measurable serum TSH.

After confirmation of the absence of methodological interferences, a differential diagnosis will distinguish resistance to thyroid hormones (RTH) and TSH-secreting pituitary adenoma. A correct diagnosis of such conditions is mandatory because each condition requires a completely different clinical management approach.[12]

14.4   RESISTANCE TO THYROID HORMONES

14.4.1   INCIDENCE AND INHERITANCE

RTH is a rare disorder and, until now, more than 1,000 cases involving about 300 different families with a wide geographic and ethnic distribution have been published.[2,5] The actual prevalence of the disease remains unknown because routine screening programs for congenital hypothyroidism based on TSH measurement cannot detect this condition. A limited survey in a laboratory measuring both TSH and total T_4 in a cohort of 80,000 newborns found a single case among 40,000 live births. Most cases (80 to 85%) are familial and the disease is inherited in an autosomal dominant fashion.

14.4.2   CLINICAL FEATURES

Goiter is present in most patients, independent of clinical symptoms. Indeed, there are no clinical signs or symptoms typical of RTH. Its wide clinical picture ranges from asymptomatic cases to subjects who exhibit manifest thyrotoxic symptoms (Table 14.3). Most RTH subjects compensate for the genetic defect at the expense of high circulating TH concentrations. The effectiveness of this compensatory mechanism is variable in each individual, in different tissues of the same individual, and during different periods of life.

Classically, RTH subjects have been divided into two subgroups according to the absence or presence of symptoms of thyrotoxicosis, i.e., generalized thyroid hormone resistance (GRTH) and selective pituitary resistance (PRTH), respectively. Patients with GRTH usually display compensated hypothyroidism, while those with PRTH exhibit variable symptoms of hyperthyroidism.[13,14] Although both forms of RTH overlap, this distinction is clinically helpful. However, TRβ mutations found in both GRTH and PRTH may be the same and in addition, patients belonging to the same family may present with either form. Indeed, PRTH patients have normal levels of sex-hormone-binding globulin, a marker of peripheral thyroid hormone action elevated in cases of hyperthyroidism, thus suggesting that insensitivity to TH action is present not only in the hypothalamius–pituitary region, but also in the liver.[15]

14.4.2.1   Goiter

Diffuse or multinodular goiter is a common finding. Goiters in RTH patients who have normal TSH levels are attributed to increased biological activity of circulating TSH molecules. In RTH patients treated with surgical ablation, goiters commonly relapse with nodular alterations and gross asymmetries and require additional surgery or radioiodine.

14.4.2.2   Cardiovascular System

Approximately 75% of RTH patients with either GRTH or PRTH exhibit palpitations and tachycardia at rest. Atrial fibrillation is present at higher frequency in patients with RTH as compared to the general population. Predominance of TRα at heart

TABLE 14.3
Testing and Clinical Features of Resistance to Thyroid Hormone (RTH)

Tissue	Tests	Clinical Features
Central nervous system	MRI: normal or pituitary incidentalomas	Attention deficit hyperactivity disorder (ADHD), hyperkinetic behavior, learning disabilities, mental retardation with IQ <60 (rare)
Eye		Color blindness only in homozygous TRβ deletion
Hearing	Sensorineural and conductive impairment	Hearing impairment, deafness (homozygous mutation and severe dominant negative mutation)
Muscles	Magnetic resonance spectroscopy: TCA/ATP synthesis uncoupling	
Bone	Reduced femur and spine BMD, normal markers of bone turnover	Stippled epiphyses, dysmorphic facies, winged scapulae (homozygous TRβ deletions), delayed bone maturation, height below 5th percentile in children, final adult height not affected
Reproductive system		Increased risk of miscarriage, intrauterine growth retardation of unaffected offspring
Metabolism	Increased REE and BMR, high LDL, impaired insulin sensitivity	Reduced BMI
Gastrointestinal		Hyperphagia (children)
Heart	Mitral valve prolapse, increased systolic cardiac performance, inadequate diastolic filling time, increased systemic vascular resistance, arterial stiffness	Tachycardia, atrial fibrillation
Immune system		Increased frequency of airway infections (pneumonia and upper airways infection)
Thyroid	Thyroid scintigraphy: normal ^{131}I uptake	Goiter

level may explain these clinical signs, as the few mutated TRβs exert less dominant negative effects on normal receptors.

Increased systolic cardiac performance associated with inadequate diastolic filling time and increased incidence of mitral valve prolapse have been reported in RTH subjects. Some indices of cardiac systolic and diastolic function (e.g., stroke volume, cardiac output, maximal aortic flow velocity) were intermediate between values in normal and hyperthyroid subjects, further supporting a partially hyperthyroid response of the heart in RTH subjects. Other parameters (e.g., ejection and shortening fractions of the left ventricle, systolic diameter, and left ventricle wall thickness) were not different. Finally, systemic vascular resistance and arterial stiffness are increased in RTH.

14.4.2.3 Central Nervous System and Hearing

Delayed developmental milestones and language disorders seem to be more frequent in RTH patients than in unaffected relatives. Mild learning disabilities (IQ <85) have been described in 30% of affected subjects, while severe mental retardation (IQ <60) is present in only 3%. It has been hypothesized that these defects are caused by uncompensated hypothyroidism at an early stage of neuroanatomical development. Some authors reported a high frequency of attention deficit hyperactivity disorder (ADHD) in their RTH cohorts. This finding has not been confirmed by other groups, but it is conceivable that low IQ accounts for ADHD manifestations.

An increased incidence of conductive or sensorineural hearing impairment has been found in RTH. The conductive defect is probably related to the susceptibility to upper airways infection in RTH children, whereas defective TRβ expression may be responsible for the cochlear dysfunction. A single kindred with deaf mutism[1] had a recessively inherited RTH due to a homozygous complete deletion of the TRβ gene. The same situation has been found in mice with targeted disruptions of the entire TRβ locus that develop profound sensorineural hearing loss, thus suggesting an important role of TH in the early developmental stages of hearing system development. Moreover, the hearing impairment may contribute to the defective speech development and language disorders found in some RTH children. Although deletion of the TRβ2 isoform produces a selective loss of M-cone photoreceptors resulting in abnormal color vision, no common color blindness has been described in RTH patients harboring heterozygous TRβ mutations.

14.4.2.4 Growth and Bone Maturation

Skeletal abnormalities, such as epiphysis abnormalities (stippled epiphyses), dysmorphic facies, and winged scapulae have been documented only in the first two cases of harboring homozygous deletion of the TRβ gene described in the literature. Delayed growth and bone maturation are present in about one-third of children with RTH. In addition, height below the 5th percentile for age and sex is a relatively common finding. However, the final adult heights did not seem affected and were no different from heights of unaffected relatives.

Preliminary data on bone mineral density, measured at the head of a femur or at the lumbar spine showed a reduction of this parameter in combination with normal markers of bone turnover. It is still debated whether these features would indicate a thyrotoxic or hypothyroid skeletal state. The prevalent expression of TRα isoforms in bone, stimulated by high TH levels, would predispose to a precocious osteoporosis and increasing risk of fracture. Conversely, the lack of correlation between bone mineral density and markers of bone turnover suggests a reduced bone formation rate resulting in a low peak bone mass. These findings are similar to those observed in childhood hypothyroidism.

14.4.2.5 Metabolism

Basal metabolic rate (BMR) has been found normal or increased, particularly in PRTH patients. However, the low body mass indices reported in about 30% of RTH children may account for the elevated BMR. Recently, an enhanced resting energy expenditure (REE) assessed by indirect calorimetry has been found in adults and children with TRβ mutations. This increase was intermediate between euthyroid and thyrotoxic subjects. In addition, RTH subjects, particularly children, have hyperphagia and enhanced energy intake that is considered a clinical feature of thyrotoxicosis.

Noteworthy, in both RTH and hyperthyroid patients, TH excess was associated with uncoupling between tricarboxylic acid cycle activity and ATP synthesis in vivo as measured by magnetic resonance spectroscopy. Indeed, mean heart rate and REE correlate in both RTH and thyrotoxicosis, suggesting a similar sensitivity of skeletal muscle and myocardium to TH. Thus, these tissues in which the TRα isoform expression is prevalent may be the major factors responsible of increased energy expenditure. Finally, reduced whole-body insulin sensitivity and dyslipidemia have been documented in a number of patients, suggesting increased cardiovascular risk in RTH.

14.4.2.6 Associated Disorders

Occasionally, RTH occurs in association with autoimmune thyroid disorders such as Graves' disease or Hashimoto's thyroiditis. However, the occurrence of anti-TPO or anti-TSH receptor autoantibodies in 70 RTH subjects was similar to that found in normal controls. The rare RTH patients who develop Graves' disease undergo a progressive increase in goiter size along with frank symptoms of thyrotoxicosis. The further elevation of TH levels causes TSH secretion to be totally inhibited. Conversely, hypothyroidism may occur in the presence of normal serum TH concentrations as consequence of Hashimoto's thyroiditis.

Coexistence of TSH-secreting pituitary adenomas (TSH-omas) and RTH has been suggested in only two cases. In theory, it has been hypothesized that the impaired TH feedback in the pituitary may lead to a continuous stimulus to thyrotropes to synthesize and secrete TSH molecules. Whether this permanent stimulus may play a role in the development of pituitary tumors remains a matter of debate. However, the pituitary lesions associated with RTH appear to be pituitary incidentalomas and not true TSH-secreting tumors.[12]

The frequency of respiratory infections (pulmonitis and infections of the upper respiratory tract) appears higher in RTH patients than in their unaffected relatives. This susceptibility has been related to reduced immunoglobulin concentrations. The linkage between the two disorders may be the presence of receptors for TH in granulocytes and lymphocytes.

Age of puberty and fertility do not seem affected by RTH. However, a retrospective study of a large family has shown a higher rate of miscarriage in mothers affected with RTH and intrauterine growth retardation of offspring unaffected by RTH, thus suggesting that intrauterine exposure to high TH levels exerts adverse effects on a fetus.RTH may have contributed to the death of only one patient homozygous for TRβ mutation. This patient had a resting pulse of 190 beats per minute and died from cardiogenic shock complicated by septicemia.

14.4.3 LABORATORY FEATURES AND DIFFERENTIAL DIAGNOSIS

Patients with RTH have elevated serum concentrations of both FT_4 and FT_3 and a normal or slightly elevated serum TSH, i.e., a biochemical phenotype that rules out all other forms of classical hyperthyroidism. No difference in the above hormones has been found between patients with RTH and those with TSH-oma.[12] PRTH patients who may exhibit signs and symptoms of hyperthyroidism no different from those seen in patients with TSH-oma show similar biochemical parameters.[4]

The measurement of glycoprotein hormone α-subunit (α-GSU) may help in differential diagnosis. In patients with TSH-omas, serum levels of α-GSU and α-GSU/TSH molar ratios are definitely elevated in more than 70 and 80% of them, respectively. Both indices in RTH patients are within normal range for age, sex, and circulating levels of gonadotropins (Figure 14.2).

To assess the degree of resistance in specific target tissues, different parameters have been proposed in vivo (basal metabolic rate, systolic time intervals, Achilles reflex time) and in vitro (sex hormone-binding globulin [SHBG], angiotensin converting enzyme [ACE], carboxy terminal telopeptide of type 1 collagen [ICTP], soluble interleukin-2 receptor [sIL-2R], osteocalcin). Table 14.4 details the parameters.

In particular, SHBG and ICTP are clearly elevated in patients with TSH-omas and normal in RTH. However, these markers seem more useful in assessing a state of severe hyperthyroidism than mild thyroid dysfunction. Nevertheless, the sensitivity and specificity of these tests can be improved when evaluated after oral administration of supraphysiological doses of T_3 (50 µg/day for 3 days, followed by 100 µg/day

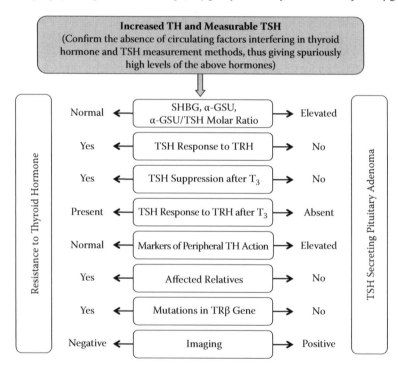

FIGURE 14.2 Flowchart for differential diagnosis of resistance to thyroid hormone (RTH) and TSH-secreting pituitary adenoma (TSH-oma). After exclusion of methodological interference, the biochemical phenotypes of both RTH and TSH-oma are confirmed. A series of clinical, biochemical, and genetic tests may be necessary to reach the final diagnosis.

TABLE 14.4
Parameters for Evaluating Peripheral Thyroid Hormone Action

Tissue	Parameters	RTH Patients	TSH-oma or Other Forms of Thyrotoxicosis
Pituitary	TSH	N/slightly ↑	N/slightly ↑
	α-GSU	N	↑
Liver	SHBG	N	↑
	Ferritin	N	↑
	Cholesterol	N/↑	↓
Skeletal muscle	CPK	N/↑	↑↑
	Ankle jerk relaxation time	N/↑	↑↑
Heart and cardiovascular system	Sleeping pulse rate	↑	↑↑
	Systolic time interval	↑	↑↑
	Diastolic isovolumetric relaxation time	↓	↓↓
Bone	Height	Short stature in childhood, normal in adults	Accelerated growth and bone maturation
	Bone age	N/delayed	Advanced
	Osteocalcin	N	↑↑
	Alkaline phosphatise	N/↑	↑↑
	Pyridinium crosslinks	N/↑	↑↑
	ICTP	N/↑	↑↑
Hematological	sIL2R	N/↑	↑↑
Lung	ACE	N/↑ in PRTH	↑↑
General	Basal metabolic rate	N/↑	↑↑

for another 3 days, and then 200 µg/day for 3 more days).[6] In RTH patients, the increases of some parameters such as SHBG, ICTP, cholesterol, creatinine kinase, ferritin, and heart rate are markedly reduced in comparison to normal subjects, thus definitively confirming resistance to TH action.

As to dynamic testing, a TRH test (intravenous injection of 200 µg TRH) has been widely used. In most patients affected with TSH-oma, TSH and α-GSU levels do not increase after TRH injection, whereas RTH subjects show normal TSH responses. An exaggerated response is found in patients who underwent thyroid ablation or were treated with antithyroid drugs.

A T_3 inhibitory test at dosages reported above or administration of T_3 for 8 to 10 days at doses of 80 to 100 µg/day may show a full inhibition of TSH levels in RTH patients, but TSH response to TRH carried out at the end of T_3 administration is still present a result not seen in control subjects. Since none of these tests has a clear diagnostic cut-off value, combining them where possible increases the specificity and sensitivity of the diagnostic process.

First-degree relatives who exhibit the same biochemical pattern of thyroid function serve as further evidence of RTH since familial cases of TSH-oma have been reported only for four families in a setting of multiple endocrine neoplasia.[1] Molecular analysis of the gene encoding TRβ can finally make a definitive diagnosis in 85 to 90% of cases of RTH (Figure 14.2). Finally, pituitary MRI should be performed in the event of unequivocal results from other tests. The presence of a pituitary lesion in combination with lack of TSH response to dynamic tests and high levels of α-GSU or α-GSU/TSH molar ratio strongly supports the diagnosis of TSH-oma. However, the detection of pituitary lesion does not definitely exclude a diagnosis of RTH because this finding is quite common (20 to 25% of MR images performed for other reasons) in the general population. These lesions should be considered pituitary incidentalomas, especially if hypothalamic–pituitary dysfunction is ruled out.

14.4.3.1 Molecular Genetics

In most subjects (nearly 85%), RTH is associated with heterozygous mutations of the TRβ gene. The mutant receptors display either reduced affinity for T_3 or impaired interaction with the cofactors (coactivators and corepressors), thus losing its ability to modulate target gene expression in different tissues. The mutations are distributed in the carboxyl terminus of TRβ. Typically, three CpG-rich hot spot regions located in the ligand-binding domain and in the contiguous hinge domain of the protein are involved. In contrast to results observed for other nuclear receptors (such as vitamin D, androgen receptor, or PPARγ), no mutations have been identified in the DNA-binding domain or in other regions of the receptor.

In about 10 to 15% of the cases with clinical and biochemical phenotypes of RTH, no mutation could be found in the TRβ gene; this situation is defined as non-TRβ RTH. It is speculated that these patients may have an abnormality of one of the cofactors or TH transporters into the cells.

To explain the presence of resistance in individuals heterozygous for the mutation, it was discovered that the mutant receptor exerts a dominant negative effect because the mutant protein inhibits the activity of the wild type β and α receptors. To exert this effect, mutant receptors must retain normal dimerization and DNA binding properties. In the original RTH family,[1] the disease segregated as an autosomal recessive trait and a deletion of exons 4 through 10 was identified. The deletion destroyed the ability of the receptor to dimerize and bind the DNA. The homozygous patient showed goiter and deaf mutism along with high TH levels. Heterozygous subjects were phenotypically normal, further supporting the concept that the presence of a single normal allele is sufficient for normal receptor function and only the presence of a mutant receptor may impair the function of the normal copy. Heterozygous mutations in regions other than the three hot spots may be clinically silent because they lack dominant negative properties.

14.4.4 Pathogenesis of Variable Resistance

As noted above, RTH subjects are clinically defined as GRTH when they display compensated hypothyroidism and classified as PRTH if they exhibit variable symptoms of hyperthyroidism. There is a significant overlap between these two forms because the symptoms are variable.

Differences in the degree of hormonal resistance are linked to the different levels of TRβ and TRα expression in different tissues. TRβ mainly is expressed in the hypothalamus, kidney, liver, anterior pituitary gland, hypothalamus, retina, and cochlea. TRα predominates in skeletal and cardiac muscles, brain, brown fat, intestine, spleen, and vascular endothelial cells. Consequently, symptoms of TH deficiency and excess may coexist. As an example, hypercholesterolemia, delayed bone maturation, growth retardation, and learning disabilities are suggestive of hypothyroidism, while weight loss, heat intolerance, hyperactivity, and tachycardia are compatible with thyrotoxicosis.

14.4.5 THERAPEUTIC APPROACHES

There is currently no definite treatment to correct the molecular defect causing RTH. In most patients, high levels of circulating free TH compensate for the resistance in peripheral tissues and those subjects are clinically euthyroid. Goiter may be the only sign of the disease. In general, the presence of hyperthyroid symptoms is the criterion to define the requirement for therapy.

For patients with signs and symptoms of thyrotoxicosis such as tachycardia and palpitations at rest, the most appropriate therapy is cardioselective β-blockers (atenolol or others). Propranolol is not appropriate because it inhibits the peripheral conversion of T_4 to T_3, thus worsening a possible hypothyroid state in some tissues. However, in the event of severe thyrotoxic symptoms that do not respond to selective β-blockers, a reduction of thyroid hormone levels may be beneficial. Antithyroid drugs are contraindicated, because the increase of TSH levels may lead to enlargement of the goiter and pituitary hyperplasia.

The administration of thyromimetic compounds, such as 3,5,3'-triiodothyroacetic acid (TRIAC), has been shown to be beneficial in both children and adult patients with RTH at the dose ranging from 1.4 to 2.8 mg/day, fractionated in twice or thrice daily administrations.[3,5,16] TRIAC, through a feedback mechanism, reduces TSH secretion, but exerts fewer thyromimetic effects on peripheral tissues. The slight decrease of circulating T_4 levels (values of T_3 are unreliable as TRIAC cross reacts in T_3 measurement methods) reduces the thyrotoxic signs and symptoms, particularly at the heart level.

The use of dopaminergic drugs and somatostatin analogs has met with limited success because TSH secretion rapidly escapes the inhibitory effects of both drugs, as the T_4 reduction triggers the much more potent stimulatory effect of TH negative feedback mechanism. Although controversial, in children with signs of growth or mental retardation, the administration of supraphysiological doses of LT_4 to overcome the high degree of resistance present in some tissues may be beneficial. Supraphysiological doses of thyroid hormones are also necessary in patients treated with total thyroidectomy for a missed diagnosis of RTH. The use of high doses of LT_4 requires careful monitoring by assessing the indices of peripheral thyroid hormone action.

Recently, TRβ-selective agonists (GC1, eprotirome) have been developed and may be beneficial for some abnormalities (dyslipidemia) found in RTH. Conversely, the development of TRα-selective antagonists may be useful in controlling symptoms of thyrotoxicosis mediated through TRα. It is conceivable that future treatments may be based on administration of small molecules that block TSH receptor activity on thyroid cell surfaces.[17] Moreover, the possible application of gene therapy to RTH patients is aimed to silence the mutated receptor or repair the mutated nucleotide responsible for the expression of the abnormal receptor protein.

14.5   DISORDERS OF THYROID HORMONE TRANSPORT

Mutations in the gene encoding the most important transporter investigated, namely the monocarboxylate transporter 8 (MCT8) gene, cause a particular form of resistance to T_3 action in the brain in a setting of a neurological syndrome characterized by severe neurodevelopmental abnormalities. This clinical situation was first described in 1944 by Allan, Herndon, and Dudley who gave the disorder the name of X-linked mental retardation. Since then, the syndrome has carried the names of the three initial finders. Only recently have abnormal thyroid function tests been discovered in such patients, a finding that leads many researchers to evaluate possible mutations in the gene encoding thyroid hormone transporter MCT8.[5,6,8]

14.5.1   INCIDENCE AND INHERITANCE

About 60 families with mutations in MCT8 have been described worldwide. Only male patients are affected as the MCT8 gene is located on chromosome Xq13.2. Carrier females show very mild thyroid dysfunction.

14.5.2   CLINICAL AND LABORATORY FEATURES

At birth, patients appear to be completely normal. However, during the first years of life, an increasingly severe hypotonia become manifest and progresses into distal spasticity and difficult head control. The final height is reduced and the body weight is extremely low, mainly due to disproportionate muscle wasting and the inability to eat properly due to difficulties in swallowing. Delayed myelination of the brain is recorded at MR in the second year of life but subsequently disappears. Adult patients are unable to sit, stand, and walk and show very low IQs (<40). Somatosensory stimuli such as the changing of clothes or lifting an affected child trigger aimless movements and characteristic paroxysms of kinesigenic dyskinesias. Not infrequent are also brisk reflexes, clonus, and nystagmus, along with true epileptic seizures[10,18] (Table 14.5).

In addition to severe psychomotor retardation, patients show several abnormalities of the hypothalamic–pituitary–thyroid axis. Serum FT_3 levels are very high, whereas FT_4 and rT_3 concentrations are clearly reduced. In contrast, serum TSH levels are high to normal or definitely high a finding that clearly supports the presence of T_3 insensitivity at hypothalamic–pituitary level. Interestingly, along with thyroid hormone resistance in the brain that mimics a state of severe hypothyroidism, the findings of high levels of SHBG and low levels of cholesterol suggest a state of peripheral hyperthyroidism in the liver. Also, the muscle wasting may be related

TABLE 14.5

Testing and Clinical Features of Defects of Thyroid Hormone Transport Caused by Mutations of MCT8 Gene (Allan-Herndon-Dudley Syndrome)

Tissue	Tests	Clinical Features
Central nervous system	Delayed myelination, leukodystrophy, white matter changes	Severe psychomotor development delay, ataxia, dysarthria, clonus, hyperreflexia, extensor plantar responses
Behavior and cognitive function	Normal Griffith's test	Mental retardation, inability to communicate, lacking gaze contact, irritability
Eyes	Normal VEP	Nystagmus, strabismus, no fixation
Hearing	Normal AEP	Auricle abnormalities (cupped ears)
Bone		Pectus excavatum, scoliosis
Muscles	Normal CPK, normal muscle biopsy	Proximal hypotonia, reduced muscle mass, spastic paraplegia and quadriplegia, inability to sit, stand, and walk
Gastrointestinal		Inability to swallow, reduced feeding, constipation

Note: VEP = visual evoked potential. AEP = auditory evoked potential. CPK = creatine phosphokinase.

to a state of hyperthyroidism at that level. Finally, the presence of a blunted response of TSH to TRH was recently reported. This observation suggests that the lack of functional MTC8 transporter may be counterbalanced at the thyrotrope level by very high serum T_3 concentrations.[19]

14.5.3 MOLECULAR GENETICS

Different types of mutations (deletions, insertions, nonsense, missense, etc.) may be found everywhere along the nucleotide sequence of MCT8 gene. There are no doubts that these mutations cause the clinical picture of the disorder. In fact, *in vitro* studies clearly show that the mutated proteins lose the ability to transport T_3 into cells. No phenotype–genotype correlation has been demonstrated except for early death.

14.5.4 PATHOGENESIS

It is well known that thyroid hormones are fundamental for brain development. Since MCT8 is the main transporter of thyroid hormone into brain neurons, it is obvious that inactivation of the transporter results in impaired CNS development, leading to severe psychomotor retardation.[8]

14.5.5 THERAPEUTIC APPROACHES

Experience in treating patients with this rare form of TH insensitivity is very modest. Today, two different approaches to MCT8 deficiency have been evaluated. The first is normalizing serum T_4 and T_3 levels with a block-and-replace regimen using a combination of propylthiouracil (PTU) and T_4. This treatment did not result in neurologic improvement, but had a marked beneficial effect on body weight and heart rate. In effect, neurologic benefit can only occur if such therapy is initiated soon after birth or even during pregnancy by administering TH analogs able to cross the placenta. The second approach is the administration of TH analogs that enter the brain cells independently of MCT8. Promising results using diiodothyropropionic acid (DITPA) have been observed in MCT8 knockout mice. Clinical trials in patients with MCT8 mutations have been initiated, and the results are (anxiously) awaited.[5,6,8]

14.6   DISORDERS OF THYROID HORMONE METABOLISM

Iodothyronine deiodinases (DIOs) constitute a family of selenocysteine-containing enzymes required for the activation or inactivation of thyroid hormones and their metabolites. Individuals with defective functions of deiodinases show distinctive abnormal patterns of thyroid function characterized by high free T_4, low free T_3, and raised reverse T_3 associated with normal or slightly elevated TSH levels. Mutations in SECIS-binding protein 2 (SBP2), a key protein that allows the incorporation of selenium in selenoproteins, cause defective production of DIOs. Because the selenoproteins are ubiquitous and multifunctional, along with abnormal thyroid function, affected individuals manifest a complex phenotype.[3,6,10]

14.6.1   INCIDENCE AND INHERITANCE

Only six families exhibiting reduced TH sensitivity due to a disorder of thyroid hormone metabolism have been described. The defect is inherited in an autosomal recessive fashion and caused by homozygous and compound heterozygous mutations in the SBP2 gene.

14.6.2   CLINICAL FEATURES

The clinical picture is multiform with patients who present a milder phenotype and others who are more severely affected (Table 14.6). Deficiencies of multiple selenoproteins have been documented in all cases. Glutathione peroxidases are markedly reduced and circulating levels of hepatic selenoprotein P are low, accounting for the low serum selenium levels recorded in these families.[10] Childhood growth retardation is a common feature in all the families described. Axial muscle dystrophy with clinical features similar to selenoprotein-related myopathy has been reported.

One subject was azoospermic, with reduced levels of testis-enriched selenoproteins that caused spermatogenic arrest. In addition, he was markedly photosensitive, with a dermal deficiency of antioxidant selenoenzymes causing increased cellular reactive oxygen species, membrane lipid peroxidation, and oxidative DNA damage. Reduction of antioxidant enzymes in immune cells was associated with impaired T cell proliferation and shortened telomeric DNA. The latter was associated with anemia and lymphopenia, similar to those observed in aplastic anemia found in telomerase deficiency. Increased adipose mass and insulin sensitivity have been described in two families.

TABLE 14.6
Testing and Clinical Features of Defects of Thyroid Hormone Metabolism Caused by Mutations of SBP2 Gene

Tissue	Tests	Clinical Features
Central nervous system	Normal MR	Growth delay (children), speech delay (hearing impairment)
Hearing	Mid- to high-frequency sensorineural hearing loss, AEP: normal, MRI: normal cochlear architecture	Mild hearing loss
Muscles	Biopsy: myopathy with type 1 fiber prevalence, increased serum CPK-MM, MRI: loss of normal spinal curvature and fatty infiltration of paraspinal muscles and Sartorius muscle groups	Axial muscular dystrophy, hypostenia, rigid spine, hypotonia
Reproductive system	Biopsy: spermatogenic maturation arrest. Azoospermia, normal testosterone, LH, and FSH	Male infertility
Metabolism	Increased insulin sensitivity, fasting hypoglycaemia, favorable serum lipid profile	Increased subcutaneous adipose tissue, normal or reduced visceral adipose tissue
Gastrointestinal	Colon biopsy: eosinophilic colitis (rare)	Colitis (rare)
Skin	Positive photosensitivity tests	Photosensitivity
Miscellaneous	Leukopenia, anemia, low serum selenium levels	

14.6.3   MOLECULAR GENETICS AND PATHOGENESIS

This defect is caused by mutations in SBP2, a factor required for the incorporation of selenocysteine during selenoprotein biosynthesis. Selenoproteins constitute a family of about 25 proteins with wide functions including metabolism of thyroid hormones (deiodinases), removal of cellular reactive oxygen species, reduction of oxidized methionines in proteins, and transport and delivery of selenium to peripheral tissues.

SBP2 mediates the incorporation of the amino acid selenocysteine during selenoprotein synthesis. A specific stem–loop (SECIS elements) in the 3'-UTR region of selenoprotein mRNAs interacts with a multiprotein complex including SBP2 and leads to selenocysteine incorporation at UGA codons.[6] Defects in this machinery result in miscoding of the UGA as a stop codon and the transcript may undergo decay. The affinity of SBP2 for SECIS elements of different mRNAs is variable and this contributes to hierarchy in selenoprotein production in cases of defective function of SBP2 or Se deficiency. In mice, complete disruption of SBP2 is embryonically lethal. In humans, the SBP2 mutations described cause a severe reduction (but not total depletion) of selenoprotein. This is probably due to the highly complex architecture of SBP2, with internal methionine residues capable of starting the synthesis of shorter protein isoforms.

14.6.4 THERAPEUTIC APPROACHES

Clinical trials with oral selenium supplementation showed raised circulating selenium concentrations without improving thyroid abnormalities. T_3 treatment was clearly beneficial for growth in two children. Tocopherols, lycopene, and other antioxidant agents may be beneficial in reducing the oxidative damage, as suggested by preliminary *in vitro* experiments.

REFERENCES

1. Refetoff, S., DeWind, L.T., and DeGroot, L.J. 1967. Familial syndrome combining deaf mutism, stippled epiphyses, goiter and abnormally high PBI: possible target organ refractoriness to thyroid hormone. *J Clin Endocrinol* 27: 279–294.
2. Refetoff, S., Weiss, R.E., and Usala, S.J. 1993. The syndromes of resistance to thyroid hormone, *Endocrinol Rev* 14: 348–399.
3. Refetoff, S. and Dumitrescu, A.M. 2007. Syndromes of reduced sensitivity to thyroid hormone: genetic defects in hormone receptors, cell transporters and deiodination. *Best Pract Res Clin Endocrinol Metab* 21: 277–305.
4. Agrawal, N.K., Goyal, R., Rastogi, A. et al. 2008. Thyroid hormone resistance. *Postgrad Med J* 84: 473–477.
5. Gurnell, M., Visser, T.J., Beck-Peccoz, P. et al. 2010. Resistance to thyroid hormone. In *Endocrinology, Adult and Pediatric,* 6th ed. Jameson, L.J. and DeGroot, L.J., Eds. Philadelphia: Saunders, Elsevier, 1745–1759.
6. Refetoff, S. and Dumitrescu, A.M. 2010. Resistance to thyroid hormone. In *Thyroid Disease Manager,* Chapter 16D (http://www.thyroidmanager.org).
7. Cheng, S.Y., Leonard, J.L., and Davis, P.J. 2010. Molecular aspects of thyroid hormone actions. *Endocrinol Rev* 31: 139–170.
8. Visser, W.E., Friesema, E.C., and Visser, T.J. 2011. Minireview: thyroid hormone transporters: the knowns and the unknowns. *Mol Endocrinol* 25: 1–14.
9. Hammes, A., Andreassen, T.K., Spoelgen, R. et al. 2005. Role of endocytosis in cellular uptake of sex steroids. *Cell* 122: 751–762.
10. Schoenmakers, E., Agostini, M., Mitchell, C. et al. 2010. Mutations in the selenocysteine insertion sequence-binding protein 2 gene lead to a multisystem selenoprotein deficiency disorder in humans. *J Clin Invest* 120: 4220–4235.
11. Gurnell, M., Halsall, D.J., and Chatterjee, V.K. 2011. What should be done when thyroid function tests do not make sense? *Clin Endocrinol (Oxf)* 74: 673–678.
12. Beck-Peccoz, P. and Persani, L. 2010. TSH-producing adenomas. In *Endocrinology, Adult and Pediatric,* 6th ed. Jameson, L.J. and DeGroot, L.J., Eds. Philadelphia: Saunders, Elsevier, 324–332.
13. Beck-Peccoz, P. and Chatterjee, V.K.K. 1994. The variable clinical phenotype in thyroid hormone resistance syndrome. *Thyroid.* 4: 225–231.
14. Beck-Peccoz, P., Persani, L., Calebiro, D. et al. 2006. Syndromes of hormone resistance in the hypothalamic–pituitary–thyroid axis. *Best Pract Res Clin Endocrinol Metab* 20: 529–546.
15. Beck-Peccoz, P., Roncoroni, R., Mariotti, S. et al. 1990. Sex hormone-binding globulin measurement in patients with inappropriate secretion of thyrotropin (IST): evidence against selective pituitary thyroid hormone resistance in non-neoplastic IST. *J Clin Endocrinol Metab* 71: 19–25.
16. Beck-Peccoz, P., Piscitelli, G., Cattaneo, M.G. et al. 1983. Successful treatment of hyperthyroidism due to non-neoplastic pituitary TSH hypersecretion with 3,5,3′-triiodothyroacetic acid (TRIAC). *J Endocrinol Invest* 6: 217–223.

17. Neumann, S., Eliseeva, E., McCoy, J.G. et al. 2011. A new small-molecule antagonist inhibits Graves' disease antibody activation of the TSH receptor. *J Clin Endocrinol Metab* 96: 548–554.

18. Biebermann, H., Ambrugger, P., Tarnow, P. et al. 2005. Extended clinical phenotype, endocrine investigations and functional studies of a loss-of-function mutation A150V in the thyroid hormone specific transporter MCT8. *Eur J Endocrinol* 153: 359–366.

19. Boccone, L., Mariotti, S., Dessì, V. et al. 2010. Allan-Herndon-Dudley syndrome (AHDS) caused by a novel SLC16A2 gene mutation showing severe neurologic features and unexpectedly low TRH-stimulated serum TSH. *Eur J Med Genet* 53: 392–395.

15 Transient Hypothyroidism

Bernadette Biondi

CONTENTS

Key words: subclinical hypothyroidism, thyrotropin, levothyroxine, transient subclinical hypothyroidism, subacute, painless or postpartum thyroiditis, untreated adrenal insufficiency, partial thyroidectomy, radioactive iodine therapy, amiodarone, radiographic contrast agents, lithium carbonate, cytokines (especially interferon-α), aminoglutetimide, ethionamide, sulfonamides and sulfonylureas, tyrosine kinase inhibitors, obesity.

15.1 DEFINITION

Transient hypothyroidism (THypo) is defined as a period of reduced mild thyroid function with elevated TSH, which is followed by a euthyroid state. Transient cases of TSH increase are frequently caused by viral or autoimmune thyroiditis, drugs that interfere with thyroid function, or toxic injury that may affect the thyroid gland.[1]

15.2 ETIOPATHOGENESIS AND EPIDEMIOLOGY

Table 15.1 details TSH increases not associated with persistent subclinical hypothyroidism. Hypo should be distinguished from other causes of physiological, false, or transient increased serum TSH levels. Autoimmune thyroiditis is frequently chronic but not always permanent. Most patients with subclinical hypothyroidism (sHypo) due to chronic autoimmune thyroiditis require lifelong thyroxine replacement therapy with increasing LT_4 doses for the progression of thyroid failure. However, spontaneous recoveries may occur in about 50% of cases.

The rate of normalization is greater in patients who have lesser degrees of serum TSH elevation and negative antithyroid antibody titers. The transient expression of TSH receptor blocking antibodies may explain the recovery of thyroid function in some cases. Some patients may become hypothyroid 4 to 8 weeks after subtotal

TABLE 15.1

Serum TSH Increases Not Associated with Persistent Subclinical Hypothyroidism

Transient subclinical hypothyroidism following subacute, painless or postpartum thyroiditis

After withdrawal of thyroid hormone therapy in euthyroid patients

Laboratory analytical problem (assay variability, heterophilic antibodies)

Recovery phase of euthyroid sick syndrome

Untreated adrenal insufficiency

Thyroid injury: partial thyroidectomy or other neck surgery, radioactive iodine therapy, external radiotherapy of head and neck

Drugs impairing thyroid function: iodine and iodine-containing medications (amiodarone, radiographic contrast agents), lithium carbonate, cytokines (especially IFNα) aminoglutetimide, ethionamide, sulfonamides and sulfonylureas, tyrosine kinase inhibitors

Thyroid infiltration (amyloidosis, sarcoidosis, hemochromatosis, Riedel's thyroiditis, cystinosis, AIDS, primary thyroid lymphoma)

Obesity

Toxic substances, industrial and environmental agents

thyroidectomy. However, thyroid function could recover several weeks or months later. The probable explanation for this mechanism may be that the remaining thyroid tissue is able to compensate and maintain normal thyroid secretion only after TSH stimulation.

Patients with Graves' hyperthyroidism after radioiodine ablation may have transient hypothyroidism for several weeks or months. Withdrawal of exogenous thyroid therapy is necessary when persistent TSH suppression develops during replacement doses of LT$_4$.

The term *thyroiditis* defines a group of thyroid disorders characterized by some form of thyroid inflammation. Transient hypothyroidism may be due to viral (subacute thyroiditis) or autoimmune disease (postpartum, painless or silent thyroiditis). Patients with thyroiditis have transient hyperthyroidism, that usually lasts only until the accumulations of T$_4$ and T$_3$ are depleted in 2 to 6 weeks. Hypothyroidism is rarely permanent.

The prevalence of postpartum thyroiditis (PPT) is about 10%.[2] About 33% of women with autoimmune thyroiditis may have transient hypothyroidism during the postpartum period, and the prevalence of PPT in type I diabetes mellitus is 25%. About 20 to 30% of women with postpartum thyroiditis have hyperthyroidism followed by transient hypothyroidism; 40 to 50% have only transient hypothyroidism during PPT.

Transient hypothyroidism may be caused by drugs such as lithium carbonate, interferon-α, interleukin-2, and those that contain iodine. Lithium may inhibit thyroid hormone release and hormone synthesis. Long-term treatment with lithium may induce subclinical hypothyroidism in about 20% of patients; this disorder is more common in patients with underlying autoimmune disease.[3]

Both iodine deficiency and excess can cause hypothyroidism. An excess of iodine may develop during treatment with cough medicines, dietary supplements, iodine-containing substances (e.g., betadine) used on the skin or vagina, drugs such as amiodarone, and radiographic contrast agents. Iodine excess can cause hypothyroidism by inhibiting iodide organification and T_4 and triiodothyronine (T_3) synthesis (Wolff-Chaikoff effect). Subjects usually "escape" quickly from this effect of iodine. However, patients with chronic autoimmune thyroiditis and those who have undergone partial thyroidectomies, radioiodine therapy, and painless, postpartum or subacute thyroiditis are at risk for iodine-induced hypothyroidism.

Amiodarone-induced hypothyroidism occurs predominantly in the first 18 months of treatment and it is more frequent in females with preexisting thyroid antibodies. Its prevalence is higher in areas of high iodine intake than in areas with lower intake (22 versus 5%, respectively).[4]

Interferon has marked immunomodulatory effects and may induce the development of autoimmune phenomena or aggravate pre-existing autoimmunity.[5,6] The prevalence of hypothyroidism in patients receiving interleukin-2 or interferon-α (IFNα) for malignant tumors or hepatitis B or C is about 5 to 20%. Two types of IFNα-induced hypothyroidism have been recognized: autoimmune and non-autoimmune. Interferon-α-induced autoimmune hypothyroidism develops in patients with positive TPO antibodies. Conversely, interferon-α-induced non-autoimmune hypothyroidism is a destructive thyroiditis responsible for an early thyrotoxic phase caused by the release of preformed thyroid hormones and a late hypothyroid phase with a complete resolution and reversible hypothyroidism.

Tyrosine kinase inhibitors that exert antiangiogenic and antitumor activities frequently affect thyroid gland function and thyroid hormone metabolism.[7] Tyrosine kinase inhibitors are used to treat a variety of disorders (e.g., gastrointestinal stromal tumors, renal cell carcinoma, and thyroid tumors). Imatinib and motesanib, sunitinib, and sorafenib therapy may induce primary hypothyroidism in many patients and may require an increase in the replacement doses of LT_4 in hypothyroid patients. Primary hypothyroidism develops in about 36 to 61% of patients treated with sunibitin and may be transient or persistent. The probability of hypothyroidism increases with the duration of treatment.

Transient TSH elevations may be caused by drugs that interfere with the central neurodopaminergic pathway, such as metoclopramide and phenothiazines. A transient increase in TSH is common in hospitalized patients during the recovery phase of euthyroid sick syndrome. TSH concentrations may be falsely increased in some assays because of the presence of heterophilic antibodies against mouse proteins.

Patients with untreated adrenal insufficiency may have high serum TSH concentrations.[8] The level of serum TSH is higher in elderly subjects than in younger ones. However, the high prevalence of increased serum TSH may not always reflect mild thyroid hormone deficiency in elderly subjects because the distribution of serum TSH shifts to higher concentrations with age, reflecting an alteration of TSH glycosylation or an altered feedback set point.

Serum TSH levels are higher in overweight and obese individuals than in lean subjects and this may falsely suggest THypo, especially in patients with negative thyroid autoantibodies.[9] However, the mild increase in serum TSH in obese subjects is usually associated with high to normal free T_3 serum levels, which indicates increased deiodinase activity as a compensatory mechanism for fat accumulation to improve energy expenditure.

TABLE 15.2

Causes of Transient Congenital Hypothyroidism

Maternal administration of antithyroid drugs

Transplacental passage of maternal TSH receptor blocking antibodies

Maternal and neonatal iodine deficiency or excess

Heterozygous mutations of THOX2 or DUOXA2

Congenital hepatic hemangioma/hemangioendothelioma

15.3 TRANSIENT CONGENITAL HYPOTHYROIDISM

Congenital hypothyroidism (CH) can be permanent or transient.[10–12] Table 15.2 lists the causes of transient CH. Permanent CH is a persistent deficiency of thyroid hormone that requires lifelong treatment. Conversely, transient CH is a temporary deficiency of thyroid hormone discovered at birth that recovers with normal thyroid hormone production. Recovery to euthyroidism typically occurs in the first few months or years of life. About 10 to 20% of newborns who are hypothyroid have temporary forms of transient CH that has several causes.

- An iodine deficiency in a newborn caused by insufficient iodine intake of the mother. Iodine deficiency is more common in European countries than in the United States, especially in preterm infants.
- TSH-receptor blocking antibodies (TRB-Abs) in pregnant women with autoimmune thyroid disease. The antibodies can cross the placenta and block the TSH receptor, affecting thyroid function of the fetus and causing hypothyroidism at birth. This may not happen in all women with autoimmune thyroid diseases. This transient form of hypothyroidism resolves in 3 to 6 months after birth when maternal antibody levels fall.
- Antithyroid drugs (propylthiouracil [PTU], methimazole) administered to pregnant hyperthyroid women. These drugs cross the placenta, causing hypothyroidism in newborns. It usually disappears several days after birth and normal thyroid function returns within a few weeks.
- Fetus or newborn exposure to high doses of iodine can cause transient hypothyroidism. This iodine exposure can result from the use of an iodine-based medication or iodine-containing antiseptics or contrast agents. The maternal administration of amiodarone may cause transient hypothyroidism in their infants. Transient hypothyroidism also occurs when iodine antiseptic compounds are used by mothers or after exposure to iodinated contrast agents. However, this may be related to the type and duration of exposure. Vaginal application of povidone or iodine during delivery or topical use of disinfectants in newborns can lead to increased serum TSH concentration and transient neonatal hypothyroidism.
- Liver hemangiomas. There are reports of congenital liver hemangiomas that produce large amounts of type 3 iodothyronine deiodinase. This produces a consumptive type of hypothyroidism in which large doses of thyroxine

are required to maintain euthyroidism. Serum T_4 levels are low, TSH is elevated, and reverse T_3 levels are also increased.
* Mutations in DUOX2 (THOX2) and DUOXA2 can lead to transient congenital hypothyroidism.

15.4 DIAGNOSIS

Table 15.3 lists diagnosis factors for THypo. A diagnosis of THypo should be verified in patients with Hashimoto's thyroiditis when LT_4 therapy is reduced during treatment for the progressive TSH decrease. In fact, in some patients a spontaneous resolution of hypothyroidism occurs because of the disappearance of TSH receptor blocking antibodies. Changes in the titers of coexisting TSH receptor that block and stimulate antibodies explain the alternating courses of hypothyroidism and hyperthyroidism that may be observed in the same subject.

Family history for thyroid disease or thyroid autoimmunity, recent delivery, previous thyroid surgery, ^{131}I therapy, and the use of specific drugs should be investigated in patients with THypo. A careful clinical examination and the determination of TPO antibodies should be performed in patients receiving drugs that may interfere with thyroid function or induce thyroid autoimmunity.

Patient with transient thyroiditis may be identified by mild symptoms of hypothyroidism preceded by an episode of mild thyrotoxicosis. Transient thyrotoxicosis may develop within 3 to 6 months after delivery as painless or postpartum thyroiditis (PPT) followed by a period of transient hypothyroidism and a return to the euthyroid state. In the early phase of the disease, a mild TSH increase may make it difficult to distinguish patients who will recover from those who will develop permanent hypothyroidism.

Long-term follow-up should be performed in these patients. A test for antithyroid peroxidase antibodies may be useful to predict the likelihood of progression to permanent overt hypothyroidism in patients with subclinical hypothyroidism or those with painless (silent) or postpartum thyroiditis.

TABLE 15.3
Diagnosis of Transient Hypothyroidism

I Level

TSH, FT_4, FT_3
AB-Tg and Ab-TPO
Thyroid Doppler ultrasound

II Level

Thyroid scan and radioiodine uptake
Erythrocyte sedimentation rate (ESR)
C-reactive protein
TSH receptor blocking and stimulating antibodies
Urinary iodine excretion

TABLE 15.4

Normal Values of Thyroid Function Tests in Childhood and Adolescence

Age	TSH (μU/mL)	TT$_4$ (μg/dL)	FT$_4$ (ng/dL)
1–4 days	1.0–10	11.0–21.5	2.2–5.3
1–4 weeks	1.7–9.1	8.2–17.2	0.9–2.3
1–12 months	0.8–8.2	5.9–16.3	0.8–1.8
1–5 years	0.7–4.5	7.3–15.0	0.8–2.1
6–10 years	0.7–4.5	6.4–13.3	1.0–2.1
11–15 years	0.7–4.5	5.5–11.7	0.8–2.0
16–20 years	0.7–4.5	4.2–11.8	0.8–2.0

The presence of antithyroid peroxidase antibodies before treatment appears to be the most significant risk factor for the development of clinical thyroid disease during treatment with lithium, interferon, or amiodarone. Elevated TPO antibodies before starting these drugs may have a positive predictive value (about 68% for IFNα) for the risk of developing autoimmune hypothyroidism. TPO antibodies may also develop de novo during IFNα treatment in 10 to 40%. Additional risk factors for thyroid disease during interferon treatment may include female gender, older age, and the presence of other autoantibodies. The addition of ribavirin to interferon therapy may increase the risk of developing hypothyroidism.

The diagnosis of transient congenital hypothyroidism should be confirmed by findings of elevated serum TSH and low free T$_4$ levels compared to normal values reported in Table 15.4; see Figure 15.1. Other diagnostic tests such as thyroid radionuclide uptake and scan, thyroid ultrasonography, or serum thyroglobulin determination can help clarify the underlying etiology of hypothyroidism, although treatment may be started without these tests.

15.5 TREATMENT

Only persistent or progressive subclinical hypothyroidism (SHypo) should be considered an early stage of thyroid disease and should be treated. Transient hypothyroidism usually requires short-term or no therapy.

Transient hypothyroidism can last a few weeks or as long as 6 months in patients with thyroiditis. Patients with minimal symptoms may not require therapy. Those with symptomatic hypothyroidism should be treated with T$_4$ for several months and then therapy should be discontinued. A normal serum TSH value 6 weeks later will confirm the recovery of thyroid function.

SHypo during treatment with lithium carbonate, iodine-containing drugs, IFNα, and interleukin-2 may disappear when these drugs are discontinued, especially in patients with negative thyroid autoantibodies. Most patients with thyroid dysfunction recover after the withdrawal of these drugs. Spontaneous normalizations of thyroid function can be expected in many patients. Interruption of interferon treatment may

Congenital Hypothyroidism: Diagnostic Algorithm

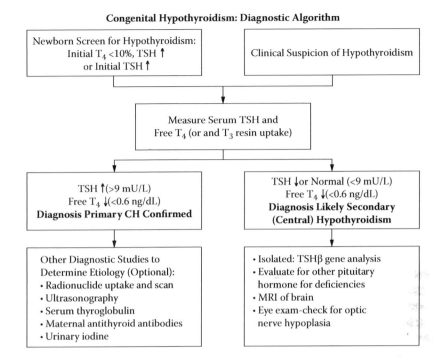

FIGURE 15.1 Diagnostic algorithm for definitive diagnosis of congenital hypothyroidism. (*Source:* Rastogi, M.V. and LaFranchi, S.H. 2010. *Orphanet J Rare Dis* 10: 5–17. With permission. http://www.biomedcentral.com/info/about/reprintsandperm)

not always be necessary if hypothyroidism develops during treatment; however, LT$_4$ therapy is recommended for patients with severe symptoms.

Levothyroxine may be considered in cases of severe congenital transient hypothyroidism. The recommended starting dose is 10 to 15 µg/kg/day. The goals of the treatment are to rapidly raise the serum T$_4$ above 130 nmol/L (10 µg/dL) and normalize serum TSH levels.

15.6 FOLLOW-UP

In women with positive TPO, thyroid function (FT$_4$ and TSH) should be assessed in the postpartum period. Women who experience postpartum thyroiditis have a 40% risk to redevelop postpartum thyroiditis after a subsequent pregnancy. About 20 to 30% of women with postpartum thyroiditis will develop permanent hypothyroidism within 5 years; the risk is higher in women with high titers of TPO antibodies.

Thyroid screening (TSH, TPO antibodies) is recommended for all patients before starting IFNα, amiodarone, or lithium therapy. If TSH is normal and TPO antibodies are negative, TSH should be monitored every 3 months during treatment with these drugs. If TPO antibodies are present, TSH monitoring every two months may be useful.

The altered thyroid hormone patterns in obese patients are reversible by weight loss. However, an increased risk of autoimmune hypothyroidism has been reported in obese subjects, suggesting the need for long-term follow-up of thyroid function. Frequent laboratory monitoring in infancy is essential to ensure an optimal neurocognitive outcome in congenital hypothyroidism. Serum TSH and FT_4 should be measured every 1 to 2 months in the first 6 months of life and every 3 to 4 months thereafter.

Screening of newborns is now routine in the United States, Canada, Western Europe, Israel, Japan, Australia, and New Zealand and is under development in Eastern Europe, South America, Asia, and Africa. It is estimated that 12 million infants are screened worldwide and 3,000 with hypothyroidism are detected annually. Additional evaluation of thyroid function is recommended when an initial blood screening test identifies a potential problem.

REFERENCES

1. Biondi, B. and Cooper, D.S. 2008. The clinical significance of subclinical thyroid dysfunction. *Endocrinol Rev* 29: 76–131.
2. Sarvghadi, F., Hedayati, M., Mehrabi, Y. et al. 2005 Follow up of patients with postpartum thyroiditis: a population-based study. *Endocrine* 27: 279–282.
3. Kleiner, J., Altshuler, L, Hendrick, V. et al. 1999. Lithium-induced subclinical hypothyroidism: review of the literature and guidelines for treatment. *J Clin Psychiatr* 60: 249–255.
4. Basaria, S. and Cooper, D.S. 2004. Amiodarone and the thyroid. *Am J Med* 118: 706–714.
5. Carella, C., Mazziotti, G., Amato, G. et al. 2004. Clinical review 169: Interferon-alpha-related thyroid disease: pathophysiological, epidemiological, and clinical aspects. *J Clin Endocrinol Metab* 89: 3656–3661.
6. Caraccio, N., Dardano, A., Manfredonia, F. et al. 2005. Long-term follow-up of 106 multiple sclerosis patients undergoing interferon-beta 1a or 1b therapy: predictive factors of thyroid disease development and duration. *J Clin Endocrinol Metab* 90: 4133–4137.
7. Desai, J., Yassa, L., Marqusee, E. et al. 2006. Hypothyroidism after sunitinib treatment for patients with gastrointestinal stromal tumors. *Ann Intern Med* 145: 660–664.
8. Betterle, C., Dal Pra, C., Mantero, F. et al. 2002. Autoimmune adrenal insufficiency and autoimmune polyendocrine syndromes: autoantibodies, autoantigens, and their applicability in diagnosis and disease prediction. *Endocrinol Rev* 23: 327–364.
9. Biondi, B. 2010. Thyroid and obesity: an intriguing relationship. *J Clin Endocrinol Metab* 95: 3614–3617.
10. Gaudino, R., Garel, C., Czernichow, P. et al. 2005. Proportion of various types of thyroid disorders among newborns with congenital hypothyroidism and normally located gland: a regional cohort study. *Clin Endocrinol (Oxf)* 62: 444–448.
11. Parks, J.S., Lin, M., Grosse, S.D. et al. 2010. The impact of transient hypothyroidism on the increasing rate of congenital hypothyroidism in the United States. *Pediatrics* 2 Suppl: S54–S63.
12. Rastogi, M.V. and LaFranchi, S.H. 2010. Congenital hypothyroidism. *Orphanet J Rare Dis* 10: 5–17.

16 Subclinical Hypothyroidism

Bernadette Biondi

CONTENTS

Key words: subclinical hypothyroidism, thyrotropin, levothyroxine, replacement therapy, prevalence, progression, cardiovascular risk, heart, symptoms, cognitive function, pregnancy, infertility, elderly.

16.1 DEFINITION

Subclinical hypothyroidism (SHypo) represents a condition of mild to moderate thyroid hormone deficiency. It is characterized by normal thyroid hormones, although at the lower limits of their normal ranges, and mild or elevated serum TSH concentrations.[1] In recent decades, the upper reference limit for TSH declined from 10 to 4.0 to 4.5 mIU/L. In the definition of SHypo, we distinguish patients with mildly increased serum TSH levels (5 to 9 mIU/L) and patients with more severely increased serum TSH levels (>10 mIU/L).

16.2 EPIDEMIOLOGY

The prevalence of SHypo has been reported to be between 4 and 10% of adult population samples.[1-3] This wide range may be due to the TSH cut-off used to define SHypo and differences in age, gender, and dietary iodine intake in the populations studied. Subclinical hypothyroidism is more frequent in areas of iodine sufficiency (4.2% in iodine-deficient areas compared to 23.9% in areas of abundant iodine intake). Iodine supplementation may increase the incidence of hypothyroidism. The prevalence of mild thyroid function is higher in women and in older populations. In the ninth decade of life the prevalence of elevated TSH is 15 to 20%.

16.3 ETIOPATHOGENESIS

The etiology of SHypo is the same as the etiology of overt hypothyroidism (Table 16.1). Chronic lymphocytic thyroiditis, an autoimmune disorder of the thyroid gland, is the most common cause of acquired persistent mild, subclinical, or overt hypothyroidism in adult patients. Subjects with family or personal histories of autoimmune endocrine diseases and non-endocrine autoimmune disorders (vitiligo, pernicious anemia, celiac disease, atrophic gastritis, multiple sclerosis, etc.) may face increased risks of developing autoimmune hypothyroidism (Table 16.2). Turner's syndrome and Down syndrome are both associated with higher than expected rates of autoimmune thyroiditis (Table 16.2).

TABLE 16.1
Common Causes of Overt Primary Hypothyroidism

Chronic autoimmune thyroiditis

Treated hyperthyroidism: radioiodine

Surgery

External radiation of neck

Iodine and iodine-containing medications

Drugs (lithium, interferon-α, tamoxifen, aminoglutetimide, serotonin reuptake inhibitors, tricyclic antidepressant agents, etc.)

TABLE 16.2
Special Population at Higher Risk of Developing Hypothyroidism

Postpartum women

Individuals with family history of autoimmune thyroid disorders

Other autoimmune endocrine conditions (type I diabetes mellitus, adrenal insufficiency, ovarian failure, etc.)

Other non-endocrine autoimmune disorders (celiac disease, vitiligo, pernicious anemia, Sjögren's syndrome, multiple sclerosis, primary pulmonary hypertension, etc.)

Down syndrome and Turner's syndrome

About 10 to 30% of patients with overt thyroid failure may have SHypo due to inadequate thyroid hormone supplementation. Patients with SHypo or overt hypothyroidism who take T_4 may become hypothyroid during the administration of drugs that decrease T_4 absorption (cholestyramine and iron salts), increase its clearance, (phenytoin and carbamazepine), or decrease T_4 to T_3 conversion (amiodarone). Other causes of primary hypothyroidism are partial thyroidectomy, radioactive iodine treatment, and external radiotherapy of the head and neck area. Some chemotherapy drugs may induce hypothyroidism.

Transient or persistent increases in serum TSH may occur after subacute, postpartum, or painless thyroiditis and after infiltrative disease (Riedel's thyroiditis, amyloidosis, hemochromatosis, and cystinosis) or infectious disorders of the thyroid gland. Several drugs (iodine-containing compounds, lithium carbonate, cytokines, and interferon) can induce persistent or transient subclinical or overt hypothyroidism, particularly in patients with underlying autoimmune thyroiditis.

Hypothyroidism may develop during treatment with aminoglutetimide, ethionamide, sulfonamides, and sulfonylureas that interfere with thyroid hormone synthesis. Persistent or transient TSH increases may develop after treatment with sunitinib and oral tyrosine kinase inhibitors. Exposure to pesticides, herbicides, industrial chemicals, and environmental chemicals may induce thyroid failure.

Germline loss-of-function mutations in one or both alleles of the TSH-receptor gene can cause SHypo. Thyrotropin receptor mutations should be considered in subjects with familial TSH increases associated with normal thyroid ultrasound and without markers of thyroid autoimmunity.

16.4 DIAGNOSIS

The diagnosis of SHypo is based on (1) personal and familial history, (2) clinical evaluation of symptoms and signs of thyroid hormone deficiency, (3) laboratory evaluation to assess hormonal patterns, (4) ultrasound of the thyroid gland, (5) evaluation of the cardiovascular effects of SHypo, and (6) lipid profile.

16.4.1 HISTORY

The diagnosis of subclinical hypothyroidism can be suspected in subjects with personal and familial histories of autoimmune disorders and previously treated thyroid disease (surgery or radioiodine; see Table 16.2). A detailed medical and pharmacological history is useful to exclude transient causes of high serum TSH due to the administration of drugs that may interfere with thyroid function.

16.4.2 SIGNS AND SYMPTOMS

Table 16.3 lists signs and symptoms of SHypo. The presence of symptoms in patients with SHypo is controversial. It is difficult to distinguish euthyroid subjects from patients with SHypo based on clinical symptoms because many symptoms are nonspecific. Age can further complicate the identification of symptoms of hypothyroidism

TABLE 16.3

Symptoms and Signs of Subclinical Hypothyroidism

Dry skin	Cold intolerance	Hoarseness
Poor memory	Puffy eyes	Fatigue
Slow thinking	Constipation	Muscle cramps
Muscle weakness		

due to the frequent association with chronic illnesses, use of drugs, and depression. The presence of symptoms (such as dry skin, poor memory, slow thinking, muscle weakness, fatigue, muscle cramps, cold intolerance, puffy eyes, constipation, and hoarseness) may be useful to identify patients who need thyroid function tests and select SHypo patients who can benefit from replacement therapy.[1] Patients who report more symptoms and more recently developed symptoms may be more likely to have thyroid hormone deficiency.

16.4.3 LABORATORY DIAGNOSIS

Table 16.4 details the three levels of laboratory diagnosis.

I level—Serum FT_4 and FT_3 concentrations are persistently at the lower limits of their normal ranges and serum TSH is mildly or more severely increased. SHypo should be confirmed by repeated tests. Ultrasound evaluation of the thyroid gland may show the typical hypoechocogenicity and ultrasound pattern that help identify individuals with thyroiditis. The thyroid gland is usually goitrous but may also be normal or atrophic.

II level—A high thyroid autoantibody titer (usually against anti-TPO and/or thyroglobulin) is associated with a persistently elevated serum TSH concentration in autoimmune thyroiditis. More than 90% of patients with chronic autoimmune thyroiditis have high serum concentrations of autoantibodies against thyroglobulin and thyroid peroxidase (thyroid microsomal antigen). Many patients also have antibodies that block the action of TSH on the TSH receptor or are cytotoxic to thyroid cells.

III level—A lipid profile is one component of this level. SHypo may be associated with an increases in total cholesterol (TC) and low density lipoprotein cholesterol (LDL-C) with inconsistent changes in serum levels of high-density lipoprotein cholesterol (HDL-C). The lipid pattern is usually deranged in SHypo individuals with serum TSH greater than 10 mIU/L, especially in smokers and in insulin-resistant

TABLE 16.4

Diagnosis of Primary Subclinical Hypothyroidism

I Level	II Level	III Level
TSH	Ab-TPO and Ab-Tg	Total cholesterol, HDL, LDL
FT_4, FT_3		Doppler echocardiography
Thyroid ultrasound		

subjects, suggesting that this evaluation should be performed in these specific subgroups of subjects.[4,5] Doppler echocardiography may be useful to detect the presence of diastolic dysfunction associated with SHypo and is characterized by slowed myocardial relaxation and impaired ventricular filling.[6] This technique is useful for elderly patients with SHypo and in the presence of underlying cardiac disease. Symptoms and signs of a pituitary mass or hypopituitarism suggest central hypothyroidism.

16.5 IMPLICATIONS OF SUBCLINICAL HYPOTHYROIDISM

16.5.1 PROGRESSION TO OVERT DISEASE

Progression from mild to overt hypothyroidism may be related to the cause of thyroid hormone deficiency, the basal TSH value, and patient age. A serum TSH level above 2 mIU/L is associated with increased probability of developing hypothyroidism, specifically in patients with positive thyroid autoantibodies.[2] The presence of positive thyroid peroxidase antibodies (TPOs) may have an important prognostic relevance for progression. The risk of hypothyroidism is higher in patients with TSH levels above 6 mIU/L and positive antibodies and is increased in elderly subjects and pregnant women.[1]

16.5.2 CARDIOVASCULAR RISK

The most consistent cardiac abnormality reported in patients with subclinical hypothyroidism is impaired left ventricular diastolic function. However, impaired systolic function can been identified with newer sensitive techniques (Doppler echocardiography, tissue Doppler, and cardiac magnetic resonance).[6] Table 16.5 lists cardiac abnormalities in SHypo. In impaired cardiac performance an effort has been documented in patients with SHypo. A higher incidence of heart failure has been reported in elderly patients with TSH levels above 7 to 10 mU/L[5] (Figure 16.1).[7]

Diastolic hypertension may develop in SHypo, especially in postmenopausal women. Impaired vascular function (increase in systemic vascular resistance, increased arterial stiffness, and endothelial dysfunction) and an altered lipid profile may increase the risks of atherosclerosis and coronary artery disease[1,4,8] (Table 16.5).

TABLE 16.5
Cardiovascular Abnormalities in Mild Thyroid Hormone Deficiency

Normal or depressed systolic function at rest

Left ventricular diastolic dysfunction at rest and during exercise

Impaired left ventricular systolic function on exercise

Increased systemic vascular resistance

Increased prevalence of diastolic hypertension

Increased arterial stiffness

Endothelial dysfunction

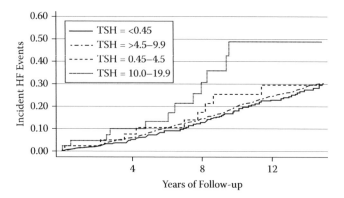

FIGURE 16.1 Subclinical hypothyroidism and risk of heart failure. (*Source:* Rodondi, N., Bauer, D.C., Cappola, A.R. et al. 2008. *J Am Coll Cardiol* 52: 1152–1159. With permission.)

A recent meta-analysis documented an increased risk of coronary heart disease (CHD) events and mortality in SHypo patients with serum TSH levels above 10 mU/L.[8]

16.6   SHYPO IN PREGNANCY

SHypo in pregnant women can represent a risk factor for pregnancy loss, preterm delivery, and placental abruption and may have deleterious effects on the intellectual development of the offspring.[1,9]

16.7   TREATMENT

Treatment of severe SHypo is recommended because of the increased risk of progression and potential adverse effects.[1,10] Treatment of persistent mild SHypo with appropriate doses of LT$_4$ to normalize serum TSH may be beneficial for reducing cardiovascular risk (Table 16.6) and is recommended in patients with TSH levels above 10 mIU/L. Small doses (i.e., 25 to 75 μg/day) are often adequate to normalize

---

TABLE 16.6

Effects of Replacement Therapy with Levothyroxine on Cardiovascular Parameters in Mild Thyroid Hormone Deficiency

Improved systolic function

Improved diastolic function at rest and during exercise

Reduction in cardiac preload

Improved endothelial function

Reduction in systemic vascular resistance

Reductions in arterial stiffness and diastolic blood pressure

Improved diastolic hypertension

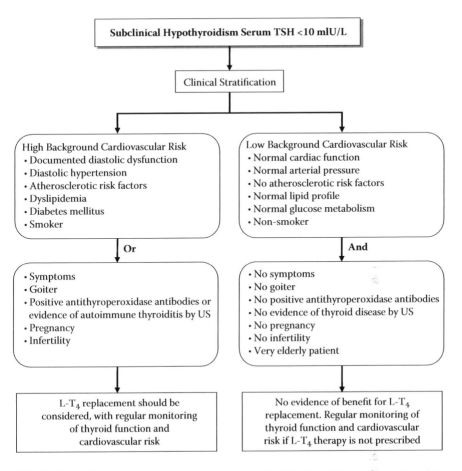

FIGURE 16.2 Indication for treatment of patients with TSH<10 mIU/L. (*Source:* Biondi, B. and Cooper, D.S. 2008. *Endocr Rev* 29: 76–131. With permission.)

serum TSH levels in SHypo (Figure 16.2). The goal of LT_4 therapy in patients with persistent SHypo is a TSH level between 1 and 2.5 mIU/L.

Conflicting opinions surround the clinical significance of mild thyroid hormone deficiency (TSH between 5 and 9 mIU/L) and there is no consensus about the TSH concentration at which treatment should be performed. It seems useful to treat mild persistent TSH increases in symptomatic patients, in those with cardiovascular risk factors, and in patients with goiters and positive thyroid antibody tests.[1,11]

Women with mild and more severe SHypo should be treated during pregnancy with LT_4. Replacement therapy should be increased during pregnancy. Furthermore, LT_4 replacement treatment should be considered in women with increased serum TSH levels who contemplate pregnancy and patients with ovulatory dysfunction and infertility because evidence indicates the potential reversibility of these dysfunctions when caused by mild thyroid failure.[1,10]

Replacement therapy is indicated in elderly patients with TSH above 10mIU/L. Therapy should be started at very low doses (12.5 to 25 μg/day) and gradually increased because of possible underlying heart disease. A reasonable target TSH level should be 3 to 4 mIU/L in individuals between 60 and 75 years and 4 to 6 mIU/L in older subjects.[1,11]

16.8 FOLLOW-UP

Periodic evaluations of serum TSH levels are required during replacement therapy with LT_4 to ensure that replacement therapy is not under- or overprescribed. A TSH test should be performed every 6 to 12 months. It is often necessary to increase the levothyroxine dosage progressively over time because of further impairment of the thyroid gland and progression to overt hypothyroidism. In cases of suppressed TSH, the levothyroxine dose should be lowered. If a low TSH persists or very low doses of LT_4 normalize thyroid function, thyroid testing should be carried out after LT_4 withdrawal to determine whether SHypo is permanent. About 50% of patients with abnormal serum TSH may be normalized after repeated testing. Approximately 20% of LT_4-treated patients have decreased serum, which usually indicates overtreatment. Physician education can improve overtreatment.

The thyroid states of women with thyroid autoimmunity should be monitored during pregnancy. TSH should be performed every 6 to 8 weeks during pregnancy and after 4 to 6 weeks if LT_4 dosage adjustment is required because of increased serum TSH levels.

The higher rate of antithyroid autoimmunity and the higher rate of progression to overt thyroid disease in subjects with TSH between 3 and 4.5 mIU/L suggest that careful follow-ups should be performed in asymptomatic patients with such serum TSH levels, especially if they have positive anti-TPO antibodies.

REFERENCES

1. Biondi, B. and Cooper, D.S. 2008. The clinical significance of subclinical thyroid dysfunction. *Endocrinol Rev* 29: 76–131.
2. Vanderpump, M.P., Tunbridge, W.M., French, J.M. et al. 1995. The incidence of thyroid disease in the community: a twenty-year follow-up of the Whickham Survey. *Clin Endocrinol* 43: 55–68.
3. Canaris, G.J., Manowitz, N.R., Mayor, G. et al. 2000. The Colorado thyroid disease prevalence study. *Arch Intern Med* 16: 526–534.
4. Danese, M.D., Ladenson, P.W., Meinert, C.L. et al. 2000. Effect of thyroxine therapy on serum lipoproteins in patients with mild thyroid failure: a quantitative review of the literature. *J Clin Endocrinol Metab* 85: 2993–3001.
5. Cappola, A.R. and Ladenson, P.W. 2003. Hypothyroidism and atherosclerosis. *J Clin Endocrinol Metab* 88: 2438–2444.
6. Biondi, B. 2007. Cardiovascular effects of mild hypothyroidism. *Thyroid* 7: 625–630.
7. Rodondi, N., Bauer, D.C., Cappola, A.R. et al. 2008. Subclinical thyroid dysfunction, cardiac function, and the risk of heart failure. *J Am Coll Cardiol* 52: 1152–1159.
8. Rodondi, N., den Elsen, W.P.J., Bauer, D.C. et al. 2010. Subclinical hypothyroidism and the risk of coronary heart disease and mortality. *JAMA* 304: 1365–1374.
9. Haddow, J.E., Palomaki, G.E., Allan, W.C. et al. 1999. Maternal thyroid deficiency during pregnancy and subsequent neuropsychological development of the child. *New Engl J Med* 341: 549–555.

10. Abalovich, M., Amino, N., Barbour, L.A. et al. 2007. Management of thyroid dysfunction during pregnancy and postpartum: an Endocrine Society Clinical Practice Guideline. *J Clin Endocrinol Metab* 92: S1–S47.
11. Biondi, B. 2009. Should we treat all subjects with subclinical thyroid disease the same way? *Eur J Endocrinol* 159: 343–345.

17 Hypothyroid Coma

Giampaolo Papi and Alfredo Pontecorvi

CONTENTS

Key words: hypothyroid coma, hypothyroidism, thyroid autoimmunity, levothyroxine substitution therapy.

17.1 DEFINITION

Hypothyroid (or myxedematous) coma is the result of a very severe, untreated hypothyroidism.[1] It is characterized by hypothermia, cardiovascular shock, and stupor that results in death if not immediately treated. It represents an endocrine emergency that should be handled in an intensive care unit. In the past, hypothyroid coma was defined as myxedematous coma because of the typical myxoedematous complication characterized by subcutaneous diffused absorption resulting from deposits of mucin and glucosaminoglycans in the interstitial and subcutaneous tissues. The myxedematous complication is very rare now and therefore the hypothyroid coma term is more appropriate.

17.2 EPIDEMIOLOGY

Hypothyroid coma manifests rarely, with a prevalence approaching 0.1% of hospitalized hypothyroid patients. It particularly affects obese female subjects aged >60 years (female:male ratio = 4:1).[5] More than 90% of cases occur in winter. Even if levothyroxine replacement therapy is quickly and appropriately given, almost half patients die.[1–6]

17.3 ETIOPATHOGENESIS

Patients display a background of thyroid hormone deficiency usually triggered by precipitating factors such as low outside temperature, systemic (mainly pulmonary) infection, cardiac insufficiency, labor, intake of anesthetics, depressants, neuroleptics, or large amounts of liquids.[1–4]

Most patients referred to emergency departments for hypothyroid coma are already followed by an endocrinologist or general practitioner for hypothyroidism due to autoimmune chronic thyroiditis, thyroidectomy, or Graves' disease treated by radioiodine (^{131}I or ^{123}I). Usually, these subjects take levothyroxine substitution therapy and may have subsequently withdrawn it on their own initiative. Rarely, the cause of a hypothyroid coma is not of primary thyroid origin and arises from reduced thyrotropin (TSH) excretion by the pituitary gland (hypopituitarism).[7]

Patients presenting with secondary hypothyroidism may have previously undergone surgery or radiotherapy due to pituitary adenoma or may be affected by a pituitary macroadenoma that overwhelms TSH-producing pituitary cells. It is important to highlight that hypothyroidism finally leading to myxedematous coma develops slowly (over months or years) in patients with chronic thyroiditis or pituitary macroadenoma. Conversely, it may occur within a few weeks in patients who have undergone thyroidectomy or hypophysectomy and do not take levothyroxine therapy. Consequently, hypothyroid coma manifests more quickly in thyroidectomized patients who withdraw levothyroxine suddenly than in subjects with previously unknown autoimmune chronic thyroiditis.

Some drugs such as amiodarone and lithium may directly cause hypothyroidism and hypothyroid coma.[3,8,9] Amiodarone is an antiarrhythmic drug that contains high amounts of iodine and induces inhibition of 5'-deiodinase activity and Wolff-Chaikoff effect. Lithium is commonly used to treat bipolar disorders; it inhibits thyroid hormone release from the thyroid and increases thyroid autoimmunity if present before therapy.[3,8] Recently, severe hypothyroidism due to impaired iodine uptake by thyrocytes that leads to coma has been described in neoplastic patients treated with tyrosine kinase-selective inhibitors.[10]

Cases of Chinese patients referred to a hospital for hypothyroid coma provoked by ingestion of raw bok choy have also been reported. Plants of the Brassicaceae family contain glucosinolate, a sulfur-containing organic anion bonded to glucose that hydrolyzes to thiocyanate, a compound known for competing with iodine. Ingestion of large amounts of Brassicaceae induces goiter and hypothyroidism.

17.4 PHYSIOPATHOLOGY

17.4.1 Thermogenesis

Thyroid hormone deficiency causes a reduction of thermogenetic activity in the human body. In hypothyroid coma, the body temperature may be reduced to 32 to

35°C. Initially, hypothermia is balanced by peripheral vessel constriction due to the enhancement of α-adrenergic and catecholamine tone; subsequently, blood volume reduction and hypovolemic shock occur.

17.4.2 CARDIOVASCULAR SYSTEM

Severe hypothyroidism and related hypothermia cause catecholamine tone elevation and consequently peripheral vessel constriction, blood volume reduction, and diastolic hypertension. These alterations represent homeostatic adaptation to reduced thermogenesis. However, persistent hypothermia finally leads to low blood pressure, extreme bradycardia, cardiomegaly, and cardiac shock.

17.4.3 RESPIRATORY SYSTEM

The respiratory system is compromised because of ventilation capacity and respiratory muscle impairment, leading to hypoxemia and hypercapnia. Reduction of ventilation capacity is also caused by superior airway obstruction, macroglossia, vocal cord edema, and pleural effusion.

17.4.4 RENAL FUNCTION AND ELECTROLYTES

Hydroelectrolyte alterations are characterized by hyponatremia and impairment of glomerular filtration. Reduction of water excretion by the kidnèys induces excess ADH secretion that consequently contributes to low serum sodium concentrations.

17.4.5 CENTRAL NERVOUS SYSTEM

Hyponatremia may provoke brain edema that compromises brain function, leading to stupor and coma. Despite hyponatremia, extracellular sodium volume is higher than normal and therefore cardiac insufficiency worsens. Brain hypoxemia derived from respiratory and cardiac insufficiency causes severely low blood pressure and a consequent reduction of brain blood inflow. Brain hypoxemia is worsened by hypothyroidism-related anemia as well.

17.5 DIAGNOSIS

The diagnosis of hypothyroid coma is based on (1) history obtained from relatives or medical reports indicating previous thyroid disease and lethargy slowly leading to coma; (2) specific signs and symptoms (Table 17.1); (3) laboratory diagnosis showing serum free thyroxine (FT_4) and tri-iodothyronine (FT_3) concentrations below the normal reference ranges; and (4) serum TSH concentrations far exceeding the normal reference range (usually >100 mIU/L). Note that in cases of hypopituitarism, serum TSH concentrations are typically low to normal[1] (Figure 17.1).

The diagnosis is relatively simple. Presenting symptoms are characterized by severe weakness and lethargia progressively evolving to coma. However, because serum thyroid hormone and TSH measurements may take hours, patients who arrive

TABLE 17.1
Symptoms and Signs Peculiar to Hypothyroid Coma

Coma status

Hypothermia (frequently severe, with body temperature <33°C)

Dyspnea

Generalized edema with yellow and dry cutis

Macroglossia

Bradycardia

Weak wrists

Reduced cardiac sounds

Overweight or obesity

Constipation

Reduced reflexes

Thin and dry hair

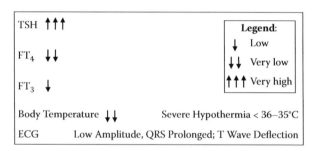

FIGURE 17.1   Diagnostic approach for hypothyroid coma.

at the emergency department should be submitted to further I level examinations in addition to serum TSH, FT_4, and FT_3 concentration measurements:

- Arterial blood gas analysis measuring hypoxemia, and hypercapnia, and possible respiratory acidosis
- Laboratory analysis revealing anemia, hyponatremia, hypoglycemia, and high serum creatine kinase, lactate dehydrogenase, transaminase, and cholesterol concentrations
- Electrocardiography demonstrating sinus bradycardia, low voltages (related to pericardial effusion), QT prolongation, and plated or inverted T waves (consequent to myocardial ischemia)
- Echocardiography invariably disclosing pericardial effusion associated with cardiomegaly, increased thickness of all cardiac walls, and reduced cardiac output
- Computed tomography (CT) of the brain, usually normal in patients with primary hypothyroidism (although long-lasting hypothyroidism promotes atherogenesis and then ischemic encephalopathy), detecting a pituitary macroadenoma or empty sella in patients with secondary hypothyroidism

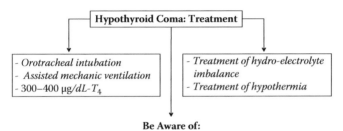

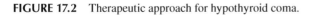

FIGURE 17.2   Therapeutic approach for hypothyroid coma.

17.6   TREATMENT

The four pillars of hypothyroid coma therapy (Figure 17.2) are described below:

- **Endotracheal intubation and assisted mechanical ventilation** with constant monitoring of blood gas parameters.
- **Levothyroxine substitution therapy** in high doses (300 to 400 μg/daily), preferably administered intravenously because of poor intestinal absorption due to severe hypothyroidism. In some countries, intravenous commercial preparations of levothyroxine are not available. In such cases, it is necessary to administer levothyroxine per os through a nasogastric tube (as a lyophilized powder in 200 to 500 μg vials) or as a galenical preparation for intravenous administration: levothyroxine is dissolved with 2 to 3 drops of NaOH 0,1 N, then diluted with 4 to 5 mL of NaCl 0,9% containing 1% albumin; the solution is passed through a 0,22 μm sterile Millipore filter and then neutralized at pH 7.4.
- **Treatment of hydroelectrolyte imbalance,** particularly hyponatremia, through water restriction. Administration of hypertonic NaCl solutions should be recommended in patients with severe hyponatremia (<120 mEq/L) only.
- **Treatment of hypothermia** through passive and gradual heating (for example, by blankets). Note that active body heating is not warranted because of the risks of vasodilatation and shock.

Assisted ventilation should seldom be prolonged for 2 weeks following the start of levothyroxine substitution therapy because of myxedematous degeneration of respiratory muscles and concurrent pulmonary complications such as pneumonitis. At the same time, treatment of precipitating factors, if any, is needed (for example, antibiotics should be administered to patients with pneumonia).

Furthermore, particular attention must be paid to concurrent diseases in the context of autoimmune polyendocrine syndromes. Specifically, hypoadrenalism due to Schmidt's syndrome (association of autoimmune adrenalitis and Hashimoto's thyroiditis) should be ruled out. Hypoadrenalism may occur as a consequence of panhypopituitarism as well. In any case, until results of a hypothalamus–pituitary–adrenal axis study are available, hydrocortisone administration (100 mg every 6 to 8 hours intravenously) is always mandatory along with levothyroxine therapy to avoid acute adrenal insufficiency.[1,6] Table 17.2 lists drugs cited in this chapter.

Death is caused by respiratory and/or cardiac (arrhythmia, acute myocardial infarction, acute pulmonary edema, cardiac shock) complications. In most cases, the latter are precipitated by high levothyroxine doses needed to treat hypothyroid coma in patients with underlying ischemic cardiomyopathy.

17.7 FOLLOW-UP

After recovery from a coma, a patient must be followed periodically as in primary hypothyroidism (see Chapter 10). Serum TSH and FT_4 should be measured every 6 months.

17.8 PROGNOSIS

The prognosis of hypothyroid coma is fatal if replacement therapy is not quickly and appropriately given. In fact, mortality is above 90% without and 40% with therapy. Prognostic negative factors are hypothermia below 35°C and severe concurrent diseases.

TABLE 17.2
Drugs Cited in Chapter 17

Drug	Dosage Forms	Dose Range
Levothyroxine (LT_4)	Tablets, capsules, solution for intravenous injection,[a] oral solution (drops)[a]	12.5 to 400 µg/day
Tri-iodothyronine (LT_3)	Tablets, solution for intravenous injection[a]	20 to 120 µg/day
$LT_4 + LT_3$	Tablets	12.5 to 400 µg/day

[a] Available only in some countries.

REFERENCES

1. Mitchell, J.M. 1989. Thyroid disease in the emergency department: thyroid function tests and hypothyroidism and myxedema coma. *Emerg Med Clin North Am* 7: 885–902.
2. Turhan, N.O., Kockar, M.C., and Inegol, I. 2004. Myxedematous coma in a laboring woman suggested a pre-eclamptic coma: a case report. *Acta Obstet Gynecol Scand* 83: 1089–1091.
3. Shaheen, M. 2009. Severe congestive heart failure patient on amiodarone presenting with myxedemic coma: a case report. *Indian Heart J* 61: 392–393.
4. Church, C.O. and Callen, E.C. 2009. Myxedema coma associated with combination aripiprazole and sertraline therapy. *Ann Pharmacother* 43: 2113–2116.
5. Kudrjavcev, T. 1978. Neurologic complications of thyroid dysfunction. *Adv Neurol* 19: 619–636.
6. Sarlis, N.J. and Gourgiotis, L. 2003. Thyroid emergencies. *Rev Endocr Metab Disord* 4: 129–136.
7. Finzi, G., Calamo, A., Chiodera, P. et al. 1991. Myxedematous coma due to transitory secondary hypothyroidism: description of a case. *Ann Ital Med Int* 6: 248–250.
8. Barbesino, G. 2010. Drugs affecting thyroid function. *Thyroid* 20: 763–770.
9. Lazarus, J.H. 2009. Lithium and thyroid. *Best Pract Res Clin Endocrinol Metab* 23: 723–733.
10. Mannavola, D. 2007. A novel tyrosine-kinase selective inhibitor, sunitinib, induces transient hypothyroidism by blocking iodine uptake. *J Clin Endocrinol Metab* 92: 3531–3534.

18 Toxic Diffuse Goiter (Basedow-Graves' Disease)

Luca Chiovato, Flavia Magri, and Mario Rotondi

CONTENTS

Key words: toxic diffuse goiter, autoimmune thyroid disease (AITD), pathophysiology, clinical symptoms, diagnosis, radioactive iodine therapy, antithyroid drugs, thyroidectomy.

18.1   DEFINITION

Toxic diffuse goiter (TDG), commonly referred to as Graves' disease in English-speaking countries or as Basedow's disease in most non–English-speaking European countries, is the underlying cause of most cases of hyperthyroidism. Hyperthyroidism is the consequence of circulating IgG antibodies directed against the thyroid-stimulating hormone (TSH) receptor (TSHR) mimicking the effects of TSH. TSHR activation induces a diffuse enlargement of the thyroid gland and an increase in thyroxine (T_4) and triiodothyronine (T_3) secretion.

TDG is often associated with a unique eye inflammatory disorder called orbitopathy and more rarely to localized infiltrative dermopathy (pretibial myxedema) and acropachy. TDG is a typical autoimmune organ-specific disease, in which both genetic background and environmental factors contribute to disrupt immune tolerance. The diagnosis of TDG is usually easy when orbitopathy is present. In other cases several clinical and laboratory features along with imaging techniques are helpful for diagnosing the disease.

18.2   EPIDEMIOLOGY

TDG affects about 0.5% of the general population and represents the most frequent cause of thyrotoxicosis, depending on regional iodine intake. The frequency of TDG depends on the different setting of evaluation, such as population sampling (age distribution or ethnic differences), iodine intake, and the diagnostic tools employed to ascertain the disease. A large survey performed in the 1970s in the United States estimated the prevalence of TDG to be 0.4%—a picture very similar to the one found in Italy (0.6%) in the Pescopagano study.

A meta-analysis of various studies published from 1965 to 1995 estimated the general prevalence of the disorder to be about 1%, making it one of the most frequent clinically relevant autoimmune disorders. A recent article estimated the incidence rates for hyperthyroidism by new-to-therapy prescriptions for antithyroid drugs in 2008.[1] By considering that this approach may be a reasonable surrogate for the actual incidence in the U.S. population and that more than 90% of patients below the age of 50 years who present with hyperthyroidism have TDG, the rates found were slightly higher than the incidence rates previously reported for Western societies (from 0.44 per 1,000 in young patients to 1.01 per 1,000 in older subjects).

Iodine intake plays a relevant role in the prevalence of TDG as shown by epidemiological surveys comparing areas of normal iodine intake versus areas of low iodine intake. In the first context, TDG accounted for 80% of cases of hyperthyroidism, while in iodine-insufficient areas only half the cases of hyperthyroidism were due to TDG.

In a comparison of two genetically similar populations that differed in iodine intake (iodine-sufficient Iceland versus iodine-deficient East Jutland in Denmark), along with a higher TDG incidence in the iodine-sufficient (20/100,000 inhabitants/ year) group than in the iodine-deficient population (15/100,000/year), the incidence of thyrotoxicosis from all causes was greater in the iodine-deficient (39/100,000/year) than iodine-sufficient (23/100,000/year) populations. Table 18.1 summarizes the prevalence and annual incidence of TDG in different geographic areas.

Similar to most autoimmune diseases, TDG is more prevalent in the female gender; the female-to-male ratio is between 5:1 to 10:1. The annual incidence is related to age, with peaks in the fourth to sixth decades of life, although TDG can be observed at any age. In children, the incidence is about 1 in 10,000 and TDG represents the most common cause of thyrotoxicosis. The concordance rate for TDG among monozygotic twins is 35%. Although ethnic differences in susceptibility to TDG are likely to exist, they have not been consistently investigated in comparative studies.

TABLE 18.1
Prevalence (A) and Annual Incidence (B) of DTG in Various Geographic Areas

(A) Prevalence

Country	%	Notes
United States	0.4	
United Kingdom	1.1–1.6	Thyrotoxicosis of all causes
Italy	0.6	
Pooled data	1	

(B) Incidence

Country	Cases per 100.000 per year	Notes
Sweden	25	High iodine intake
New Zealand	15	After full iodine supplementation
Great Britain	23	After full iodine supplementation
Iceland	20	After full iodine supplementation
Denmark	15	Low iodine intake

18.3 PATHOGENESIS

TDG is an organ-specific autoimmune disorder with involvement of both T and B cell-mediated immunity against thyroid antigens. The human TSH receptor (TSHR) is the principal autoantigen of TDG. It is a G-protein linked receptor, with seven transmembrane domains employing c-AMP and phosphoinositol pathways for signal transduction. It is expressed not only in the thyroid, but also in many other cells such as fibroblasts, adipocytes, lymphocytes, and muscle cells.

The primary requirement for a specific autoimmune (humoral or cell-mediated) response is T cell infiltration of the inflamed organ. Activated T cells both in the peripheral circulation and in the thyroid gland were described in TDG. Intrathyroidal T cells in TDG are predominantly of the T_H1 subtype, as assessed by their cytokine and chemokine profiles; this is also true for TSHR-responsive clones.[2]

Because thyroid hyperfunction and follicular cell growth in TDG are due to the presence of TSHR antibodies (TRAbs), this T_H1 dominance may seem unexpected. However, it is known that T_H1 cells may also induce antibody production and that TRAbs are more often of the IgG1 subclass that is induced selectively T_H1 cells. This initial T_H1 predominance progresses toward a T_H2 immune phenotype in long-standing TDG.

In TDG, the binding of TRAbs to TSH receptors causes activation of adenylate cyclase. Consequences of this binding are the induction of thyroid growth, increased vascularity, and increased rates of thyroid hormone production and secretion. Most patients with TDG display positivity for TRAbs with stimulating activity. Other varieties of TRAbs may also be present: a receptor antibody that acts as a TSH antagonist (blocking TRAbs) or a neutral form of antibody with no functional effect on receptors. Blocking TRAbs may be coincident with the stimulating type and may also predominate in certain patients after treatment with radioactive iodine, antithyroid drugs, or surgery. TRAbs are thought to bind to discontinuous conformational epitopes in the leucine-rich repeat region of the extracellular domain of the TSHR, similarly to TSH. Since many patients have all three antibodies (stimulating, blocking, and neutral TRAbs) the degree of thyroid stimulation depends on the relative concentration and bioactivity of the different autoantibodies.

TRAbs are unique human disease-specific antibodies in that they are detected only in patients with TDG, in contrast with thyroglobulin antibodies (TgAbs) and thyroid peroxidase antibodies (TPOAbs) that have high prevalence even in the general elderly population. With a sensitive assay, TRAbs with thyroid-stimulating activity are detectable in 90 to 100% of untreated hyperthyroid patients with TDG. The serum levels of TRAbs are decreased by treatment of the disease and may predict recurrence when they persist. Over time, TRAbs with blocking activity may become the more prevalent type, contributing to the hypothyroid evolution of TDG.

18.3.1 RISK FACTORS

TDG is considered a multifactorial disease in which a complex interplay of genetic, hormonal, and environmental factors lead to the loss of immune tolerance to thyroid antigens and to the initiation of a sustained autoimmune reaction.

18.3.1.1   Genetic Susceptibility

Heredity has a great influence on the development and the subsequent course of TDG as demonstrated by the increased incidence of other autoimmune disorders in members of patients' families and by the observation that monozygotic twins have higher concordance rates of TDG than dizygotic twins.

The CTLA-4 gene that codes for a modulator of the second signal to T cells influences the predisposition for development of thyroid autoantibodies. Furthermore, susceptibility to TDG may be due to the presence of multiple genetic loci, confirming the polygenic and complex features of this disease. An association with the HLA region has been proposed (e.g., increased frequency of the HLA DR3 and DQA10501 haplotypes in Caucasians), but the HLA region provides less than 5% of genetic susceptibility. Thus, the contributions of CTLA4 and HLA to genetic susceptibility to TDG are small. Several other genes have also been shown to confer susceptibility to AITD and can be classified into two groups: (1) immune regulatory genes such as CD40, protein tyrosine phosphatase-22, and CD25; and (2) thyroid-specific genes such as thyroglobulin and TSHR genes.

The search for thyroid-specific genetic susceptibility revealed only small influences exerted by polymorphisms in the thyroglobulin and TSHR genes. The influence of individual genes on the development of TDG, when assessed in a population, appears to be weaker than would be expected from data showing a strong genetic susceptibility to TDG. As a result, more remains to be learned about TDG specificity in relation to genetic susceptibility.[3]

18.3.1.2   Environmental Factors

18.3.1.2.1   Infection

Over the years, both experimental and epidemiologic evidence suggested that infections may play a role in the pathogenesis of TDG. The possible role of infection in the development of thyroid autoimmunity via bystander effects or molecular mimicry (i.e., cross reactions of microbial antigens with self-antigens) has been extensively proposed. It has been suggested that TDG may be associated with infectious agents (e.g., *Yersinia enterocolitica, Leishmania*, and *Mycoplasma*), but no study meets the necessary criteria to firmly prove this hypothesis.

Infections of the thyroid gland (e.g., subacute thyroiditis or congenital rubella) are associated with thyroid autoimmunity. Nevertheless, a causative role of infectious agents has not been definitively demonstrated in TDG despite the observation of AITDs induced in experimental animals by certain viral infections.

18.3.1.2.3   Stress

TDG commonly becomes evident after severe emotional stress. Clinical studies support the view that major stress may be associated with the onset of TDG. Many patients with TDG have histories of major stress in the 12 months before disease onset. The hypothesis is that, following the general condition of immune suppression induced by stress, a rebound of the immune system resulting in greater immune activity than normal occurs and may initiate disease if individuals are genetically susceptible. This event may precipitate the onset of autoimmune hyperthyroidism. It is interesting to note that in cross-sectional studies, an increase in the prevalence of TDG was reported among refugees during World War II in Germany, but not during the civil unrest in Ireland or during the German occupation of Belgium. This suggests that the stressful events of personal life may be more important than social stresses.

18.3.1.2.4 Gender

TDG has a higher prevalence in women than in men (7:1 to 10:1). The disease tends to be more common after puberty. These data, along with the fact that androgens, in contrast to estrogens, may actually suppress autoimmune thyroiditis, suggests that female sex steroids may be responsible for this gender-related difference. It was also proposed that factors on the X chromosome may explain the female preponderance to TDG. This consideration comes from the observation that TDG continues to occur after menopause and also occurs in many men. When the disease develops in men, it tends to occur at a later age, is more severe, and is accompanied more often by orbitopathy.

A linkage analysis in families with TDG located a putative TDG susceptibility locus on the long arm of the X chromosome. Women have two X chromosomes and thus receive twice the gene dose. However, larger studies did not confirm the existence of a locus on the X chromosome linked to TDG. The phenomenon of X chromosome inactivation (XCI) has also been invoked in autoimmune diseases. Female cells may inactivate either one of the two X chromosomes to variable degrees in different tissues, leading to potentially differing immune responses.

18.3.1.2.5 Pregnancy

Severe TDG is uncommon during pregnancy. Hyperthyroidism is associated with an increased risk of pregnancy loss and pregnancy complications. Data indicate that excessive thyroid hormone has a direct toxic effect on a fetus. Successful pregnancy is associated with a shift toward a T_H2 predominance of the immune response, which prevents rejection of the fetal allograft. Therefore, TDG tends to ameliorate in the course of pregnancy, mainly because both T cell and B cell functions are diminished under the influence of local placental factors and regulatory T cells.

After delivery, a rebound from this immunological deviation occurs and may contribute to the development of postpartum AITDs. However, the role of pregnancy as a risk factor for development of TDG in susceptible women is still controversial. Early observations reported that as many as 30% of young women have histories of pregnancy in the 12 months before the onset of TDG, indicating that postpartum is a major risk factor for developing the disease. A more recent study demonstrated that, at least in an iodine-deficient area, the prevalence[4] of TDG developing postpartum was lower—around 7% after correcting for age and parity status. In this context, further studies are required to elucidate the issue.

18.3.1.2.6 Iodine and Drugs

Iodine excess and iodine-containing drugs such as amiodarone and contrast media may precipitate the onset of TDG or its recurrence in susceptible individuals. In an iodine-deficient population, the pharmaceutical use of iodine is most likely to precipitate thyrotoxicosis simply by allowing TRAbs to effectively stimulate the formation of more thyroid hormone. A direct effect of iodine on the immune system was also demonstrated. Iodine may damage thyroid cells directly and release thyroid antigens to the immune system.

Several clinical and experimental studies support the notion that the therapeutic use of Type I interferons (interferon-α for chronic HCV-related hepatitis and malignancies, and interferon-β for multiple sclerosis) are associated with the occurrence of TDG. More recently, a novel clinical entity, the so-called immune reconstitution syndrome, was described.[5] TDG may develop as a consequence of immune reconstitution in three clinical settings: (1) bone marrow transplantation from a donor with TDG may cause the disease to appear in the recipient; (2) treatment with alemtuzumab for multiple sclerosis or other pathological conditions may lead to the development of TDG during the phase of naive T cell expansion following therapeutic lymphocyte depletion; and (3) TDG may occur during the phase of CD4+ T cell expansion following highly active antiretroviral therapy for HIV infection. The mechanisms responsible for reconstitution of TDG are at present unclear, but it is likely that TDG may be an aspect of a broader spectrum of immunoregulatory disturbances that may arise after immune reconstitution.

18.3.1.2.7 Thyroid Damage

There is no evidence that radiation exposure is a risk factor for TDG. Nevertheless, TDG may appear in patients treated with radioactive iodine for multinodular goiters. Radioactive iodine may also cause the onset or worsening of orbitopathy. Evidence indicates that thyroid autoantibodies are more prevalent in populations exposed to radioactive fallout. Claims of increased rates of autoimmune thyroiditis in these populations have been made.

TDG was also reported to appear after ethanol injections for the treatment of autonomous thyroid nodules. Similar to radioactive-iodine induced TDG, this phenomenon was interpreted as arising from a massive release of thyroid antigens, thereby triggering an autoimmune response to TSHRs in predisposed individuals.

18.3.1.2.8 Smoking

A number of studies provided evidence associating smoking and thyroid diseases including TDG. Retrospective analysis shows that smokers face an increased risk of TDG and orbitopathy, and also relapsing hyperthyroidism after antithyroid drug withdrawal. These findings may be explained both by direct effects of smoking metabolites on the immune system or by damage to thyrocytes induced by smoking metabolites that may determine exposure of thyroid antigens to the immune system. Table 18.2 lists risk factors for the development of TDG.

18.4 PATHOPHYSIOLOGY

In TDG, both the function and the growth of the thyroid are controlled by TRAbs that act as abnormal stimulators. Their stimulating action leads to suppression of the normal regulatory mechanisms of thyroid function. The resulting hyperfunction leads to suppression of TSH secretion reflected by undetectable serum TSH. In cases

TABLE 18.2
Risk Factors for Development of TDG

Genetic factors	CTLA-4
	HLA DR 3
	DQA10501 haplotypes
	Genes coding for thyroid-specific molecules
Infections	Yersinia enterocolitica
	Leishmania
	Mycoplasma
	Infections of thyroid gland
Stress	Emotional stress
Female gender	Estrogens
	X chromosome
	X chromosome inactivation
Pregnancy/postpartum	Rebound after pregnancy immunosuppression
Iodine	Drugs (amiodarone)
	Contrast media containing iodine
Thyroid damage	Radiation exposure
	Ethanol injection
	Radioactive iodine treatment
Smoking	Smoking metabolite damage to immune system
	Smoking metabolite damage to thyrocytes
Drugs	Immunomodulators
	Immune reconstitution syndrome

of disease remission, when the stimulator is withdrawn, normal TSH secretion and regulation of thyroid function are restored. The proportion of total plasma T_4 and T_3 in the free (or unbound) state is increased because of (1) a decrease in the concentration of thyroxine-binding globulin (TBG) and (2) an increase in the concentration of T_4.

The chronic hyperstimulation of the gland results in an almost doubled molar ratio of T_3 to T_4 in thyroglobulin. In iodine-deficient areas, T_3 is frequently the major secretory product, so that serum T_3 levels are increased while serum T_4 concentration is within the normal range (T_3 thyrotoxicosis).

18.5 CLINICAL ASPECTS

A wide range of clinical manifestations of overt hyperthyroidism due to diffuse toxic goiter may be divided into those common to other thyroid disorders (but usually more prominent and severe) and those specific to diffuse toxic goiter, each contributing to a clinical picture that can rarely be mistaken when both possibilities are present.[6]

Table 18.3 summarizes the main signs and symptoms of untreated TDG. The severity and the duration of the disease along with patient age are important determinants of the spectrum of manifestations of thyrotoxicosis. Precipitating events such as

TABLE 18.3
Signs and Symptoms of Untreated TDG

Symptoms	Signs
Common to Other Causes of Thyrotoxicosis	
Hyperactivity, altered mood, insomnia	Tachycardia, atrial fibrillation
Heat intolerance	Fine tremor, hyperreflexia
Palpitations	Warm, moist skin
Fatigability	Muscle weakness and wasting
Dyspnea	Congestive (high-output) heart failure
Weight loss	Periodic paralysis
Increased stool frequency	Psychosis
Oligomenorrhea, amenorrhea, erectile dysfunction	Increased bone turnover, osteoporosis, fracture
Specific for TDG	
Diffuse goiter	
Orbitopathy	
Pretibial myxedema	
Acropachy	

trauma, infection, surgery, or childbirth may induce a thyroid storm (treated in detail in Chapter 24). This life-threatening condition is characterized by tachycardia, atrial fibrillation, congestive heart failure, hyperpyrexia, psychosis, and coma.

18.5.1 THYROID GLAND

The thyroid gland is usually enlarged, soft, and symmetrical (Figure 18.1), although nodular glands can be seen, especially in geographic areas of iodine deficiency where

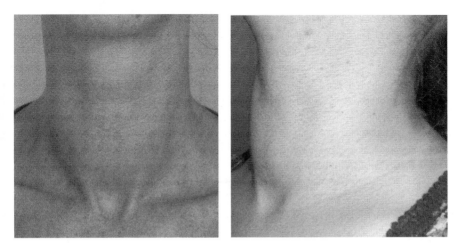

FIGURE 18.1 Diffuse symmetrical goiter in patient with toxic diffuse goiter.

preexisting nodular goiters are common. Goiter size is widely variable, and some patients, especially elderly people, even have glands of normal size. The pyramidal lobe is often palpable and sometimes thrills and bruits resulting from increased blood flow may be apparent on the gland.

18.5.2 SKIN AND APPENDAGES

The skin of a thyrotoxic patient is warm, thin, and moist; palmar erythema is common. Dermatographism and pruritus are often reported along with urticaria. Vitiligo as an independent autoimmune skin disease may coexist. Hair and nails are friable. Diffuse alopecia of mild degree is often observed.

Pretibial myxedema is a unique feature of diffuse toxic goiter related to the immune system disorder (Figure 18.2). It consists of a localized area of indurated non-pitting edema that usually affects the pretibial surfaces, feet, or areas of trauma. Dermopathy occurs in 1 to 2% of patients, usually in the presence of severe orbitopathy. Pretibial swelling is caused by the inordinate accumulation of hyaluronic acid in the subcutaneous layers of the involved areas, similar to the diffuse myxedematous changes of hypothyroidism and also by a chronic inflammatory infiltrate similar to that observed in the orbit. The cause of pretibial myxedema is unknown, but most studies support the hypothesis of an autoimmune disorder because of the ectopic expression of thyroidal antigens, possibly TSHRs, or the presence of cross-reacting antigens localized to restricted regions of the skin.

Thyroid acropachy is observed in fewer than 1 in 1,000 patients. It is characterized by clubbing and soft tissue swelling of the last phalanxes of the fingers and

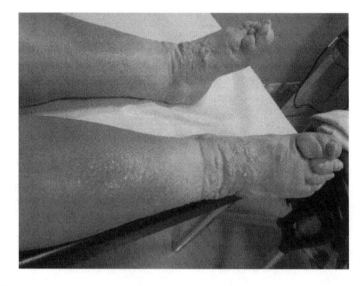

FIGURE 18.2   Pretibial myxedema in a patient with toxic diffuse goiter.

toes, similar to that observed in chronic respiratory insufficiency. Increased glycosaminoglycan deposition in the skin and subperiosteal new bone formation are present. The pathogenesis and the link with the immunological changes of TDG are unknown, but it is believed that they may be similar to the those for orbitopathy and pretibial myxedema.

18.5.3 CARDIOVASCULAR SYSTEM

The cardiovascular signs and symptoms are the most profound and clinically relevant features of diffuse toxic goiter (DTG). Thyroid hormone effects on the heart are mediated by the regulation of the expression of key structural and regulatory genes and by extranuclear nongenomic effects. Table 18.4 shows the cardiovascular effects of diffuse toxic goiter. The most common heart-related symptoms are tachycardia and palpitations. Atrial fibrillation or flutter can occur in up to 10 to 15% of patients, especially if elderly. Recently, the prevalence rate for atrial fibrillation was found to be significantly lower than previously described (less than 2%), probably as the result of earlier diagnosis and treatment of DTG.

Thyrotoxicosis induces enhanced cardiac contractility and cardiac output. These changes, combined with sinus tachycardia or atrial fibrillation, can produce left ventricular dysfunction and heart failure. Indeed, signs and symptoms of heart failure may develop and edema of the lower extremities is often found in elderly patients. Overall, vascular resistance is decreased because of peripheral vasodilatation. Increased cardiac workload causes increased oxygen consumption that may in turn precipitate angina pectoris in the presence of preexisting coronary artery disease.

Peripheral edema can be observed in the absence of overt heart failure. A high prevalence of pulmonary artery hypertension in diffuse toxic goiter is described and some signs of heart failure such as neck vein distension and peripheral edema may be related to right heart dysfunction. Figure 18.3 summarizes the effects of thyroid hormones on the heart and peripheral vasculature leading to decreased systemic vascular resistance and increased resting heart rate, blood volume, and left ventricular contractility. Dyspnea on exertion or at rest and chest pain may also be present and may depend on both left and right heart failure as well as a decrease of skeletal muscle function.[7]

TABLE 18.4

Cardiovascular Effects of DTG

Tachycardia and palpitations	Atrial fibrillation
Dyspnea on exertion	Peripheral edema
Increased cardiac output	Heart failure
Chest pain	Decrease of vascular resistance

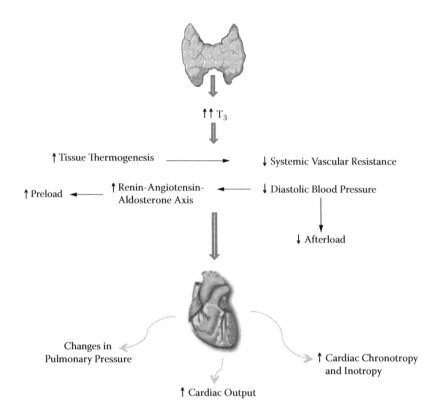

FIGURE 18.3   Effects of thyroid hormone excess on cardiovascular hemodynamics.

On physical examination, the heart of a thyrotoxic patient is characterized by resting tachycardia. Heart sounds are accentuated. A systolic murmur may be heard on the precordium, sometimes related to associated mitral valve prolapse. Arrhythmias can range from sporadic premature beats to atrial fibrillation. Electrocardiographic findings are nonspecific and include sinus tachycardia with ST elevation, QT shortening, and PR prolongation. Ischemic changes can be found when underlying coronary artery disease is present.

18.5.4   GASTROINTESTINAL TRACT

Appetite increase is common, but may not be adequate to maintain weight in thyrotoxicosis and is due to increased catabolism. Vomiting as a direct effect of thyroid hormone on gastrointestinal motility, thyroid hormone stimulation of a chemoreceptor trigger zone in the central nervous system, and increased adrenergic activity have been proposed as GI findings.

Up to 25% of patients with hyperthyroidism have mild-to-moderate diarrhea with frequent bowel movements. These symptoms can be associated with some degree of malabsorption and steatorrhea that may contribute to weight loss. Patients with TDG have a fivefold added risk for being celiac when compared to sex- and age-matched controls.

Mild elevations of liver enzymes are often detected in thyrotoxic patients. These findings must to be taken into account when patients are treated with antithyroid drugs, because they can be mistaken for adverse reactions to thionamides.

18.5.5 Nervous System

Mood and anxiety disorders, insomnia and sometimes cognitive dysfunction are commonly present in patients with DTG. Patients appear restless and agitated, they complain about fatigue and asthenia, logorrhea is often present, and concentration ability is decreased. These symptoms may be confused with true manic or bipolar disorders. In some cases, nervous signs take the form of apathetic thyrotoxicosis (severe apathy, lethargy, and pseudodementia—a profile more commonly observed in elderly patients.

The peripheral nervous system is also deeply affected. Fine distal tremor is an almost universal finding and can be easily observed at the eyelids. Deep tendon reflexes are brisk and relaxation time is shortened. The characteristic stare of a thyrotoxic patient is due to autonomic hyperstimulation of the elevator muscle of the lid and can also be found in the absence of orbitopathy. Although hyperactivity of the adrenergic nervous system is considered the main pathogenetic factor, the persistence of some neurological symptoms after successful treatment of hyperthyroidism suggests that other mechanisms such as autoimmunity may also be involved.

18.5.6 Muscles

Thyrotoxic patients frequently report muscle weakness, easy exhaustion, and in more severe cases, muscle atrophy of variable degrees. Fewer than 1% of patients with TDG have classic myasthenia gravis, although ocular myasthenia gravis may be more frequent. The pathogenic significance of this association is not known, but it is important to remember that thyrotoxic myopathy can worsen the muscular symptoms of myasthenia.

In some patients, thyrotoxicosis can precipitate crises of periodic hypokalemic paralysis, a syndrome clinically identical to familial periodic paralysis in which thyrotoxicosis of various causes is invariably present. The association with certain HLA haplotypes and the presence of mutations of ionic (potassium) channel genes has been observed in patients with periodic hypokalemic paralysis.

18.5.7 Skeletal System

Thyrotoxicosis results in increased bone turnover, shortening of the bone remodelling cycle, and reduced bone mass density. Untreated, long-standing thyrotoxicosis is included in the FRAX calculator to estimate the 10-year probability of fractures. The population at higher risk is represented by postmenopausal women whose suppressed TSH concentrations are associated with threefold to fourfold increased risks of fracture. Treatment of thyrotoxicosis rapidly normalizes the levels of bone turnover markers and/or reduced bone mass density, although some evidence reported that the increased risk of fracture persists for at least 5 years after initial diagnosis and treatment.

18.5.8 HEMATOPOIETIC SYSTEM

Mild leukopenia with relative lymphocytosis may be observed in patients with DTG and must be distinguished from antithyroid drug-induced leukopenia or agranulocytosis. Pernicious anemia occurs in a small minority of patients with TDG, while circulating autoantibodies to gastric parietal cells are found in a much higher percentage of cases and are signs of associated gastric autoimmunity. Aplastic anemia, autoimmune thrombocytopenic purpura, and other nonimmunologic alterations in hemostasis have also been reported.

18.5.9 REPRODUCTIVE SYSTEM

In females, thyrotoxicosis, particularly if leading to severe weight loss, is often associated with oligomenorrhea or amenorrhea. Fertility is decreased, but pregnancy can still occur. Thyrotoxicosis in pregnancy is associated with increased incidence of miscarriage, low-birth-weight infants, and preeclampsia.

Gynecomastia may develop in men; erectile dysfunction and reduced sperm count are not infrequent. The circulating estradiol level is increased, probably because of increased peripheral aromatization of testosterone. In both sexes, sex hormone–binding globulin (SHBG) is increased. In males, these changes are responsible for an increase of total testosterone, but unbound and bioavailable testosterone levels remain in the normal range. All these changes are reversible with treatment of thyrotoxicosis.

18.5.10 METABOLIC CHANGES

The increased metabolic rate and heat production induced by thyrotoxicosis result in a significant weight loss despite normal or increased caloric intake, a moderate rise in body temperature that is partially compensated for by increased sweating and heat intolerance. Increased (but inefficient) mitochondrial oxygen consumption is the main mechanism responsible for these symptoms.

Thyrotoxicosis leads to hyperglycemia via increased glucose absorption, hyperinsulinemia, high free fatty acid levels, and increased peripheral glucose transport and metabolism. The increased hepatic glucose output constitutes a major element in the induction of hyperinsulinemia, glucose intolerance, and peripheral insulin resistance (Table 18.5).

Type I diabetes mellitus may be associated with TDG within polyglandular autoimmune syndromes, but thyrotoxicosis may precipitate subclinical diabetes and worsens glycemic control in preexisting type 1 diabetes mellitus and also induces diabetic ketoacidosis. Serum cholesterol and triglyceride levels are decreased in thyrotoxicosis, mainly because of decreases in low-density lipoproteins (LDLs) in spite of an increase of hepatic lipogenesis. Cholesterol conversion to bile acid in the liver is enhanced and LDL receptors on adipocytes increase as well. Thyroid function may alter adipokines such as leptin, adiponectin, and resistin.

TABLE 18.5
Metabolic Changes Induced by Thyrotoxicosis

↑ Glucose turnover and gastrointestinal absorption

↑ Hepatic glucose output

↑ Plasma glucose and insulin levels

↑ Peripheral tissue glucose uptake

↑ Peripheral insulin resistance

Protein metabolism is altered during thyrotoxicosis, with both increased synthesis and degradation. In most cases, however, degradation predominates and causes negative nitrogen balance.

18.5.11 TDG-ASSOCIATED ORBITOPATHY

TDG-associated orbitopathy is a distinctive manifestation of DTG (Figure 18.4). It is an inflammatory disorder of the orbit related to a central pathophysiologic event of autoimmune disease. Orbitopathy is examined in detail in Chapter 26. Briefly, the eye bulb is pushed forward and proptosis or exophthalmos results, often asymmetrically. Venous congestion causes swelling and edema of the periorbital tissue. Inflammatory changes also involve the extraocular muscles and may cause diplopia. Retraction, edema, and lid swelling are also typical.

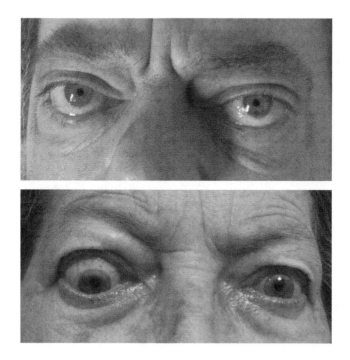

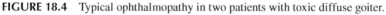

FIGURE 18.4   Typical ophthalmopathy in two patients with toxic diffuse goiter.

The conjunctival mucosa is injected and edematous (chemosis). Lagophthalmos (incomplete palpebral closure) and lacrimal gland dysfunction may combine to cause drying of the mucosal and corneal surfaces and consequent irritation and (less often) corneal ulceration. Photophobia, burning sensation, retrobulbar pain, tearing, and sandy sensation are common symptoms. Optic neuropathy resulting from optic nerve compression by inflamed and swollen extraocular muscles at the orbital apex may occur in the most severe cases and cause reduction or loss of vision. When the proptosis is extremely severe, subluxation of the bulb outside the orbit may occur.

Clinical signs or symptoms of orbitopathy are present in about 50% of patients with DTG. The degree of orbitopathy is widely variable and it may coincide with, follow, or precede thyrotoxicosis.

18.6 DIAGNOSIS

18.6.1 CLINICAL DIAGNOSIS

In moderate or severe TDG, the clinical diagnosis is straightforward because patients present with signs and symptoms of thyrotoxicosis, diffuse goiter, and ophthalmopathy. In some patients, the thyroid may not be enlarged and orbitopathy may not be clinically evident. In elderly people, the symptoms of hyperthyroidism are typically less evident. These exceptions account for the need to confirm clinical diagnosis by an accurate laboratory workup.

18.6.2 HORMONE MEASUREMENT

Suspicion of hyperthyroidism is usually confirmed by the assessment of a thyroid hormone profile. Laboratory findings show undetectable serum TSH levels and elevated FT_4 and FT_3 concentrations in I level investigations. TSH is the most useful test because in mild thyrotoxicosis only the pituitary hormone may be low in spite of normal TSH concentrations (so-called subclinical hyperthyroidism).

Low serum TSH levels may also be observed in a number of other non-autoimmune conditions such as factitious thyrotoxicosis, toxic adenoma, nodular toxic goiter, and other conditions of extrathyroidal origin, such as non-thyroidal illnesses and endogenous or exogenous corticosteroid excess. Therefore, parallel measurement of thyroid hormone levels is recommended in all patients to ensure correct interpretation of low serum TSH concentrations.

In TDG, the serum-free T_4 and T_3 are more increased compared to total T_4 and T_3 levels. The serum T_3 concentration may be proportionally more elevated than the serum T_4 level. In patients with severe accompanying non-thyroidal illnesses and those taking amiodarone, the conversion of T_4 to T_3 may be impaired, resulting in a normal free T_3 associated with a high free T_4 (T_4 thyrotoxicosis). Occasionally, especially in iodine-deficient countries, the discrepancy between T_4 and T_3 levels is exaggerated, with the serum T_4 concentration normal and the serum T_3 concentration elevated (T_3 thyrotoxicosis).

Because suppressed serum TSH has other causes such as major depression or hypothalamus–pituitary disease and because an increase in the serum concentration of total T_4 may also result from an increase of TBG levels, the estimated free T_4 concentration or the free T_4 index should also measured along with TSH. Circulating thyroglobulin concentrations are high in hyperthyroidism and low in factitious thyrotoxicosis. Measurement of thyroglobulin in serum, although not routinely recommended, may be useful for differential diagnosis of thyrotoxicosis in patients with no goiter or orbitopathy.

18.6.3   CIRCULATING AUTOANTIBODIES

Quantitation of TRAbs confirms the clinical diagnosis of TDG and serves as a useful indicator of the degree of disease activity. Table 18.6 summarizes the main indications to TRAb assay in clinical practice.[8] Routine measurement of TRAbs will reveal any antibody that binds to TSHRs. Although these assays do not explore the biological activity of TRAbs, a positive result in a hyperthyroid patient is almost pathognomonic of TDG. Although by no means necessary, tests for circulating TgAbs and TPOAbs may be useful to confirm thyroid autoimmunity.

Determination of these antibody titers as II level investigations provides indirect supporting evidence for TDG. More than 95% of patients have positive assays for TPOAbs and about 50% reveal positive TgAb assays. In chronic autoimmune thyroiditis, the prevalence of positive TgAb assays is higher. On the other hand, these antibodies can be detected in a relatively high percentage (up to 25%) of normal subjects, especially elderly women and patients with other non-autoimmune thyroid disorders such as nodular goiter or thyroid carcinoma. Positive assays prove

---

TABLE 18.6

Indications for TRAb Assay

Prediction of relapse of TDG after antithyroid drugs

Diagnostically intriguing conditions:

- Subclinical hyperthyroidism with diffuse goiter
- Hyperthyroidism associated with nodular goiter in iodine-deficient area
- Differentiation between silent and toxic diffuse goiter
- Thyrotoxicosis in pregnancy
- Euthyroid orbitopathy (of limited value)
- Follow-up of differentiated thyroid cancer associated with TDG
- Differentiation of type 1 versus type 2 amiodarone-induced thyrotoxicosis

Prediction of fetal-neonatal hyperthyroidism:

- Previous child with neonatal hyperthyroidism
- TDG disease in mother:

    Euthyroid postablation

    Hypothyroid postablation while on levothyroxine therapy

    On antithyroid drug therapy, requiring high dose in third trimester

Prediction of transient neonatal hypothyroidism:

- Previous child with transient neonatal hypothyroidism
- Autoimmune atrophic thyroiditis on levothyroxine replacement

that autoimmunity is present, but they are not pathognonomic of TDG. Therefore, tests for TPOAbs and TgAbs have limited diagnostic value and must be considered complementary to a diagnosis. During therapy with antithyroid drugs, the titers of TRAbs, TPOAbs, and TgAbs characteristically decrease and the changes persist during remission. A rise in thyroid antibody titers is commonly observed following radioactive iodine treatment.

18.6.4 THYROID RADIOIODINE UPTAKE (RAIU) AND SCAN

RAIU is typically elevated in TDG. However, determining RAIU is not useful in the diagnosis of clinically evident TDG. Measuring RAIU is useful in the differential diagnosis of thyrotoxicosis (Section 18.6.6). Normal ranges for RAIU vary according to the status of iodine supply in the population. In iodine-replete countries, the upper limit of normal 24-hour RAIU is around 25%, whereas it may reach 40% in areas with mild to moderate iodine deficiency. RAIU results can also be used before radioiodine treatment of hyperthyroidism to calculate the dose needed.

A thyroid scintiscan with radioactive iodine (usually ^{123}I) or Tc^{99m} typically shows a symmetrically increased gland (Figure 18.5). RAIU and thyroid scintiscan, like other radioisotopic in vivo procedures, are absolutely contraindicated during pregnancy.

18.6.5 THYROID ULTRASOUND (US)

In hyperthyroid TDG, the echoic pattern of the thyroid undergoes diffuse changes. The tissue, possibly because of reduced colloid content, increased thyroid vascularity, and lymphocytic infiltration, becomes hypoechoic. This pattern, especially when

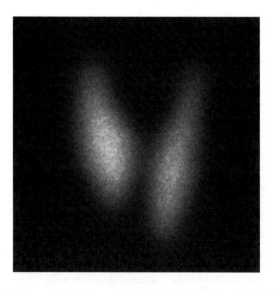

FIGURE 18.5 Tc^{99m} thyroid scintiscan in patient with TDG showing diffuse and increased uptake of radionuclide by thyroid gland.

TABLE 18.7

First- and Second-Level Investigations Required for Diagnosis of TDG

Assay	Finding	Diagnostic Accuracy
	I Level	
TSH	Reduced	Good
FT$_4$	Increased	Good
FT$_3$	Increased	Good
TRAbs	Positive	Excellent
	II Level	
Thyroid ultrasound	Thyroid size: mostly increased; normal pattern rare; hypoechogenic pattern; increased vascularity	Good
Radioactive iodine uptake (RAIU)	Increased, producing homogeneous and symmetric distribution	Good

diffuse, is almost pathognomonic of thyroid autoimmunity. US also allows accurate measurement of thyroid size—a detail that may help in the decision-making process when definitive treatment is planned.

Markedly increased signals indicating hypervascularization that appear in color flow-Doppler (CFD) evaluation indicate hyperthyroid TDG as opposed to painless thyroiditis characterized by a low blood flow. CFD evaluations of the thyroid gland can also be useful to differentiate the hyperthyroidism of TDG from amiodarone-induced thyrotoxicosis, subacute thyroiditis, and factitious thyrotoxicosis. For this reason, CFD evaluation may become a valid substitute for RAIU when these conditions are included in a differential diagnosis.

Coexistent thyroid nodules are easily detected by US. Non-functioning nodules should be evaluated for the presence of thyroid cancer by means of fine-needle aspiration cytology. Whether papillary thyroid cancer is more aggressive when associated with TDG is still a matter of debate. Table 18.7 illustrates the diagnostic approach to a thyrotoxic patient.

18.6.6 DIFFERENTIAL DIAGNOSIS

A patient with all the major manifestations of TDG—thyrotoxicosis, goiter, and infiltrative orbitopathy—does not pose a diagnostic problem. In some patients, however, one of the major manifestations may dominate the clinical picture, no other manifestations may be present, or the disorder may mimic another disease.[9]

The diffuse goiter of TDG may rarely be confused with goiters of other thyroid diseases if thyrotoxicosis is present. Very low values of RAIU in association with thyrotoxicosis signal factitious thyrotoxicosis, ectopic thyroid tissue, subacute "viral" thyroiditis, or the thyrotoxic phase of autoimmune (silent) thyroiditis (Table 18.8). A low value may also alert a clinician to unsuspected iodine-induced hyperthyroidism in which production of hormone by the thyroid gland is increased, for example, following contrast medium or amiodarone administration.

TABLE 18.8

RAIU Differential Diagnosis of TDG from Other Causes of Thyrotoxicosis

Thyrotoxicosis associated with normal or elevated RAIU over neck	Toxic diffuse goiter
	Toxic adenoma or toxic nodular goiter
	Trophoblastic disease
	TSH-secreting pituitary adenoma
	Resistance to thyroid hormone (T_3 receptor mutation)
Thyrotoxicosis associated with near-absent RAIU over neck	Painless (silent) thyroiditis
	Amiodarone-induced thyroiditis
	Subacute (granulomatous, De Quervain's) thyroiditis
	Iatrogenic thyrotoxicosis
	Factitious ingestion of thyroid hormone
	Extensive metastases from follicular thyroid cancer (very rare)

When TDG is in a latent or inactive phase and thyrotoxicosis is absent, a goiter may require differentiation from Hashimoto's thyroiditis or simple nontoxic goiter as possible diagnoses. The goiter of Hashimoto's disease is somewhat lobulated and firmer and rubbery compared with that of TDG. Serum levels of thyroid antibodies are generally higher in Hashimoto's disease but may not be helpful in distinguishing individual patients. In the absence of thyrotoxicosis, the diffuse goiter of TDG cannot be distinguished from non-toxic or simple goiter. An abnormally low serum TSH concentration and the presence of TRAbs indicate underlying TDG, but their absence does not exclude quiescent disease.

18.7 THERAPY

Correction of thyroid hormone overproduction can be achieved through three treatment options: antithyroid drugs (ATDs), radioactive iodine therapy, and thyroidectomy. Selection of a treatment differs in various countries. In the United States, radioactive iodine is the preferred choice, while in Europe and in Japan, ATDs or surgery are most commonly offered. Treatment is also based on patient choice and logistics concerns. Table 18.9 summarizes the main factors indicating or contraindicating a particular treatment modality.

18.7.1 ANTITHYROID DRUGS

18.7.1.1 First Line Therapy

Thionamides, specifically methimazole (MMI), carbimazole, and propylthiouracil (PTU), are the first line antithyroid drugs used to treat hyperthyroidism due to their actions as inhibitors of the organification of iodine and the coupling of iodothyrosines that block the synthesis of thyroid hormones. High dose PTU has the additional effect of partially inhibiting the conversion of T_4 to T_3 in peripheral tissues, but this effect is of limited clinical value. Other effects may depend on immunosuppression resulting in disease remission. Whether this effect is caused by the drug per se or

TABLE 18.9

Factors Indicating or Contraindicating Treatment Modality

	Indication	Contraindication
Antithyroid drug therapies	High likelihood of remission Elderly patients with limited longevity High surgical risk Previous radiation or neck surgery Moderate to severe orbitopathy	Known major adverse reactions
^{131}I therapy	High surgical risk Previously radiation or neck surgery Female planning pregnancy within 12 months High-volume surgeon unavailable	Pregnancy or lactation Coexisting suspicious thyroid nodule or cancer Female planning pregnancy within 12 months Inability to comply with radiation safety guidelines
Surgery	Symptomatic compression Coexisting suspicious thyroid nodule or cancer Moderate to severe orbitopathy Female planning pregnancy within 4 to 6 months	Major comorbidities Pregnancy (absolute contraindication in first and third trimesters)

by the induced euthyroidism is still debated. Carbimazole, a prodrug of MMI, is the preferred ATD in the U.K. PTU and MMI are most commonly used in the United States, Europe, and Asia. MMI is at least 10 times more potent than PTU. Table 18.10 compares the pharmacologic properties of the two major thionamides.

Higher doses of ATDs are sometimes administered continuously and combined with levothyroxine in doses to maintain euthyroid levels (block-and-replace therapy). However, this approach is not generally recommended because it results in a higher rate of ATD side effects. ATDs may be used as a primary therapy to restore and maintain euthyroidism or as a preparative therapy. Table 18.11 shows the principal clinical uses of ATDs. Side effects of MMI and PPU ATDs are reported in 5% of patients although a higher rate of side effects for PTU is often reported. Most side effects are considered minor but in rare cases they may be potentially life threatening. Minor and serious side effects of ATDs are reported in Table 18.12.

Fulminant hepatic necrosis under PTU therapy, sometimes fatal or requiring liver transplantation has been reported. For this reason, PTU is not to be prescribed as a first line agent in children or adults. PTU is recommended instead of MMI during the first trimester of pregnancy or in individuals who experienced severe adverse effects on MMI. The duration of ATD treatment should be 12 to 18 months. Longer periods of treatment may be considered for patients not in remission who refuse or have contraindications for other modalities of treatment.

Remission, defined as normal serum TSH, FT_4, and FT_3 levels for 1 year after discontinuation of ATD therapy, is achieved in about 20 to 30% of patients in the United States and in 40 to 50% of European and Japanese patients. Patients with mild disease, small goiters, and low levels of TSHR antibodies (TRAbs) may have remission rates over 50%, making ATD use more favorable in this group of patients.

TABLE 18.10
Pharmacological Properties of Thionamides: Comparison of Methimazole and Propylthiouracil

Property	Methimazole	Propylthiouracil
Relative potency	10–50	1
Administration route	Oral	Oral
Absorption	Almost complete	Almost complete
Binding to serum proteins	Negligible	80%
Serum half-life (hours)	4–6	1–2
Duration of action (hours)	>24	12–24
Transplacental passage	Low	Lower
Levels in breast milk	Low	Lower
Inhibition of T_4/T_3 conversion	No	Yes
Dosing	1 or 2 times daily	2 or 3 times daily
Initial dosage[a]	10–30 mg	100–300 mg

[a] Dose adjustments usually not necessary in children, elderly, or patients with impaired liver or hepatic function.

TABLE 18.11
Clinical Use of Antithyroid Drugs

Primary Treatment for Hyperthyroidism	Preparative Therapy
To achieve remission	Pretreatment before radio-ablative therapy
In pregnancy	Before thyroid surgery
In children and adolescents	
In severe orbitopathy	

The factors associated with decreased remission rate, both during ATD therapy and after withdrawal, are reported in Table 18.13. Other drugs may be used as symptomatic or adjuvant therapies (Table 18.14).

18.7.1.2   Second Line Therapy

Beta-adrenergic antagonist drugs are always indicated for elderly patients with thyrotoxicosis or patients with severe tachycardia or coexistent cardiovascular diseases. Because of the significant side effects associated with the long-term use of glucocorticoids and the effectiveness of alternative treatments, the use of these drugs for managing TDG is not justified except in cases of orbitopathy and dermopathy.

Iodine-containing compounds and inorganic iodine (as Lugol's solution or a saturated solution of potassium iodide [SSKI]) exert transient antithyroid actions that last a few days or weeks. Therefore, these agents are ideally used in emergency situations when rapid control of thyrotoxicosis is needed, in preparation for thyroid

TABLE 18.12
Side Effects of Antithyroid Drugs

Overall prevalence = 5 %

Minor side effects[a,b]

    Urticaria, skin rash, pruritus

    Arthralgia

    Fever

    Gastrointestinal complaints

    Changes in taste and smell

    Arthritis

    Transient granulocytopenia

Major side effects[a,b]

    Agranulocytosis (absolute granulocyte count < 500/mL)

    Hepatotoxicity: cholestatic hepatitis (MMI), cytotoxic hepatitis (PTU)

    Vasculitis

[a] Cross reactivity between MMI and PTU » 50%.

[b] Side effects of MMI are dose-related; side effects of PTU are less clearly dose-related.

TABLE 18.13
Factors Associated with Decreased Remission Rate during and/or after Antithyroid Drug Therapy

Severe Hyperthyroidism	Thyroid Nodularity on US Imaging
Large goiter	High intrathyroidal blood flow (Doppler US)
High serum T_3/T_4 ratio	High TRAbs at onset of disease or at end of antithyroid drug therapy
Youth	Male sex
Smoking	Long duration of symptoms before treatment
Orbitopathy	Family history of autoimmune thyroid disease

TABLE 18.14
Symptomatic or Adjuvant Therapies

Drug	Goal
Beta-adrenergic antagonist	Decrease tachycardia, palpitation, tremor, anxiety, and sweating
Glucocorticoid	Block conversion of T_4 to T_3 (high doses)
Inorganic iodine	Inhibit iodide oxidation and organification and thyroglobulin proteolysis (thus decreasing preformed thyroid hormone release)
Organic iodine-containing compounds	Inhibit T_4-deiodinase activity
Potassium perchlorate	Competitively inhibit intrathyroidal iodide transport
Lithium carbonate	Inhibit T_4 and T_3 release and possibly their synthesis

surgery, or rarely while waiting for the effect of radioactive iodine therapy. In the latter case, these drugs may also be used to prevent or correct the transient thyrotoxicosis caused by the release of preformed thyroid hormone that may occur after radioactive iodine therapy.

In conjunction with thionamides, perchlorate has been successfully used as a tool for depleting the thyroidal iodine overload in amiodarone-induced hyperthyroidism, while lithium carbonate can be used in cases of severe thyrotoxicosis in persons allergic to iodine or caused by amiodarone. Pretreatment with lithium before radioactive iodine therapy enhances the activity of ^{131}I necessary to cure hyperthyroidism. However, this approach is not widely used.

18.7.2 RADIOACTIVE IODINE THERAPY

Radioactive iodine is the preferred therapy of TDG in the United States. It is a safe and cost-effective treatment intended to cause permanent hypothyroidism in most patients. The isotope of choice is ^{131}I which, after oral administration, is completely absorbed, rapidly concentrated, oxidized, and organified by thyroid follicular cells. The ionizing effects of beta particles destroy thyroid cells and elicit an early inflammatory response, necrosis of follicular cells, and vascular occlusion. These early effects are followed by chronic inflammation and fibrosis leading to thyroid atrophy and hypothyroidism. The exposition to radioactive iodine therapy induces severe changes of thyroid cytology, resembling those of thyroid carcinoma. Therefore, fine-needle aspiration, if necessary, should be performed before ^{131}I therapy.

Before and after ^{131}I therapy, ATD treatment should be considered to avoid the complications due to worsening of thyrotoxicosis, particularly in elderly patients with significant comorbidities such as poorly controlled diabetes mellitus, atrial fibrillation, and cerebrovascular or pulmonary diseases. If given as pretreatments, ATDs should be discontinued 3 to 5 days before the administration of radioactive iodine and restarted 3 to 7 days later. Among ATDs, PTU treatment before ^{131}I increases the radioresistance of the thyroid. The effect of MMI is unclear. Iodine-containing multivitamins and high-iodine diets should be avoided for at least 7 days before ^{131}I administration.

Hypothyroidism can be achieved by administering a fixed single activity (usually 10 to 15 mCi) or by calculating the activity based on the size of the thyroid and its ability to trap iodine, using the following equation:

$$\text{Dose (mCi)} = \frac{\text{Estimated thyroid weight (g)} \times \text{planned dose (μCi/g)}}{\text{Fractional 24-hour radioiodine uptake} \times 1{,}000}$$

Hypothyroidism, regarded as the goal of radioactive iodine therapy, is observed in about 80% of patients when an activity >150 μCu/g is delivered. Table 18.15 summarizes the causes associated with failure of radioactive iodine therapy. Hypothyroidism may occur between 2 and 6 months after therapy; thus, the timing of thyroid hormone replacement should be determined by results of thyroid function tests. Due to the relatively long time lapse from radioactive iodine

TABLE 18.15

Factors Associated with Failure to Cure Hyperthyroidism after Radioactive Iodine Therapy

Youth	Prior exposure to antithyroid drugs
Large thyroid gland (>60 ml)	High ^{131}I uptake with 24-hour value lower than 3- to 6-hour value
Severe thyrotoxicosis	Recurrence of toxic diffuse goiter

therapy and onset of hypothyroidism, a second dose of ^{131}I should not be given for 6 to 12 months.

Short-term adverse effects of radioactive iodine consist of transient exacerbation of mild to moderate preexisting orbitopathy, usually controlled with a short course of oral corticosteroids. When severe orbitopathy is present, specific treatment with high-dose oral or intravenous corticosteroids and/or external radiation therapy should be started soon after radioactive iodine treatment. A long-term increase in cardiovascular and cerebrovascular death rate has been reported after radioactive iodine therapy, most probably related to hyperthyroidism rather than to the therapy.

There is no evidence of increased mortality from cancer after radioactive iodine therapy with the exception of small bowel cancer cited in one study. However, a dose-related increase in cancer incidence, especially of the stomach, kidney, and breast commencing 5 years after ^{131}I therapy has been described. Based on these findings and on data extrapolated after the Chernobyl accident, many authorities (including ourselves) discourage the use of ^{131}I in patients younger than 16 to 18 years.

Because of transplacental passage and passage into breast milk, pregnancy and breastfeeding are absolute contraindications to ^{131}I therapy. Pregnancy should be avoided during the first 6 to 12 months after ^{131}I therapy, and planned when euthyroidism is restored. A pregnancy test should be performed 48 hours before a therapeutic or diagnostic radioactive procedure for all premenopausal sexually active women. Every country has radiation protection rules regarding radioactive iodine therapy that must be followed.

18.7.3 SURGERY

Near-total and total thyroidectomy are the surgical procedures. Thyroidectomy is more costly than ATD or radioactive iodine therapy. However, the risks of recurrence are 0% and 8% for total thyroidectomy and near-total thyroidectomy, respectively. Recurrence of hyperthyroidism is particularly undesirable because a second operation is technically more difficult than the first one and involves greater risk of complications. With few exceptions, such patients should be treated with radioactive iodine therapy. Indications for thyroid surgery in diffuse toxic goiter are reported in Table 18.16.

Patients undergoing surgery should be euthyroid. A course of thionamide treatment is recommended to restore and maintain euthyroidism and deplete intrathyroidal stores of hormones that may be released during surgery. The preoperative administration (10 days) of inorganic iodine (3 to 5 drops three times a

---

TABLE 18.16

Indications for Surgery in DTG

Patient preference

Large goiter

Coexisting suspicious thyroid nodule or cancer

Children and adolescents

Pregnant women (second trimester)

---

day) induces involution of the gland and a reduction in vascularity. When emergency surgery is needed, oral cholecystographic agents represent the fastest way to obtain euthyroidism.

Specific complications of thyroid surgery are thyroid storm (now extremely rare), bleeding, injury to the recurrent laryngeal nerve, and hypoparathyroidism. In the hands of an experienced high-volume thyroid surgeon, permanent hypocalcemia is less than 2% and permanent recurrent laryngeal nerve injury occurs in <1%. Bleeding necessitating reoperation occurs in 0.3 to 0.7% of cases. Mortality after thyroidectomy is extremely rare, between 1 in 10,000 and 5 in 10,000,000.

Postoperative routine supplementation with oral calcium and calcitriol decreases the development of hypocalcemic symptoms. This supplementation may be continued or tapered according to serum calcium and/or PTH levels. Following thyroidectomy, levothyroxine should be started at a daily dose appropriate for the patient's weight (1.7 µg/Kg body weight/day), and serum TSH measured 6 to 8 weeks postoperatively.

18.7.4 TDG AND PREGNANCY

In a pregnant woman with TDG, ATD therapy should be used. PTU was generally preferred in pregnancy because of the rare teratogenic effect associated with MMI (aplasia cutis and choanal or esophageal atresia). Recently, a rare but potentially fatal PTU hepatotoxicity led the U.S. Food and Drug Administration to recommend that PTU be reserved for patients in their first trimesters of pregnancy or those who are allergic to or intolerant of MMI. The ATD dose in pregnancy should be the lowest possible to keep maternal FT_4 in the upper level of the normal range for pregnancy and avoid fetal hypothyroidism particularly in the second and third trimesters when the fetal thyroid has begun to function.

Pregnancy is an absolute contraindication to radioactive iodine therapy. When thyroidectomy is necessary during pregnancy, it should be performed during the second trimester to avoid the increased risks of miscarriage and of premature delivery that may occur in the first and second trimesters, respectively.

The block-and-replace regimen is not recommended in pregnancy, because much more thionamide than levothyroxine will cross the placenta and cause fetal hypothyroidism. Iodine is avoided because of the risk of fetal hypothyroidism and goiter caused by the greater sensitivity of the fetal thyroid to the Wolff-Chaikoff effect. The use of beta-blockers is controversial in pregnancy, but these drugs may be allowed for short treatment periods.

Both MMI and PTU are secreted in breast milk in small amounts (MMI more than PTU). MMI doses up to 20 mg daily have been documented not to affect infant thyroid function.[10]

18.7.5 TDG in Children and Adolescents

Children and adolescents with TDG may be treated with ATDs, radioactive iodine therapy, or thyroid surgery. Although long-term remission after ATD occurs in only a small minority of pediatric patients, MMI therapy for 1 to 2 years is still considered the first line treatment for most children. Only MMI should be used in children, since PTU is associated with very high risks of hepatotoxicity and liver failure. The MMI dose for a pediatric population ranges from 0.1 to 1 mg/kg/day. The overall rate of side effects to ATDs (minor and major) in children is reported to be 6 to 35% (Table 18.17).

The duration of MMI therapy should be 1 to 2 years. The remission rate after cessation of therapy is low (20 to 30%), particularly if the thyroid gland is large, the child is younger than 12 years, not Caucasian, serum TRAb levels are above normal on therapy, or FT_4 levels are elevated at diagnosis (>4 ng/dL; 50 pmol/L).

The high failure rate of standard trials of ATD therapy in children and adolescents with diffuse toxic goiter implies that MMI therapy should either be continued for extended periods or definitive therapy should be proposed. Radioactive iodine, when administered at a sufficiently high dose, is an effective treatment option in the pediatric population. However, the increased rates of thyroid nodules and thyroid cancer observed in young children exposed to radiation from nuclear fallout at Hiroshima and after the Chernobyl nuclear reactor explosion raised concerns about this therapy.

To date, long-term studies did not show long-term side effects of radioactive iodine therapy in terms of thyroid cancer and genetic damage in adults treated with ^{131}I as children or adolescents. However, the number of treated patients and the duration of follow-up are still insufficient to allow definitive conclusions. It is important to emphasize that larger (>150 µCi/g of thyroid tissue) rather than smaller activities of ^{131}I must be administered in children to achieve hypothyroidism and avoid the risk of thyroid neoplasia due to residual radiated thyroid tissue.

Surgery is an acceptable form of therapy for TDG in children. Indications for surgery are summarized in Table 18.18. Before surgery, children should be rendered euthyroid with a short course of MMI. Near-total or total thyroidectomy is the recommended procedure.

TABLE 18.17
Side Effects of Methimazole in Pediatric Population

Pruritic rash	Fever or pharyngitis (suggesting agranulocytosis)
Arthralgias, myalgias	Jaundice, dark urine, acolic stools (suggesting hepatotoxicity)
Abdominal pain, nausea	Fatigue

TABLE 18.18
Indications for Surgery in Pediatric Patients with TDG

Suspicious nodules or cancer

Very young children (<5 years) in whom ^{131}I is contraindicated

Presence of high-volume thyroid surgeon

Large thyroid gland (>60 g)

Poor response to [131]I

TABLE 18.19
Factors in Pathogenesis of Thyroid Storm

Abrupt cessation of antithyroid drugs

Thyroid or nonthyroidal surgery in inadequately treated patient

Acute illness

After radioactive iodine therapy (rare)

Use of iodine-containing contrast agents (rare)

18.7.6 THYROID CRISIS (OR STORM)

Thyroid storm is an acute and severe life-threatening complication of thyrotoxicosis with a high mortality rate if not immediately recognized and treated aggressively. Precipitants of thyroid storm in a patient with previously compensated thyrotoxicosis are summarized in Table 18.19.

Symptoms suggestive for thyroid storm are tachycardia, arrhythmias, congestive heart failure, hypotension, hyperpyrexia, agitation, delirium, psychosis, stupor and coma, as well as nausea, vomiting, diarrhea, and hepatic failure. Treatment includes procedures to normalize body temperature, sustain peripheral circulation, and prevent shock. All means (beta-adrenergic blockade, antithyroid drug therapy, inorganic iodide, corticosteroids) should be used to reduce the levels of circulating thyroid hormones. Iodinated contrast agents are probably the fastest way to obtain a significant reduction in circulating T_3.

18.8 PROGNOSIS

Untreated TDG can lead to significant morbidity, disability, and even death. However, the long-term history also includes spontaneous remission in some cases and eventually spontaneous development of hypothyroidism if autoimmune thyroiditis coexists and destroys the thyroid gland. When effective thyroid treatment is started, the general response is mostly favorable: physical symptoms resolve, vitality returns, and mental processes again become efficient.

However, symptom relief is usually not immediate and is achieved over time as the circulating thyroid hormone levels return to normal range. This may require 4 to

6 weeks after initiation of treatment with antithyroid drugs that do not block the release of preformed thyroid hormones deposited in thyroid follicles. In addition, not all symptoms may resolve at the same time. Prognosis also depends on the duration and severity of the disease before starting treatment.

Evaluation of TRAb titers is useful in predicting the outcomes for patients with TDG who are treated with antithyroid drugs. Persisting TRAbs at high levels indicate a poor remission rate after withdrawal of medical therapy.

18.9   FOLLOW-UP

Adequate follow-up must be carried out after any kind of treatment of TDG (Table 18.20). Periodic clinical and biochemical evaluation of thyroid status is needed for patients taking ATDs, and it is essential that the patients understand the importance of regular evaluation. Assessments of serum free T4 and free T3 should be obtained about 4 weeks after initiation of therapy, then every 4 to 8 weeks until euthyroidism is achieved. The dose of medication should be adjusted accordingly.

After a patient is euthyroid, biochemical testing and clinical evaluation can be undertaken at intervals of 2 to 3 months. Serum TSH may remain suppressed for several months after starting therapy and is therefore not a good parameter for monitoring therapy early in the course. Measurement of TRAb levels prior to stopping antithyroid drug therapy is suggested, as it helps predict which patients can be weaned from the medication; normal levels indicate greater chance for remission. Patients are considered in remission if they maintain normal serum TSH, FT_4, and T_3 concentrations for 1 year after discontinuation of ATDs.

TABLE 18.20
In Vitro and in Vivo Investigations in Follow-Up of TDG

Assay	Finding
Laboratory Studies	
TSH	May be suppressed ≥2 months, even when normal serum levels of T_4 and T_3 are restored by ATD or radioactive iodine treatment; when TSH returns to normal range, TSH is best parameter for monitoring and adjusting therapy
FT_4	Effective for monitoring response to therapy
FT_3	Effective for monitoring response to therapy
TRAb	Persistent elevation correlates with disease activity; remission usually accompanied by decrease in antibody titers; not usually necessary for monitoring
Imaging Studies	
Thyroid US	Not routinely used; helpful for evaluation of nodules and vascularization
RAIU	Usually used to measure uptake in planning of ^{131}I treatment
Neck CT or MR	Useful only in cases of signs or symptoms of obstruction
Orbital imaging	Useful only in cases of worsening orbitopathy

Early or late recurrence after drug withdrawal is always possible, but nearly 90% of the relapses of hyperthyroidism occur within the first 2 years after ATD withdrawal. In addition, there is always the threat that the orbitopathy may worsen even when patient progress seems favorable. Lower remission rates have been described in men, smokers (especially men), and patients with large goiters. Persistently high levels of TRAbs and high thyroid blood flow as assessed by CFD are also associated with higher relapse rates. These patients should be assessed more frequently and at shorter intervals after antithyroid drugs are discontinued.

Conversely, patients with mild disease, small goiters, and negative TRAbs have a remission rates over 50%, making the use of antithyroid medications potentially more favorable in this group. When antithyroid drugs are discontinued, thyroid function testing should continue to be monitored at 1- to 3-month intervals for 6 to 12 months for an early diagnosis of relapsing hyperthyroidism. Thyroid ultrasound may be useful; other imaging studies are not usually performed. Patients should be counseled to contact their treating physicians if symptoms of hyperthyroidism are recognized.

Patients who undergo near-total thyroidectomy should have replacement levothyroxine therapy after the procedure. Thyroid failure is also seen after ^{131}I therapy. Early or late hypothyroidism may also occur in patients with TDG who experience long-lasting remissions after medical therapy. Table 18.21 lists all drugs cited in this chapter.

TABLE 18.21
Drugs Cited in This Chapter

Drug	Dosage	Notes
	Antithyroid Drugs	
Methimazole	5–60 mg/day	
Propylthiouracil	50–600 mg/day	Not available in some countries
	Beta Blockers	
Propranolol	10–40 mg three or four times a day	
Atenolol	25–100 mg one or two times a day	
Metoprolol	25–50 mg four times a day	
Nadolol	40–160 mg daily	
Esmolol	IV pump: 50–100 mg/kg/min	In intensive care unit
Supersaturated potassium iodide	1 or 2 drops (50 mg iodide/drop) three times a day	
Potassium iodide (Lugol's solution)	5–7 drops (8 mg iodide/drop) three times a day	
Iopanoic acid and sodium iodate	0.5–1 g/day	Not available in most countries
Lithium	450–900 mg/day	
Perchlorate	50–1500 mg/day	

REFERENCES

1. Emiliano, A.B., Governale, L., Parks, M. et al. 2010. Shifts in propylthiouracil and methimazole prescribing practices: antithyroid drug use in the United States from 1991 to 2008. *J Clin Endocrinol Metab* 95: 2227–2233.
2. Rotondi, M., Chiovato, L., Romagnani, S. et al. 2007. Role of chemokines in endocrine autoimmune diseases. *Endocr Rev* 28: 492–520.
3. Tomer, Y. 2010. Genetic susceptibility to autoimmune thyroid disease: past, present, and future. *Thyroid* 20: 715–725.
4. Rotondi, M., Cappelli, C., Pirali, B. et al. 2008. The effect of pregnancy on subsequent relapse from Graves' disease after a successful course of antithyroid drug therapy. *J Clin Endocrinol Metab* 93: 3985–3988.
5. Weetman, A. 2009. Immune reconstitution syndrome and the thyroid. *Best Pract Res Clin Endocrinol Metab* 23: 693–702.
6. Brent, G.A. 2008. Clinical practice: Graves' disease. *New Engl J Med* 12: 2594–2605.
7. Biondi, B. And Kahaly, G.J. 2010. Cardiovascular involvement in patients with different causes of hyperthyroidism. *Nat Rev Endocrinol* 6: 431–443.
8. Zöphel, K., Roggenbuck, D., and Schott, M. 2010. Clinical review about TRAb assay's history. *Autoimmun Rev* 9: 695–700.
9. Bahn, R.S., Burch, H.B., Cooper, D.S. et al. 2011. Hyperthyroidism and other causes of thyrotoxicosis: Management Guidelines of the American Thyroid Association and American Association of Clinical Endocrinologists. *Thyroid* 21: 593–646.
10. Negro, R., Beck-Peccoz, P., Chiovato, L. et al. 2011. Hyperthyroidism and pregnancy: an Italian Thyroid Association (AIT) and Italian Association of Clinical Endocrinologists (AME) joint statement for clinical practice. *J Endocrinol Invest* 34: 225–231.

19 Toxic Multinodular Goiter

Giorgio Napolitano and Fabrizio Monaco

CONTENTS

Key words: autonomously functioning thyroid nodule, hot nodule, hyperthyroidism, subclinical hyperthyroidism, atrial fibrillation, apathetic syndrome, iodine deficiency, radioiodine treatment.

19.1 DEFINITION

Toxic multinodular goiter (TMNG), also named Plummer's disease according to Henry Stanley Plummer who first described a "non-hyperplastic toxic goiter" in 1913, is a cause of hyperthyroidism due to the presence of one or more autonomously functioning thyroid nodules that are usually mixed with other hypo- or normally functioning thyroid nodules. Thyroid scintigraphy shows the coexistence of areas of different uptake levels (increased, hot and reduced, cold nodules).

TMNG is also defined by suppressed TSH values that indicate thyroid autonomy (independence from TSH stimulus) and differentiate the condition from nontoxic multinodular goiter. As TMNG usually develops on a long-standing goiter and the overall functional status is determined by the balance of the properties of the coexisting nodules, it is important to understand that the clinical condition of a patient is not static and may change over time.

19.2 EPIDEMIOLOGY

TMNG is more frequent in iodine-deficient regions where it can be the most frequent cause of hyperthyroidism. Indeed, in iodine-deficient areas of Denmark, thyroid autonomy accounts for 60% of hyperthyroid patients, with TMNG five times more frequent than single toxic nodules. In iodine-sufficient areas, thyroid autonomy is responsible for <10% of hyperthyroidism[1] (Figure 19.1). TMNG has a prevalence of 1 to 8 cases/10^6 inhabitants and is more frequent in iodine-deficient areas.

However, thyroid autonomy can be demonstrated (by thyroid scan) in 40% of patients with non-toxic multinodular goiters and thus more patients are at risk to develop TMNG. This observation is also supported by the evidence of increased prevalence of TMNG following an increase in iodine intake from iodine-containing drugs or use of radiographic contrast agents. An increased prevalence of TMNG after iodine supplementation has been described in old studies. However, after 15 years of salt supplementation with iodine, a 73% decrease of TMNG has been registered in Switzerland.[2] TMNG frequency increases with age; it is usually detected 40 and 60 years of age and 50% of patients are older than 60. Patients with TMNG are usually 10 years older than patients with Graves' disease. As with most thyroid diseases, TMNG is more frequent in women (female:male ratio = 4:1 to 10:1).

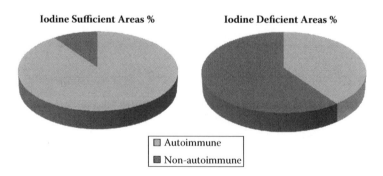

Iodine Sufficient Areas %   **Iodine Deficient Areas %**

☐ Autoimmune
■ Non-autoimmune

FIGURE 19.1   Frequency of autoimmune and non-autoimmune hyperthyroidism in iodine-sufficient and iodine-deficient areas.

19.3 ETIOLOGY

Epidemiological data clearly show that iodine deficiency, sex, age, and duration of goiter are the main determinants for TMNG. A sequence of three steps that lead to nodular development and thyroid autonomy has been proposed[2-4] (Figure 19.2).

The first step is based on the thyroid hyperplasia favored by iodine deficiency and with minor impact by goitrogens. A growth-promoting effect is likely to be played by estrogens as well. They have been shown in vitro to stimulate growth and proliferation of rat thyroid cells (FRTL-5). In this setting of increased cell proliferation a higher number of cell mutations are likely. H_2O_2 and free radical production that usually accompanies thyroid cell proliferation would cause DNA damage and increase cell mutations. The high replication rate would also interfere with mutation-repairing mechanisms, further facilitating damages to genes involved in thyroid cell growth and function.

Those somatic mutations that confer constitutive activation (independently of TSH binding) of the cAMP pathway cause an increase of thyroid cell function and proliferation, thus initiating focal growth (step 2). Mutation of TSH receptor (TSHr) and Gsα protein activates the cAMP pathway and have indeed been detected in TMNG (mutations of TSHr are more frequent than those of Gsα).

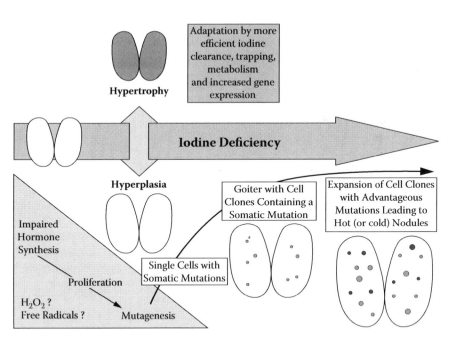

FIGURE 19.2   Hypothesis for development of thyroid autonomy. Iodine deficiency increases mutagenesis and, following hyperplasia, some clones develop; according to the type of mutation (i.e.. activating the TSHr pathway or leading to dedifferentiation). "hot" or "cold" nodules develop.

The main role of activating mutations in the pathogenesis of TMNG is confirmed by the observation that different mutations can coexist within the same goiter; each one is responsible for different nodules (encapsulated adenomas or unencapsulated hyperplastic adenomatous nodules). Moreover, mutations of genes responsible for thyroid growth but not function (i.e., genes stimulating only proliferation like those in the *ras* cascade) have been detected in nonfunctioning (cold) nodules. In a proliferating thyroid, growth factors (IGF-1, TGF-β1, EGF) are overexpressed and favor the proliferation of mutated cells that will form small clones (step 3).

19.4   NATURAL COURSE

Two correlated aspects of TMNG must be followed over its natural course: nodule growth and thyroid function. Increasing volumes of thyroid nodules have been described in both iodine-sufficient and -deficient areas. In different studies with 3- to 5-year follow-ups, an increase (>30% of initial volume) of thyroid nodules was reported in 30 to 50% of patients. Several studies have shown that the increased nodular volume is critical to the development of hyperthyroidism and that a volume equal to or greater than 16 mL is frequently associated with hyperthyroidism.

In TMNG, hyperthyroidism has been shown to be correlated to dimensions of hyperfunctioning nodules and age. The correlation is corroborated by old studies performed at the Mayo Clinic showing that (1) 60% of patients 60 or more years of age with multinodular goiters (MNGs) were hyperthyroid, (2) the average duration of goiter before developing hyperthyroidism was 17 years, and (3) the longer the duration of goiter, the higher the risk of becoming hyperthyroid. Finally, studies report the onset of overt hyperthyroidism in 10% of patients with previous euthyroid MNG during 7 to 12 years of follow-up and the development of thyroid autonomy (as shown by suppressed TSH levels) in 8 to 9% of patients with previously normal thyroid function tests in a 5-year follow-up.

All these data confirm that in MNG patients, the progression first to subclinical and then to overt hyperthyroidism is a slow phenomenon developing over years. However two possible intervening factors may change the fate of a goiter. Excessive amounts of iodine intake, for example, after administration of contrast agents or iodine-containing drugs such as amiodarone will hasten the progression to thyroid autonomy and clinical hyperthyroidism. Iodine contamination has been indeed evidenced in 54% of non-autoimmune hyperthyroidism. Conversely, in a small percentage of patients, hemorrhagic and necrotic phenomena within nodules may significantly reduce the number of thyroid cells and thus slow the progression toward hyperthyroidism.

19.5   CLINICAL FEATURES

Symptoms of TMNG are dependent on the volume of the thyroid gland and the severity of thyrotoxicosis. About half of the patients seek initial assistance for symptoms related to the goiter, 25% for thyrotoxicosis, and the remainder for specific symptoms.[5] A patient may consult a doctor because of a lump in the neck without clinical manifestation. In a different scenario, an increase in thyroid size may cause

TABLE 19.1
Presenting Symptoms of Patients with TMNG

	Symptom	%
Compressive symptoms	Choking	40
	Dysphagia	35
	Dyspnea	25
Cardiac symptoms	Tachycardia	65
	Atrial fibrillation	30
	Angina	2–3
	Heart failure	1–3

symptoms likely to result from pressure, for example, coughing, choking, difficulty in swallowing, and dyspnea (Table 19.1).

Compressive symptoms have been reported in 20% of patients.[6] Rarely enlargement of the thyroid may affect a recurrent laryngeal or phrenic nerve, causing palsy or compression of a sympathetic nerve leading to Horner's syndrome characterized by the classic triad of miosis (i.e., constricted pupils), partial ptosis, and loss of hemifacial sweating (i.e., anhydrosis). Very rarely, acute airway obstruction may occur. An alternative presentation is due to a sudden increase in the size of all or part of the gland along with pain and tenderness. In such cases, bleeding within a thyroid nodule may be documented by ultrasound. Usually symptoms subside within few days. In all these clinical presentations, the discovery of low or suppressed TSH, FT_3 and FT_4 within the normal range (i.e., subclinical hyperthyroidism) is very common and usually no clinical signs of hyperthyroidism are present.

Table 19.2 lists the prevalence of symptoms and signs of hyperthyroidism observed in TMNG patients. The most frequent signs or symptoms are tachycardia, asthenia, agitation, weight loss, and heat intolerance. Note, however, that the clinical course of TMNG is often insidious, slow, and spans years. Symptoms can be ignored for long time, especially in elderly patients who may be affected by the so-called "apathetic syndrome" combining weight loss, anorexia, tachycardia, and general weakness with apathy and depression. Although the classical description of hyperthyroidism fits only a small proportion of patients (usually under 50 years old) with TMNG, all signs and symptoms (especially those affecting the cardiovascular system) related to thyrotoxicosis have been described. However, differences exist among patients affected by TMNG and Graves' disease.

19.5.1 CARDIOVASCULAR SYSTEM

Tachycardia is responsible for palpitations, the most frequent symptoms of thyroid hormone excess in young patients. Increased heart rate along with increased preload with low systemic vascular resistance leading to increased stroke volume cause high cardiac output. Despite their high cardiac output state, however, hyperthyroid patients have reduced exercise tolerance because of the inadequate increase in cardiac output during physical exercise.

TABLE 19.2

Prevalence of Symptoms and Signs of Hyperthyroidism Observed in TMNG

Symptom or Sign	%
Tachycardia	65–75
Weight loss	50–60
Asthenia	50–60
Emotional disturbance	45–55
Increased sweating	40–50
Heat intolerance	30–45
Hyperkinetic behavior	30–40
Polydipsia	26–35
Tremor	25–35
Atrial fibrillation	25–35
Diarrhea	10–12
Polyphagia	5–7
Leg edema	5–7

Studies comparing cardiovascular function in Graves' and TMNG patients showed significant differences. The maximal work rate was significantly reduced in untreated patients with hyperthyroidism (P <0.0001), especially in those with toxic multinodular goiters.[7] Compared to Graves' patients, those with TMNG had decreased forced vital capacity and oxygen uptake per heartbeat and decreased left ventricular ejection fraction as shown by echocardiography. Results were probably influenced by the different ages of the two groups of patients.

As to cardiac arrhythmia issues, atrial arrhythmias, dysfunctions of the sinus nodes, and supraventricular ectopic activities are more frequent in hyperthyroid patients. Prevalence of supraventricular arrhythmia is higher in patients with TMNG than in those with Graves' disease (80% versus 15% respectively). Atrial fibrillation is the most common cardiac complication in hyperthyroid patients, especially in elderly individuals, and develops in 10 to 28% of patients with thyrotoxicosis compared to 0.5 to 9.0% of the general population. It increases with age (31% of patients 40 years of age or older versus 0% of patients under 40) and in elderly hyperthyroid patients can cause a progressive increase in left atrial size.

Atrial fibrillation is more frequent in patients with TMNG (43%) than in those with Graves (10%) and is more common in males than females.[7] Atrial fibrillation can be categorized as paroxysmal (recurrent episodes lasting less than 1 week) or persistent (recurrent episodes lasting more than 1 week). In patients with overt or subclinical hyperthyroidism, it is usually persistent and must be considered an important adverse cardiovascular event because the consequences of atrial fibrillation can be detrimental to the heart.

The risk of persistent atrial fibrillation is high in patients with TMNG, because of their advanced age and because they usually experience several years of subclinical hyperthyroidism before diagnosis. Coexistence of ischemic heart disease, congestive heart failure, or heart valve disease is frequently associated with atrial fibrillation (1.8-fold, 3.9-fold, and 2.6-fold increases, respectively). Atrial fibrillation is a risk factor for cardiovascular or cerebrovascular disease, whose frequency has been investigated in a hyperthyroid population. Cardiovascular disease was more frequent in patients with both Graves' disease and TMNG. However, the increased frequency of cardiovascular disease in autoimmune hyperthyroidism is age-dependent and only present in patients over 45 years old. In TMNG patients, the risk of cardiovascular disease is increased at all ages with increased risk of cerebrovascular disease only for patients aged 65 years or older. Congestive heart failure is a further cardiovascular complication of hyperthyroidism. It is more common in patients above 60 years of age with long-term hyperthyroidism (therefore in TMNG) and in individuals with preexisting atrial fibrillation.

19.5.2 GASTROINTESTINAL APPARATUS

Unlike Graves' disease, all the symptoms due to the association of other autoimmune disorders such as atrophic gastritis or celiac disease are missing in TMNG. However, the signs and symptoms due to increased levels of thyroid hormones are still present although usually less serious. Intestinal motility is accelerated with a 50% time reduction of food transit through jejunum and colon, thus leading to diarrhea. Weight loss is dependent on the duration and severity of hyperthyroidism.

Dysphagia is related to the size of the nodule and/or gland and is therefore more frequent in patients suffering from TMNG (especially those with a long history of goiter) than in those affected by Graves' disease, which usually causes only a limited increase of volume. Liver function is mildly impaired in most patients and hyperbilirubinemia can be observed in exceptional cases; it is likely to be due to increased erythrocyte turnover during hyperthyroidism. Slightly increased transaminases are a common feature as is the observation of high γGT levels.

19.5.3 BONES, JOINTS, AND CALCIUM METABOLISM

The association of hyperthyroidism and osteoporosis has been known for at least 50 years and occurs more frequently in postmenopausal women and elderly patients. Recent evidence indicates that reduction of bone mass density (BMD) occurs even when thyroid hormones are in the upper normal range and it is associated with increased risk of non-vertebral fractures.[8]

Osteoporosis must be therefore evaluated even in patients whose subclinical hyperthyroidism remains stable. However, diagnosis and treatment of hyperthyroidism will reverse the increased risk of fracture that will equal the risk in control populations 3 years after treatment. Calcium metabolism results in accelerated turnover with increased osteoclastic activity. Calcium and phosphorus excretion in urine is increased, while serum calcium and phosphate are usually within normal ranges. However, moderate hypercalcemia is not rare. Alkaline phosphatase may be elevated in thyrotoxicosis and may further increase after therapy because of the increase of bone isoenzymes.

19.5.4 Skin

Although symptoms associated with autoimmunity such as vitiligo or pretibial myx-edema that play central roles in cutaneous involvement of Graves' disease are miss-ing, symptoms related to overactivity of the vasomotor system are part of the clinical pictures of TMNG patients. The skin is warm and moist and looks thin and soft. Perspiration is excessive, even after moderate exercise and suggestive of a hyper-metabolic state. Although warm and moist hands can be found in other conditions, cold and dry hands almost always exclude hyperthyroidism.

19.5.5 Neuromuscular System

The central and autonomous nervous system are involved in hyperthyroidism. Increased irritability, nervousness, insomnia, and tremors are only some of the com-plaints. The fine tremor (one of the cardinal signs) varies widely in intensity, with a frequency of about 8 to 10 tremors per second. Encephalopathy has been reported in extreme hyperthyroidism and is very uncommon in TMNG.

Muscular weakness is a common feature but must be carefully analyzed by specific questioning. Myopathy has been observed in 10% of TMNG patients and resembles myasthenia gravis. Thyrotoxic periodic paralysis is a rare complication in Europe and America and more frequent in the Far East. Symptoms are similar to those of periodic hypokalemic paralysis, usually appear after physical stress or exposure to cold, and may be provoked by a carbohydrate-rich diet.

19.5.6 Specific Presentations

As mentioned before, atrial fibrillation is a common feature of TMNG patients, espe-cially those 60 years of age or older. It can be the initial symptom of the so-called apathetic syndrome that combines weight loss, anorexia, apathy, and weakness and mimics a depressive disorder. The syndrome may appear as non-specific, since most of the common symptoms of hyperthyroidism in young patients, such as hyperpha-gia, tachycardia, warm skin, and increased perspiration, are missing, and may be confused with melancholia. Note that subclinical hyperthyroidism (see Chapter 23) is typical of TMNG; the name implies that clinical manifestations are missing or very mild and the diagnosis is based on laboratory tests. It has been detected in up to 40% of patients with TMNG and can persist for a long time.

19.6 DIAGNOSIS

19.6.1 Clinical

Patients who consult thyroid centers for hyperthyroidism in several cases turn out to be euthyroid and are affected by anxiety state or neurotic personality. Tachycardia, palpitations, tremor, and hyperhydrosis are common to both psychiatric and hyper-thyroid patients. Weight loss is not unique to thyrotoxicosis and is also associated with neoplasia, chronic infections, and pheochromocytoma. It also occurs in severe diabetes mellitus in conjunction with hyperphagia.

Several other conditions such as Paget's disease, arteriovenous fistulas, lead intoxication, and Addison's disease exhibit symptoms resembling hyperthyroidism and must be ruled out before a clinical diagnosis of hyperthyroidism is accepted. An old but useful tool for diagnosing hyperthyroidism is Crooks' clinical index[9] (Table 19.3). Note, however, that in patients with mild hyperthyroidism, such as elderly patients with TMNG, the clinical index score is often within the euthyroid range.

TABLE 19.3
Clinical Index for Hyperthyroidism

Symptom or Sign	Present	Absent	Symptom or Sign	Present	Absent
Dyspnea on effort[a]	+1		Bruit over thyroid[i]	+2	−2
Palpitation[b]	+2		Exophthalmos[j]	+2	
Tiredness[c]	+2		Lid retraction[k]	+2	
Preference for heat[d]		−5	Lid lag[l]	+1	
Preference for cold[d]	+5		Hyperkinetic movements[m]	+4	−2
Excessive sweating[e]	+3		Finger tremor[n]	+1	
Nervousness[f]	+2		Hot hands[o]	+2	−2
Appetite increased	+3		Moist hands[o]	+1	−1
Appetite decreased		−3	Fibrillation	+4	
Weight increased[g]		−3	Pulse rate < 80 per minute		−3
Weight decreased[g]	+3		Pulse rate 80–90 per minute	0	
Palpable thyroid[h]	+3	−3	Pulse rate >90 per minute	+3	

Source: Crooks, J., Murray, I.P.C., and Wayne, E.J. 1959. *Q J Med* 28: 211–234.

Note: Euthyroid: Fewer than 11 points. Doubtful: 11–19 points. Hyperthyroid: 20 or more points.

[a] Age must be taken into account.
[b] At rest or on light effort.
[c] Unusual exhaustion after familiar effort.
[d] Question patient, e.g., What type of weather do you prefer? How do you feel in a warm room?
[e] Thermal and emotional sweating.
[f] Irritability, easy loss of temper, tenseness.
[g] At least 3 kg within up to 1 year.
[h] Palpable and visible.
[i] High pitched systolic or to-and-from.
[j] Sclera visible between lower lid and iris with patient looking straight ahead.
[k] Sclera visible between upper lid and iris with patient looking straight ahead.
[l] Area of sclera appears or increases when patient's eyes are fixed on examiner's finger moving downward.
[m] Rapid, jerky (overreactive) movements on dressing and undressing.
[n] Patient's eyes closed, outstretched, separated fingers; ignore coarse tremor.
[o] Compared to hands of examiner and considering ambient temperature.

19.6.2 LABORATORY

TSH is by far the most useful test for detecting hyperthyroidism. It shows the highest sensitivity and specificity in the evaluation of hyperthyroidism and serves as the first screening test (Table 19.4). However, free T_4 (FT_4) assay in addition to TSH strongly improves the accuracy of diagnosis and discriminates between subclinical and overt hyperthyroidism. Remember that FT_4 and TSH have an inverse log-linear relationship. Thus, small changes of FT_4 result in great modifications of TSH. TSH and FT_4 determinations are therefore the first line investigations.

Elevation of FT_4 and free T_3 (FT_3) are not uncommonly dissociated, i.e., only FT_3 is elevated. This situation, called T_3 toxicosis, is observed in 10 to 40% of TMNG patients and is typically encountered in iodine-deficient areas. It probably reflects predominant T_3 secretion by a nodule. Therefore, in patients with TMNG, diagnosis of hyperthyroidism relies on TSH and FT_4 as well as FT_3 determinations (Table 19.4). It must be emphasized that the FT_3 and FT_4 assays commonly used in non-reference laboratories are estimates. This means that the bound and free fractions of the iodothyronines are not separated before testing (this result is obtained by equilibrium dialysis, ultrafiltration, and gel filtration[10]); as a consequence, assays are binding protein-dependent to some extent.

In this context, assays estimating FT_3 are less validated than those evaluating FT_4 and therefore less reliable. Measurement of total T_3 is therefore preferred in some labsoratories.[11] Measurement of thyroid antibodies (antithyroglobulin antibodies [Tg-Abs] and thyroid peroxidase antibodies [TPO-Abs]) is not usually necessary as a first line test.

In iodine-deficient areas, however, differential diagnosis between TMNG and Graves' disease may be difficult if ophthalmopathy is absent and/or nodules are present (25 to 35%) in Graves' patients. Detection of TSH-receptor antibodies (TSHr-Abs) that are causative of Graves' disease and are absent in TMNG may discriminate the two diseases, especially in those patients, such as women who are pregnant or

TABLE 19.4
Diagnostic Investigation for TMNG

	I Level Tests	Accuracy	II Level Tests	Accuracy
Laboratory	TSH	Excellent	TSHr-Ab	Poor
	FT_4	Excellent	Tg-Ab	Poor
	FT_3	Good	TPO-Ab	Poor
			Urinary iodine excretion	Poor
Imaging	Scintigraphy (^{99m}Tc, ^{131}I, or ^{123}I)	Excellent	X-ray scan	Good
	Ultrasound	Good	Color Doppler flow	Poor
			Suppression scintigraphy	Poor
			CT scan	Poor
			MR scan	Poor

breastfeeding and cannot undergo thyroid scintigraphy (see below). Urinary iodine excretion can be measured if iodine contamination is suspected.

19.6.3 IMAGING

Identification of hyperfunctioning nodules in a thyroid is based on thyroid scintigraphy performed by administering either ^{99m}pertechnate (^{99m}Tc) or radioactive iodine (mainly ^{123}I or ^{131}I). The scintigraphy materials are transported within the thyrocytes by the sodium–iodide symporter (NIS). ^{99m}Tc is not organified and radioactive iodine shows organification within the gland. ^{99m}Tc is inexpensive, has a short half-life (6 hours), and causes negligible radiation; it usually produces an image with higher background. ^{99m}Tc is administered intravenously and the image is recorded within 20 minutes of injection. Radioactive iodine has several limitations including low availability, high cost, and significant radiation; it produces semifunctional information—iodine uptake, usually increased in TMNG patients.

Several studies have shown comparable diagnostic values of the different isotopes. Discordance between ^{99m}Tc and radioiodine uptake may be observed in <10% of patients. In these cases, ^{99m}Tc may show hot nodule(s) that appear "cold" when radioiodine is used. However, if scanning is repeated at a later time, it will appear that the surrounding tissue is not suppressed and a nodule is not really "hot."

A characteristic image of TMNG shows one or more "toxic" nodules and the surrounding parenchyma completely (Figure 19.3a) or partially (Figure 19.3b) suppressed. Nodules may be delineated clearly and compatible with palpation or ultrasound pattern or they may yield more "patchy" images with only partial correspondence to palpable nodules.

If autonomy is strongly suspected in a still euthyroid patient, suppression scintigraphy can be used. It consists of thyroid scintigraphy, as previously described, anticipated by the exogenous administration of thyroid hormone (usually LT_4 at doses of 75 μg/day for 15 days, then 150 μg/day for 2 more weeks). The hormone will suppress any uptake from non-autonomous tissues and unmask thyroid autonomy. As previously mentioned, thyroid scintigraphy is contraindicated during pregnancy and breastfeeding and is useless if a patient has been exposed to iodine, as in the case of administration of contrast agents or iodine-containing drugs.

Ultrasound does not add information about hyperfunctioning nodule(s), but it is of great value in detecting all coexisting lesions. This information becomes critical when further diagnostic and therapeutic decisions must be made. It orients toward the need for a fine need aspiration biopsy (FNAB) and yields necessary information if surgery is chosen for final treatment. More details on FNAB and ultrasound are available in Chapter 2 discussing non-toxic multinodular goiter and Chapter 6 discussing single thyroid nodules.

When thyroid scintigraphy is contraindicated, ultrasound with color Doppler flow may provide useful information. Increased intranodular flow is characteristic of hyperactivity. X-ray scan, computed tomography, and magnetic resonance imaging are not necessary to diagnose TMNG but they are useful in presurgical planning for patients with large or intrathoracic goiters.

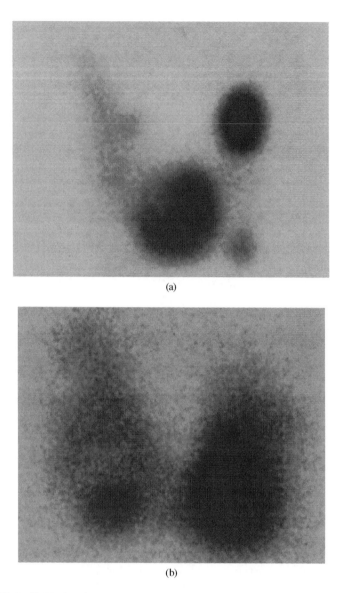

(a)

(b)

FIGURE 19.3 ^{99m}Tc thyroid scintigraphy in TMNG showing the presence of "hot" nodules and complete (a) or partial (b) suppression of extranodular tissue.

19.7 TREATMENT

Treatment for TMNG includes medical, surgical, and radioiodine options. The optimal choice is radical: ^{131}I treatment or surgery. However, medical treatment is required in preparation for radical therapy and in several situations its long-term use can be considered or advised. Therefore, ^{131}I administration, surgery, and medical treatment must all be considered first line therapeutic options.

19.7.1 RADIOIODINE

[131]I is the one of the radical options for treatment of TMNG. It has an 80% rate of success after the first administration and euthyroidism is reached after 3 months in 50 to 60% and after 6 months in 80% of patients. On the other hand, hypothyroidism has a prevalence of 3% after 1 year, 31% after 8 years, and 64% after 24 years[11] and is more common in younger patients (under 50 years old).

Several factors can suggest or advise against radioiodine treatment in comparison to surgery.[12] The main factors are listed in Table 19.5. In general, ^{131}I is indicated for middle-age and elderly patients, for small to moderate size goiters, in patients with significant comorbidities, and whenever an affordable surgeon (performing an adequate number of thyroidectomies) is not available. It has absolute contraindications for women who are pregnant or breastfeeding and should be strongly discouraged when pregnancy is planned within 6 to 12 months, when the risk of thyroid cancer (in coexisting nodules) has not been ruled out, and when a patient cannot comply with radiation safety rules.

Moreover, since studies following the Chernobyl accident revealed increased risk of thyroid cancer in pediatric populations, the use of I^{131} in patients under 14 years old must be avoided. From a patient view, the possibility of avoiding hospitalization, scarring in the anterior neck, and risks of long-time surgical complications support the choice of I^{131}, while the need for a longer time to achieve euthyroidism will play against it.

Side effects of radioiodine treatment are mainly local pain, swelling of thyroid, and drooling. Worsening of hyperthyroidism due to destructive thyroiditis is very rare. As to increased risk of cancer, population-based studies have not shown increased risk of thyroidal, hematologic, or reproductive neoplasia. The aim of radioiodine treatment is to treat thyrotoxicosis; therefore, a single dose of ^{131}I should be sufficient to resolve the hyperthyroidism. However, in some centers, a standard dose (370 to 740 MBq or 10 to 20 mCi) is administered; other centers tailor doses to deliver a certain ^{131}I activity (150 to 200 μCi corrected for 24-hour uptake) per gram of tissue.

In this context, the Marinelli formula (Table 19.6), which takes into account uptake and half-life, is frequently used. In general, the dose needed to treat TMNG

TABLE 19.5
Recommendations and Contraindications to Radioiodine Treatment of TMNG Patients

Recommendations	Contraindications
Middle-aged and elderly patients	Pregnancy, breastfeeding
Small to moderate goiter	Desire for pregnancy within 6–12 months
Significant non-thyroidal disease	Coexisting nodule with risk of neoplasia
Affordable surgeon not available	<14 years old
Possibility of avoiding hospitalization and scarring	Non-compliance with radiation safety protocols
	Longer time to achieve euthyroidism

TABLE 19.6
Marinelli Formula for Calculating ^{131}I Dose

$$A = \frac{5,829 \times D_t \times nm}{U_{max} \times T_{1/2eff}}$$

Note: A = activity to be administered; D_t = adsorbed dose; nm = weight of nodule in grams; U = maximum uptake; $T_{1/2eff}$ = effective half-life in target tissue.

TABLE 19.7
Precaution Requirements and Recommendations after ^{131}I Treatment

Restriction	Time Unit	Dose Administered			
		10 mCi	15 mCi	20 mCi	30 mCi
Sleep in separate bed	Days	3	6	8	11
Sleep in separate bed from pregnant adults, children, infants	Days	15	18	20	23
Return to work (after)	Days	1	1	2	5
Maximize distance from pregnant individuals	Days	1	1	2	5
Avoid attendance in public places	Days	1	1	1	3
Recommendations for safe travel by public transportation					
Travel hours without exceeding limits: day 0	Hours	5.9	3.9	2.9	2.0
Travel hours without exceeding limits: day 1	Hours	9.2	6.1	4.6	3.1
Travel hours without exceeding limits: day 2	Hours	13.0	8.7	6.5	4.3
Travel hours without exceeding limits: day 3	Hours	—	10.6	8.0	5.3

Source: Modified from Sisson, J.C., Freitas, J., MdDougall, I.R. et al. 2011. *Thyroid* 21: 335–346.

is higher than that for Graves' disease; therefore, radiation safety precautions may be cumbersome[13] (Table 19.7). A fringe activity of ^{131}I is a decrease of thyroid volume; a 30 to 40% reduction after 3 years has been shown. In this respect the use of low dose (0.03 mg) recombinant human TSH (rhTSH) has been shown to increase the downsizing effect of ^{131}I while reducing the risk of side effects.[14] However, further studies, showing that this procedure does not increase the risk of exacerbating the hyperthyroidism are needed before the use of rhTSH becomes a standard procedure.

Several cautions must be observed before ^{131}I is administered.[13] The most important is to rule out the possibility of thyroid cancer. It has been shown that non-functioning nodules within TMNG have a 9% prevalence of thyroid cancer that is very close to the 10.5% level found for non-toxic multinodular goiters. Therefore, FNAB must be considered for coexisting cold nodules (for more details on selection of nodules, see Chapter 6). The next decision is the optimal therapy to be used immediately before radioiodine is administered. A general consensus favors the use of β-blockers in all patients above 60 years old and those with concomitant cardio-vascular disease. Prevention of posttreatment tachyarrhythmia is the rationale for their use at doses and modalities, which will be detailed later (Table 19.11).

The use of antithyroid drugs in preparation for ^{131}I therapy is more controver-sial. From one side, a slight increase of TSH has been shown to maximize radioio-dine uptake (RAIU) and efficacy. The other side suggests that an increase of TSH before radioiodine treatment can accelerate the onset of hypothyroidism and lead to destruction of perinodular tissue.[11] Furthermore, in most patients, the use of beta blockers is sufficient to prevent most adverse effects. The use of antithyroid drugs (mainly MMI) is thus suggested for elderly patients and those with cardiovascular disease who face increased risk if hyperthyroidism worsens. In a posttreatment set-ting, antithyroid drug administration may be necessary because 3 to 6 months must usually pass before euthyroidism is achieved.

19.7.2 SURGERY

Near-total or total thyroidectomy is the best surgical option. It treats TMNG in >99% of patients without need for further therapy and hyperthyroidism is resolved within a few days. However, it must be emphasized that hypothyroidism appears in most patients. Several factors may influence the choice between surgery and ^{131}I treatment. The main factors (including patient preference) that are favorable or unfavorable for surgery are listed in Table 19.8.

In general, large volume goiters (especially those causing compressive symp-toms), retrosternal extension, fear of thyroid neoplasia in coexisting cold nodules, or need for rapid control of hyperthyroidism are the most relevant features suggest-ing surgery. Old age and coexisting non-thyroid diseases (especially neoplastic, car-diac, or pulmonary) are the main reasons for avoiding surgery.[4,11] Pregnancy is not an absolute contraindication although surgery should be performed only in the late second trimester when prompt control of hyperthyroidism is required and medical treatment is unadvisable. Indeed, surgery within the first trimester presents risk of teratogenic effects and fetal loss; in the third trimester, an increased risk of preterm labor is present.

TABLE 19.8
Recommendations and Contraindications to Surgery for TMNG Patients

Recommendations	Contraindications
Large goiter (± compressive symptoms)	Old age
Retrosternal extension	Non-thyroidal diseases (especially cardiovascular,
Coexisting cold uncertain nodule	neoplastic, or pulmonary)
Rapid control of hyperthyroidism	Esthetic concerns
Experienced surgeon (>100 operations/year)	
Fear of radioactive exposure	

From a patient perspective, need for rapid control of hyperthyroidism and fear of radioactive exposure are the main issues supporting surgery, while esthetic concerns advise against surgery. Few complications surround thyroid surgery; <2% of permanent hypoparathyroidism and recurrent laryngeal nerve injury follow near-total or total thyroidectomy. It has been clearly shown that an experienced surgeon who performs more than 100 surgeries per year has the least occurrence of complications. Surgeons who perform fewer than 30 thyroidectomies per year may be likely to face complications. There is no significant difference between near-total, total, and subtotal thyroidectomies in relation to percentage of complications. However, the latter procedure is affected by a higher rate of recurrence, requiring more frequent second interventions that in turn are affected by a threefold to tenfold increased risk of complications.

Before surgery is performed, euthyroidism must be achieved and therefore antithyroid drugs with or without beta-blocking agents must be administered until the day of surgery. Indeed, one of the most hazardous complications of thyroid surgery is the thyroid storm, a life-threatening event characterized by exacerbation of hyperthyroidism. Its frequency is decreased by 90% since patients undergoing thyroid surgery are previously rendered euthyroid. If antithyroid drugs cannot be used, association of beta-blocker agents such as propranolol, and either dexamethasone (0.5 to 2 mg p.o. tid), inorganic iodide (Lugol's solution 5% I_2, 5 to 8 drops p.o. tid), or saturated solution of potassium iodide (10% KI 1 to 2 drops p.o. tid) have been shown to reduce perioperative complications.

Note that the standard use of inorganic iodide, as suggested in the past, is not recommended if a patient has been rendered euthyroid because of the risk of exacerbating hyperthyroidism. Calcium (1,000 to 2,000 mg p.o. per day) and calcitriol (0.5 mg p.o. per day) may be prophylactically administered after surgery or alternatively after determination of serum calcium and PTH (see Section 19.9). Levothyroxine (1.2 to 1.7 mg/kg body weight p.o. per day) must be started the day after surgery and its dose must be tailored according to TSH (Section 19.9). Lower doses should be used initially in elderly patients.

19.7.3 MEDICAL TREATMENT

Medical treatment is based on the administration of antithyroid drugs and beta-adrenergic blocking agents.

19.7.3.1 Antithyroid Drugs

Restoration of long-lasting euthyroidism should not be expected in TMNG patients after a course of treatment with thionamide drugs (propylthiouracil [PTU], carbimazole, or methimazole [MMI]; see Table 19.9). Indeed these drugs can control thyrotoxicosis but their suspension ends in relapse of the disease. Therefore, long-term (lifelong) medical treatment of TMNG is not usually advisable. This option is appropriate only in special cases, such as patients who have short estimated life spans, absolute contraindications to surgery, or refuse radioiodine treatment.[11]

TABLE 19.9
Antithyroid Drugs

	Plasma Half-Life (hrs)	Daily Oral Dose (mg/day)		Doses/Day
		Initial	Maintenance	
Propylthiouracil	1–1.5	300–600	50–100	3 (later 2)
Methimazole	3–7	30–40	2.5–15	2 (later 1)
Carbimazole	3–7	45–60	2.5–20	2 (later 1)

Usually, antithyroid drugs are considered the first line treatment in all thyrotoxic patients because they alleviate the hazards (especially when cardiac disease is present) of hyperthyroidism and are meant as a preparation for subsequent radical therapy in TMNG patients. Initial dosage is typically 30 mg/day of MMI, 40 to 50 mg/day of carbimazole, and 300 mg/day of PTU (Table 19.9). Dosages are then tailored according to clinical symptoms and FT_4 and TSH levels. Higher dosages do not result in faster resolution of hyperthyroidism and are hampered by more frequent adverse effects including agranulocytosis, cholestasis, immunoallergic hepatitis, and even fulminant hepatic necrosis[12] (Table 19.10). Low dose (5 to 10 mg/day) MMI treatment should be considered for patients with subclinical hyperthyroidism (see Chapter 23 for a more complete discussion), especially those with coexisting cardiac disorders and reduced bone density; alternatively or conjointly, beta-blocking drugs can be evaluated.

TABLE 19.10
Side Effects of Antithyroid Drugs

Mainly or Exclusively with Methimazole/Carbimazole	Common to All Drugs	Mainly or Exclusively with Propylthiouracil
Major		
Cholestasis	Polyarthritis	Immunoallergic hepatitis
Insulin autoimmune syndrome (described in Asian patients)	Agranulocytosis	Fulminant hepatic necrosis
	Thrombocytopenia and aplastic anemia	ANCA-positive vasculitis
Minor		
Abnormal sense of taste or smell	Skin reactions (including urticarial and macular reactions)	
Sialadenitis	Gastrointestinal effects (including gastric distress and nausea)	
	Arthralgias	

TABLE 19.11

Beta-Adrenergic Receptor Blockers

Drug	Dose	Frequency	Notes
Propranolol	10–40 mg	3–4/day	Inhibits T_4/T_3 conversion at high doses
Atenolol	25–100 mg	2–4/day	β1-selective
Metoprolol	25–50 mg	4/day	β1-selective
Esmolol	50–100 mg/Kg/minute (intravenous)		In intensive care units

19.7.3.2 Beta-Adrenergic Blocking Agents

Recent guidelines from the American Thyroid Association, subsequently approved by the European and Latin American Thyroid Associations and by the most prominent endocrine societies worldwide,[11] established that: "Beta-adrenergic blockade should be given to elderly patients with symptomatic thyrotoxicosis and to other thyrotoxic patients with resting heart rates in excess of 90 bpm or co-existent cardiovascular disease" and "beta-adrenergic blockade should be considered in all patients with symptomatic thyrotoxicosis." Furthermore, beta blockers have to be considered in preparation for surgery and [131]I.

Propranolol, atenolol, metoprolol, and esmolol have been suggested (Table 19.11). Propranolol, beyond its beta-blocking activity, is also useful because it partially inhibits T_4 conversion into T_3. At recommended doses, these drugs are not (or only partially) β1 selective and therefore should not be used in patients with bronchospastic asthma. Alternatively, calcium channel blockers, such as verapamil (120 mg po bid) and diltiazem (60 to 120 mg po twice or thrice a day) can be orally administered for controlling heart rate.

19.7.4 Alternative Options

Percutaneous ethanol injection (PEI), and thermal and radiofrequency ablation have been considered as alternatives for treating TMNG and may be considered second line choices. PEI is the most studied alternative procedure; it is based on the necrosis of thyroid tissue that follows the injection of ethanol at 95% within a nodule. At least four to eight sessions are required before results are satisfying. PEI has a success rate estimated close to 90% and a major complication rate of 3%.[1,2] Side effects include local pain, fever, transient paralysis of the laryngeal nerve, hematoma, and jugular vein thrombosis. At present, the use of PEI in the treatment of TMNG has been almost abandoned and is confined to the treatment of cystic thyroid nodules.

Insufficient data are presently available for thermal and radiofrequency ablation and these procedures must still be considered experimental. They may be alternatives to surgery and their main advantage is the possibility of confining treatment to hyperfunctioning nodules, thus preserving the perinodular tissue and decreasing the risk of subsequent hypothyroidism.

19.8   PROGNOSIS

TMNG has a very good prognosis with a very high success rate when treatment is readily administered.[14] More caution must be reserved for older patients, those subject to cardiac failure, and the very rare cases that develop thyroid storm.

19.9   FOLLOW-UP

Follow-up of TMNG patients differs based on the chosen treatment (Table 19.12). Follow-up of patients treated with I[131] is initially aimed at evaluating the success of the treatment. TSH, FT_4, and FT_3 should be evaluated 1 to 2 months after radioiodine therapy and at the same intervals thereafter until stable results are obtained. TSH and thyroid hormone levels are therefore used also to taper antithyroid drug therapy if it becomes necessary after ^{131}I treatment.

If euthyroidism has not been achieved 6 months after radioiodine, a new ^{131}I treatment must be considered. However, since slower progression toward euthyroidism has been described, a further period with MMI administration may be considered.[11] Onset of hypothyroidism has been described in up to 64% of patients in a 24-year period; therefore, TSH and FT_4 evaluation must be performed at least annually (or according to clinical suspicion). If hypothyroidism develops and levothyroxine treatment is established, the initial dose must be lower than that required for full replacement because of possible residual secretion from the thyroid.

Determinations of serum calcium and intact PTH 6 and 12 hours after surgery should evaluate the possibility that hypoparathyroidsm has developed. Steady calcium levels >7.8 mg/dL would allow patient's discharge. On the contrary, low PTH levels would indicate the need for calcium and calcitriol supplementation. If prophylactic administration

TABLE 19.12
Follow-Up

	Test	Initial	Thereafter
Medical treatment	TSH	Every 4 months[a,b]	Every 6 months
	FT_4	Every 4 months[a,b]	Every 6 months
	FT_3	Every 4 months[a,b]	Every 6 months
	US	—	Annually
Surgery	Calcium	6 and 12 hours post-op	Every 6 months
	PTH	6 and 12 hours post-op	Every 6 months
	TSH	6–8 weeks post-op[a]	Annually
[131]I	TSH	Every 6–8 weeks[a]	Annually[c]
	FT_4	Every 6–8 weeks[a]	Annually[c]
	FT_3	Every 6–8 weeks[a]	—

[a]   Until euthyroidism is achieved.
[b]   After 6–8 weeks if dose is changed.
[c]   Or according to clinical suspicion of hypothyroidism.

of calcium and calcitriol is chosen, PTH must be determined. Supplementation can be tapered only when PTH levels are appropriate for serum calcium levels.

TSH levels are used to tailor levothyroxine therapy and should be assessed every 6 to 8 weeks after surgery and until stability has been achieved; annual determination is sufficient after that.

If antithyroid treatment (with or without beta blockers) has been selected, evaluation of TSH, FT_4. and possibly FT_3 must be performed every 4 months; any change in the dosage of the drug must be assessed after 6 to 8 weeks. Ultrasound is usually performed each year to evaluate change in sizes of thyroid nodules (hyperfunctioning and non-functioning). Table 19.13 lists drugs discussed in this chapter.

TABLE 19.13
List of Drugs Cited in This Chapter

Drug	Dose	Daily Frequency
Propylthiouracil	25–200 mg	2 or 3 times
Methimazole	2.5–20 mg	1 or 2 times
Carbimazole	2.5–30 mg	1 or 2 times
Dexamethasone	0.5–2 mg	3 times
Propranolol	10–40 mg	3 or 4 times
Atenolol	25–100 mg	2 or 4 times
Metoprolol	25–50 mg	4 times
Esmolol	50–100 mg/Kg/minute (intravenous)	In intensive care units
Verapamil	120 mg	2 times
Diltiazem	60–120 mg	2
Calcium gluconate	1000–2000 mg	1
Calcitriol	0.5 mg	1
Levothyroxine	1.2–1.7 µg/Kg body weight	1

REFERENCES

1. Santarelli, L. and Monaco, F. 2007. Nodulo autonomo e gozzo multinodulare tossicco o malattia di Plummer. In *Malattie della Tiroide*, Monaco, F., Ed. Rome: Societa Edizione Universo, 421–456.

2. Fuhrer, D., Krohn, K., and Paschke, R. 2005. Toxic adenoma and toxic multinodular goiter. In *Werner & Ingbar's The Thyroid: A Fundamental and Clinical Text*, 9th ed., Braverman, L.E. and Utiger, R.D., Eds. Philadelphia: Lippincott, Williams & Wilkins, 508–518.

3. Krohn, K., Fuhrer, D., Bayer, Y. et al. 2005. Molecular pathogenesis of euthyroid and toxic multinodular goiter. *Endocr Rev* 26: 504–524.

4. Hegedus, L., Paske, R., Krohn, K. et al. 2010. Multinodular goiter. In *Endocrinology. Adult and Pediatric*, 6th ed., Jameson, J.L. and DeGroot L.J., Eds. Philadelphia: Saunders, Elsevier, 1636–1649.

5. Orgiazzi, J. and Mornex, R. 1993. Toxic nodular goiter. In *Thyroid Diseases: Clinical Fundamentals and Therapy*, Monaco, F. et al., Eds. Boca Raton: CRC Press, 63–80.

6. Porterfield, J.R., Thompson, G.B., Farley, D.R. et al. 2008. Evidence-based management of toxic multinodular goiter (Plummer's disease). *World J Surg* 32: 1278–1284.

7. Biondi, B. and Kahaly, G.J. 2010. Cardiovascular involvement in patients with different causes of hyperthyroidism. *Nature Rev Endocrinol* 6: 431–443.

8. Murphy, E., Gluer, C.C., Reid, D.M. et al. 2010. Thyroid function within the upper normal range is associated with reduced bone mineral density and an increased risk of nonvertebral fractures in healthy euthyroid postmenopausal women. *J Clin Endocrinol Metab* 95: 3173–3181.

9. Crooks, J., Murray, I.P.C., and Wayne, E.J. 1959. Statistical methods applied to the clinical diagnosis of thyrotoxicosis. *Q J Med* 28: 211–234.

10. Spencer, C.A. 2003. Thyroid testing in the new millennium. *Thyroid* 13: 2–126.

11. Bahn, R.S., Burch, H.B., Cooper, D.S. et al. 2011. Hyperthyroidism and other causes of thyrotoxicosis: management guidelines of the American Thyroid Association and American Association of Clinical Endocrinologists. *Thyroid* 21: 593–646.

12. Cooper, D.S. 2005. Antithyroid drugs. *New Engl J Med* 352: 905–917.

13. Sisson, J.C., Freitas, J., McDougall, I.R. et al. 2011. Radiation safety in the treatment of patients with thyroid diseases by radioiodine [131]I: practice recommendations of the American Thyroid Association. *Thyroid* 21: 335–346.

14. Kahaly, G.J., Bartalena, L., and Hegedus, L. 2011. The American Thyroid Association/ American Association of Clinical Endocrinologists guidelines for hyperthyroidism and other causes of thyrotoxicosis: a European perspective. *Thyroid* 21: 585–591.

20 Pretoxic and Toxic Autonomous Nodule

Giorgio Napolitano and Fabrizio Monaco

CONTENTS

Key words: Autonomous nodule, "hot" nodule, hyperthyroidism, subclinical hyperthyroidism, atrial fibrillation, TSH receptor mutation, GSα mutation, iodine deficiency.

20.1 DEFINITION

The term *autonomously functioning thyroid nodule* (AFTN) describes the clinical presentation of thyroid autonomy—a condition characterized by production of thyroid hormones independently from thyrotropin (TSH) stimulation and in the absence of TSH receptor (TSHr) stimulating antibodies. The AFTN can be single in the context of the thyroid or can coexist with other functioning and non-functioning nodules (in the latter case, see Chapter 19 describing toxic multinodular goiter).

Because of its function independent of TSH, the AFTN progressively increases production of thyroid hormones and consequently leads to suppression of TSH levels and quiescence of extranodular tissue. According to the levels of thyroid hormones, it can be categorized as a pretoxic (PTN) nodule or toxic (TN) nodule if thyroid hormones are within or above the normal range and the nodule is without or with clinical signs and symptoms, respectively.

20.2 EPIDEMIOLOGY

Epidemiological data strongly support the idea that AFTNs are more common in iodine-deficient areas where they account for up to 44% of untreated hyperthyroidism in comparison to 1.5% in iodine-sufficient areas[1] (Table 20.1). Indeed, in countries with mild to moderate iodine deficiency, thyroid autonomy (both TN and TMNG) is responsible for 60% of cases of hyperthyroidism; correction of iodine deficiency through salt supplementation programs has been shown to decrease the incidence of thyroid autonomy.

The incidence of TN has been estimated in Sweden to be 4.8 per 100,000/year. TN represents 5 to 10% of all solitary nodules and the female:male ratio in patients with TN is 4:1 to 6:1. Interestingly the ratio is significantly higher for PTN: 14:1. Age has a significant effect in the progression of a nodule from non-toxic to toxic. Hyperthyroidism is present in >50% of patients 60 years of age or older, but only in 10 to 15% of younger patients. Nodule size is a significant factor as well. Only 2% of nodules with a diameter <2.5 cm are toxic while this percentage rise up to 42% in nodules ≥2.5 cm.

TABLE 20.1
TN Frequency in Various Countries

	% TN
Europe	
Austria	44.5
England	3.7
Finland	18
France	24
Germany	19.7
Greece	9.5
Italy	11.4
Switzerland	33
North America	
Cleveland (Ohio)	1.6
New York (New York)	1.5
Rochester (New York)	15.8
Southfield (Michigan)	2
Oceania	
Tasmania (Australia)	17

20.3 PATHOGENESIS

Histological classification of hyperfunctioning thyroid nodules distinguishes two types: monoclonal and polyclonal. In the first case, we observe almost identical cells within the nodule. In the latter situation, cells of different sizes and characteristics coexist in the same nodule. However, differences may reflect changes during growth or secondary phenomena such as hemorrhages and calcifications.

One proposal is that hyperfunctioning nodules originate from a single clone and through its growth develop a follicular adenoma (if the nodule is encapsulated) or an adenomatous nodule (if the capsule is missing). Cells originating from this clone will have special features to facilitate growth and function (see below).[1-3] TSH regulates both growth and function of thyroid cells through the binding to its receptor and this event preferentially leads to stimulation of adenylyl cyclase via the Gsα protein.

More than 20 years ago, it was suggested that mutations affecting the cyclic AMP (cAMP) cascade would cause constitutive activation (independent of TSH binding to its receptor and in the absence of TSHr-stimulating antibodies) of thyrocytes and be responsible for its autonomous function. It is now clear that somatic mutations affecting the genes involved in the cAMP pathway are indeed responsible for thyroid autonomy and therefore for the formation and growth of TN.

Two major sites of mutation have been identified in the genes codifying for the TSHr and the Gsα proteins; together they are detected in ~60% of TN. Although high variabilities among studies have been shown, TSHr mutations are more frequent (~50% of TN) than those affecting the Gsα protein (~10%). Mutations of the TSHr gene have been initially located within the third intracellular loop and in the sixth transmembrane domain. Subsequent studies, however, found a wider range of localizations covering the entire transmembrane region and the carboxy terminal region of the extracellular domain.

It is of interest to remember that different activating mutations have been associated with different morphological and functional responses. In the remaining ~40% of TNs that have not been identified for TSHr or Gsα mutation, a monoclonal origin is strongly suspected because of studies of X chromosome inactivation on nodules from female patients. It is therefore conceivable that mutations affecting different genes (such as other G-protein subunits, protein kinase A, and phosphodiesterase) may be responsible for TN.

Epidemiological data have shown that thyroid autonomy is more frequent in areas with iodine deficiency, which is thus supposed to be a predisposing factor for the development of TN. A brief description of the cascade of events leading to the formations of autonomous nodules following iodine deficiency is depicted in Chapter 19 (Section 19.3). In summary, iodine deficiency (and goitrogens) may cause thyroid hyperplasia, thus increasing the cell replication rate and risk of accidental mutation.

If such mutations confer constitutive activation of the cAMP pathway, they will cause focal growth and facilitate the development of small clones with special features. In vivo cells from hyperfunctioning clones have different properties from cells of the surrounding tissue. They are characterized by up-regulation of the sodium–iodide symporter (NIS) gene expression that explains the increased iodide uptake and the high thyroperoxidase protein level that contributes to the increased thyroid hormone production.

20.4 NATURAL COURSE

The total amount of T_3 and T_4 produced by the thyroid gland is determined by the sum of the hormones produced by each follicle. Therefore, if some follicles synthesize and secrete high amounts of thyroid hormones, compensatory down-regulation of the remaining follicles will prevent the onset of hyperthyroidism. However, when the number of hyperactive follicles exceeds the compensatory capacity of the remaining tissue, hyperthyroidism will develop (Figure 20.1).

This simple concept explains several features of the natural history of the TN. Indeed, thyroid scintigraphy can show the sequence of events previously described. At the beginning, the AFTN is surrounded by isotope uptake in the remaining follicles, thus giving evidence for residual activity. As soon as the AFTN grows, the surrounding tissue becomes "silent" and no residual uptake can be registered. However, at this point, a patient may still be euthyroid. A further increase in thyroid hormone production (usually secondary to further enlargement of the AFTN) will then shift the patient to the hyperthyroid state.[1,2]

This sequence of events explains two typical features of TN: the slow progression toward hyperthyroidism and its correlation with the size of the nodule. Several studies evaluating progression of TN toward hyperthyroidism have reported an annual incidence ~4% of thyrotoxicosis in previously euthyroid patients. Hyperthyroidism has been detected in 93.5% of patients with TNs >3 cm with a 20% risk of developing thyrotoxicosis in 6 years for still-euthyroid patients. The risk was only 2% in patients having TNs <2.5 cm.

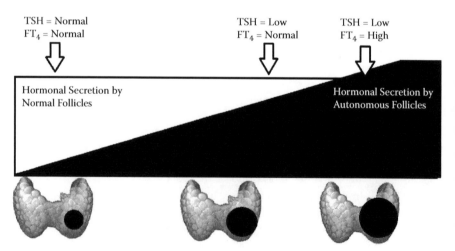

TSH = Normal
FT_4 = Normal

TSH = Low
FT_4 = Normal

TSH = Low
FT_4 = High

Hormonal Secretion by Normal Follicles

Hormonal Secretion by Autonomous Follicles

FIGURE 20.1 Pathogenesis of hyperthyroidism in toxic nodular goiter. In the slow process of growth, production of thyroid hormones is increasingly due to the actions of autonomously functioning thyroid follicles, while remaining tissue decreases its share of thyroid hormones. As the number of autonomously functioning follicles increases, hyperthyroidism develops.

The slow progression towards hyperthyroidism can be reversed (i.e., fastened) by the use of high quantities of iodide via administration of contrast agents or iodine-containing drugs such as amiodarone. Conversely, hemorrhagic and degenerative phenomena within the nodule may cause its loss of function and reinstate the physiological regulation of the pituitary–thyroid axis; such an occurrence has been registered in 4% of patients in an observation period of 6 years.[1]

20.5 CLINICAL FEATURES

Patients with TN can be asymptomatic for many years. Indeed, compressive symptoms are less frequent than in toxic multinodular goiter and signs of hyperthyroidism are absent in most patients for several years. Mechanical symptoms are not common presenting features in TN; hoarseness and dysphagia are usually reported by patients with very large nodules that are already under treatment for hyperthyroidism.

Onset of thyrotoxicosis is usually insidious and slow and patients experience few symptoms of hyperthyroidism. Asthenia, agitation, heat intolerance, and weight loss are the most frequent complaints. If the prevalence of symptoms in TN patients is compared to that observed in Graves' disease patients (Table 20.2), it appears that most symptoms are more prevalent in the latter disease. However, atrial fibrillation is more frequent in TN due to the older ages of patients.[4,5] Cardiovascular manifestations predominate and may be the sole indications of hyperthyroidism; therefore, along

TABLE 20.2
Comparative Prevalence of Symptoms and Signs of Hyperthyroidism

	Toxic Nodule	Graves' Disease
Tachycardia	4	5
Atrial fibrillation	1	0
Arterial bruit	1	2
Weight loss	3	5
Asthenia	3	4
Muscular weakness	0	2
Increased sweating	3	3
Heat intolerance	2	4
Polyphagia	0	0
Accelerated bowel movements	0	1
Polydipsia	2	4
Hyperkinetic behavior	2	4
Tremor	2	2
Leg edema	0	1

Note: Legend: 0 = 0 to 15%; 1 = 16 to 30%; 2 = 31 to 45%; 3 = 46 to 60%; 4 = 61 to 75%; 5 = >75%.

with atrial fibrillation, conditions such as paroxystic tachyrhythmia, cardiac failure, and worsening of preexisting cardiac insufficiency must be systematically evaluated.

As explained in Chapter 19, apathetic syndrome is an unusual form of hyperthyroidism characteristically encountered in elderly patients suffering from TN or toxic multinodular goiter. It is usually characterized by the presence of only one main symptom such as weight loss, anorexia, apathy, or weakness in the absence of the most revealing symptoms of hyperthyroidism such as hyperphagia, tachycardia, warm skin, and increased perspiration. Patients are often misdiagnosed as having melancholia.

Subclinical hyperthyroidism is characterized by low TSH levels and thyroid hormones within normal ranges (for a more comprehensive review see Chapter 23) and is frequently observed in TN. Although symptoms are missing by definition, mild forms of signs typical of hyperthyroidism can still be found. Tachycardia and supraventricular premature contractions are commonly registered in TN patients. Decreased bone mineral density has been shown in women with low TSH along with an increased risk of hip and vertebral fracture during 3.7 years of follow-up.[6]

20.6 DIAGNOSIS

Diagnosis of TN is based on three steps aimed to (1) identify the nodule via neck palpation and ultrasound, (2) demonstrate subclinical or overt hyperthyroidism based on medical history and laboratory tests, and (3) identify the localized autonomous area by thyroid scintigraphy.

20.6.1 CLINICAL

Medical history and careful neck palpation are the main steps of clinical evaluation in most patients with TN. The history is intended to discover the few signs of hyperthyroidism developed over several years. Palpation focuses on the identification of a nodule in one of the lobes while the remaining tissue is not palpable. Palpation gives also information about changes within a nodule; increases in size and tenderness indicate intranodular necrosis, hemorrhage, and formation of a cyst.

20.6.2 LABORATORY

TSH is the first screening test (Table 20.3) because it is the most useful way of detecting hyperthyroidism; low (>0.1 to 0.4 µUI/mL) or suppressed (<0.1 µUI/mL) values are noted. As one of the aims is to distinguish subclinical from overt hyperthyroidism, free T_4 (FT_4) assay in addition to TSH strongly improves the accuracy of diagnosis.

An inverse log-linear relation between FT_4 and TSH is physiologically present and therefore small changes of FT_4 result in much greater modifications of TSH.[7,8] In 5 to 46% of TN patients, isolated elevations of FT_3 serum concentration and FT_4 levels within normal range are observed. This phenomenon known as T_3 toxicosis is typical of iodine-deficient areas. Diagnosis of hyperthyroidism is based therefore on TSH, FT_4, and FT_3 determinations (Table 20.3).

TABLE 20.3
Diagnostic Investigation for Autonomous Nodule

	I Level	Accuracy	II Level	Accuracy
Clinical	Medical history	Excellent		
	Neck palpation	Excellent		
Laboratory	TSH	Excellent	TSHr-Ab	Poor
	FT$_4$	Excellent	Tg-Ab	Poor
	FT$_3$	Good	TPO-Ab	Poor
Imaging	Scintigraphy (^{99m}Tc or ^{131}I/^{123}I + iodine uptake)	Excellent	X-ray scan	Good
	Ultrasound	Good	Color Doppler flow	Good
			Suppression scintigraphy (± iodine uptake)	Good
			CT scan	Poor
			MR scan	Poor

As previously discussed in Chapter 19, the commonly used FT$_3$ and FT$_4$ assays represent estimates (i.e., the bound and free fractions of the iodothyronines are not separated before testing) and FT$_3$ is a less reliable measurement than FT$_4$. Measurement of total T$_3$ (TT$_3$) is therefore preferred in some laboratories. Thyroid antibodies (antithyroglobulin [Tg-Abs], thyroid peroxidase [TPO-Abs], and TSH-receptor [TSHr-Abs] are not routinely tested; however, TSHr-Abs may be determined in pregnant and breastfeeding women who cannot undergo thyroid scintigraphy (see below) whenever a clinical picture is not discriminating with Graves' disease. Tg-Ab and TPO-Ab assays may be performed when suspicion of chronic autoimmune thyroiditis must be excluded (see below).

20.6.3 IMAGING

Scintigraphy is the key test for detecting thyroid autonomy. According to the natural course of the disease, different images can be visualized. In the first phase, the AFTN nodule is revealed by a slightly or definitely increased uptake in comparison to the surrounding tissue. In this phase, the nodule can be defined, according to the difference of uptake, "warm or hot." More precisely, it is defined pretoxic, because the patient is still euthyroid or, according to the German literature, "compensated."

In the following phase, the nodule becomes a unique area of uptake of the tracer (Figure 20.2), and is defined as hot or toxic because the patient has hyperthyroidism (subclinical or overt) or is "decompensated." ^{99m}Pertechnate (^{99m}Tc), ^{123}I, and ^{131}I are the most common tracer elements. ^{99m}Tc is the most frequently used because it is inexpensive, has a short half-life (6 hours), and causes negligible radiation. It is administered intravenously and the image is recorded within 20 minutes. Its main disadvantages are the lack of organification when it is transported within the cells and the inability to use its uptake by the thyroid as a measure of thyroid function.[8]

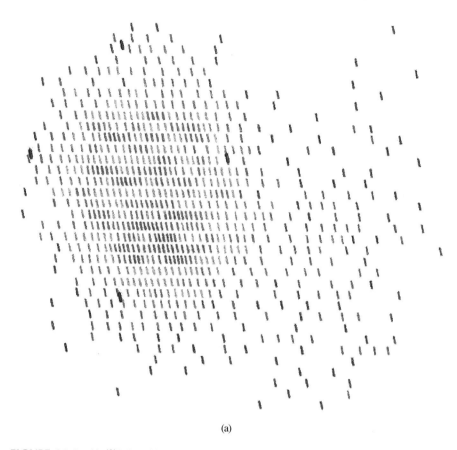

(a)

FIGURE 20.2   (a) [131]I thyroid scintigraphy in thyroid autonomy showing hot nodule and complete suppression of extranodular tissue; (b) ultrasound image of same nodule.

Due to the difference with radioiodine tracers (^{123}I and ^{131}I) that are both transported and organified within thyroid cells, a 5 to 8% discordance may be observed and a hot nodule revealed by ^{99m}Tc may be cold when radioiodine is used. However, an additional scan after ^{99m}Tc will show uptake also in the surrounding tissue and therefore indicate the nodule is not really hot.

Radioiodine compounds have several limitations, including low availability (^{123}I), high price, and long half-lives; ^{131}I is less expensive. They are orally administered and the images are recorded 4 to 24 hours later. Radioiodine compounds yield semi-functional information—the measure of iodine uptake, usually increased in TN (Figure 20.3a). Iodine uptake information is useful in uncommon cases in which the scintigraphic image (unique area of uptake) is not related to TN and involves compensatory hyperplasia of intact tissue in chronic autoimmune thyroiditis or to thyroid hemiagenesis.

Iodine uptake measurement can also be used in cases in which autonomy is strongly suspected, for example, a patient with a warm nodule whose surrounding

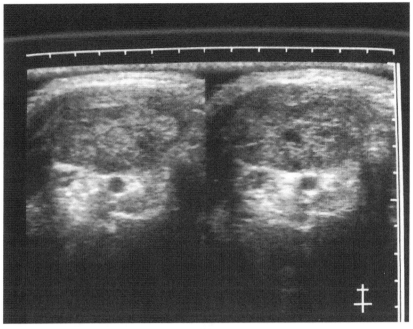

(b)

FIGURE 20.2 (continued)

tissue still functions. A "suppression" scintigraphy (based on the preventive administration of LT_4 at a dose of 75 µg/day for 15 days and then 150 µg/day for 2 more weeks, or T_3 doses of 25 µg thrice a day for 10 days) with a measure of uptake will show a complete disappearance of the extranodular tissue and only a minor uptake reduction (Figure 20.3b).

Ultrasound should be used as a verification of neck palpation; it also adds information about all possible coexisting lesions and confirms the integrity of the surrounding tissue. This information becomes critical when further diagnostic and therapeutic decisions must be made. Ultrasound is therefore used to evaluate the possible presence of other nodules on one side and exclude the possibility that the scintigraphic image is the result of the absence of contralateral lobe (thyroid) hemiagenesis.

Color Doppler flow analysis may provide useful information showing increased intranodular flow when thyroid scintigraphy is contraindicated. Fine needle aspiration biopsy (FNAB) is not only useless as a diagnostic tool in TN, but may also be misleading. Indeed, the presence of malignant neoplasia in AFTN is almost exceptional and differentiation of follicular adenoma and carcinoma is presently impossible with FNAB. X-ray, computed tomography, and magnetic resonance imaging are usually unnecessary but may be useful for presurgical planning for patients with very large nodules.

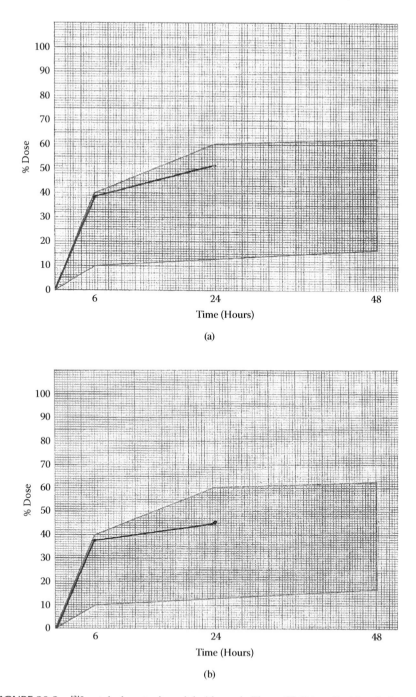

(a)

(b)

FIGURE 20.3   [131]I uptake by a toxic nodule (shown in Figure 20.2) basally (a) and after suppression with T$_3$ (b), 25 µg tid for 10 days; the uptake is only slightly reduced.

20.7   TREATMENT

No treatment of a TN is needed as long as euthyroidism is present. Similar to toxic multinodular goiter, medical, surgical, and radioiodine (^{131}I) options must be considered for hyperthyroid patients.[1,2,9] However, while radioiodine and surgery are radical choices, medical treatment is only temporary and thyrotoxicosis will relapse as soon as the treatment is suspended. For a more complete discussion on dosage, administration methods, and special features of the three options, see Chapter 19 (Section 19.7).

In this section, the specifics of treatment for TN will be discussed. Along with surgery and ^{131}I therapy as first line treatments, percutaneous ethanol injection (PEI) and thermal and radiofrequency ablation must be considered as alternative and second line options. They may acquire a greater relevance for TN because they are intended to preserve the extranodular tissue. At present, however, they require larger studies before definite conclusions about their utility can be drawn.

20.7.1   RADIOIODINE

^{131}I is the first line treatment. It is safe and effective, with a success rate of 85 to 100% in TN and a risk of recurrence or relapse of hyperthyroidism ranging from 0 to 30%, according to different reviews.[1,2,9] Furthermore, volume shrinkage of 35% after 3 months and 45% after 2 years has been reported. Hypothyroidism, originally reported to be absent after ^{131}I, has been subsequently revealed in up to 36% of cases after a 16.5-year follow-up.

Two main factors contribute to the onset of hypothyroidism: the presence of thyroid autoantibodies and uptake in the surrounding tissue. The presence of thyroid antibodies is associated with the onset of hypothyroidism in 18% of patients, compared to 1.4% when antibodies are absent. ^{131}I uptake in surrounding tissues is a further complicating factor. If radioiodine treatment is performed when patients are hyperthyroid (and extrathyroidal tissue is silent), only 1.5% develop hypothyroidism compared to 9.7% in euthyroid patients.[1]

For this reason, the use of antithyroid drugs in preparation for ^{131}I therapy has been questioned by some authors. Although a slight increase of TSH maximizes radioiodine uptake, an increase of TSH before radioiodine treatment can lead to destruction of perinodular tissue.[9] Choosing the best therapeutic option between ^{131}I and surgery is based on several factors; the pros and cons of radioiodine treatment are listed in Table 20.4. Absolute contraindications are pregnancy or breastfeeding, and ^{131}I should be strongly discouraged when a patient expresses desire for pregnancy in the near future.

^{131}I can be administered as a fixed dose (usually 10 to 20 mCi) or based on a calculated dose (150 to 200 µCi per gram/uptake). Available data do not show significant differences in outcome and onset of hypothyroidism, but they show that a calculated dose allows a lower ^{131}I activity to achieve the same result. MMI administration may be necessary posttreatment since euthyroidism is achieved 3 to 6 months after ^{131}I administration.

TABLE 20.4
Recommendations and Contraindications to Radioiodine Treatment of TN Patients

Recommendations	Contraindications
Elderly patients	Pregnancy, breastfeeding
Small to moderate nodule	Desire for pregnancy within 6 to 12 months
Significant non-thyroidal disease	Longer time to achieve euthyroidism
Affordable surgeon not available	<14 years old
Possibility to avoid hospitalization and scarring	Non-compliance with radiation safety protocols

20.7.2 SURGERY

Hemithyroidectomy (lobectomy) is the best surgical option, provided that a preliminary ultrasound has shown integrity of the contralateral lobe. This procedure can resolve hyperthyroidism in most patients and has a very low incidence of complications. However, hypothyroidism develops in ~5% of patients, possibly because of the contemporaneous presence of thyroid autoimmunity, as indicated by detectable TPO-Abs and Tg-Abs.

Table 20.5 lists recommendations and contraindications to choosing surgery as a first line treatment.[8,9] As in cases of toxic multinodular goiter, an experienced surgeon (performing >100 operations per year) is strongly advisable; however, this suggestion is less compelling in TN because data have not shown statistical differences in outcomes between high- and low-volume surgeons.[9] Before surgery, hyperthyroidism must be controlled and a patient must be euthyroid. Antithyroid drugs with or without β-adrenergic blocking agents must be administered until the day of surgery.

Because the contralateral lobe and two parathyroid glands are to be preserved, no prophylactic treatment with LT$_4$ or calcium and calcitriol has to be administered. Although no conclusive data show that LT$_4$ treatment after surgery can prevent the appearance of a new nodule in the contralateral lobe, several authors suggested such a possibility. This decision must be tailored for each patient, based mainly on age and risk of cardiovascular disease and osteoporosis.

TABLE 20.5
Recommendations and Contraindications to Surgery in TN Patients

Recommendations	Contraindications
Large nodule (± compressive symptoms)	Old age
Retrosternal extension	Non-thyroidal diseases (especially cardiovascular, neoplastic, or pulmonary)
Rapid control of hyperthyroidism	
Experienced surgeon (>100 operations/year)	
Fear of radioactive exposure	

20.7.3 MEDICAL TREATMENT

Medical treatment is based on the administration of antithyroid drugs (methimazole [MMI], carbimazole, and propylthiouracil [PTU]) and β-adrenergic blocking agents. Antithyroid drugs can be used as a first option in patients with short estimated life spans, patients who refuse radioiodine treatment, or present absolute contraindications to surgery. Antithyroid drugs are considered the initial options for all thyrotoxic patients because they alleviate the hazards of hyperthyroidism and are meant as preparations for subsequent radical therapy.[9,10] β-adrenergic blocking agents should be considered in all patients with symptomatic thyrotoxicosis, resting heart rates above 90 bpm, or coexisting cardiovascular disease.

20.7.4 ALTERNATIVE OPTIONS

Percutaneous ethanol injection (PEI) was proposed in the mid-1990s as an alternative to radioiodine treatment of AFTN. It has been subsequently used also to treat solid and cystic non-functioning nodules. It is based on injection of a 95% ethanol solution that causes nodule shrinkage secondary to coagulative necrosis and thrombosis of small intranodular blood vessels. Most of the data available are based on uncontrolled trials and show resolution of hyperthyroidism in almost 100% of patients with a nodule having volumes <15 mL and a success rate similar to I^{131} in larger nodules.[11]

Nodule shrinkage was similar in the two groups of patient (treated with either PEI or ^{131}I). However, multiple injections are necessary to achieve euthyroidism, and adverse effects such as pain, ethanol seepage outside the nodule, transient thyrotoxicosis, hematoma, jugular vein thrombosis, and recurrent laryngeal nerve damage are not uncommon. At present PEI is the treatment choice for recurrent cystic nodules. For TN, PEI should be considered only when both surgery and ^{131}I have been refused or are contraindicated.

Ultrasound-guided percutaneous laser thermal ablation has been proposed since 2000 as an alternative treatment of hyperfunctioning and non-functioning thyroid nodules. It is based on the insertion, under ultrasound control, of 14- to 21-gauge spine needles. A 300-μm diameter quartz optical fiber is advanced through the sheath of the needle. A laser with output power of 3 to 5 W is then used. The few data available show a 50 to 70% reduction of the volume of the nodule and an increase of TSH in 31% of patients after 6 months.[11,12] Patients experienced burning cervical pain, shoulder pain, and temporary dysphonia that took up to 2 months to resolve and were shown to be associated to cord palsy.

The main limitation of laser thermal ablation at present is the inability to identify the true boundaries of the laser-induced tissue damage and poor correlation with echogenic zones observed on real-time ultrasonography. More data are necessary before considering thermal laser ablation an alternative to surgery and ^{131}I. However, it has attractive features and it acts only on hyperfunctioning nodules, thus decreasing their size and avoiding hypothyroidism because the technique does not affect perinodular tissue.

Radiofrequency ablation has been recently proposed in patients not suitable for surgery or [131]I. It is based on the introduction through a 17- or 18-gauge needle of one internally cooled electrode and then ablation is started with the application of 30 to 80 W of power.[13] In a preliminary report on treatment of nine patients with TN, six were euthyroid after 6 months, two were still toxic, and one (positive for thyroid antibodies) developed hypothyroidism. Nodules were reduced by 70% at 6-month follow-ups. Most patients complained of mild neck pain, sometimes radiating to the head or shoulders. However, no major complications such as voice change, hematoma, infection, or dysphonia were described. At present, radiofrequency ablation for TN is only experimental.

20.8 PROGNOSIS

TN has a very good prognosis. With treatment, most previously hyperthyroid patients become and remain euthyroid and only a minority develop hypothyroidism that is easily controlled by LT$_4$. Note that a large number of patients never develop hyperthyroidism and need only regular control.

20.9 FOLLOW-UP

Follow-up of TN patients is dependent on functional status and possible choice of treatment (Table 20.6). If a patient is euthyroid, evaluation of FT$_4$ and TSH every 6 months and annual ultrasound are needed. In cases of subclinical hyperthyroid patients who are not receiving treatment, evaluation of TSH, FT$_4$, and FT$_3$ should be performed every 4 months, particular for the elderly.

If antithyroid treatment has been selected along with annual ultrasound evaluation, TSH, FT$_4$, and possibly FT$_3$ should be determined every 4 months. Any change in the dosage of a drug must be assessed after 6 to 8 weeks. Serum calcium and intact PTH assay, 6 and 12 hours after surgery, should confirm the functional integrity of the remaining parathyroids. TSH and FT$_4$ must be assessed 6 to 8 weeks after surgery and then annually to detect possible onset of hypothyroidism. TSH should be also tested every 6 months if LT$_4$ treatment is administered. TSH, FT$_4$, and FT$_3$ should be evaluated 1 to 2 months after radioiodine therapy and at the same intervals thereafter to evaluate the success of the treatment.

TSH and thyroid hormone levels are used also to taper antithyroid drug therapy if necessary after ^{131}I treatment. If a patient is still hyperthyroid 6 months after radioiodine administration, surgery or a new ^{131}I treatment must be considered. Although the onset of hypothyroidism has been described in a minority of TN patients treated with I[131], TSH and FT$_4$ evaluation must be performed at least annually (or according to clinical suspicion). If levothyroxine treatment is established because of hypothyroidism, the suggestion is to start with a dose lower than usual because of possible residual areas of autonomy in the contralateral lobe. Table 20.7 lists drugs cited in this chapter.

TABLE 20.6
Follow-Up of TN Patients Based on Functional Status and Treatment

	Test	Initial Follow-Up	Thereafter
Euthyroidism (no treatment)	TSH	Every 6 months	Every 6 months
	FT$_4$	Every 6 months	Every 6 months
	US	Annually	Annually
Subclinical hyperthyroidism	TSH	Every 4 months	Every 4 months
(no treatment)	FT$_4$	Every 4 months	Every 4 months
	FT$_3$	Every 4 months	Every 4 months
	US	Annually	Annually
Medical treatment	TSH	Every 4 months[a,b]	Every 6 months
	FT$_4$	Every 4 months[a,b]	Every 6 months
	FT$_3$	Every 4 months[a,b]	Every 6 months
	US	—	Annually
Surgery	Calcium	6 and 12 hours post-op	—
	PTH	6 and 12 hours post-op	—
	TSH	6 to 8 weeks post-op[a]	Annually
I[131]	TSH	Every 6 to 8 weeks[a]	Annually[c]
	FT$_4$	Every 6 to 8 weeks[a]	Annually[c]
	FT$_3$	Every 6 to 8 weeks[a]	—

Note: US = ultrasound.
[a] Until euthyroidism is achieved.
[b] After 6 to 8 weeks if dose is changed.
[c] Or according to clinical suspicion for hypothyroidism.

TABLE 20.7
List of Drugs Cited in This Chapter

Drug	Dose	Daily Medication Frequency
Propylthiouracil	25–200 mg	2 or 3 times
Methimazole	2.5–20mg	1 or 2 times
Carbimazole	2.5–30 mg	1 or 2 times
Propranolol	10–40 mg	3 or 4 times
Atenolol	25–100 mg	2 to 4 times
Metoprolol	25–50 mg	4
Verapamil	120 mg	2
Diltiazem	60–120 mg	2
Levothyroxine	1.2–1.7 µg/kg body weight	1

REFERENCES

1. Hennemann, G. 2010. Autonomously functioning thyroid nodules and other causes of thyrotoxicosis. In *Endocrinology. Adult and Pediatric*, 6th ed. Jameson, J.L. and DeGroot, L.J., Eds. Philadelphia: Saunders, Elsevier, 1572–1582.
2. Fuhrer, D., Krohn, K., and Paschke, R. 2005. Toxic adenoma and toxic multinodular goiter. In *Werner & Ingbar's The Thyroid: A Fundamental and Clinical Text*, 9th ed., Braverman, L.E. and Utiger, R.D., Eds. Philadelphia: Lippincott Williams & Wilkins, 500–518.
3. Krohn, K., Fuhrer, D., Bayer, Y. et al. 2005. Molecular pathogenesis of euthyroid and toxic multinodular goiter. *Endocr Rev* 26: 504–524.
4. Biondi, B. and Kahaly, G.J. 2010. Cardiovascular involvement in patients with different causes of hyperthyroidism. *Nature Rev Endocrinol* 6: 431–443.
5. Orgiazzi, J. and Mornex, R. 1993. Toxic nodular goiter. In *Thyroid Diseases: Clinical Fundamentals and Therapy*, Monaco, F. et al., Eds. Boca Raton: CRC Press, 63–80.
6. Murphy, E., Gluer, C.C., Reid, D.M. et al. 2010. Thyroid function within the upper normal range is associated with reduced bone mineral density and an increased risk of nonvertebral fractures in healthy euthyroid postmenopausal women. *J Clin Endocrinol Metab* 95: 3173–3181.
7. Spencer, C.A. 2003. Thyroid testing in the new millennium. *Thyroid* 13: 2–126.
8. Santarelli, L. and Monaco, F. 2007. Nodulo autonomo e gozzo multinodulare tossicco o malattia di Plummer. In *Malattie della Tiroide*, Monaco, E., Ed. Rome: Societa Edizione Universo, 421–456.
9. Bahn, R.S., Burch, H.B., Cooper, D.S. et al. 2011. Hyperthyroidism and other causes of thyrotoxicosis: management guidelines of the American Thyroid Association and American Association of Clinical Endocrinologists. *Thyroid* 21: 593–646.
10. Cooper, D.S. 2005. Antithyroid drugs. *New Engl J Med* 352: 905–917.
11. Filetti, S., Durante, C., and Torlontano, M. 2006. Nonsurgical approaches to the management of thyroid nodules. *Nat Clin Pract Endocrinol Metab* 2: 384–394.
12. Kahaly, G.J., Bartalena, L., and Hegedus, L. 2011. The American Thyroid Association/American Association of Clinical Endocrinologists guidelines for hyperthyroidism and other causes of thyrotoxicosis: a European perspective. *Thyroid* 21: 585–591.
13. Baek, J.H., Moon, W.J., Kim, J.S. et al. 2009. Radiofrequency ablation for the treatment of autonomously functioning thyroid nodules. *World J Surg* 33: 1971–1977.

21 Rare Forms of Thyrotoxicosis

Enrico Macchia, Fausto Bogazzi,
Luca Tomisti, and Enio Martino

CONTENTS

Key words: thyrotoxicosis, amiodarone, TSH-secreting pituitary adenoma, thyrotoxicosis factitia.

21.1 AMIODARONE-INDUCED THYROTOXICOSIS

21.1.1 DEFINITION

Amiodarone-induced thyrotoxicosis (AIT) is a challenging complication occurring on average in 10% of patients during chronic therapy. Two main forms of AIT may be identified: type 1, occurring in patients with underlying thyroid diseases, and type 2 occurring in patients with normal glands. Type 1 AIT is a form of true iodine-induced hyperthyroidism triggered by excess iodine released by amiodarone metabolism unveiling latent Graves' disease or functional autonomy. Type 2 AIT is a drug-induced destructive thyroiditis arising from the cytotoxic effect of amiodarone on thyroidal follicular cells. The coexistence of destructive phenomena and increased thyroid hormone (TH) synthesis are key features of the mixed (or undefined) forms of AIT.[1,2]

21.1.2 PHARMACOLOGY

Amiodarone is a benzofuranic iodine-rich class III antiarrhythmic drug used for treating various arrhythmic disturbances. Its structural formula is similar to that of thyroid hormone (Figure 21.1) and, as expected, amiodarone and its main metabolite, desethylamiodarone, exert thyromimetic action. In fact, amiodarone and desethylamiodarone can bind to thyroid hormone receptor as a weak competitor, thus reducing thyroid hormone effect. These actions contribute to the hypothyroid-like effect observed in euthyroid subjects tasking this therapy, including transient increase of TSH and reduced expression of thyroid hormone-sensitive genes.

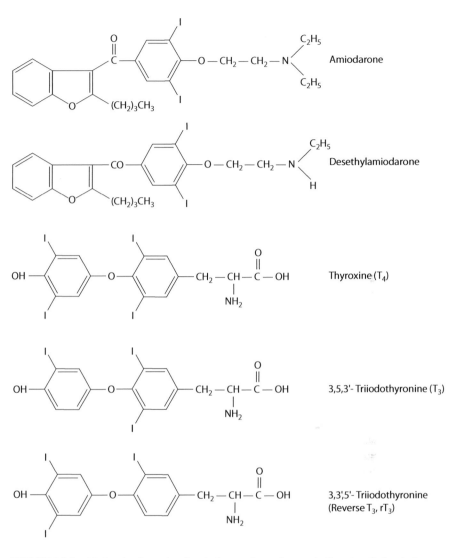

FIGURE 21.1 Molecular formula of amiodarone, its main metabolite, desethylamiodarone, and thyroid hormone, showing their similar structures.

Amiodarone is highly lipophilic and this accounts for its varied tissue distribution (adipose tissue, lung, and thyroid) and its long-lasting storage. Amiodarone metabolism occurs mainly through N-dealkylation, leading to the main active metabolite, desethylamiodarone. In addition, amiodarone may undergo deiodination and glucuroconjugation; excretion is mainly through biliary excretion. The average half-lives of amiodarone and desethylamiodarone are 40 days and 57 days, respectively and account for their long-lasting effects.

TABLE 21.1
Effects of Amiodarone on Thyroid Function

Mechanism	Effects	Thyroid Function Tests
Inhibition of type I 5'-deiodinase	Increased T_4	T_4 increased/high normal
	Decreased T_3	T_3 decreased/low normal
	Increased rT_3	
Inhibition of type II 5'-deiodinase	Decreased pituitary T_3 generation	Increased TSH (short term)
Inhibition of TH entry into cells	Decreased peripheral T_3 production	Decreased T_3/increased TSH
Interaction with TH receptor	Decreased transcription of TH-sensitive genes	Peripheral hypothyroidism
Thyroid cytotoxicity	Leakage of preformed TH	Increased T_4 and T_3
		Decreased TSH

21.1.3 EFFECTS ON THYROID HORMONE TESTS

Amiodarone exerts effects on thyroid function tests in all patients. About 1 to 2 months after the start of amiodarone therapy, a transient increase in serum TSH concentrations occurs because of an inhibitory effect of amiodarone on intracellular T_4 transport and pituitary iodothyronine type 2 deiodinase activity. Both effects (reduced entry of T_4 into cells and reduced metabolism of T_4) lead to (1) lower intracellular T_3 content and (2) lower T_3 binding to its cognate pituitary receptor, reducing thyroid hormone inhibitory effect on TSH gene transcription.

Conversely, during long-term therapy (>3 months), TSH returns to the normal range, serum-free T_4 and reverse T_3 concentrations increase, and serum-free T_3 concentrations decrease due to the inhibitory effect of amiodarone on hepatic iodothyronine type 1 deiodinase activity. Thus, euthyroid subjects on chronic amiodarone therapy frequently have slightly increased T_4, low to normal T_3, and normal TSH (Table 21.1).

21.1.4 EPIDEMIOLOGY OF AMIODARONE-INDUCED THYROID DYSFUNCTIONS

The prevalence of amiodarone-induced thyroid diseases is influenced by environmental iodine supplies. In iodine-sufficient areas, hypothyroidism is more frequent (on average 13%) than thyrotoxicosis (2%), whereas in iodine-deficient areas, thyrotoxicosis is more frequent (10 to 12%) than hypothyroidism (7%). Interestingly, during recent decades, it has been reported that prevalence of type 1 AIT did not change whereas the prevalence of type 2 dramatically increased; the practical consequence is that endocrinologists are mainly faced with amiodarone-induced destructive thyroiditis.[3]

21.1.5 PATHOGENESIS

Under a standard dose of amiodarone (on average, 200 mg/day), patients are exposed to a 7-g iodine load, largely exceeding the recommended daily allowance (150 to 200 μg). When exposed to large amounts of iodine, normal thyroids respond with an intrinsic autoregulatory mechanism leading to an acute block of thyroid hormone (TH) synthesis (Wolff-Chaikoff effect). As a consequence, a TH decrease leads to a TSH increase. The thyroid usually escapes the iodine-induced block of TH synthesis by reducing iodine transport. The reduced intracellular iodine concentrations are thus no longer sufficient for maintaining the Wolff-Chaikoff effect. Failure to escape the Wolff-Chaikoff effect is responsible for amiodarone- (and iodine)-induced hypothyroidism in patients without autoimmune thyroiditis.

Excessive iodine is the cause of type 1 AIT, a form of iodine-induced hyperthyroidism in which iodine load unveils underlying thyroid autonomy or latent Graves' disease (Jod-Basedow phenomenon). In such patients, the iodine load triggers increased TH synthesis in glands, creating a potential for hyperthyroidism.

On the other hand, amiodarone and desethylamiodarone have pro-apoptotic and cytotoxic effects on follicular epithelial cells. Thyroid cell cultures undergo increased apoptosis following amiodarone or desethylamiodarone exposure through an iodine-independent cytochrome-c release mechanism. In addition, amiodarone directly induces cytotoxic effects in follicular cells, but excess iodine released by the drug may contribute to its toxic action.

Histopathological studies of animals and AIT patients who underwent thyroidectomies showed disruption of thyroid structure, including follicular damage, reduced numbers of mitochondria, increased numbers of lysosomes and dilation of endoplasmic reticulum and lympho-plasma cellular infiltrate, in keeping with drug-induced thyroid damage similarly to that occurring in subacute thyroiditis. The above mechanism is responsible for the development of type 2 AIT, which is a drug-induced destructive thyroiditis.

21.1.6 CLINICAL PRESENTATION

Overall clinical features of AIT patients are indistinguishable from those of patients with spontaneous hyperthyroidism and other forms of thyrotoxicosis. However, some specific aspects should be considered: (1) thyrotoxicosis may occur in older patients with apathetic features: reduced appetite, absence of distal tremors, depression; (2) thyrotoxicosis may worsen underlying cardiac disease and particular attention is required when arrhythmias are no longer well-controlled in elder patients taking amiodarone; (3) thyrotoxicosis may increase degradation rates of vitamin K-dependent coagulation factors. Indeed, patients with atrial fibrillation who use anticoagulants and amiodarone and exhibit unexplained increased sensitivity to warfarin should lead their physicians to suspect thyrotoxicosis.

Differentiation of the two main forms of AIT is crucial, although challenging, because therapeutic options and outcomes greatly differ.

21.1.7 DIAGNOSIS

Patients with type 1 AIT present typical features of increased TH synthesis: underlying thyroid disease, positive thyroid antibody (including TSH receptor antibodies in patients with Graves' disease), increased thyroid vascularization on color flow Doppler sonography, and normal to increased thyroidal radioactive uptake in spite of iodine load. Conversely, findings in patients with type 2 AIT are those of thyrotoxicosis,

TABLE 21.2
AIT Diagnostic Tests

Test	Diagnostic Accuracy
I Level	
Serum FT_4, FT_3, TSH	+
Serum Tg-Ab, TPO-Ab, TR-Ab	+/–
Thyroid US (+ ECD pattern evaluation)	++
24-hour RAIU	++
II Level	
^{99m}Tc MIBI scan	?
Urinary iodide excretion	+

TABLE 21.3
Differential Diagnosis of AIT

	Type 1	Type 2
T_4/T_3 ratio	Usually <4	Usually >4
CFD pattern (thyroid vascularity)	Increased	Normal
Thyroidal RAIU	Normal to increased	Low to suppressed
Underlying functional autonomy	Present	Absent
Spontaneous remission	No	Possible
Thionamides and $KClO_4$	Effective	Ineffective
Glucocorticoids	Ineffective	Effective
Late hypothyroidism	No	Possible

Note: Thyroidal RAIU = thyroidal ^{131}-I uptake. CFD: color flow Doppler.

i.e., increased circulating thyroid hormone without evidence of increased glandular production: absence of thyroid disease and thyroid autoimmunity, low to suppressed thyroidal RAIU, and no increase in thyroid vascularization on color flow Doppler sonography (Table 21.2).

Mixed forms of AIT in which destructive phenomena superimpose to increased TH synthesis may exist. The use of a technetium (^{99m}Tc) Sestamibi scan may help identify these AIT forms, although its use is still under investigation. Indeed, consensus exists on the differentiation of the two main forms of AIT using standard procedures, and this has practical consequences for therapeutic options (Table 21.3).

21.1.8 TREATMENT

Management of AIT patient warrants strict cooperation between cardiologist and endocrinologist: In fact, treatment of AIT cannot be separated from cardiac functioning, requirements for amiodarone continuation, and differentiation of AIT types.

Based on different pathogenic mechanisms, type 1 and type 2 AIT should be managed using different drug regimens. Classically, medical therapy of type 1 AIT is devoted to controlling increased TH synthesis and release. Thus, thionamides and, when feasible, potassium perchlorate (to block thyroidal iodine uptake) are combined. High doses of methimazole (40 to 80 mg/day or equivalent propylthiouracil) are usually necessary because of the resistance of iodine embedded in thyroid glands to thionamides. Potassium perchlorate (600 to 1000 mg/day) treatment should not exceed 30 to 40 days. Conversely, the primary goal of medical therapy of type 2 AIT is to restore functional properties of damaged follicular cells using glucocorticoids (i.e., prednisone at initial dose of 5 to 7 mg/kg/day). Glucocorticoids are gradually tapered until euthyroidism restoration.[4,5]

Type 1 AIT patients have underlying thyroid disease that requires definitive therapy that does not differ from therapy of patients with spontaneous hyperthyroidism. Note that the time required to restore euthyroidism in some type 2 AIT patients may be exceptionally long. In both situations, medical therapy may be replaced by total thyroidectomy or radioiodine therapy. Radioiodine therapy is not feasible in the short run due to iodine contamination and/or follicular cell damage. Recently radioiodine therapy has been used in a few patients with AIT; in those cases, high radioactive iodine doses (on average 80 mCi) were used, sometimes employing rhTSH to increase iodine uptake. The latter procedure is not recommended because of significant and harmful increases of serum thyroid hormones.

Patients who have unstable control of underlying heart disease, those with extremely long predicted cure times, those taking medical therapy for recurrent or resistant thyrotoxicosis should be considered for total thyroidectomy. Restoration of euthyroidism with iopanoic acid, when feasible, before surgery and careful management of clinical conditions of AIT patients significantly reduce the reported surgical risks (Figure 21.2). A collaborative team of experienced endocrinologist, surgeon, and anesthetist is necessary.

21.1.9 Follow-Up

Patients with AIT should be closely followed up. Specifically, those with type 2 AIT should be followed after glucocorticoid withdrawal to monitor subsequent hypothyroidism development.

21.1.10 Screening

A general approach may be drawn from various guidelines: baseline evaluation including FT_4, FT_3, TSH, Ab-Tg, and Ab-TPO and thyroid echography and a follow-up assessment every 6 months measuring serum TSH (minimal evaluation) and FT_4 and FT_3 (complete evaluation). Measurement of serum antithyroid antibody is not recommended during follow-up because amiodarone therapy is not usually associated with development of thyroid autoimmunity.

During amiodarone therapy, changes in thyroid function tests (transient increases of serum TSH concentrations, increases in serum T_4 and rT_3, and reduced serum T_3 levels) may not reflect thyroid abnormalities. In addition, undetectable serum TSH

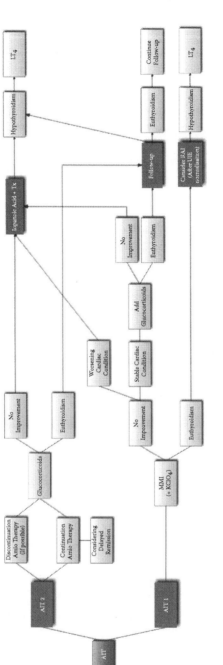

FIGURE 21.2 Proposed flowchart for managing patients with amiodarone-induced thyrotoxicosis. Medical therapy is usually the first therapeutic option for both types. If amiodarone therapy must be continued, a delay in euthyroidism restoration should be considered because of more frequent thyrotoxicosis recurrence. Subsequent management will depend on response to initial medical therapy, cardiac condition, and time needed to restore euthyroidism. In selected patients, total thyroidectomy may be considered as a first line therapeutic option (see text for details).

suggesting subclinical thyrotoxicosis spontaneously reverts in about half of AIT patients and usually does not require medical action.

21.2 IODINE-INDUCED THYROTOXICOSIS

While AIT is by far the most relevant form of iodine-induced thyrotoxicosis on clinical grounds, an excess of iodine acquired through diet or from iodine-containing compounds or other sources may lead to thyrotoxicosis. Iodinated contrast media are the most frequent causes of iodine load. Mechanisms leading to iodine-induced thyrotoxicosis do not differ from those described for type 1 AIT.

21.2.1 CLINICAL PRESENTATION

The clinical presentation does not differ from presentations for other conditions of TH excess including goiter or autoimmune thyroid disease in some patients.

21.2.2 DIAGNOSIS

The diagnostic considerations are no different from those for other forms of thyrotoxicosis. Increased urinary iodine excretion confirms a diagnosis of iodine-induced thyrotoxicosis.

21.2.3 TREATMENT

On average, iodine-induced thyrotoxicosis spontaneously remits in almost 50% of patients although remission requires several weeks.

21.3 LITHIUM-INDUCED THYROTOXICOSIS

Lithium is widely used to treat patients with bipolar disorders. Lithium has many effects on thyroid physiology because it concentrates in the thyroid with a threefold or fourfold ratio with plasma. Following lithium administration, thyroidal radioiodine uptake increases or reduces in humans. The major action of lithium is inhibition of thyroid hormone release due to TSH-dependent inhibition of tubulin polymerization.

Indeed, goiter is the most frequent thyroid abnormality during lithium therapy due to the initial inhibition of thyroid hormone secretion rate leading to a slight TSH increase and thyroid enlargement. In addition, lithium may exert direct proliferative action on follicular cells, contributing to the development of goiter.[6]

Hyperthyroidism may develop quickly or several years after therapy initiation. Graves' disease, toxic nodular goiter, and painless thyroiditis may be forms of hyperthyroidism associated with lithium therapy. Besides Graves' disease and toxic nodular goiter, a few patients on lithium therapy may develop lithium-associated silent thyroiditis. In a retrospective study, silent thyroiditis associated with lithium therapy had a higher incidence (1.3 to 2.7 cases per 1,000 person-years) than in the general population (0.03 to 1.2).

This form of thyrotoxicosis is due to transient lithium-induced destructive thyroiditis as supported by absent to low thyroidal iodine uptake. It spontaneously remits in most patients and leads to hypothyroidism in a few. Management of patients with lithium-associated hyperthyroidism with underlying Graves' disease or toxic nodular goiter is no different from managing patients with spontaneous hyperthyroidism.

21.4 THYROTOXICOSIS FACTITIA

21.4.1 CLASSIFICATION AND ETIOLOGY

Thyrotoxicosis factitia is caused by surreptitious intake of excessive amounts of exogenous thyroid hormones. The ingested thyroid hormone is most frequently thyroxine, but triiodothyronine or a mixture of the two hormones may be responsible for the occurrence of the syndrome. Table 21.4 shows the possible sources of exogenous thyroid hormones. Excess intake may derive from medical prescriptions (iatrogenic thyrotoxicosis), accidental (or suicidal) ingestion, surreptitious ingestion (thyrotoxicosis factitia), and inadvertent ingestion of a food contaminated by the thyroid gland (so-called hamburger thyrotoxicosis).[7]

21.4.2 CLINICAL FEATURES

Thyrotoxicosis factitia is usually observed in psychiatrically disturbed patients; they are almost invariably women who have psychoneurotic disturbances such as obsessive preoccupation with body weight, gender identity conflict, hysterical personality, and emotional instability. The clinical picture does not differ from that of classical spontaneous hyperthyroidism. Patients complain of tachycardia, tremors, loss of weight, increased perspiration, heat intolerance, extreme anxiety, nervousness, and insomnia. Goiter and ophthalmopathy are absent as are the thyroid pain and tenderness commonly observed in subacute thyroiditis. Cardiac and bone complications may occur, more often in elderly patients, as consequences of prolonged excess TH ingestion.

21.4.3 DIAGNOSIS

Laboratory evaluation shows typical increases of free thyroxine and triiodothyronine levels and undetectable TSH concentrations; circulating thyroid antibodies are absent.

TABLE 21.4
Exogenous Thyroid Hormone Origins

1   Iatrogenic thyrotoxicosis
2   Accidental (or suicidal) thyrotoxicosis
3   Surreptitious ingestion of thyroid hormones (thyrotoxicosis factitia)
4   Inadvertent ingestion of thyroid hormones ("hamburger thyrotoxicosis")

Thyroidal radioactive uptake is typically very low or suppressed. Likewise, color flow Doppler sonography reveals absent increase vascularity. Serum thyroglobulin concentration is characteristically markedly reduced or undetectable in thyrotoxicosis factitia; accordingly, its measurement is a useful tool for differentiating thyrotoxicosis factitia from other thyrotoxic conditions associated with low RAIU values.[8]

Table 21.5 shows the main differential characteristics of various thyrotoxic conditions. If a patient denies the surreptitious TH intake, it may be necessary to hospitalize her or him to interrupt deliberated thyroid hormone ingestion. Under strict medical controls, rapid improvement of thyrotoxicosis is usually observed. However, for a full recovery, psychiatric aid or counseling is mandatory.

TABLE 21.5

Typical Clinical Features of Graves' Disease, Subacute Thyroiditis, Thyrotoxicosis Factitia, and Amiodarone-Induced Thyrotoxicosis Types 1 and 2

Parameter	Graves' Disease	Subacute Thyroiditis	Thyrotoxicosis Factitia	AIT Type 1	AIT Type 2
Serum TH levels	Increased	Biphasic (increased → decreased)	Fluctuating	Increased	Increased
Serum Tg	Normal or increased	Increased	Low or undetectable	Increased	Increased
Underlying thyroid disease	Yes	Yes	Usually absent	Yes	No
Thyroid ultrasound	Diffuse goiter	Diffuse or nodular goiter	Normal (hypoechoic) gland	Diffuse or nodular goiter	Normal (hypoechoic) gland
CFDs	Increased vascularity	Normal or reduced vascularity	Normal or reduced vascularity	Increased vascularity	Normal vascularity
Thyroidal RAIU	High	Low	Low	Low or normal/ increased	Low or absent
Serum thyroid antibody	Present	Occasionally present	Usually absent	Sometimes present	Usually absent
Pathogenesis	Autoimmunity	Destructive thyroiditis	Surreptitious ingestion of TH or analogs	Iodine-induced hyperthyroidism	Destructive thyroiditis
Therapy	Thionamides	Corticosteroids	TH withdrawal	Thionamides (plus $KClO_4$)	Corticosteroids
Urinary iodine excretion	Usually normal	Usually normal	Normal or elevated	Elevated	Elevated
Pelvic RAIU	Absent	Absent	Absent	Absent	Absent
Duration	Lasting	Transient	Unpredictable	Lasting	Transient

21.5 HYPERTHYROIDISM ARISING FROM THYROTROPIN SECRETION: TSH-SECRETING PITUITARY TUMORS

21.5.1 INTRODUCTION

Thyroid stimulating hormone tumors (TSHomas) are rare, accounting for only 1 to 2% of pituitary tumors, with an approximate prevalence of one case per million individuals. The mean estimated latency between first symptoms and the diagnosis of TSHoma ranges from 2 to 6 years and is shorter for microadenoma.[9]

Hyperthyroidism resulting from oversecretion of TSH by a pituitary tumor was first identified in 1960. Since then, over 400 documented cases of TSHomas causing central hyperthyroidism have been published. Men and women are affected almost equally. TSHomas are rarely associated with multiple endocrine neoplasia type I (MEN 1) and McCune-Albright syndrome. TSH-secreting adenomas can secrete TSH alone (72%) or co-secrete other hormones such as growth hormone (GH; 16%), prolactin (PRL; 11%), and occasionally gonadotropins (FSH/LH) as well. This may be because GH- and PRL-secreting cells share several transcription factors with thyrotrophs, such as Pit-1 and Prop-1. An ectopic TSH-producing tumor has also been reported.[10]

21.5.2 ETIOLOGY AND PATHOGENESIS

The cells of TSHomas exhibit two major features that distinguish them from normal thyrotrophs: (1) excessive cellular proliferation and (2) autonomous TSH production that is unresponsive to normal regulatory controls. Evidence suggests that some TSHomas may also secrete TSH molecules that have enhanced biological potency. As a result, the thyroid gland enlarges and produces excess amounts of hormones, causing clinical thyrotoxicosis.

TSHomas probably arise from the monoclonal expansion of a single transformed cell. Several experimental data suggest earlier cells such as the Pit-1-dependent stem cells as sources of the neoplasms in at least some tumors. Some TSHomas seem to consist of two cell populations, one that produces intact TSH molecules and one that produces only α-subunits, suggesting that certain neoplastic cells have lost the ability to make the TSH β-subunit. This is most likely the result of a secondary modification that occurs some time after the initial transformation and impairs TSH production capability without altering synthesis in affected cells.

21.5.3 PATHOLOGY

These neoplasms are invasive, but mostly benign, and metastases are exceedingly rare. TSH-secreting tumors present positive immunostaining for the α-subunit and TSH as well as for Pit-1 and GATA-2 in most cells. Clinically silent TSHomas can occur and are usually detected incidentally or because of mass effect. Immunostaining reveals the adenoma subtype.

21.5.4 CLINICAL PRESENTATION

The clinical presentation of TSHomas depends on the quantity, rhythm, and biological potency of the TSH produced and the size of the tumor. Symptoms may be due to tumor size (headache, visual field abnormalities, cranial nerve palsies) and/or hormone excess (weight loss, irritability, palpitations, cardiac arrhythmias, and goiter).

A relatively long period of hyperthyroidism, initially thought to be Graves' disease and treated accordingly, often precedes the correct diagnosis of central hyperthyroidism. Seventy to 90% of TSH-secreting tumors are macroadenomas and more than 60% are also locally invasive. When the adenoma co-secretes other hormones, signs or symptoms of acromegaly or hyperprolactinemia may also be present.

21.5.5 EVALUATION AND DIAGNOSIS

Circulating T_4, T_3, TSH (by high-sensitivity assay), and α-subunit should be measured. The diagnosis should be suspected in any patient with increased serum levels of free T_4 and T_3 associated with a non-suppressed or elevated serum TSH value. Other conditions such as abnormal thyroid hormone-binding proteins, anti-TH autoantibodies, and heterophilic antibodies interfering with the measurement of TSH may exhibit deceptively similar laboratory findings. Therefore, their preliminary exclusion is necessary. This is best accomplished by measuring free thyroid hormone concentrations by methods similar to equilibrium dialysis and adding normal murine serum to the immunoradiometric TSH assay to exclude the presence of heterophile antibodies. If the free thyroid hormone levels are still elevated and true TSH is not suppressed, the differential diagnosis is narrowed to include RTH and TSHomas.

In some patients with familial RTH due to mutations in the β isoform of the thyroid hormone (TH) receptor, the hypothalamus—pituitary feedback mechanism shows a higher resistance to TH action than that of peripheral tissues such as the heart. As the pituitary is selectively resistant to TH, the set point of the pituitary for TH is fixed at a higher level of circulating TH. These patients may therefore present thyrotoxic symptoms and goiter associated with high serum TH and detectable serum TSH. In these cases, patient family histories are crucial since RTH is inherited in an autosomal dominant pattern.

Consequently, in patients with TSHomas, serum TSH levels fail to increase after the intravenous administration of TRH and always remain detectable after high doses of exogenous TH (T_3 suppression tests for 10 days). Serum α-subunit and β-subunit/TSH molar ratio (α-subunit in g/L divided by TSH in U/L multiplied by 10) are nearly always elevated, although α-subunit values must be carefully matched for sex and age. Parallel measurement of an α-subunit at each point during the TRH test represents an additional useful diagnostic tool.

In vivo markers, such as the basal metabolic rate (BMR) and cardiac systolic time intervals (STIs), and in vitro indices including SHBG, ferritin, angiotensin-converting enzyme (ACE), bone GLA protein (BGP), and soluble interleukin-2 receptors (sILR) facilitate the differential diagnosis and are normal in cases of RTH and elevated in TSHomas. Diagnostic accuracy may be improved by measuring in vivo and in vitro markers both before and after the administration of supraphysiologic doses of T_3. A lack of significant changes after T_3 is consistent with RTH. A further helpful method for differentiating the two conditions in vivo is thyroid color flow Doppler sonography.

PRL and IGF1 levels must also be measured to exclude hyperprolactinemia or acromegaly associated with hyperthyroidism.

High-resolution computed tomography (CT) and nuclear magnetic resonance (MR) imaging are the major tools for the visualization of TSHomas. Most TSHomas are diagnosed at the stage of visible adenomas, sometimes with suprasellar extension or sphenoidal sinus invasion. When an MR of the pituitary is unable to detect an adenoma, inferior petrosal sinus sampling for TSH can be a useful option.

Scintigraphy with radio-labelled octreotide (Octreoscan) can identify TSHomas expressing somatostatin receptors but it lacks specificity. Octreoscan may still be useful to localize ectopic TSHomas.

21.5.6 TREATMENT

The first principle for treating TSHomas is the careful establishment of a correct diagnosis. Patients with TSHomas are sometimes erroneously diagnosed as having Graves' disease. Inappropriate treatment of such patients with subtotal thyroidectomy or radioiodine administration fails to cure the underlying disorder and also seems to be associated with subsequent pituitary tumor enlargement and increased risk of invasiveness into adjacent tissues. Therapy for TSHomas must be directed at significantly reducing the pituitary tumor mass and the associated TSH hypersecretion.

The treatment of choice in most cases is surgical removal of the tumor using the transphenoidal approach. Surgery is recommended as first line treatment, although surgical cure occurs only in about half of the patients, mainly because the tumors may be large, locally invasive with the involvement of cavernous sinus, and structurally fibrotic. The rarity of this kind of tumor, however, has prevented large controlled studies. In a recent large series study, surgery cured the disease in over 50% of cases.

Radiation has mostly been employed as adjunctive therapy to surgery, principally when surgery was not curative. However, no large series studies report treatment of TSH-secreting tumors with radiotherapy alone.

Medical therapy with long acting somatostatin analogues (SSAs) such as octreotide long acting release (LAR) or lanreotide autogel is an effective approach. Treatment with these analogues leads to a reduction of TSH and its α-subunit secretion in most cases and often to a normal thyroid function. Visual field improvement occurred in two-thirds of patients, and reduction in tumor size was demonstrable in about a third of them. Dopamine agonists such as bromocriptine on the contrary failed to control TSH-secreting adenomas, except those co-secreting PRL where tumor shrinkage was observed.

A few cases showed resistance to SSA treatment or side effects that required the discontinuation of therapy. Furthermore, in most patients with mixed TSH/GH hypersecretion, symptoms of acromegaly were clearly reduced by SSA treatment. In addition, SSA has utility as a preoperative strategy to reduce tumor size and as a complement to radiotherapy in patients not cured by surgery. Radioiodine, thyroidectomy, and antithyroid medications are targeted to the thyroid gland rather than to the pituitary source of the disease. Both also abolish the residual negative feedback of T_3 on TSH and may lead to increased TSH production. Because SSAs lower TSH, β-subunit, and TH, they are recommended as first line drugs in the initial control of hyperthyroidism due to TSH-secreting tumors because their onset of action is faster than other therapeutic approaches.

21.6 THYROTOXICOSIS ASSOCIATED WITH TROPHOBLASTIC TUMORS: HYDATIDIFORM MOLE AND CHORIOCARCINOMA

21.6.1 INTRODUCTION

Mild to severe thyrotoxicosis in pregnancy is caused by chorionic gonadotropin-secreting tumors that belong to the neoplastic group of gestational trophoblastic diseases first described in 1955.[11] Thyrotoxicosis may develop in men with chorionic tumors of the testes, usually with metastatic disease.[12]

21.6.2 DEFINITION

Gestational trophoblastic diseases include a heterogeneous group of neoplastic disorders that develop from the trophoblastic epithelium of the placenta characterized by excessive hCG secretion. Based on histopathological, cytogenetic, and clinical features, gestational trophoblastic diseases are classified in five distinct groups: complete (CHM) and partial (PHM) hydatidiform mole, invasive mole, choriocarcinoma, placental site trophoblastic tumor, and miscellaneous trophoblastic lesions. These disorders show varying potential for local invasion and metastases but generally respond extremely well to chemotherapy.

21.6.3 EPIDEMIOLOGY

Complete hydatidiform moles and partial hydatidiform moles occur in approximately 1 in 1,500 and 1 in 750 pregnancies, respectively. Most cases end in miscarriage during the first trimester. The prevalence of choriocarcinoma is approximately 1 in 50,000 pregnancies, about one half occurring in patients with previously diagnosed hydatidiform moles.

21.6.4 PATHOGENESIS OF THYROTOXICOSIS

Thyrotoxicosis is due to the tumoral production of large amounts of hCG that bind to TSH receptors and display intrinsic thyroid-stimulating activity.

TABLE 21.6

Symptoms and Signs of Hydatidiform Moles

Symptoms or Signs	Complete mole (%)	Partial mole (%)
Vaginal bleeding	97	73
Enlarged uterus	51	4
Thecal lutein cyst over 6 cm	50	0
Preeclampsia	27	3
Hyperemesis	26	0
Thyrotoxicosis	7	0

21.6.5 CLINICAL PRESENTATION

Signs of thyrotoxicosis may be present only in a complete mole and are infrequent (7%). Partial moles are usually discovered upon the first signs of a miscarriage. Vaginal bleeding remains the most common presenting symptom. Hyperthyroidism associated with choriocarcinoma is extremely rare in men (Table 21.6).

21.6.6 DIAGNOSIS

Pelvic ultrasound usually revealing the absence of a fetus (in cases of complete moles) and characteristic swollen villi that produce a snowstorm-like pattern or multicystic appearance and very high levels of hCG associated with increased serum thyroid hormone and absent thyroidal RAIU suggest diagnosis.

21.6.7 TREATMENT

Removal of the tumor and/or effective chemotherapy results in the disappearance of the excess hCG and consequently of the thyrotoxicosis.

21.6.8 FOLLOW-UP

After evacuation of the uterus, a patient should be carefully monitored for the potential development of persistent intrauterine or metastatic GTD. The key is the serial determination of β-hCG in the patient's serum.

21.7 STRUMA OVARII

21.7.1 DEFINITION

Struma ovarii (SO) is a very rare cause of thyrotoxicosis due to an ovarian teratoma containing hyperfunctioning autonomous thyroid tissue. To fulfill the definition of SO, the ectopic thyroid tissue contained in the teratoma should be more than 50% or should at least be able to cause thyrotoxicosis. Struma ovarii without associated thyrotoxicosis is much more common and may be discovered accidentally during surgery for an ovarian tumor.

21.7.2 Epidemiology

Struma ovarii was first described in 1889. Fewer than 500 cases have been reported in the literature and fewer than 30 caused thyrotoxicosis. Most struma ovarii are benign; fewer than 3% are malignant.[13]

21.7.3 Pathology

The histological criteria for malignancy are uncertain. Malignancy criteria include papillae lined by cells with overlapping ground-glass nuclei, and capsular and blood vessel invasion or dissemination. The absence of capsular invasion and vascular invasion suggest a better prognosis. About one third of malignant struma ovarii metastasize and may spread to the peritoneum (causing peritoneal seeding and ascites) or to abdominal lymph nodes, liver, lung, mediastinum, bone, and brain.

21.7.4 Pathogenesis of Thyrotoxicosis in Struma Ovarii

Two possible pathogenetic mechanisms are possible. The ovarian tumor may autonomously produce a significant amount of TH and cause thyrotoxicosis, or ovarian strumal hyperfunction is caused by the autoimmune phenomena from the concomitant Graves' disease.

21.7.5 Clinical Presentation

Clinically, most cases of struma ovarii are silent or present with vague symptoms, similar to other ovarian tumors. Only a few patients show symptoms of hyperthyroidism. Thyrotoxic crisis is a rare but life-threatening complication that may follow the excision of struma when thyrotoxicosis was not diagnosed preoperatively.

21.7.6 Diagnosis

Struma ovarii should be considered in a patient with thyrotoxicosis, low radioiodine or 99mpertechnetate (Tc) uptake over the thyroid, and a pelvic mass. Laboratory studies show suppressed serum TSH, increased serum TH and Tg, and absent antithyroid autoantibodies if autoimmune thyroiditis or Graves' disease is not associated with the struma.

21.7.7 Treatment

Surgery is the treatment of choice to excise the functional ovarian teratoma. Since the ectopic thyroid tissue is potentially malignant, alternative treatment with radioiodine is neither appropriate nor curative.

Once malignancy has been histologically demonstrated, no current consensus exists on the surgical and postoperative treatments of patients with a malignant SOs. After the initial surgery, treatment options include further pelvic surgery with total abdominal hysterectomy and bilateral salpingo-oophorectomy, and thyroidectomy.

REFERENCES

1. Martino, E., Bartalena, L., Bogazzi, F. et al. 2001. The effects of amiodarone on the thyroid. *Endocr Rev* 22: 240–254.
2. Bogazzi, F., Bartalena, L., Gasperi, M. et al. 2001.The various effects of amiodarone on thyroid function. *Thyroid* 11: 511–519.
3. Eskes, S.A. and Wiersinga, W.M. 2009. Amiodarone and thyroid. *Best Pract Res Clin Endocrinol Metab* 23: 735–751.
4. Bogazzi, F., Bartalena, L., and Martino, E. 2010. Approach to the patient with amiodarone-induced thyrotoxicosis *J Clin Endocrinol Metab.* 95: 2529–2535.
5. Gammage, J.A.F. 2007. Treatment of amiodarone-associated thyrotoxicosis. *Nat Clin Pract Endocrinol Metab* 3: 662–666.
6. Lazarus, J.H. 2009. Lithium and thyroid. *Best Pract Res Clin Endocrinol Metab* 23: 723–733.
7. Kopp, P. 2010. Thyrotoxicosis of other etiologies. In *Thyroid Disease Manager,* Chap. 13. http://www.thyroidmanager.org/Chapter13/chapter13.pdf.
8. Cohen, J.H., Ingbar, S.H., and Braverman, L.E. 1989. Thyrotoxicosis due to ingestion of excess thyroid hormone. *Endocr Rev* 10: 113–124.
9. Beck-Peccoz, P., Persani, L., Mannavola, D. et al. 2009. TSH-secreting adenomas. *Best Pract Res Clin Endocrinol Metab* 23: 597–606.
10. Rouach, V. and Greenman, Y. 2011. Thyrotropin-secreting pituitary tumors. In *The Pituitary*, 3rd ed., Melmed, S., Ed. Amsterdam: Elsevier, Chap. 17.
11. Goldstein, D.P. and Berkovitz, R.S. 2008. Gestational trophoblastic disease. In *Abeloff's Clinical Oncology*, 4th ed., Abeloff, M.D., Ed. Churchill Livingstone Elsevier.
12. Oosting, S.F., de Haas, E.C., Links, T.P. et al. 2010. Prevalence of paraneoplastic hyperthyroidism in patients with metastatic non-seminomatous germ-cell tumors. *Ann Oncol* 21: 104–108.
13. Yassa L., Sadow P., and Marqusee, E. 2008. Malignant struma ovarii. *Nat Clin Pract Endocrinol Metab* 4: 469–472.

22 Transient Hyperthyroidism

Bernadette Biondi

CONTENTS

Key words: subclinical hyperthyroidism (exogenous and endogenous), thyrotropin, Hashimoto's thyroiditis, silent thyroiditis, postpartum thyroiditis, autoimmune transient neonatal hyperthyroidism, thyrotoxicosis factitia, iodine-induced hyperthyroidism, amiodarone-induced thyroiditis.

22.1 DEFINITION

Transient hyperthyroidism is caused by a self-limiting serum excess of thyroid hormones and low TSH, lasting a few weeks to a few months and returns spontaneously to normal. TSH concentration is inversely log-linearly proportional to thyroid hormone excess; minimal changes in serum thyroid hormone levels may suppress serum TSH. It is important to differentiate persistent subclinical hyperthyroidism from other causes of transient TSH suppression.

22.2 ETIOPATHOGENESIS AND EPIDEMIOLOGY

Several causes of low or undetectable serum TSH may not reflect the presence of persistent subclinical hyperthyroidism.[1-3]

22.2.1 NON-AUTOIMMUNE CAUSES OF ADULT TRANSIENT HYPERTHYROIDISM

Table 22.1 lists the causes of transient subclinical hyperthyroidism. The hypothalamus–pituitary–thyroid axis may remain suppressed during treatment with antithyroid drugs in overt and subclinical hyperthyroidism and after complete resolution of

---

TABLE 22.1

Causes of Transient Subclinical Hyperthyroidism

Autoimmune Causes

Hashimoto's thyroiditis

Silent thyroiditis

Postpartum thyroiditis

Autoimmune transient neonatal hyperthyroidism

Non-autoimmune Causes

Acute and subacute thyroiditis

During treatment of overt hyperthyroidism with antithyroid drugs

After radioiodine treatment

Thyrotoxicosis factitia

Iodine-induced hyperthyroidism

Drug administration (amiodarone-induced thyroiditis)

Gestational transient thyrotoxicosis

Hyperemesis gravidarum

---

hyperthyroidism with radioiodine. This may explain why the normalization of serum TSH may occur in treated hyperthyroid patients after 2 or 3 months.[4]

In adult subjects, thyrotoxicosis can result from the destruction of thyroid follicles and thyrocytes in various forms of thyroiditis.[5] Acute, subacute, and chronic thyroiditis may be characterized by transient, self-limiting hyperthyroidism. TSH suppression in these inflammatory disorders is caused by thyroid destruction with the release of thyroid hormone into circulation. The thyrotoxic phase may be followed by transient or permanent hypothyroidism.

Transient TSH suppression may usually occur after acute suppurative thyroiditis, a rare infectious disease commonly associated with pyriform sinus fistula, especially in children. Immunosuppressed patients and organ-transplant patients are predisposed to recurrent episodes of suppurative thyroiditis. Subacute thyroiditis is characterized by a viral infection by adenovirus, coxsackievirus, Epstein-Barr, and influenza viruses. It is characterized by thyroid pain, tenderness, and transient thyrotoxicosis. Thyroid function usually normalizes within 12 to 18 months and permanent hypothyroidism may develop in 5% of cases.

Thyrotoxicosis factitia may develop after the iatrogenic ingestion of exogenous thyroid hormone by psychiatric patients or after the improper use of thyroid hormone in obese patients to lose weight or treat depression. Thyrotoxicosis can also be induced by excessive thyroid hormone intake due to the consumption of meat containing bovine thyroid tissue,[6] as reported in the United States and called "hamburger thyrotoxicosis." Excessive intake of iodine, drugs, or other iodine-containing compounds may lead to thyrotoxicosis.[7,8]

Iodine-induced thyrotoxicosis (IIT) may occur in patients from endemic goiter areas, patients with multinodular goiters who live in non-endemic areas, individuals with Graves' disease, and those without apparent thyroid disease. Patients with multinodular goiters are particularly prone to developing IIT. The prevalence of IIT is increased in endemic iodine-deficient areas after iodination of salt or administration of iodized oil. This risk is estimated between 2 and 7%, with increased risks for elderly patients with multinodular goiter.

The natural course of the disease is usually mild and recovery is spontaneous. Several studies suggest that chronic excessive iodine intake may modulate thyroid autoimmunity, leading to thyrotoxicosis in genetically susceptible individuals. IIT may often develop several weeks after exposure to iodine contrast agents. Transient subclinical thyrotoxicosis may be frequently induced in elderly patients with multinodular goiter; this risk is low after coronary angiography and prophylactic therapy with antithyroid drugs is not recommended in unselected patients.

Amiodarone, a benzofuranic drug containing 75 mg iodine per 200 mg tablet, is an anti-arrhythmic agent used to treat ventricular and supraventricular arrhythmias.[9] Amiodarone may induce thyrotoxicosis in about 10% of patients living in iodine-deficient areas. The prevalence of amiodarone induced thyrotoxicosis (AIT) has been reported as 0.003% to 11.5%. The mechanism of AIT may be due to the iodine released during the metabolism of the drug (AIT Type I) or to the induction of a destructive thyroiditis (AIT Type 2).

Suppressed serum TSH may be observed at the end of the first trimester of pregnancy because of structural homology of placental hCG, which may induce thyroid stimulation.[10,11] Gestational transient thyrotoxicosis caused by stimulating the TSH receptor through hCG occurs in about 1.4 % of pregnant women, particularly when hCG levels exceed 70,000 to 80,000 IU/L. This disorder is usually transient and limited to the first 3 to 4 months of gestation. Suppressed serum TSH may be present in women with hyperemesis gravidarum or trophoblastic disease. Hyperemesic patients have significantly greater mean serum levels of hCG, free T_4, total T_3, and estradiol, and lower serum TSH concentrations compared to controls. The degree of biochemical hyperthyroidism and hCG concentration correlate directly with the severity of vomiting.

22.2.2 AUTOIMMUNE CAUSES OF ADULT TRANSIENT HYPERTHYROIDISM

Hashimoto's thyroiditis, silent thyroiditis and postpartum thyroiditis (PPT) represent important causes of transient hyperthyroidism and hypothyroidism[1,5] (see Table 22.1). Silent thyroiditis can be considered a silent form of subacute thyroiditis or an unusual presentation of chronic lymphocytic thyroiditis with unknown or well-defined cause factors. The pathological diagnosis in both cases is characterized by lymphocytic infiltration. Thyrotoxic symptoms may occur during the first 1 to 4 weeks after diagnosis of silent thyroiditis, although they are usually mild.

TSH may remain suppressed after 1 to 6 weeks in about 60% of patients. Enlargement of the thyroid gland may develop, but it is associated with low thyroid radioiodine uptake, while thyroglobulin (Tg) concentration may increase. Usually this destructive process is self-limited and normal thyroid function is restored within 12 to 18 months, although transient hypothyroidism may develop. Permanent hypothyroidism occurs in fewer than 20% of patients. Thyrotoxic symptoms during the postpartum period may be related to a recurrence of GD or PPT. This last disorder is a destructive process during the first 12 months postpartum with a prevalence of 3 to 17%. This disease is threefold higher in patients with type 1 diabetes and in women with previous episodes of PPT.

22.2.3 AUTOIMMUNE TRANSIENT NEONATAL HYPERTHYROIDISM

Graves' disease has an estimated incidence of about 2 in 1,000 pregnancies. Transient autoimmune neonatal hyperthyroidism is rare and occurs in fewer than 2% of new-born offspring of mothers with histories of Graves' disease.[12] This transient form of hyperthyroidism may be caused by transplacental passage of stimulating TSH receptor autoantibodies. Antibody-induced neonatal hyperthyroidism usually disappears within the first few months of life. Occasionally, thyroid function may fluctuate with elevated or decreased hormone levels because of the concomitant presence of stimulating and blocking antibodies.

22.3 DIFFERENTIAL DIAGNOSIS OF TRANSIENT SUBCLINICAL HYPERTHYROIDISM

Table 22.2 details diagnosis of this condition. In the presence of suppressed TSH, it is important to exclude the recent administration of an iodinated contrast agent or excessive iodine exposure. If necessary, 24-hour radioactive iodine uptake (RAIU) measurement and thyroid scan will differentiate the increased uptake in patients with Graves' disease, the presence of warm or hot nodules in multinodular goiters, and autonomously functioning thyroid adenoma.

The absence of uptake is typical of a hyperthyroid phase of thyroiditis and may be observed in patients who take exogenous thyroid hormone or iodine-containing preparations. The T_4 to T_3 ratio is higher in Graves' disease than in thyroiditis.

TABLE 22.2

Diagnosis of Transient Thyrotoxicosis

I Level

TSH, FT_4, FT_3

T_4/T_3

Tg-Ab and TPO-Ab

TSHR-Ab

Doppler ultrasound of thyroid

II Level

Thyroid scan and radioiodine uptake

Erythrocyte sedimentation rate (ESR)

C-reactive protein

Tg

TSHR-Ab

Serum interleukin-6

Urinary iodine excretion

Urinary iodine excretion is increased in iodine-induced thyrotoxicosis. A suspicious intake of thyroid hormone should be suspected in patients with thyrotoxicosis, low radioiodine uptake, low Tg, and absence of goiter. TSH receptor antibodies are negative in PPT and this may permit the differential diagnosis of GD during the thyrotoxic period. Leukocytosis and elevated erythrocyte sedimentation rate (ESR) and C-reactive protein levels are observed in acute and subacute thyroiditis. Serum interleukin-6 may be useful to differentiate iodine-induced thyrotoxicosis (Type 1) and destructive thyroiditis (Type 2), since it is only elevated in Type 2. Color Doppler may show hypervascularization in Type 1 and amiodarone-induced thyrotoxicosis and hypovascularity in Type 2.

22.4 TREATMENT OF TRANSIENT SUBCLINICAL HYPERTHYROIDISM

Treatment is dictated by the etiological factors (Table 22.3). In patients with thyroiditis, treatment with antithyroid drugs is inappropriate because the thyroid is not overactive. Beta blockers may decrease palpitations and reduce shakes and tremors. Thyrotoxicosis symptoms are usually mild and sedatives are sufficient to control the symptoms.

If permanent hypothyroidism develops, the patients should be treated with thyroid hormone replacement therapy as primary hypothyroidism is treated. Anti-inflammatory medications such as aspirin and ibuprofen are often adequate to control thyroidal pain in mild cases of subacute thyroiditis. More serious cases may need temporary treatment with steroids (for example, 40 mg prednisone for a week, followed by progressive tapering for 2 to weeks) to control inflammation. Treatment of acute thyroiditis requires therapy with antibiotics based on the causative agent.

Patients with AIT I are preferably treated with thionamides (initially 40 to 60 mg methimazole/day followed by gradual adjustment of the dose). In selected patients, treatment with potassium perchlorate ($KClO_4$; 1 g/day for 4 to 6 weeks) can also be considered. Potassium perchlorate may cause aplastic anemia and its use should be limited to patients who cannot be controlled by methimazole or are allergic to thionamides. Patients with AIT Type 2 generally respond to glucocorticoids.

TABLE 22.3
Treatment of Transient Thyrotoxicosis

Autoimmune thyrotoxicosis	Asymptomatic patients: no treatment
	Symptomatic patients: β blockade
Non-autoimmune thyrotoxicosis	Withdrawal of drugs inducing thyrotoxicosis when possible
	Asymptomatic patients: no treatment
	Symptomatic or high-risk (elderly, cardiac patients): β-blockade, MMI or PTU
Subacute thyroiditis	Salicylates, non-steroidal anti-inflammatory drugs, corticosteroids
Type I AIT	MMI, potassium perchlorate
Type II AIT	Corticosteroids
Acute thyroiditis	Antibiotics

Prednisone (0.5 to 0.7 mg/Kg body weight daily) can be used for several months. Since the distinction between AIT Type I and Type II is difficult and may be unclear and some patients have mixed forms of AIT, these therapies may be combined if necessary. Antiemetics are necessary for women with hyperemesis.

22.5 FOLLOW-UP

Patients with transient thyrotoxicosis who recover spontaneously should be examined annually (FT_4 and TSH levels) to determine potential risk of hypothyroidism.

REFERENCES

1. Biondi, B. and Cooper, D.S. 2008. The clinical significance of subclinical thyroid dysfunction. *Endocr Rev* 29: 76–131.
2. Davies, T.F. and Larsen, P.R. 2003. Transient hyperthyroidism. In *Williams' Textbook of Endocrinology,* 10th ed., Polonsky, J. et al., Eds. Philadelphia: W.B. Saunders, 407.
3. Napolitano, G. and Monaco, F. 1993. Transient hyperthyroidism. In *Thyroid Disease: Clinical Fundamentals and Diagnosis*, Monaco, F. et al., Eds. Boca Raton: CRC Press.
4. Kubota, S., Tamai, H., Ohye, H. et al. 2004. Transient hyperthyroidism after withdrawal of antithyroid drugs in patients with Graves' disease. *Endocrine J* 51: 213–217.
5. Fatourechi, V., Aniszewski, J.P., Eghbali, G.Z. et al. 2003. Clinical features and outcome of subacute thyroiditis in an incidence cohort: Olmsted County, Minnesota study. *J Clin Endocrin Metab* 88: 2100–2105.
6. Parmar, M.S. and Sturge, C. 2001. Recurrent hamburger thyrotoxicosis. *CMAJ* 169: 415–417.
7. Roti, E. and Uberti, E.D. 2001. Iodine excess and hyperthyroidism. *Thyroid* 11: 493–500.
8. Burgi, H. 2010. Iodine excess. *Best Pract Res Clin Endocrinol Metab* 24: 107–115.
9. Martino, E., Bartalena, L., Bogazzi, F. et al. 2001. The effects of amiodarone on the thyroid. *Endocr Rev* 22: 240–254.
10. Radetti, G., Zavallone, A., Gentili, L. et al. 2002. Foetal and neonatal thyroid disorders. *Minerva Pediatr* 54: 383–400.
11. Zakarija, M. and McKenzie, J.M. 1983. Pregnancy-associated changes in the thyroid-stimulating antibody of Graves' disease and the relationship to neonatal hyperthyroidism. *J Clin Endocrinol Metab* 57: 1036–1040.
12. Higuchi, R., Kumagai, T., Kobayashi, M. et al. 2001. Short-term hyperthyroidism followed by transient pituitary hypothyroidism in a very low birth weight infant born to a mother with uncontrolled Graves' disease. *Pediatrics* 107, E57.

23 Subclinical Hyperthyroidism

Bernadette Biondi

CONTENTS

Key words: subclinical hyperthyroidism (exogenous and endogenous), thyrotropin, levothyroxine, replacement therapy, thyroid cancer, thyroid autonomy, thyrotropin suppression, prevalence, progression, cardiovascular risk, heart, bone, osteoporosis, symptoms, elderly.

23.1 DEFINITION

Subclinical hyperthyroidism (SHyper) is defined as serum free thyroxine (FT_4) and free triiodothyronine (FT_3) concentrations at upper levels but within their respective reference ranges in the presence of low or undetectable serum thyrotropin-stimulating hormone (TSH) levels.[1] *Subclinical hyperthyroidism* is a misnomer and inappropriate term because patients with this disorder may have specific symptoms of mild thyroid hormone excess.[1] In fact, thyroid hormones are sufficiently increased to suppress TSH and induce adverse tissue effects.[1] Highly sensitive and specific TSH assays allow experts to distinguish mild SHyper when a serum TSH level is low, but still detectable (0.1 to 0.4 mIU/L), from a more severe condition in which TSH is undetectable and fully suppressed (<0.1 mIU/L; see Table 23.1).

TABLE 23.1

Definition of Subclinical Hyperthyroidism and Minimally Suppressed TSH

Patients with mildly low but still detectable serum TSH (0.1 to 0.4 mIU/L)

Patients with undetectable serum TSH level (<0.1 mIU/L)

23.2 ETIOPATHOGENESIS AND EPIDEMIOLOGY

The most common cause of SHyper is an excessive LT_4 replacement therapy in hypothyroid patients or intentional TSH suppressive therapy with LT_4 for differentiated thyroid cancer (exogenous SHyper).[1] This condition is present in about 20 to 40% of patients receiving levothyroxine (LT_4) therapy[2] (Table 23.2).

Endogenous SHyper is commonly associated with autonomous thyroid function. Graves' disease (GD), toxic multinodular goiter (TMNG), and toxic nodule (TN) represent the most frequent causes of this disorder. The prevalence of endogenous SHyper is between 0.7 to 9% in relation to the degree of TSH suppression, cause of the disease, patient age, and sensitivity of the methods used to measure serum TSH concentrations.[3]

In a cross-sectional study of 25,862 subjects in Colorado (U.S.), SHyper (TSH <0.3 mIU/L) was found in 0.9% of 24,337 individuals and was present in 20.7% of the 1,525 individuals taking thyroid hormone preparations.[2] The prevalence of functional autonomy was 6.4 % in the Italian Pescopagano survey that defined SHyper as a TSH level <0.4 mU/L.[4] The prevalence of SHyper increased with age in this iodine-deficient population and reached a peak of 15.4% in subjects above the age of 75 years.

Graves' disease, an autoimmune cause of endogenous SHyper, is prevalent in young and middle-aged patients and in areas of high iodine intake. Conversely, thyroid autonomy due to toxic multinodular goiter (TMNG) and toxic nodule (TN) represents the most frequent cause of endogenous SHyper in elderly patients and in areas where iodine intake is low.[3] In patients with GD, endogenous SHyper is a transient disease that may resolve spontaneously without treatment or may progress to overt disease.[3]

TABLE 23.2

Causes of Persistent Overt and Subclinical Hyperthyroidism

Endogenous Causes

Graves' disease

Autonomously functioning thyroid adenoma

Toxic multinodular goiter

Exogenous Causes

Intentional TSH suppression in patients with
  differentiated thyroid cancer

TABLE 23.3
Causes of Low Serum TSH Other Than
Subclinical Hyperthyroidism

Non-thyroidal illness
Psychiatric illness
Administration of drugs (dopamine, glucocorticoids)
Pituitary or hypothalamic insufficiency

The natural history of TMNG is characterized by progressive development of thyroid autonomy over many years with persistent SHyper and potential progression to overt disease that is more frequent in patients with undetectable serum TSH levels than in patients with low serum TSH.[3] Since subclinical hyperthyroidism is only detected as a TSH abnormality, the exclusion of transient causes of TSH suppression and diseases should be performed before diagnosing persistent SHyper (Table 23.2). Transient TSH suppression usually occurs during subacute, silent, or postpartum thyroiditis.[1]

Diseases other than subclinical hyperthyroidism, specifically non-thyroidal illness and psychiatric illness, may be associated with low serum TSH levels (Table 23.3). Some drugs (e.g., high-dose steroids, dopamine or dobutamine, and amiodarone) may cause subclinical and overt hyperthyroidism. Pituitary dysfunction is characterized by persistently decreased serum TSH concentration but low or low–normal serum thyroid hormone levels are present.[1] An isolated reduction in serum TSH is frequent during the first trimester of pregnancy.[1] About 1 to 3% of elderly people (between 60 and 80 years or older) exhibit serum TSH <0.4 mIU/L and blunted TSH responses to TRH because of the reduced TSH secretion by the pituitary gland.[1] However, in elderly subjects FT_3 levels are decreased due to the reduced peripheral conversion of T_4 to T_3.

23.3 DIAGNOSIS

The diagnosis of SHyper should include (1) a clinical evaluation of symptoms and signs of thyroid hormone excess or signs of autoimmune thyroid disease such as ophthalmopathy; (2) a detailed medical and pharmacological history to exclude transient causes of low serum TSH; (3) a typical hormonal pattern of SHyper (FT_4 and FT_3 at the upper limit of the normal range and TSH decreased); (4) radioiodine uptake that can confirm the diagnosis of SHyper and guide the choice of definitive treatment; (5) evaluation of the cardiovascular effects of SHyper; and (6) evaluation of bone risk in elderly patients with SHyper.

23.3.1 CLINICAL EVALUATION: SYMPTOMS AND SIGNS

Table 23.4 lists signs and symptoms of SHyper. Some studies assessed the presence of symptoms and signs of hyperthyroidism in patients with SHyper. They reported that patients with SHyper, especially those with undetectable serum TSH, may have specific

TABLE 23.4

Symptoms and Signs of Subclinical Hyperthyroidism in Young and Middle-Aged Patients

Palpitations	Nervousness
Heat intolerance	Anxiety
Tremors	Reduced feeling of well-being
Impaired exercise tolerance	Impaired quality of life
Sweating	

but less severe symptoms and signs of overt hyperthyroidism with higher prevalence of palpitations, tremors, heat intolerance, reduced exercise tolerance, sweating, nervousness, anxiety and reduced feelings of wellbeing compared with normal subjects.[1]

Older subjects with endogenous SHyper frequently have few of the classic symptoms of hyperthyroidism and this may explain why they are misdiagnosed. The predominant symptoms and signs of hyperthyroidism in the elderly often reflect cardiac dysfunction such as heart failure, atrial fibrillation, or angina. Affective disorders (particularly depression in females and mania in males) were found more prevalent in elderly patients with SHyper and suppressed serum TSH.[2] The risk of dementia and Alzheimer's was increased in some studies of patients with SHyper.[1]

23.3.2 HISTORY

A careful physical examination, detailed medical history, and analysis of thyroid hormone patterns may be helpful in diagnosing this condition. Patient history should carefully cover previous treatments such as the administration of drugs (e.g., dopamine, glucocorticoids, amiodarone, contrast media, other iodine-containing medication, and iodine-containing foods), severe chronic illnesses, and pituitary or hypothalamic insufficiency. Thyroid hormone levels are usually low in non-thyroidal illness, although serum TSH is low and may be detected with a third-generation TSH assay.

23.3.3 LABORATORY DIAGNOSIS

Table 23.5 lists the three levels of laboratory diagnosis.

I level—Serum FT_4 and FT_3 concentrations are at the upper limits of their normal ranges and serum TSH concentration is persistently low–undetectable (<0.1 μU/mL) in SHyper. FT_4 levels can be 10 to 25% higher when measured in specimens drawn within 3 to 4 hours of the morning LT_4 dose in patients who receive TSH suppressive therapy.[6] FT_3 levels are usually at the upper limits of the normal range in patients with endogenous SHyper.[1,2]

II level—Thyroid autoantibody testing (e.g., thyroid peroxidase antibodies [TPO-Abs], TSH-receptor antibodies [TR-Abs], or thyroid-stimulating immunoglobulins [TSIs]) may be of use in patients with GD. However, antithyroid antibodies may be negative in about 10% of GD patients. Thyroid ^{99m}Tc scintigraphy can confirm the diagnosis of SHyper by mapping areas of the thyroid gland that accumulate the

TABLE 23.5
Diagnosis of Subclinical Hyperthyroidism

I Level	II Level	III Level[a]
TSH, FT$_4$, FT$_3$	TSHR-Ab	ECG
Doppler ultrasound	Thyroid radioiodine uptake and thyroid scan	Holder ECG
	Computed tomography	Doppler echocardiography
	Magnetic resonance	Bone mineral density
	Fine needle aspiration biopsy	

[a] In selected patients.

radioactive drug. Radioiodine 24-hour uptake should be considered before definitive therapy; if RAI uptake is low, other treatment modalities should be considered.

Doppler ultrasound of the thyroid gland permits assessment of the gland volume and the sizes and characteristics of the thyroid nodules. Computed tomography (CT) without contrast agents or magnetic resonance (MR) should be considered to assess the extension of a large goiter and evaluate suspected airway compression.

Fine needle aspiration biopsy (FNAB) should be performed to evaluate scintigraphically hypofunctioning nodules larger than 1 to 1.5 cm and nodules with suspicious sonographic features.

III level—Electrocardiography and/or Holter ECG should be performed in patients complaining about persistent symptoms and signs of adrenergic overactivity or suspicious symptoms of atrial arrhythmias and paroxysmal or persistent atrial fibrillation. Doppler echocardiography should be performed to assess cardiac morphology and function in high-risk thyroid cancer patients, who will receive long-term TSH suppressive therapy and in elderly patients with endogenous SHyper, especially those with underlying cardiac disease.

Bone mineral density (BMD) scanning should be performed in postmenopausal women, elderly men, and patients with risk factors for osteoporosis during long-term TSH suppressive therapy for high-risk thyroid cancer and after the diagnosis of long-term untreated endogenous SHyper.

23.4 IMPLICATIONS OF SHYPER

Patients with long-term SHyper may progress to overt hyperthyroidism. Long-term untreated SHyper may induce the development of adverse cardiovascular risk factors and exert negative effects on bone structure and metabolism. Increased cardiovascular mortality and increased risk of bone fracture have been reported in SHyper, particularly in elderly patients and those with comorbidities.

23.4.1 PROGRESSION OF SHYPER TO OVERT DISEASE

The risk of progression to overt hyperthyroidism is higher in patients with GD than in patients with TMNG. Patients with low serum TSH rarely progress to overt disease.

However, the risk of progression is 2 to 5% per year in patients with undetectable serum TSH.

23.4.2 CARDIOVASCULAR RISK

Some studies demonstrated increased prevalence of symptoms and signs of adrenergic overactivity in young and middle-aged patients with exogenous and endogenous SHyper.[1] Sinus tachycardia, atrial premature beats, and atrial fibrillation (AF) are frequent complications of overt and subclinical hyperthyroidism.[1,2] An increase in the average heart rate with reduced heart rate variability was found in some studies in young patients with SHyper and undetectable serum TSH. These effects can be explained by the electrophysiological action of the thyroid hormone that increases the systolic depolarization and diastolic repolarization rate and decreases the action potential duration and refractory period of the atrial myocardium and the atrial–ventricular nodal refractory period.

Long-term untreated SHyper may induce changes in cardiac morphology and function because of the increased cardiac workload. The clinical consequences of untreated SHyper in young-middle aged patients are characterized by increased left ventricular mass that may impair diastolic filling.[1,5,6] These effects represent a negative prognostic factor for cardiovascular mortality and morbidity in the general population.

Increased risk of AF (twofold to threefold increased risk compared to euthyroid age-matched subjects) was associated with the onset of SHyper in subjects 60 years or older with low and undetectable serum TSH levels in the Cardiovascular Health Study and in the Framingham Study over 10 to 13 years of follow-up[7,8] (Figure 23.1).

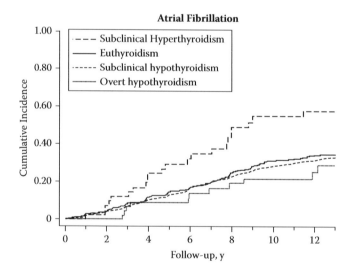

FIGURE 23.1 Subjects with TSH <0.1 had nearly twice the risk of developing atrial fibrillation. The hazard ratio for atrial fibrillation in the subgroup of patients with low serum TSH concentrations was 1.85 (95% confidence interval, 1.14 to 3.00). (*Source:* Sawin, C.T. et al. 1991. *Arch Intern Med* 151: 165–168. With permission.)

The hypercoagulable state induced by SHyper may represent an important factor for the increased risk of stroke in patients with AF, especially in the presence of cardiac disease. Conflicting results have been reported on the cardiovascular mortality of patients with exogenous and endogenous subclinical hyperthyroidism.[9] Elderly patients and those with comorbidities face increased likelihood of death (overall hazard ratio for mortality of 1.4, 95% confidence interval, 1.1 to 1.8 in a recent meta-analysis of eight studies) that may progressively increase 10 years after the diagnosis of SHyper.[10]

23.4.3 BONE RISK

A decrease in bone mineral density (BMD) was reported in postmenopausal women with endogenous SHyper, specifically in cortical bone-rich sites, whereas little evidence indicates effects on bone in premenopausal women.[1] The effects of exogenous SHyper on BMD are less clear and more debated. In a cohort study of 686 women aged 65 years or older followed for approximately 4 years, undetectable serum TSH was associated with a fourfold increase in vertebral fractures and a threefold increased risk of hip fracture.[11]

23.5 TREATMENT

23.5.1 EXOGENOUS SUBCLINICAL HYPERTHYROIDISM

The goal of LT_4 treatment in low-risk patients with differentiated thyroid cancer and no evidence of disease is to maintain the TSH level in the normal range because TSH suppression therapy does not affect the outcomes in these patients.[6] Clinicians must consider the clinical stage, patient age, and any underlying comorbidities before starting TSH suppressive therapy.

Long-term treatment with LT_4 suppressive therapy should be considered in patients with intermediate and high risks of differentiated thyroid cancer before the assessment of the complete remission of the disease.[6] In the elderly, the beneficial effects of TSH suppression on cancer growth should be balanced with the increased cardiovascular risk.[6] In young patients with exogenous subclinical hyperthyroidism, the administration of beta-blocking drugs may prevent or counteract the negative cardiac effects of long-term TSH suppression in symptomatic subjects during LT_4 therapy. The dosage of the beta blockade should be guided by heart rate control.[5,6]

23.5.2 ENDOGENOUS SUBCLINICAL HYPERTHYROIDISM

Persistent SHyper should be documented by repeatedly subnormal or undetectable serum TSH levels and normal free thyroid hormone levels. Today the treatment and management of SHyper in still debated, although clinicians are more prone to treat persistent SHyper in advanced age.[1,12,13] Young asymptomatic patients with low serum TSH should be followed without treatment due to the low risk of progression to overt hyperthyroidism and the absence of cardiac and bone risks.

Increased cardiovascular risk, increased risk of osteoporosis, and progression to overt disease are all linked to subclinical hyperthyroidism, particularly in elderly

TABLE 23.6
Advantages and Disadvantages of Therapeutic Options

Therapy	Advantages	Disadvantages
Medical (12 to 18 months)	Young- to middle-aged patients with low undetectable serum TSH	Recurrence in GD; persistent disease in TMNG and TN
Radioactive iodine	Long-term successful therapy; appropriate for elderly patients, SHyper with persistent undetectable serum TSH, underlying cardiac disease; contraindications to surgery	Hypothyroidism, low-severe active orbitopathy in GD
Surgical (near or total thyroidectomy)	Long-term successful therapy; appropriate in presence of airway compression	Hypothyroidism in 95 to 100%, surgical complications

patients with persistent undetectable serum TSH and in patients with cardiovascular or bone risk factors. Treatment of SHyper should be considered in these conditions (Table 23.6). In older patients with or without AF, ablative therapy with ^{131}I is the preferred option, mainly in patients with toxic multinodular goiters or solitary toxic nodules, since spontaneous remission is unlikely.

In patients with Graves' disease, treatment with antithyroid drugs or radioiodine (RAI) is appropriate. Elderly patients with TMNG or TN and those with cardiovascular disease are at an increased risk of complications after RAI due to the worsening of hyperthyroidism. These patients should be treated with antithyroid drugs before RAI therapy until euthyroidism is achieved. Antiresorptive therapy should be considered in postmenopausal women with endogenous SHyper, patients with osteoporosis, and subjects with risk factors for bone loss.

23.6 FOLLOW-UP

Table 23.7 lists follow-up measures. Serum TSH concentration should be regularly monitored in patients with endogenous SHyper to evaluate whether the disease is

TABLE 23.7
Follow-Up Measures

Measure	At Baseline Evaluation	3 months	6 months	After RAI	After Surgery
Clinical examination	+	+	+	+	+
TSH at baseline evaluation	+	+	+	+	+
FT$_3$, FT$_4$	+	+	+	+	+
TSHR-Ab	–	+	+	+	–
Thyroid scan and radioiodine uptake	+	–	–	–	–
Thyroid ultrasound	+	–	–	+	+

persistent or progressive. This is particularly true before pursuing definitive treatment with radioiodine or surgery. The patient's thyroid function (TSH, T_3, and T_4) should be monitored after 4 to 6 weeks and monitoring should be repeated at regular intervals until stable results are obtained after RAI or antithyroid drug treatment.[12] Because of the progressive risk of clinical or subclinical hypothyroidism, long-term clinical and laboratory follow-up are required at least once a year in patients with SHyper after RAI.[12] Levothyroxine in replacement doses should be started after total thyroidectomy.

REFERENCES

1. Biondi, B. and Cooper, D.S. 2008. The clinical significance of subclinical thyroid dysfunction. *Endocr Rev* 9: 76–131.
2. Canaris, G.J., Manowitz, N.R., Mayor, G. et al. 2000. The Colorado thyroid disease prevalence study. *Arch Intern Med* 160: 526–534.
3. Biondi, B. and Kahaly, G. 2010. Cardiovascular involvement in patients with different causes of hyperthyroidism. *Nat Rev Endocrinol* 6: 431–443.
4. Aghini-Lombardi, F., Antonangeli, L., Martino, E. et al. 1999. The spectrum of thyroid disorders in an iodine-deficient community: the Pescopagano survey. *J Clin Endocrinol Metab* 84: 561–566.
5. Biondi, B., Fazio, S., Carella, C. et al. 1994. Control of adrenergic overactivity by β-blockade improves quality of life in patients receiving long term suppressive therapy with levothyroxine. *J Clin Endocrinol Metab* 78: 1028–1033.
6. Biondi, B. and Cooper, D.S. 2010. Benefits of thyrotropin suppression versus the risks of adverse effects in differentiated thyroid cancer. *Thyroid* 20: 135–146.
7. Sawin, C.T., Geller, A., Kaplan, M.M. et al. 1991. Low serum thyrotropin (thyroid-stimulating hormone) in older persons without hyperthyroidism. *Arch Intern Med* 151: 165–168.
8. Cappola, A.R., Fried, L.P., Arnold, A.M. et al. 2006. Thyroid status, cardiovascular risk, and mortality in older adults. *JAMA* 295: 1033–1041.
9. Biondi, B. 2010. Cardiovascular mortality in subclinical hyperthyroidism: an ongoing dilemma. *Eur J Endocrinol* 162: 587–589.
10. Haentjens, P., Van Meerhaeghe, A., Poppe, K. et al. 2008. Subclinical thyroid dysfunction and mortality: an estimate of relative and absolute excess all-cause mortality based on time-to-event data from cohort studies. *Eur J Endocrinol* 159: 329–341.
11. Bauer, D.C., Ettinger, B., Nevitt, M.C. et al. 2001. Study of Osteoporotic Fractures Research Group: risk for fracture in women with low serum levels of thyroid-stimulating hormone. *Ann Intern Med* 134: 561–568.
12. Bahn, R.S., Burch, H.B., Cooper, D.S. et al. 2011. Thyrotoxicosis and hyperthyroidism: management guidelines of the American Thyroid Association and American Association of Clinical Endocrinologists. *Thyroid* 21: 593–646.
13. Wartofsky, L. 2011. Management of subclinical hyperthyroidism. *J Clin Endocrinol Metab* 96: 59–61.

24 Thyrotoxic Crisis

Giampaolo Papi and Alfredo Pontecorvi

CONTENTS

Key words: thyroid crisis, thyroid storm, hyperthyroidism, thyrotoxicosis.

24.1 THYROID CRISIS

24.1.1 DEFINITION

Thyroid crisis, also known as thyroid storm, represents the acute, extreme consequence of severe thyrotoxicosis.[1,2] It is characterized by very severe signs and symptoms of hyperthyroidism: high fever, tachycardia, dehydration, diarrhea, and mental confusion.

24.1.2 EPIDEMIOLOGY

The prevalence of thyroid crisis averages 0.1 to 2.0% of hospitalized thyrotoxic subjects. It occurs at any age and is more frequent in the female gender. Unlike hypothyroid coma, it occurs during any season of the year.

24.1.3 ETIOPATHOGENESIS

The most common cause is Basedow-Graves' disease, followed by toxic nodular goiter or in a thyrotoxic patient as a complication of a major stress such as surgery or trauma. As hypothyroid coma, thyroid crisis is frequently triggered by typical precipitating factors that occur when patients are already affected by overt

389

(occasionally, subclinical) hyperthyroidism.[1,2] The main triggering factors are surgery (particularly thyroidectomy); iodide compound intake or radioiodine (^{131}I or ^{123}I) therapy in patients with Graves' disease or autonomously functioning thyroid nodules; trauma (mainly in the neck area); systemic infections; delivery; and severe emotional stress.[3,4]

Fortunately, thyroid crisis is a rare event mostly affecting hyperthyroid patients who have not been adequately treated, have withdrawn thyrostatic therapy on their own initiative, or have undergone surgery.[1–4] Why serum FT_4 and FT_3 concentrations in thyroid crisis patients are as high as in hyperthyroid patients without thyroid crises is still a matter of debate.

Indeed, the clinical picture characteristic of thyroid crisis is not related to thyroid hormone levels.[5] Nonetheless, patients presenting with thyroid storm have larger numbers of ubiquitous catecholamine binding sites than hyperthyroid subjects who do not develop it. The most common etiopathogenetic hypothesis is that in the presence of both greater availability of adrenergic receptors and a reduction of thyroid hormone binding to thyroid hormone binding (TBG) globulin, a catecholamine leak provoked by an acute event (triggering factor) finally precipitates thyroid crisis.

Pregnancy and the postpartum period present high risks of thyroid storm occurrence.[6] Indeed, on the one hand, the altered coagulation state peculiar to pregnancy may be worsened by thyrotoxicosis (see Section 24.1.4 below); on the other hand, immune system modulation (called remodulation in the postnatal phase) may cause new-onset autoimmune hyperthyroidism or reawake a previous (preconception) hyperthyroidism.

Recent radioiodine treatment of severely hyperthyroid patients (subjects manifesting marked signs and symptoms of thyrotoxicosis, suppressed TSH, markedly elevated free T_4 and/or free T_3, and elevated radioactive iodine uptake) represents a risk factor for the development of thyroid crisis.[7] However, it has been demonstrated that it is safe to administer ^{131}I to patients who are severely hyperthyroid without fear of thyroid storm, provided beta-blockade drugs are used to control the signs and symptoms.[8]

Furthermore, external radiation therapy to treat neck neoplasm may cause thyroid follicle rupture and subsequent leakage of large amounts of preformed thyroid hormones into the systemic blood circulation, precipitating thyroid crisis. The same mechanism underlies severe thyrotoxicosis and thyrotoxic coma seldom provoked by acute or subacute thyroiditis.[9] In contrast, the etiopathogenesis of thyroid storm in patients with partial hydatidiform moles can be ascribed to thyroid hyperfunction showing high 24-hour RAIU following beta-HCG follicular cell stimulation.[10] Anecdotal cases of accidental or voluntary thyroid hormone ingestion unleashing thyroid crisis have been reported.

24.1.4 Diagnosis

The diagnosis of thyroid storm is based on (1) the history of thyroid disease and presence of triggering factors; (2) typical signs and symptoms; see Table 24.1; and (3) laboratory examinations.

TABLE 24.1

Symptoms and Signs Specific to Thyroid Crisis

Fever

Unreasonable anxiety, confusion, delirium up to coma state

Tachyarrhythmia (particularly atrial fibrillation)

Tachypnea and dyspnea

Congestive heart failure up to cardiac shock

Lerman-Means scratch (pleuro-pericardiac sound)

Increased systolic versus diastolic blood pressure ratio

Hyperhydrosis and skin hyperemia

Generalized tremors

Diarrhea

Nausea and vomiting

24.1.4.1 Clinical Diagnosis

Thyroid crisis presents as multiorgan failure in most cases.[1,4–6] The organs mainly affected by thyroid hormone excess are the heart (tachyarrhythmia ranging from sinus tachycardia to atrial fibrillation is invariably present), nervous system, gastrointestinal tract, and liver.[1,4–6] Fever is also frequent. A positive history for recent trauma in the neck area should always be explored in patients without histories of thyroid disease.[2] Occasionally, the clinical picture of apathetic thyrotoxicosis occurs.

24.1.4.2 Laboratory Diagnosis

Serum FT_4 and FT_3 concentrations exceeding the normal reference ranges and undetectable (<0.1 mIU/L) TSH levels are present. Besides altered thyroid function, slight elevation of serum bilirubin (seldom associated with jaundice) and transaminase and low total cholesterol values are frequently detected. Nonetheless, an altered coagulation state, in particular, antithrombin deficiency and increased levels of factor VIII, has been observed in patients with thyroid storm, sometimes inducing disseminated intravascular coagulation.

24.1.5 TREATMENT

Figure 24.1 depicts treatment of thyroid crisis. Treatment relies on a number of drugs.

24.1.5.1 First Line Therapy

Thyrostatics—Methimazole (15 to 20 mg every 6 hours) or propylthiouracil (up to 1000 mg daily) is administered. Propylthiouracil should be preferred because it reduces the T_4 to T_3 peripheral deiodination.

Beta-blockers—Propranolol (1 to 2 mg intravenously or 40 to 80 mg per os every 8 hours) is the drug of choice because, on the one hand, it contrasts the increased binding of catecholamine to beta-adrenergic receptors; on the other hand, it reduces the T_4 to T_3 peripheral deiodination.

Specific Therapy
A. Methimazole 60-80 mg/d *or*   Propylthiouracyle up to 1 g/d
B. Propranolol 120-240 mg/d   Lugol solution *or*   Potassium iodide solution *or*   Sodium iodide
D. Hydrocortisone 300-400 mg/d
E. Lithium carbonate 900-1200 mg/d

Support Therapy
A. Repolarizing electrolyte solutions
B. Paracetamol
C. Phenobarbital
D. Cardiac support therapy in case of   congestive heart failure

FIGURE 24.1   Specific and support therapy in patients with thyroid crisis.

Large iodine amounts—Lugol's solution (10 drops three times daily) or saturated potassium iodide solution (5 drops three times daily) per os or intravenous sodium iodide (500 to 1,000 mg daily) inhibits thyroid hormone leakage by the gland.

Glucocorticoids—Intravenous hydrocortisone (100 mg every 6 to 8 hours) reduces the T_4 to T_3 peripheral deiodination.

24.1.5.2   Second Line Therapy

Lithium carbonate (300 mg every 6 to 8 hours) inhibits thyroid hormone leakage by the thyroid gland. Extracorporeal plasmapheresis is an additional tool for removing circulating thyroxine in patients who do not respond quickly to conventional standard therapy.

Additional support therapy should include liquids (particularly repolarizing electrolyte solutions), antipyretics (e.g., paracetamol), and phenobarbital (plays a sedative role and reduces serum FT_4 and FT_3 concentrations by increasing thyroid hormone metabolism). If congestive heart failure is present, cardiac support therapy is also mandatory. Furthermore, heparin therapy is indicated in individuals with atrial fibrillation; however, changes in patients with thyroid storm may lead to heparin resistance and pro-coagulation state. Moreover, high body temperatures must be reduced by cooled mattresses and cold poultices.

24.1.6   Follow-Up

Immediately after the acute phase, it is necessary to measure serum TSH, FT_4, FT_3, and antithyrotropin receptor (TSHR-Ab), antithyroglobulin (Tg-Ab), and antithyroperoxidase (TPO-Ab) autoantibodies to identify the thyroid disease responsible for the crisis so that it may be treated adequately and prevent thyroid crisis recurrence.

24.1.7   Prognosis

Thyroid crisis is unfavorable in almost 80% of cases unless it is treated quickly and adequately.[4] Indeed, contrary to what happens to patients with hypothyroid coma, adequate therapy reduces thyroid crisis mortality to less than 10%.[5] Table 24.2 lists dosages of all drugs cited in this chapter.

TABLE 24.2
Drugs Cited in This Chapter

Drug	Dosage	Notes
Antithyroid Drugs		
Methimazole	5 to 80 mg/day	
Propylthiouracil	50 to 1,000 mg/day	Not available in some countries
Beta Blockers		
Propranolol	10 to 80 mg tid or qid	
Atenolol	25 to 100 mg/once or tid	
Metoprolol	25 to 50 mg qid	
Nadolol	40 to 160 mg/day	
Esmolol	IV pump 50 to 100 mg/kg/min	In intensive care unit
Other Drugs		
Supersaturated potassium iodide	1 to 2 drops (50 mg iodide/drop) tid	
Potassium iodide (Lugol's solution)	5 to 7 drops (8 mg iodide/drop) tid	
Iopanoic acid and sodium ipodate	0.5 to 1 g/day	Not available in most countries
Lithium	450 to 900 mg/day	
Perchlorate	50 to 1,500 mg/day	

REFERENCES

1. Nayak, B. and Burman, K. 2006. Thyrotoxicosis and thyroid storm. *Endocrinol Metab Clin North Am* 35: 663–686.
2. McKeown, N.J., Tews, M.C., Gossain, V.V. et al. 2005. Hyperthyroidism. *Emerg Med Clin North Am* 23: 669–685.
3. Dillmann, W.H. 1997. Thyroid crisis. *Curr Ther Endocrinol Metab* 6: 81–85.
4. Burch, H.B. and Wartofsky, L. 1993. Life-threatening thyrotoxicosis: thyroid storm. *Endocrinol Metab Clin North Am* 22: 263–277.
5. Trasciatti, S., Prete, C., Palummeri, E. et al. 2004. Thyroid storm as precipitating factor in onset of coma in an elderly woman: case report and literature review. *Aging Clin Exp Res* 16: 490–494.
6. Molitch, M.E. 1992. Endocrine emergencies in pregnancy. *Baillieres Clin Endocrinol Metab* 6: 167–191.
7. Kadmon, P.M., Noto, R.B., Boney, C.M. et al. 2001. Thyroid storm in a child following radioactive iodine (RAI) therapy: a consequence of RAI versus withdrawal of antithyroid medication. *J Clin Endocrinol Metab* 86: 1865–1867.
8. Vijayakumar, V., Nusynowwitz, M.L., and Ali, S. 2006. Is it safe to treat hyperthyroid patients with I-131 without fear of thyroid storm? *Ann Nucl Med* 20: 383–385.
9. Sherman, S.I. and Ladenson, P.W. 2007. Subacute thyroiditis causing thyroid storm. *Thyroid* 17: 283.
10. Chiniwala, N.U., Woolf, P.D., Bruno, C.P. et al. 2008. Thyroid storm caused by a partial hydatidiform mole. *Thyroid* 18: 479–481.

25 The Thyroidologist in the Intensive Care Unit (ICU)

Antonio Bianchi and Alfredo Pontecorvi

CONTENTS

Key words: critical illness, sick euthyroid syndrome (SES), non-thyroidal illness syndrome (NTIS), low T_3 syndrome.

25.1 INTRODUCTION

Critical illness is defined as any life-threatening condition requiring the support of failing vital organ functions and is often associated with alterations in thyroid hormone concentrations in patients with no previous histories of thyroid diseases. For these reasons, the thyroidologist should be familiar with the thyroid axis changes in intensive care unit (ICU) patients. This chapter reviews the effects of critical illness on the function of the hypothalamus–pituitary–thyroid axis and on thyroid hormone metabolism, focusing on the so-called sick euthyroid syndrome (SES).

25.2 DEFINITION

A thyroidologist in an ICU frequently observes sick euthyroid syndrome (SES) or low T_3 syndrome, defined more recently as non-thyroidal illness syndrome (NTIS). It is a condition characterized by low total and free serum levels of triiodothyronine

TABLE 25.1

Alterations of Thyroid Axis in Critical Illness, Central and Primary Hypothyroidism

Disease	Free T_3	Free T_4	Reverse T_3	TSH
Mild critical illness	↓	N	↑	N
Moderate illness	↓↓	N, ↑↓	↑↑	N, ↓
Severe or chronic illness	↓↓↓	↓	↑, N	↓↓
Recovery from illness	↓	↓	↑	↑
Central hypothyroidism	↓	↓	N, ↓	↓, N
Primary hypothyroidism	↓↓	↓	↓	↑

(T_3) and high levels of reverse T_3 (rT_3) with normal or low levels of thyroxine (T_4) and normal or low levels of thyroid-stimulating hormone (TSH).

NTIS includes a wide variety of abnormalities, but the changes in thyroid function constitute a continuum, with the abnormalities becoming progressively more severe in parallel with the patient's clinical condition (Table 25.1). We can divide this condition into three main NTI syndromes: (1) low T_3 syndrome in which T_3 falls acutely (in hours), with normal or high T_4 and normal TSH levels; (2) low T_3 and T_4 syndrome in which, after a more severe and prolonged illness, both T_3 and T_4 fall; low T_3, T_4, and (3) TSH syndrome in which a reduction of TSH levels to subnormal or undetectable levels is suggestive of the most severe form of NTIS.[1–3]

25.3 EPIDEMIOLOGY

Laboratory tests of thyroid function may be abnormal in 11 to 70% of hospitalized patients and in up to 90% of critically ill patients. With increasing illness severity, both free T_3 and free T_4 levels are depressed and this pattern occurs in 30 to 50% of ICU patients.[1–7]

25.4 ETIOPATHOGENESIS AND PHYSIOPATHOLOGY

In ICU, the thyroid hormone concentrations are affected by a variety of non-thyroidal stresses that include infectious diseases and sepsis, malignancy, myocardial infarction and heart failure, major surgery, severe malnutrition, burns, trauma, gastrointestinal bleeding, and acute central nervous system disease. As a physiological response to any acute event, serum levels of T_3 decrease (normally within 2 hours), rT_3 increases, whereas T_4 and TSH can briefly rise and subsequently return to normal range.

The magnitude of T_3 drop within 24 hours after an insult has been found to reflect the severity of illness and inversely correlate with mortality. The low T_3 levels persist beyond TSH normalization and, in very severe illness, T_4 levels may also decrease. The etiology of the NTIS is clearly multifactorial and the pathogenetic mechanisms involve both peripheral and central factors, and the common medications used in ICU (Figure 25.1).

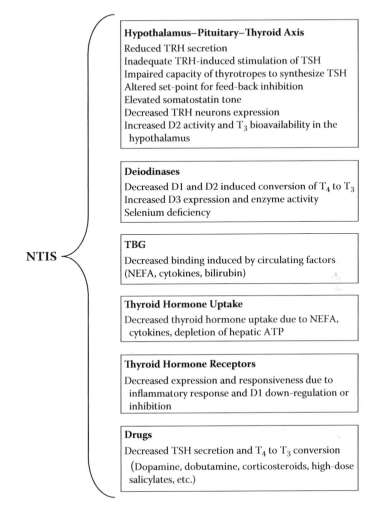

NTIS

Hypothalamus–Pituitary–Thyroid Axis
Reduced TRH secretion
Inadequate TRH-induced stimulation of TSH
Impaired capacity of thyrotropes to synthesize TSH
Altered set-point for feed-back inhibition
Elevated somatostatin tone
Decreased TRH neurons expression
Increased D2 activity and T_3 bioavailability in the
  hypothalamus

Deiodinases
Decreased D1 and D2 induced conversion of T_4 to T_3
Increased D3 expression and enzyme activity
Selenium deficiency

TBG
Decreased binding induced by circulating factors
(NEFA, cytokines, bilirubin)

Thyroid Hormone Uptake
Decreased thyroid hormone uptake due to NEFA,
  cytokines, depletion of hepatic ATP

Thyroid Hormone Receptors
Decreased expression and responsiveness due to
  inflammatory response and D1 down-regulation or
  inhibition

Drugs
Decreased TSH secretion and T_4 to T_3 conversion
(Dopamine, dobutamine, corticosteroids, high-dose
salicylates, etc.)

FIGURE 25.1   Etiology of NTIS is multifactorial and the pathogenetic mechanisms involve peripheral and central factors. Hypothalamus–pituitary–thyroid axis abnormalities play a role in the pathogenesis of NTIS.

25.4.1   PERIPHERAL FACTORS IN NTIS

The thyroid produces T_4 in larger quantities than the biologically active T_3. Although released from the thyroid in a T_4:T_3 ratio of about 17:1, the circulating levels of each hormone are also determined by extrathyroidal conversion of T_4 to T_3, which in healthy humans accounts for more than 80% of T_3 production. At an early stage of critical illness, low T_3 levels are mainly caused by decreased peripheral conversion of T_4 to T_3.

The peripheral metabolism of thyroid hormone involves three deiodinases: D1, D2, and D3. These enzymes constitute a family of membrane selenoproteins that selectively remove iodide from T_4 and its derivatives, activating or inactivating these hormones. D1 and D2 have enzymatic outer-ring deiodination (ORD) activity (5′ deiodination), which is considered an activating pathway forming T_3, whereas D3 catalyzes inner-ring deiodination (IRD), which is an inactivating pathway (5 deiodination). D1 is expressed in the thyroid, liver, and kidneys, and is the main source of circulating T_3. D2 is expressed in the brain, anterior pituitary, thyroid, and skeletal muscles, and is important for local T_3 production. Skeletal D2 also contributes to circulating T_3. D3 is present in the brain, skin, placenta and pregnant uterus, and in various fetal tissues. It is the main inactivating enzyme; it catalyzes the conversion of T_4 in rT_3 and of T_3 in T_2 (3,3′-diiodothyronine) and thereby is able to protect tissues from excess thyroid hormone.

For many years, the main accepted factors contributing to the low serum T_3 and high serum rT_3 levels observed in acute critical illness were the down-regulation of hepatic and renal D1 activity, the loss of muscle D2 activity and the induction of D3 in muscles and liver. The trigger of these changes in deiodinase expression and activity has been attributed to an increase in serum glucocorticoids and proinflammatory cytokines (IL-1, IL-6, TNF-α) that often occurs in NTIS. Recent evidences confirm in effect that, in critical illness, D3 expression occurs in skeletal muscle and liver— tissues that usually do not express the deiodinase in adults, and that expression of D3 was found to be positively correlated with rT_3 in serum and negatively correlated with serum T_3.

On the other hand, the validity of these conclusions has now been challenged and some have argued that modifications of deiodinase expression in NTIS may be a consequence of the changes that occur in T_3 and T_4, rather than the causes of these hormonal changes, at least in acute illness. This hypothesis is supported by studies on both D3 knockout mice and D1/D2 knockout mice subjected to treatment with lipopolysaccharide (LPS). In these mice, the changes in T_3 and T_4 that occurred in response to LPS were essentially no different from the changes seen in wild-type animals.

Furthermore, recent studies show that levels of D2 deiodinase gene expression and activity are increased in the prolonged but not in acute phase of critical illness. Other potential mediators of NTIS at tissue level have been described. It has been suggested that the expression of the selenoenzymes D1, D2 and D3 may be limited by low selenium supplies in critically ill patients, and that this represents a mechanism for the pathogenesis of the low T3 seem in the NTIS. However, there is little evidence to support this view.

It seems more likely that the low selenium status seen in acute and chronically ill patients results from diminished concentrations of selenoproteins in plasma as a consequence of the acute phase response. Further mechanisms include low concentrations of thyroid hormone binding proteins and inhibition of hormone binding, transport, and metabolism. Thyroid hormones are bound reversibly to thyroxine-binding globulin (TBG), transthyretin (previously known as thyroxine-binding pre-albumin), and albumin. TBG transports most of thyroid hormone in blood. Transthyretin and TBG are acute phase proteins and their concentrations can fall markedly in a wide range of illnesses.

This acute fall of plasma binding proteins may thus lead to the changes in plasma total T3 and T4 and this observation supports the hypothesis that total thyroid hormone concentration during acute NTIS is mainly due to changes in the serum binding capacity of thyroid hormones as a result of the acute phase response. On the other hand, free hormones changes are of a more modest nature than changes of total thyroid hormone. In acute critical illness, free T4 may appear low, normal, or raised even in the same sample, depending on assay method. Free T3 changes are more blunted than total T3. However, in critically ill patients, the serum binding capacity for thyroid hormone is significantly decreased because many substances (NEFA, bilirubin, cytokines), accumulate in patients with hepatic and renal failure and may compete with thyroid hormone-binding proteins.

Finally, two other mechanism are involved in pathogenesis of NTIS: the cellular uptake of thyroid hormones and the thyroid hormone receptors (THRs). The cellular uptake of thyroid hormones is not simply the result of passive diffusion across the lipid bilayer, but involves ATP-dependent transport processes. Current evidence thus suggests that down-regulation of thyroid hormone transporters does not occur in NTIS, and other mechanisms must be responsible for the impaired uptake of thyroid hormone in critical illness.

Such mechanisms may include depletion of hepatic ATP. The presence in plasma of substances such as NEFA and cytokines that impair hepatic uptake of thyroid hormone and accumulate in the plasma of patients with renal or liver dysfunction inhibit cellular transport of T4. Thyroid hormone action is largely dependent on binding to THRs, which are ligand-regulated transcription factors that bind to thyroid hormone response elements (TREs) in target genes. THRs reside in both the nucleus and cytoplasm. Some authors observed that THRs may participate in the pathogenesis of NTIS by decreasing the responsiveness to thyroid hormones, via down-regulation of hormone expression caused by inflammatory response.[1-3,6-7]

25.4.2   Central Factors in NTIS

Prolonged illness is characterized by different changes within the thyroid axis. Pulsatile TSH secretion is reduced and serum levels of T_3 and T_4 are low. These findings are in line with a predominantly central origin: reduced TRH secretion, inadequate TRH-induced stimulation of TSH, impaired capacity of thyrotropes to synthesize TSH, an altered setpoint for feedback inhibition, and elevated somatostatin tone. The pathogenesis of these alteration is still not understood. Specific groups of TRH neurons situated in the paraventricular nucleus (PVN) of the hypothalamus are required to promote TSH synthesis in the pituitary and regulate thyroid hormone synthesis.

In humans, a loss of TRH gene expression in PVN samples taken postmortem from patients with prolonged illnesses who died with serum biochemistry typical of NTIS was observed. Finally, another hypothesis is that intracerebral increased D2 expression and activity observed in NTIS may promote the conversion of T_4 to T_3 in the mediobasal hypothalamus and directly inhibit hypophysiotropic TRH neurons in the PVN, whereas T_3 circulating in the portal capillary system may suppress TSH secretion. This finding may explain the inappropriately low or normal TSH and impaired TSH pulsatility characteristically observed in NTIS.[1-3,6.7]

TABLE 25.2
Drugs Causing Abnormal Thyroid Function Tests in ICU

Drug	Physiopathological Mechanism
Glucocorticoids	Low serum TBG
Salicylates, furosemide, heparin	Decreased T_4 binding to TBG
Phenytoin, carbamazepine, rifampin, phenobarbital	Increased T_4 clearance
Amiodarone, glucocorticoids, iodinated contrast agents, propylthiouracil, beta blockers	Impaired conversion of T_4 to T_3
Dopamine, dobutamine, glucocorticoids, octreotide	Suppression of TSH secretion

25.4.3 DRUGS

Several pharmacologic agents frequently administered to critically ill patients may alter TSH and thyroid hormone levels independently of systemic illness, further complicating the clinical picture. Corticosteroids, dopamine, and dobutamine suppress TSH release and conversion of T_4 to T_3, whereas the use of pharmacologic agents, such as estrogen, oral contraceptives, high-dose salicylates, phenytoin, furosemide, fenclofenac, and carbamazepine alters thyroid hormone binding to TBG and may also result in deranged thyroid hormone concentrations.

Amiodarone can cause hypothyroidism or hyperthyroidism. Initially, it usually causes a decrease in T_3 via inhibition of 5′ deiodinase, with a transient reciprocal increase in TSH. When amiodarone induces thyrotoxicosis, the condition can be subclinical, manifested by low TSH in the setting of normal levels of thyroid hormones or as overt thyrotoxicosis with low TSH and elevated levels of thyroid hormones. In diabetic patients taking metformin, a modest decrease of TSH has been reported. Chronic alcoholic patients may have nocturnal TSH surges suppressed and a blunted TSH response to TRH.[1–3,6,7] Table 25.2 summarizes the medications used in ICU and their mechanisms of action.

25.5 DIAGNOSIS

Clinical signs of hypothyroidism are not easily interpreted in critically ill patients and it is difficult to judge whether hypothyroidism is present on clinical grounds. Many of these patients are febrile, have clouded mental status, extensive edema, sepsis, severe cardiac or pulmonary diseases, and in general display features that may easily mask evidence of hypothyroidism. Even their laboratory tests may be suspect. Starvation and critical illness can induce alterations in cholesterol, liver enzymes, TBG, and basal metabolic rate.

Typically, a subject affected by NTIS is a severely ill patient in whom clinical findings of hypothyroidism are either absent or masked by other disorders, with low total T_4 and free T_4, low or normal TSH, and low total and free T_3 (Table 25.1). Measurements of reverse T_3 were considered useful in differentiating NTIS (high rT_3) from secondary hypothyroidism (low TSH) that should be associated with low rT_3. Subsequent studies, however, showed that rT_3 does not accurately distinguish the two states (Table 25.1). Serum cortisol should be measured. Transient, apparently central, hypoadrenalism is an unusual but recognized phenomenon in severe illness. Cortisol should be above 20 μg/dL, and commonly is above 30. If below 20, ACTH should be drawn and the patient should be given supportive cortisol therapy.

When thyroid function is examined in ICU, we recommend obtaining at least a complete thyroid panel including free T_3, free T_4, TSH, and antithyroid antibodies. Obviously, if possible, it should be better also to assay total T_3 and T_4. During critical illness, the presence of low T_3 or T_4 levels with a normal or low TSH is strongly suggestive of NTIS. If T_4 is below 4 μg/dL in this setting, the diagnosis of NTIS associated with a potentially fatal outcome, may be assumed. However, true hypothyroidism can produce similar results.

TSH levels may be high, normal, or low in the setting of NTIS. If TSH is at least 20 mU/L, primary hypothyroidism is likely. If TSH is normal or only mildly elevated (<20 mU/L), low free T_4 levels, a thyroid goiter, or antithyroid antibodies suggest primary hypothyroidism. Finally, if TSH levels are low, anterior pituitary hormone status should be further assessed and hypothyroidism secondary to hypothalamic or pituitary lesion should be excluded. Low (or low–normal) cortisol levels and abnormalities in prolactin secretion suggest pituitary dysfunction. It should be remembered that transient hypogonadotropic hypogonadism is common in critically ill patients. Therefore, assessment of the gonadal axis is usually not helpful in this setting, but FSH and LH measurements in postmenopausal women as signs of pituitary function are very useful. Finally, it is important to remember that secondary hypothyroidism is extremely rare without a prior history of pituitary or hypothalamic dysfunction. If necessary hypothalamus–pituitary anatomy can be evaluated by MR imaging.

As a general rule, establishing a diagnosis of the NTIS based on a single day's thyroid function tests (TFTs) is not advisable. Most often, repeat TFT interpretation after 3 to 5 days in the setting of an evolving clinical course in ICU is required to firmly establish the diagnosis.[1–3,6,7]

25.6 THERAPY

Many authors have considered the altered serum thyroid hormone levels in NTIS as a transient adaptive response of an organism to minimize metabolic demands during a stressful event. However, whether NTIS represents a protective and appropriate adaptation to an acute insult or a maladaptive response to illness that needs correction remains a matter of controversy. Goals of thyroid hormone therapy in NTIS are to reduce morbidity and mortality and avoid muscle weakness or wasting and adverse cardiovascular effects induced by subclinical hypothyroidism.

To date, another controversial issue is whether direct administration of T_3 or T_4 to raise T_3 levels has clinical benefits. Multiple studies have investigated the effect of thyroid hormone replacement therapy in NTIS during certain clinical situations such as caloric restriction, cardiac disease, acute renal failure, brain-dead potential organ donors, and burn patients. Treating patients with NTIS seems not to be harmful, but no strong evidence indicates replacement therapy is beneficial and much of the literature on the treatment of NTIS encourages further randomized controlled trials on large numbers of patients.

An extremely prudent approach is needed if treatment is given. In our opinion, according to DeGroot[3] and on the basis of our experience, the target groups in whom thyroid hormone administration should be considered are patients with NTIS, usually moderate and severe or chronic illness, patients with very low T_4 levels (under 4 µg/dL), and patients with clear hypothyroidism based on known disease, treatment with dopamine, or elevated TSH. If therapy is to be given, it cannot be thyroxine alone, since this fails to promptly elevate T_3 levels. Experimental administration of hypothalamic releasing factors in patients with NTIS appears to be safe and effective in improving metabolism and restoring the anterior pituitary pulsatile secretion in the chronic phase of critical illness. However, this promising strategy needs to be explored further.

Therefore, treatment should include oral or intravenous T_3 at a replacement level of approximately 40 to 50 µg/day, given in divided doses every 8 or 12 hours. It may be appropriate to give slightly higher doses such as 60 to 75 µg/day for 3 to 4 days to increase the body pool more rapidly, followed by replacement doses as described. After these 3 to 4 days, it is appropriate to start replacement with T_4. Serum levels of T_4 and T_3 should be followed at frequent intervals (every 48 hours) and dosages adjusted to achieve a serum T_3 level at least low normal prior to the next scheduled dose. If treatment is successful, T_3 administration can gradually be reduced and thyroxine administration can be increased to replacement levels as deiodination increases. Because of the marked diminution in T_4 to T_3 deiodination and shunting of T_4 toward rT_3, replacement with T_4 may initially only lead to elevation of rT_3 and have very little effect on T_3 levels or physiologic action. In this situation, continued administration of T_3 is preferred.[1,3,8]

25.7   PROGNOSIS

In patients with severe systemic illnesses, low serum T_3 and T_4 levels have significant prognostic value and are associated with increased mortality and morbidity. Extensive literature about NTIS in ICUs and critically ill patients show that the degree of reduction in serum T_3 is predictive of poor prognosis in patients with acute myocardial infarction, congestive heart failure, sepsis, respiratory failure with mechanical ventilation, acute stroke, and a variety of intensive care settings. Evidence suggests that low T_3 is an independent predictor of survival, as are elevated rT_3 and decreased T_3/rT_3. Some authors observed that the probability of death is 50% when serum T_4 is less than 4 µg/dL and increases to 80% when serum T_4 is less than 2 µg/dL.[3,7,9]

25.8   FOLLOW-UP

In the ICU, if hormonal replacement treatment started in the presence of prolonged or severe critical illness, thyroid function tests (TFTs) should be performed every 48 to 72 hours. After recovery, only patients suspected of previous thyroid dysfunction and suspicion of pituitary dysfunction following traumatic brain injury (TBI) and subarachnoid hemorrhage (SAH) after exclusion of hypothalamus–pituitary

TABLE 25.3

ICU Diagnostic Tests for NTIS

I level (if thyroid disease is suspected)	fT_3, fT_4, TSH (T_3, T_4), ACTH, plasma cortisol, antithyroid antibodies
II level (if pituitary dysfunction is suspected)	FSH,[a] LH,[a] estrogen,[a] IGF-I, ACTH, plasma cortisol, hypothalamus–pituitary MRI
Screening	fT_3, fT_4, TSH (T_3, T_4)

[a] Only in postmenopausal women.

disease must be followed periodically by clinical examination and at least every 6 months for 2 years should undergo complete thyroid or pituitary function tests.[10]

25.9 SCREENING

In assessing thyroid function screening in ICU, in our opinion, important general principles must be considered. First, thyroid function tests should not be assessed in seriously ill patients unless (1) thyroid dysfunction or (2) pituitary dysfunction, such as in the case of traumatic brain injury (TBI) and subarachnoid hemorrhage (SAH) that are conditions at high risk for the development of hypopituitarism[10] (Table 25.3).

When hypothyroidism of an ICU patient is suspected clinically and evaluation suggests central hypothyroidism, the probability of NTIS is much higher than pituitary or hypothalamic disease. When thyroid dysfunction is suspected in critically ill patients, measurement of serum TSH alone or with free T_4 is inadequate to evaluate thyroid function. It is mandatory to obtain a complete panel of thyroid function test including free T_3, free T_4, and TSH (Table 25.3).

REFERENCES

1. Adler, S.M. and Wartofsky, L. 2007. The non-thyroidal illness syndrome. *Endocrinol Metab Clin North Am* 36: 657–672.
2. Marino, P. 2007. Adrenal and thyroid dysfunction. In *ICU*, 3rd ed. Philadelphia: Lippincott Williams & Wilkins, 872–882.
3. DeGroot, L.J. 2010. Non-thyroidal illness syndrome: a form of hypothyroidism. In *Endocrinology, Adult and Pediatric*, 5th ed., Jameson, J.L. and DeGroot, L.J., Eds. Philadelphia: Elsevier, Saunders, 1628–1634.
4. Iglesias, P., Muñoz, A., Prado, F. et al. 2009. Alterations in thyroid function tests in aged hospitalized patients: prevalence, aetiology and clinical outcome. *Clin Endocrinol (Oxf)* 70: 961–967.
5. Tognini, S., Marchini, F., Dardano, A. et al. 2010. Non-thyroidal illness syndrome and short-term survival in a hospitalised older population. *Age Ageing* 39: 46–50.
6. Economidou, F., Douka, E., Tzanela, M. et al. 2011.Thyroid function during critical illness. *Hormones (Ath)* 10: 117–124.
7. Pappa, T.A., Vagenakis, A.G., Alevizaki, M. 2011. The non-thyroidal illness syndrome in the non-critically ill patient. *Eur J Clin Invest* 41: 212–220.

8. Bello, G., Paliani, G., Annetta, M.G. et al. 2009. Treating non-thyroidal illness syndrome in the critically ill patient: still a matter of controversy. *Curr Drug Targets* 10: 778–787.

9. Bello, G., Pennisi, M.A., Montini, L. et al. 2009. Non-thyroidal illness syndrome and prolonged mechanical ventilation in patients admitted to the ICU. *Chest* 135: 1448–1454.

10. Schneider, H.J., Kreitschmann-Andermahr, I., Ghigo, E. et al. 2007. Hypothalamopituitary dysfunction following traumatic brain injury and aneurysmal subarachnoid hemorrhage: a systematic review. *JAMA* 298: 1429–1438.

26 Thyroid Orbitopathy

Luigi Bartalena and Maria Laura Tanda

CONTENTS

Key words: thyroid orbitopathy, Graves' orbitopathy, Graves' ophthalmopathy, thyroid–eye disease, thyroid-associated ophthalmopathy, glucocorticoids, TSH receptor, orbital radiotherapy, rituximab, smoking.

26.1 DEFINITION

Thyroid orbitopathy (also known as Graves' orbitopathy, Graves' ophthalmopathy, thyroid–eye disease, and thyroid-associated ophthalmopathy) defines the ocular signs and symptoms associated with thyroid disease, most commonly Graves' disease.[1] *Orbitopathy* seems to be a preferable term because the condition is primarily an orbital rather than ocular disease.

26.2 EPIDEMIOLOGY

Thyroid orbitopathy is a rare disease. As illustrated in Table 26.1, age-adjusted annual incidence in the general population is around 16 women/100,000 and 3 men/100,000.[2] Although women are more frequently affected, the disease tends to be more severe and occur at more advanced ages in men.[2]

Ethnic factors may play a role, as a lower prevalence of orbitopathy has been reported in Asians compared to Caucasians.[2] Thyroid orbitopathy may develop at any age, but a bimodal peak occurs in the fifth and seventh decades. The disease is less frequent than it was in the past. This may be due both to earlier diagnosis and treatment of hyperthyroidism and orbitopathy and a decrease in smoking habits. Cigarette smoking is, in fact, an important risk factor for the occurrence of thyroid orbitopathy and its progression to more severe forms.[3]

Most patients with thyroid orbitopathy have concomitant Graves' hyperthyroidism. Thyroid orbitopathy may, however, rarely develop in patients with no previous or current history of hyperthyroidism (euthyroid Graves' disease) or even in patients with hypothyroid chronic autoimmune (Hashimoto's) thyroiditis.[4] (Table 26.1). About half of Graves' patients apparently have no orbital disease although orbital imaging often demonstrates subclinical involvement of orbital structures. Among the remaining Graves' patients, thyroid orbitopathy is moderate to severe in 20 to 30% and sight-threatening in 3 to 5%[5] (Table 26.1).

Graves' hyperthyroidism and orbitopathy develop in 85% of cases concomitantly or within 18 months of each other.[5] Less frequently, the orbitopathy may occur long before or after hyperthyroidism (Table 26.1). The natural history of thyroid orbitopathy is incompletely understood. However, orbital involvement seems to progress over time to more severe forms in about 15% of cases, remains unchanged in 65%, or spontaneously improves in 20%[4] (Table 26.1).

TABLE 26.1
Epidemiology of Thyroid Orbitopathy

Incidence	16/100,000/year (women); 3/100,000/year (men)
Prevalence in patients with Graves' disease	Around 50% (moderate to severe in 20 to 30%, sight-threatening in 3 to 5%)
Age of onset	Peaks in fifth and seventh decades
Gender effect	More frequent in women; men tend toward more severe forms and at more advanced ages
Ethnic factors	Less frequent in Asians than in Caucasians
Thyroid status	Most commonly associated with hyperthyroidism; infrequent in euthyroid or hypothyroid patients
Eye involvement	More frequently bilateral; may be asymmetrical or unilateral
Natural history	Progression in 15%; remission in 20%; no change in 65%

26.3 PATHOGENESIS

Substantial evidence supports the autoimmune origin of thyroid orbitopathy. To the best of current knowledge, the close link between thyroid disease and orbital disease may be explained by the occurrence of autoimmune reactions directed against one or more antigens shared by the thyroid gland and orbital tissue.[6,7]

According to this hypothesis, autoreactive T lymphocytes directed against the thyrotropin receptor and possibly the insulin-like growth factor-1 receptor or other thyroid antigens may reach the orbit. After antigen presentation by macrophages and B lymphocytes, a cascade of events triggered includes stimulation of orbital fibroblast proliferation and function, differentiation of preadipocyte fibroblasts into adipocytes, secretion of a number of cytokines automaintaining the ongoing reactions, infiltration of extraocular muscles, and increased production of hydrophilic glycosaminoglycans.[6,7]

Thyroid orbitopathy results from a complex interplay of yet poorly defined genetic factors and environmental (exogenous) factors including cigarette smoking, thyroid dysfunction, high serum TSH receptor antibody levels, and radioiodine treatment for Graves' hyperthyroidism.[1] In addition to cigarette smoking (see above), both hyperthyroidism and hypothyroidism influence the course of thyroid orbitopathy, making restoration of euthyroidism a high priority in Graves' patients with orbitopathy (Table 26.2).

TABLE 26.2
Risk Factors for Occurrence and Progression of Thyroid Orbitopathy

Factor	Evidence	Action
Cigarette smoking	More frequent in smokers than in non-smokers	Quit smoking
	Severe forms more frequent in smokers	
	Response to treatment lower and delayed in smokers	
	Decreased occurrence of exophthalmos and diplopia in former smokers than in current smokers	
Thyroid dysfunction	Improvement of orbitopathy with correction of hyperthyroidism	Restore euthyroidism promptly and maintain it stably
	More severe forms in patients with uncontrolled hyperthyroidism	
	Possible onset during uncontrolled hypothyroidism	
Radioiodine treatment for hyperthyroidism	Progression of preexisting orbitopathy	Cautious use of radioiodine
	Possible de novo occurrence, mostly in smokers	Steroid prophylaxis in patients with active orbitopathy
TSH receptor antibodies	Independent risk factor for severe forms of orbitopathy	Restore euthyroidism promptly and maintain it stably
		Thyroid ablation?

High serum TSH receptor antibody levels constitute an independent risk factor for the occurrence of severe forms of thyroid orbitopathy[8] (Table 26.2). Radioiodine treatment causes progression or de novo occurrence of orbitopathy in about 20% of patients, particularly smokers.[9] This untoward effect, however, may be almost universally prevented by low-dose oral prednisone given concomitantly with radioiodine[10] (Table 26.2).

26.4 PATHOPHYSIOLOGY

The expansion of the orbital fibroadipose tissue and edema due to the attraction of glycosaminoglycan to water are responsible for the common manifestations of thyroid orbitopathy. Because of the rigid bony structure of the orbit, the globe is displaced forward (exophthalmos or proptosis).

Exophthalmos may be responsible for the incomplete closure of eyelids at night (lagophthalmos). Periorbital soft tissues and conjunctiva are swollen because of orbital inflammation and venous and lymphatic congestion. The infiltration of the extraocular muscles (and secondary muscle damage) induce extraocular muscle dysfunction heralded by the most disturbing symptom: diplopia. Strabismus results from muscle fatty degeneration and fibrosis. The increased orbital tissue volume may cause optic nerve compression, particularly posteriorly at the orbital apex. This is in turn responsible for different degrees of optic nerve dysfunction and loss of vision.

26.5 CLINICAL FEATURES

Although thyroid orbitopathy is more commonly bilateral, asymmetrical and even unilateral forms are not infrequent (Table 26.1). This may pose diagnostic problems, particularly in patients who have no overt thyroid dysfunction or thyroid-directed autoimmunity.[1] In these cases, other causes of exophthalmos or ocular involvement (Table 26.3) must be carefully investigated and ruled out.

26.5.1 SIGNS

In typical Graves' patients with little or no orbital involvement, the only ocular sign may be upper eyelid retraction and stare (Figure 26.1) present in most patients at the onset of hyperthyroidism. This is due to sympathetic overactivity, but may also reflect the participation of eyelid muscles in the inflammatory process, as occurs with extraocular muscles (Table 26.4). Upper lid retraction due to overstimulation of the Muller's muscle commonly improves with restoration of euthyroidism.

Lower lid retraction is observed in patients with exophthalmos. Soft tissue changes frequently occur in thyroid orbitopathy. These include upper palpebral or periorbital swelling, with eyelid erythema in the active phases (see below) of the disease (Figure 26.2). In some cases, soft tissue changes may be extremely severe and persist for a long time. Conjunctiva may also be inflamed and erythematous (Figure 26.2). Conjunctival edema (chemosis) may be relevant and lead to conjunctival prolapse across the lower eyelid (Figure 26.2). Caruncle edema is another expression of conjunctival involvement and a marker of active inflammation.

TABLE 26.3

Main Causes of Enlarged Extraocular Muscles and/or Exophthalmos (Other Than Thyroid Orbitopathy)

Cushing's syndrome

Obesity

Orbital pseudotumor

Idiopathic myositis

Orbital cellulitis

Orbital lymphoma

Orbital meningioma

Leukemia

Rhabdomyosarcoma

Metastases (breast cancer, melanoma, lung cancer, pancreatic cancer, seminoma, carcinoid)

Vascular causes (arteriovenous malformations, carotid cavernous fistula, angioma)

Systemic manifestations of amyloidosis, sarcoidosis, vasculitis

Wegener's granulomatosis

Eosinophilic granuloma

Cysts

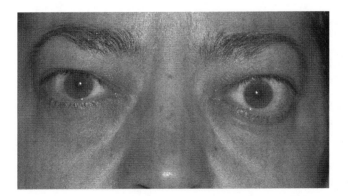

FIGURE 26.1 Patient with mild thyroid orbitopathy. Note mild upper and lower lid retraction in left eye and mild exophthalmos in left eye.

Exophthalmos is the forward eyeball displacement (Figure 26.3). This causes globe exposure with incomplete eye closure at night (lagophthalmos; Figure 26.4) and may be responsible for secondary corneal damage ranging from punctate keratopathy to corneal ulcer and perforation. Severe cases of exophthalmos may rarely be responsible for globe subluxation ("popping out") that may cause optic nerve stretching and damage. Extraocular muscle involvement may cause muscle dysfunction and limitation of ocular movements that in turn are responsible for diplopia (double vision).

TABLE 26.4
Signs of Thyroid Orbitopathy

Sign	Cause
Upper eyelid retraction	Overstimulation or inflammation of eyelid muscle
Exophthalmos	Increased orbital volume (extraocular muscles and/or adipose tissue)
Lower lid retraction	Exophthalmos
Periorbital swelling, eyelid erythema	Soft tissue and conjunctival inflammation and congestion
Conjunctival hyperemia and chemosis (conjunctival edema)	Conjunctival inflammation and congestion
Abnormal ocular motility, strabismus	Extraocular muscle inflammation/fibrosis
Corneal abnormalities	Eyeball exposure (due to exophthalmos and/or lid retraction; poor Bell's phenomenon)
Optic nerve involvement	Compression or stretching of optic nerve

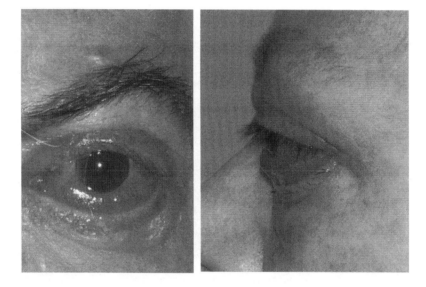

FIGURE 26.2 Two patients with severe inflammatory changes. Note mild periorbital edema, eyelid erythema, conjunctival hyperemia, marked chemosis, edema of caruncle.

Although all extraocular muscles may be affected, the inferior rectus muscle and the medial rectus muscle are most commonly involved. Thus, elevation and abduction are the eye movements most frequently impaired (Figure 26.5). Strabismus can be present, particularly when fibrotic changes occur in the muscles. The most serious manifestation of thyroid orbitopathy is dysthyroid optic neuropathy that may in rare cases lead to permanent blindness. This may be caused by compression of the optic nerve, particularly at the orbital apex, by the increased orbital content (fibroadipose tissue, swollen extraocular muscles), or by stretching of the nerve when

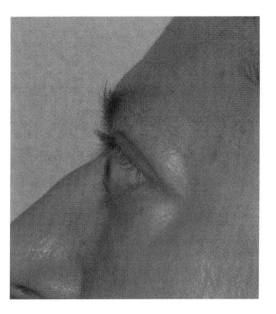

FIGURE 26.3 Marked exophthalmos and upper and lower lid retraction. Absence of relevant inflammatory soft tissue changes.

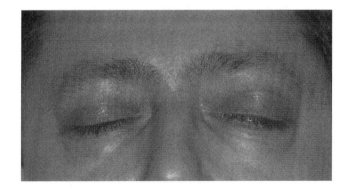

FIGURE 26.4 Lagophthalmos (incomplete eyelid closure).

exophthalmos is particularly severe. A useful mnemonic tool for the evaluation of the different signs of thyroid orbitopathy is represented by the NOSPECS classification of eye changes (Table 26.5).

26.5.2 SYMPTOMS

Symptoms of thyroid orbitopathy are widely variable. Eyeball and corneal exposure due to exophthalmos and/or lid retraction are often associated with inflammatory symptoms such as lacrimation, photophobia, grittiness, or sandy sensation (Table 26.6). Patients may complain of these symptoms particularly when awakening

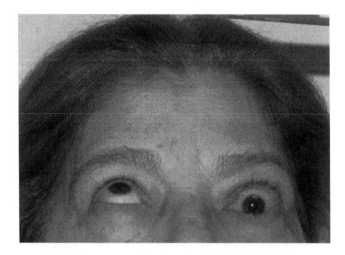

FIGURE 26.5   Marked limitation in upward gaze in the left eye.

TABLE 26.5
Abridged NOSPECS Classification of Thyroid Orbitopathy

Class	Definition	Degree of Involvement
0	No signs or symptoms	—
1	Only signs	—
2	Soft tissue involvement	0: absent a: minimal b: moderate c: marked
3	Proptosis (exophthalmos)	0: absent a: minimal b: moderate c: marked
4	Extraocular muscle involvement	0: absent a: minimal b: moderate c: marked
5	Corneal involvement	0: absent a: minimal b: moderate c: marked
6	Sight loss (due to optic nerve compression)	0: absent a: minimal b: moderate c: marked

TABLE 26.6

Symptoms of Thyroid Orbitopathy

Symptom	Cause
Lacrimation	Eyeball and corneal exposure
Photophobia	Eyeball and corneal exposure
Grittiness (sandy sensation)	Eyeball and corneal exposure
Diplopia	Extraocular muscle dysfunction
Pain in or behind eye	Inflammation of orbital and periorbital tissues or muscle inflammation (pain with eye movements)
Blurring	Dysthyroid optic neuropathy that does not clear with blinking
Sight loss	Dysthyroid optic neuropathy or corneal opacity
Abnormal color vision	Dysthyroid optic neuropathy

TABLE 26.7

Forms of Subjective Diplopia (Double Vision)

Form	Definition
Absent	No double vision
Intermittent	Present only when patient is fatigued or awakens
Inconstant	Present only at extremes of gaze
Constant	Present also in primary and/or reading positions (may be correctable with prisms)

in the morning if they have lagophthalmos responsible for corneal drying during the night.

If the limitation of extraocular muscle function is asymmetrical, diplopia develops (Table 26.7). It may be intermittent if present only when a patient awakens in the morning or is tired in the evening, inconstant, if present only at extremes of gaze, or constant if present also in primary gaze and/or in reading position (Table 26.6). Pain in or behind the eyes may be present, either spontaneous or evoked by eye movements. Dysthyroid optic neuropathy may cause different degrees of visual field defects and visual loss up to blindness. Subtle optic nerve involvement should be suspected if a patient cites blurring that does not clear with blinking or a decrease in color vision (Table 26.6). Patients often mention exacerbation of symptoms and signs in recent weeks or months. This an important feature underscoring that the disease is in a progressive phase (see Section 26.6.2).

26.5.3 QUALITY OF LIFE

Fully blown thyroid orbitopathy is an invalidating and disfiguring disease. Marked inflammatory signs and symptoms and exophthalmos, diplopia, blurred vision, and evident decrease in visual acuity are all manifestations that profoundly affect the quality of life.[11] A striking feature of the disease is that the quality of life during

TABLE 26.8
Signs and Symptoms Requiring Referrals to Specialists

Urgent Referral

Unexplained decrease in visual acuity
Change in intensity or quality of color vision
Eyeball subluxation
Corneal opacity
Poor Bell's phenomenon
Disk swelling

Non-urgent Referral

Photophopia, grittiness, or lacrimation that does not improve with
  lubricant use in recent weeks
Pain in or behind eyes, worsening in recent weeks
Change in eye appearance over recent weeks
Appearance or worsening of diplopia (double vision)
Tilting of head to avoid diplopia

Source: Bartalena, L. et al. 2008. *European Journal of Endocrinology*
158: 273–285. With permission.

daily activities, social activities, and working activities is often profoundly impaired also in patients who have milder forms of the disease, both in terms of ocular appearance and visual functioning.[11]

26.5.4 REFERRALS TO SPECIALIZED CENTERS

If a patient is not first seen in a specialized center, it is important to establish whether he or she should be referred to a specialized center and whether the referral is urgent or non-urgent. While Graves' patients with no symptoms or signs of thyroid orbitopathy should not be referred to specialists, all other Graves' patients should be referred when feasible to specialists or preferably to specialized thyroid–eye clinics.[3] Referral is urgent in cases of unexplained worsening of visual acuity, deterioration in the intensity or quality of color vision, or in rare instances of globe subluxation because these manifestations may be expressions or causes dysthyroid optic neuropathy (Table 26.8).

Referral is non-urgent for all other conditions, but should be considered if a patient shows evidence of progression of symptoms and/or signs in recent weeks or months or symptoms cannot be controlled with local measures (see Section 26.7).

26.6 DIAGNOSIS AND ASSESSMENT

Diagnosis of thyroid orbitopathy is simple when a patient has a clear-cut diagnosis of Graves' disease and ocular involvement is bilateral and symmetrical. Diagnosis is more difficult in patients with euthyroid Graves' disease or asymmetrical or unilateral ocular involvement. In these cases, orbital imaging by CT scan or MRI is

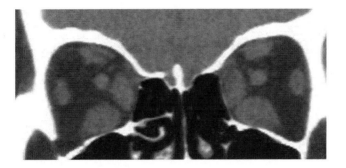

FIGURE 26.6 Coronal section of orbital CT scan. Note swollen inferior recti and medial recti muscles. The optic nerve is not compressed by enlarged muscles.

necessary to exclude other causes of exophthalmos or other signs mimicking thyroid orbitopathy (Table 26.3). Typical imaging findings include an increase in orbital fat volume and swollen extraocular muscles. The increased extraocular muscles typically show sparing of tendon insertions. All muscles may be affected, but inferior and medial recti are more frequently involved. Some patients show predominant increases of fat tissue and others display more pronounced extraocular muscle involvement (Figure 26.6).

26.6.1 ASSESSMENT

Evaluation of soft tissue changes should take advantage of the use of a downloadable color atlas from the website of the European Group on Graves' Orbitopathy (EUGOGO, www.eugogo.eu). The atlas allows a more precise and less subjective grading of eyelid and conjunctival abnormalities.

Eyelid aperture (width of the mid-pupil vertical fissure) is measured with a ruler. The patient should be in a relaxed state with distant fixation (Table 26.9). Exophthalmos is measured by a Hertel exophthalmometer. It is important to record the intercanthal aperture to allow comparison of measurements in different situations and assess the natural course of the disease or the effects of treatment. Normal exophthalmometer readings show racial, age, and gender variations. In general, values below 20 mm are normal, but specialized centers should have their reference values based on the normal population.

To evaluate extraocular muscle dysfunction, in addition to subjective methods (Table 26.7), objective methods, such as the Lancaster red–green test, prism cover test, orthoptic evaluation of monocular ductions, and determination of the field of binocular single vision field are fundamental to assess motility (Table 26.9). Corneal involvement, secondary to corneal exposure, can be assessed by fluorescein staining and slit lamp examination. Lagophthalmos and the absence of Bell's phenomenon (upward eyeball rotation on attempted eye closure) represent risk factors for the occurrence of corneal ulcers.

Evaluation of the optic nerve requires determination of best-corrected visual acuity, color sensitivity, pupillary responses, perimetry, and fundoscopy (Table 26.9).

TABLE 26.9
Assessment of Thyroid Orbitopathy

Feature	Assessment Method
Soft tissue changes (Class 2 NOSPECS)	Evaluate soft tissue changes comparing them with pictures in disease color atlas (www.eugogo.eu)[a]
Eyelid width	Measure eyelid aperture (distance between eyelid margins) with ruler; patient should sit relaxed and look in primary position with distant fixation[a]
Exophthalmos (Class 3 NOSPECS)	Measure eyeball protrusion with Hertel exophthalmometer, using same intercanthal aperture for serial measurements[a]
Extraocular muscle dysfunction (Class 4 NOSPECS)	First line assessment: subjective diplopia score (see Table 26.7)[a]
	Second line assessment: objective evaluation of motility (monocular ductions, determination of binocular single vision field)
Intraocular ocular pressure	Tonometry
Corneal involvement (Class 5 NOSPECS)	Evaluate corneal status (fluorescein test, slit lamp)
Sight loss due to optic neuropathy (Class 6 NOSPECS)	First line assessment: assess best-corrected visual acuity, color vision, fundus oculi (fundoscopy), presence or absence of relative afferent pupillary defects
	Second line assessment (suspicion of dysthyroid optic neuropathy): visual field, visual evoked potential, orbital imaging
Orbital inflammatory status (activity)	Calculate CAS (see Table 26.10)[a]
Quality of life	Use disease-specificity quality of life questionnaire (www.eugogo.eu)[a]

[a] Assessment can be performed in office by a general practitioner or endocrinologist without assistance from an ophthalmologist.

Visual evoked potentials may be useful in doubtful or subclinical forms. Measurement of intraocular pressure should also be performed, because this is often increased in upward gaze because of frequent inferior rectus muscle involvement and tightness. Evaluation of the quality of life is important, because this may help plan a therapeutic strategy. Quality of life in patients with thyroid orbitopathy can be assessed by validated disease-specific questionnaires downloadable from the EUGOGO website.

Two main features of thyroid orbitotopathy must be considered when assessing patient: activity and severity of the disease. Thyroid orbitopathy progresses through different phases; the first (active phase) is characterized by active inflammation due to ongoing autoimmune reactions in the orbital space followed by occurrence of the clinical manifestations of disease. Then inflammation tends to stabilize (static phase) and slowly remit (remission phase) to reach a status of complete inactivation (burnt-out disease). Sometimes an orbitopathy may reactivate. The time required to reach the inactive phase is not precisely known, but it is believed to be 1 to 2 years.

When the orbital inflammatory process flares, clinical manifestations of the disease that reflect its severity also tend to progress, then stabilize, and eventually subside. Complete remission of clinical manifestations is almost impossible in patients who develop moderate to severe forms of the orbitopathy.

26.6.2 ACTIVITY

Assessment of the activity of thyroid orbitopathy is difficult and controversial. Several tools such as MRI, ultrasound of the orbit, measurement of urinary glycosaminoglycans, and octreoscan have been proposed. None of them has sufficient sensitivity and specificity or cost:benefit effectiveness for use in clinical practice.

One useful tool to assess activity of thyroid orbitopathy in daily practice is the Clinical Activity Score (CAS). CAS, in its revised definition, consists of seven item: (1) eyelid edema, (2) eyelid erythema, (3) conjunctival injection, (4) chemosis, (5) caruncle edema, (6) spontaneous ocular pain, and (7) pain with eye movements (Table 26.10). One point is given to each item present; accordingly, CAS scoring ranges from 0 (no activity) to 7 (maximal activity). Thyroid orbitopathy is considered active if CAS is equal to or greater than 3 of the 7 points.[3] CAS is imperfect because it is based on a binary (absent versus present) evaluation; accordingly, it does not allow a precise grading of the severity of the different inflammatory manifestations, However, it can be easily calculated in the office and help predict the response to subsequent immunosuppressive treatment.

TABLE 26.10
Clinical Activity (CAS) Scoring

Sign of Symptom	Score
Eyelid edema	Absent: 0
	Present: 1
Eyelid erythema	Absent: 0
	Present: 1
Conjunctival hyperemia	Absent: 0
	Present: 1
Conjunctival edema (chemosis)	Absent: 0
	Present: 1
Caruncle edema	Absent: 0
	Present: 1
Spontaneous ocular pain	Absent: 0
	Present: 1
Pain with eye movements	Absent: 0
	Present: 1
Sum of individual scores = CAS score	0: No activity
	1 or 2: Inactive
	3 to 7: Active

TABLE 26.11

Classification of Thyroid Orbitopathy Based on Severity

Grade of Severity	Corneal Breakdown and/or Dysthyroid Optic Neuropathy	Other Objective and Subjective Features
Sight-threatening	Present	May be present or absent
Moderate to severe	Absent	One or more of following: lid retraction ≥2 mm, exophthalmos ≥3 mm, moderate to severe soft tissue changes, inconstant or constant diplopia, relevant impairment of quality of life
Mild	Absent	Less severe features: lid retraction <2 mm, exophthalmos <3 mm, mild soft tissue changes, no or intermittent diplopia[a]

[a] Impairment of quality of life may be relevant also in patients with mild orbitopathy due to changes in visual appearance or visual function.

26.6.3 SEVERITY

Severity of thyroid orbitopathy is also difficult to define. The disease can be mild, moderate to severe, or very severe (sight-threatening).[3] This classification stems from an overall evaluation of the different components of the disease (Table 26.11). While diagnosis of sight-threatening forms due to dysthyroid optic neuropathy and/or corneal breakdown, is relatively straightforward, the distinction between moderate to severe and mild forms is not always easy because it is not based exclusively on objective parameters (Table 26.11). In addition, what a physician judges mild may not be considered mild from the patient's view because of the influence of thyroid orbitopathy on the quality of life.

26.6.4 IMAGING

Imaging plays an important role for a refined evaluation of orbital status. It is most commonly carried out by CT or MR scan, both in longitudinal and coronal sections. Imaging may demonstrate swelling of extraocular muscles (with sparing of tendon insertion; Figure 26.6) and/or an increase in retrobulbar fibroadipose tissue. As previously noted, orbital imaging is mandatory when thyroid orbitopathy is unilateral or asymmetrical (Table 26.3). In cases of suspicious dysthyroid optic neuropathy, orbital imaging may evidence compression or stretching of the optic nerve. Compression is most commonly observed at the orbital apex (apical crowding).

26.7 THERAPY

Because the course of orbitopathy and its development are affected by exogenous factors, the first step in any patient with Graves' disease, independent of the absence or presence of the orbitopathy, its severity, and activity, is to control risk factors associated with its occurrence or progression (Table 26.2). Accordingly, patients should be urged to quit smoking. If necessary, smoking patients should be referred to specialized stop-smoking groups or organizations.[8]

Euthyroidism should be promptly restored and stably maintained although the optimal treatment of hyperthyroidism in patients with thyroid orbitopathy remains a dilemma (see below). If radioiodine is the selected treatment for hyperthyroidism, most patients should receive steroid prophylaxis using low-dose oral prednisone to avoid possible radioiodine-associated progression or de novo occurrence of the orbitopathy.[10] A reduction in TSH receptor antibody levels can usually be achieved by treatment with antithyroid drugs or thyroidectomy, while radioiodine treatment is usually associated with a transient (but not short-lived) increase in antibody levels.[12]

26.7.1 Mild Thyroid Orbitopathy

Most patients with mild thyroid orbitopathy require only local measures such as artificial tears (if lacrimation is excessive or eyes are dry), ointments (particularly at night if lagophthalmos is present), dark lenses (to avoid excessive exposure to light and control photophobia), and prisms (to control mild diplopia); see Table 26.11. A recent randomized, placebo-controlled study has shown that a 6-month course of sodium selenite (200 μg/day, equivalent to 92 μg of selenium) is effective in controlling mild ocular manifestations and preventing progression to more severe forms.[13]

In selected cases of mild *and* active orbitopathy, immunosuppressive treatment as for moderate to severe disease may be justified if the quality of life is severely impaired.[3] Rehabilitative surgery to correct exophthalmos or eyelid malposition may be proposed as needed or requested by a patient, only after the disease has been stably inactive for at least 6 months (Table 26.12).

26.7.2 Moderate to Severe Orbitopathy

In these patients, the treatment plan depends on the activity of the disease. In patients with active disease (CAS equal to or more than 3) glucocorticoids represent the first line treatment for their anti-inflammatory and immunosuppressive actions[3] (Table 26.11). Glucocorticoids can be administered via different routes. Local (retrobulbar or subconjunctival) injections are less effective than systemic glucocorticoids. Oral glucocorticoids are effective but intravenous glucocorticoids are usually more effective and better tolerated.[14] Oral glucocorticoid treatment requires high starting doses (80 to 100 mg of prednisone or equivalent steroids). The daily dose is then slowly tapered at 1- to 2-week intervals and the drug is withdrawn after 4 to 6 months.

Intravenous glucocorticoids are given as weekly slow (2- to 3-hour) infusions of methylprednisolone for 12 weeks. The best therapeutic regimen remains to be established, but the most common schedule employs a cumulative dose of 4.5 g (six weekly infusions of 500 mg followed by six weekly infusions of 250 mg).[14] In view of the potential adverse effects of intravenous glucocorticoids, particularly liver toxicity, the current recommendation is not to exceed a cumulative dose of 8 g per cycle of therapy.[3]

TABLE 26.12
Management of Thyroid Orbitopathy

Degree of Severity	First Line Treatment	Second Line Treatment
Mild	Local measures (artificial tears, ointments, dark lenses, prisms) as needed; selenium (6-month course of 200 µg sodium selenite)	Rehabilitative surgery (orbital decompression, eye muscle surgery, eyelid surgery) for residual cosmetic or functionally relevant changes when disease has been inactive at least 6 months
Moderate to severe	Glucocorticoids (intravenous > oral > locally injected) if disease is active; local measures as needed	Disease still active: second course of intravenous or oral glucocorticoids combined with orbital radiotherapy; alternatives: low-dose oral glucocorticoids combined with cyclosporine, or rituximab (experimental); rehabilitative surgery (orbital decompression, eye muscle surgery, eyelid surgery) as needed when disease has been inactive at least 6 months
Sight-threatening	Corneal breakdown: eyelid temporary closure plus intensive local care; dysthyroid optic neuropathy: high-dose intravenous methylprednisolone (1 g for 3 consecutive days, repeat next week)	Poor response to first line treatment in 2 weeks: prompt orbital decompression; good response to first line treatment: continue intravenous glucocorticoids; rehabilitative surgery (orbital decompression, eye muscle surgery, eyelid surgery) for residual cosmetic or functionally relevant changes when disease has been inactive at least 6 months

Orbital radiotherapy is a second line treatment and is effective, particularly in patients with motility disorders[3] (Table 26.11). It is, however, less effective than glucocorticoids and is presently not used often as a first line treatment. The combination of orbital radiotherapy (usually 10 to 20 Gy per eye in ten fractions over a 2-week period) with oral glucocorticoids is more effective than either treatment alone. Evidence that the combination with intravenous glucocorticoids provides an advantage over intravenous glucocorticoids alone is lacking.[3]

In the event of glucocorticoid failure, a second course of intravenous glucocorticoids combined with orbital radiotherapy is a possible option.[15] When glucocorticoids fail and the orbitopathy is still active, other possible second line treatments are (1) a combination of oral glucocorticoids and cyclosporine or (2) rituximab, a CD20-positive B cell depleting agent. The use of the latter drug has not yet been validated by randomized clinical trials.[16] Other treatments, proposed over time, such as somatostatin analogues, intravenous immunoglobulins, azathioprine, and cyclophosphamide are presently not recommended because evidence of their effectiveness is lacking.

In patients with inactive disease, medical treatment plays no role and is not effective. These patients may require multiple surgical operations, i.e., orbital (and/or fat) decompression to reduce exophthalmos, squint surgery to correct strabismus, and eyelid surgery to correct malposition or cosmetic abnormalities. If all three procedures are needed, they should be performed in the above order, because possible side effects of each step can affect the following step[3] (Table 26.12).

26.7.3 Sight-Threatening Thyroid Orbitopathy

This is an endocrine emergency because of dysthyroid optic neuropathy or corneal breakdown or both. Immediate treatment for corneal lesions is needed with lubricants and temporary corneal closure (moisture chambers, blepharorraphy, tarsorraphy, botulinum toxin injections). Dysthyroid optic neuropathy should be treated with high doses of intravenous methylprednisolone (e.g., 1 g for 3 consecutive days, to be repeated the next week).[3] See Table 26.11. If, however, the response is absent or poor within 2 weeks, the patient should be promptly submitted to orbital decompression to prevent irreversible damage of the optic nerve.

26.7.4 Treatment of Hyperthyroidism in Patients with Thyroid Orbitopathy

Management of Graves' hyperthyroidism in patients with thyroid orbitopathy represents an unsolved dilemma.[17] Antithyroid drugs have no direct effect on the course of an orbitopathy, but may have indirect beneficial effects related to control of hyperthyroidism.

The same conclusion can be reached concerning thyroidectomy. The use of radioiodine is more controversial, because, as already noted, radioiodine may cause in some patients (mainly smokers) the onset or exacerbation of thyroid orbitopathy,[18] This adverse effect can, however, be almost universally prevented by a short course of low-dose oral prednisone.[10] In patients with mild (active or inactive) orbitopathy, the choice of treatment for hyperthyroidism is independent of the eye disease and should be made on the basis of established criteria (age, goiter size, first episode versus recurrence of hyperthyroidism, and other factors; Table 26.13).

In patients with moderate to severe orbitopathy, eye disease must be treated promptly, because the effectiveness of treatment is inversely related to the duration of eye disease. Management of concomitant hyperthyroidism in these patients should be conservative (antithyroid drugs) for some experts or ablative (radioiodine, thyroidectomy, or a combination of the two treatments) for others. The rationale for ablative treatment is to remove most of the autoreactive T lymphocytes and antigens shared by the thyroid and the orbit, because the removal may be beneficial for the course of the orbitopathy. Supporters of antithyroid drug treatment give priority to the management of the orbitopathy and postpone the definitive treatment of hyperthyroidism (if necessary) until thyroid orbitopathy is inactive. For the time being, we have no evidence demonstrating the superiority of the conservative approach or the ablative approach.[17]

TABLE 26.13
Treatment for Concomitant Hyperthyroidism in Patients with Thyroid Orbitopathy

Degree of Thyroid Orbitopathy	Treatment for Orbitopathy	Treatment for Hyperthyroidism
Mild, active	Local measures	Antithyroid drugs (MMI, PTU)
		Radioiodine with steroid prophylaxis
		Thyroidectomy
Mild, inactive	Local measures	Antithyroid drugs (MMI, PTU)
		Possible rehabilitative surgery
		Radioiodine (no steroid prophylaxis if no risk factors for radioiodine-associated progression of orbitopathy)
Moderate to severe, active*	Glucocorticoids (preferably intravenous)	Antithyroid drugs (MMI, PTU)
		Radioiodine
		Thyroidectomy
Moderate to severe, inactive	Rehabilitative surgery, as needed	Antithyroid drugs (MMI, PTU)
		Radioiodine (no steroid prophylaxis if no risk factors for radioiodine-associated progression of orbitopathy)
		Thyroidectomy
Sight-threatening	High-dose intravenous glucocorticoids	Antithyroid drugs (MMI, PTU) (treatment of orbitopathy has priority)

[a] No sufficient evidence is available to establish the superiority of conservative treatment (antithyroid drugs) over ablative approach (thyroidectomy, radioiodine, combination of both) in final outcome of orbitopathy.

26.8 PROGNOSIS

Mild thyroid orbitopathy often improves spontaneously and may not need specific treatment. Most patients with moderate to severe orbitopathy, even if they respond well to medical (immunosuppressive) treatment, ultimately require some kind of rehabilitative surgery (orbital decompression, squint surgery, eyelid surgery) to correct residual invalidating manifestations. Sight-threatening orbitopathy has a good prognosis as to recovery of normal visual acuity if treated promptly with high doses of intravenous glucocorticoids and/or orbital decompression. After this initial aggressive approach, further treatment will depend on whether the disease is still active and will not differ from treatment of moderate to severe forms.

26.9 FOLLOW-UP

Patients whose thyroid orbitopathy has been treated medically and/or surgically should be followed periodically (every 6 months) for the first 1 to 2 years to assess the long-term outcome of treatment and the possible, although extremely rare, event of a flare-up of the disease. Long-term follow-up of Graves' patients with orbitopathy will then not differ from treatment of patients without orbitopathy and consists of annual controls.

REFERENCES

1. Bartalena, L. and Tanda, M.L. 2009. Clinical practice: Graves' ophthalmopathy. *New England Journal of Medicine* 360: 994–1001.
2. Daumerie, C. 2010. Epidemiology. In *Graves' Orbitopathy: A Multidisciplinary Approach.*, 2nd ed., Wiersinga, W.M. and Kahaly, G.J., Eds. Basel: Karger, 33–39.
3. Bartalena, L., Baldeschi, L., Dickinson A. et al. 2008. Consensus statement of the European Group on Graves' orbitopathy (EUGOGO) on management of GO. *European Journal of Endocrinology* 158: 273–285.
4. Pearce, S. and Kendall-Taylor, P. 2010. Natural history. In *Graves' Orbitopathy: A Multidisciplinary Approach*, 2nd ed., Wiersinga, W.M. and Kahaly, G.J., Eds. Basel: Karger, 77–87.
5. Bartalena, L., Pinchera, A., and Marcocci, C. 2000. Management of Graves' ophthalmopathy: reality and perspectives. *Endocrine Reviews* 21: 168–199.
6. Bahn, R.S. 2010. Mechanisms of disease: Graves' ophthalmopathy. *New England Journal of Medicine* 362: 726–738.
7. Smith, T.J. 2010. Pathogenesis of Graves' orbitopathy: a 2010 update. *Journal of Endocrinological Investigation* 33: 414–421.
8. Bartalena, L. 2010. Prevention. In *Graves' Orbitopathy. A Multidisciplinary Approach*, 2nd ed., Wiersinga, W.M. and Kahaly, G.J., Eds. Basel: Karger, 248–254.
9. Acharya, S.H., Avenell, A., Philip, S. et al. 2008. Radioiodine therapy (RAI) for Graves' disease (GD) and the effect on ophthalmopathy: a systematic review. *Clinical Endocrinology* 69: 943–950.
10. Lai, A., Sassi, L., Compri, E. et al. 2010. Lower dose prednisone prevents radioiodine-associated exacerbation of initially mild or absent Graves' orbitopathy: a retrospective cohort study. *Journal of Clinical Endocrinology & Metabolism* 95: 1333–1337.
11. Wiersinga, W.M. 2010. Quality of life. In *Graves' Orbitopathy. A Multidisciplinary Approach*, 2nd ed., Wiersinga, W.M. and Kahaly, G.J., Eds. Basel: Karger, 211–220.
12. Laurberg, P., Wallin, G., Tallstedt, L. et al. 2008. TSH-receptor autoimmunity in Graves' disease after therapy with anti-thyroid drugs, surgery, or radioiodine: a 5-year prospective randomized study. *European Journal of Endocrinology* 158: 69–75.
13. Marcocci, C., Kahaly, G.J., Krassas, G.E. et al. 2011. Selenium and the course of mild Graves' orbitopathy. *New England Journal of Medicine* 364: 1920–1931.
14. Zang, S., Ponto, K.A., and Kahaly, G.J. 2011. Intravenous glucocorticoids for Graves' orbitopathy: efficacy and morbidity. *Journal of Clinical Endocrinology & Metabolism* 96: 320–332.
15. Bartalena, L. 2010. What to do for moderate-to-severe and active Graves' orbitopathy if glucocorticoids fail. *Clinical Endocrinology* 73: 149–152.
16. Hegedus, L., Smith, T.J., Douglas, R.S. et al. 2011. Targeted biological therapies for Graves' disease and thyroid-associated ophthalmopathy. *Clinical Endocrinology* 74: 1–8.
17. Bartalena, L. 2011. The dilemma of how to manage Graves' hyperthyroidism in patients with associated orbitopathy. *Journal of Clinical Endocrinology & Metabolism* 96: 592–599.
18. Tanda, M.L., Lai, A., and Bartalena, L. 2008. Relation between Graves' orbitopathy and radioiodine therapy for Graves' hyperthyroidism: facts and unsolved questions. *Clinical Endocrinology* 69: 845–847.

27 Thyroid Diseases in Pregnancy

Francesco Vermiglio, Mariacarla Moleti, and Francesco Trimarchi

CONTENTS

Key words: thyroid and pregnancy, gestational transient thyrotoxicosis, hypothyroidism in pregnancy, hyperthyroidism in pregnancy.

27.1 INTRODUCTION

Thyroid disorders are generally more frequent in females than in males, in particular during the child-bearing period. Not surprisingly, therefore, these disorders are common clinical problems in pregnant women.

Management of thyroid disease in pregnancy involves specific problems, primarily but not exclusively related to the significant changes in maternal thyroid economy during pregnancy. These changes, for instance, make the non-pregnant population reference ranges of thyroid function parameters invalid for pregnant women. For this reason, the use of gestational and trimester-specific reference ranges is strongly recommended for interpreting thyroid results during pregnancy. In addition, the natural course of some thyroid diseases may be affected by pregnancy. In fact, some thyroid diseases may become evident or worsen during pregnancy, whereas other conditions such as Graves' disease usually improve during pregnancy and relapse in the postpartum period. Finally, pregnancy imposes some therapeutic limitations, mostly related to possible effects of drugs used on fetal thyroid function.

Because of these specific considerations, the management of pregnant women with thyroid disease requires special care, bearing in mind that both maternal thyroid disease per se and related treatments may adversely affect the newborn's health.

27.2 THYROID PHYSIOLOGY DURING PREGNANCY

Starting from the first weeks of pregnancy, some events combine to exert complex effects on maternal thyroid function.[1] During the first trimester, the thyroid gland is directly stimulated by chorionic gonadotropin (hCG) that acts as a thyrotropic agonist, thus inducing near the end of the first trimester a transient increase in free thyroid hormone levels. This event is mirrored by a transient decrease in serum TSH concentrations, with thyrotropin levels falling below the lower limit of the reference range in some cases (about 20% of pregnancies).

Under the effects of high concentrations of circulating estrogens, serum thyroxine binding globulin (TBG) levels significantly increase from the first trimester of pregnancy and remain high until term. The increase in TBG concentrations is responsible for an increase in total T_4 and T_3 concentrations, and is accompanied by a contextual decrease in free thyroid hormone levels (~10 to 15%). This decrease is partially offset by an increase in thyroid hormone output (about 50% over gestation) induced by TSH, the concentrations of which, following the first trimester, shows a slight but definite trend toward an increase in response to decreased serum free thyroid hormone levels.

The increased hormone production by the maternal thyroid gland is designed to reach a new equilibrium state (and ultimately guarantee maternal euthyroidism), and can be achieved provided that the gland is both anatomically and functionally intact and iodine intake is adequate to the increased demands of pregnancy. Table 27.1 summarizes the main changes in maternal thyroid function parameters observed over the course of gestation.

TABLE 27.1
Main Changes in Thyroid Function Parameters Observed during Gestation in Iodine-Replete Pregnant Women

Parameter	Observed Changes
TSH	Transient decrease at early pregnancy; slight increase from early second trimester until term
Total T_4, Total T_3	Progressive increase from early pregnancy to mid-gestation (~50%); plateau thereafter
Free T_4, Free T_3	Slight increase at very early pregnancy; then progressive decrease until term (~10 to 15%)

The following sections will discuss the most common thyroid disorders observed in pregnant women. The disorders are classified as follows:

Thyroid diseases associated with altered thyroid function
    Thyroid insufficiency during pregnancy
    Thyroid hyperfunction during pregnancy
Thyroid diseases not associated with altered thyroid function
    Non-toxic nodular thyroid disease (including thyroid cancer)

Other thyroid diseases not included in this list, such as acute and subacute thyroiditis, Riedel's thyroiditis, central hypothyroidism, generalized or selective resistance to thyroid hormones (rare during pregnancy or usually diagnosed before pregnancy), and postpartum thyroiditis are discussed in detail in other chapters of this book.

27.3 THYROID DISEASES ASSOCIATED WITH ALTERED THYROID FUNCTION

27.3.1 THYROID INSUFFICIENCY DURING PREGNANCY

27.3.1.1 Definition

A pregnant woman can be diagnosed as suffering from hypothyroidism when TSH values exceed the normal upper limit for pregnancy (>2.5 to 3.0 mIU/L) and FT_4 levels fall within (subclinical hypothyroidism [SCH]) or below (overt hypothyroidism [OH]) the normal range for the pregnant state.[2] According to the latest guidelines of the American Thyroid Association (ATA) for the diagnosis and management of thyroid disease during pregnancy, women with TSH levels of 10.0 mIU/L or greater, regardless of FT_4 levels, are also considered to have OH. SCH is defined as a serum TSH level between 2.5 and 10 mIU/L with normal FT_4 concentration.[3]

A state of thyroid hypofunction may predate the establishment of a pregnancy or can occur for the first time during pregnancy in women who were previously euthyroid.

The latter condition is referred to as *gestational hypothyroidism*, a term that emphasizes the close pathogenetic relationship between pregnancy-related events and the onset of maternal thyroid failure.

27.3.1.2 Epidemiology

Thyroid hormone insufficiency is by far the most common thyroid function disorder that can occur during pregnancy, although its prevalence varies considerably in different regions of the world. In iodine-replete regions, prevalence is estimated to be 0.3 to 05% for OH and 2 to 3% for SCH. A much higher prevalence is reported from studies in countries where iodine intake is inadequate or definitely insufficient.[2,4]

27.3.1.3 Etiopathogenesis

As noted above, hypothyroidism can occur before pregnancy or occur during pregnancy (gestational hypothyroidism). In the first case, the causes are the same as the causes of hypothyroidism in adults, discussed elsewhere in this book and listed in Table 27.2.

Iodine deficiency (ID) is the main cause of gestational hypothyroidism on a worldwide basis. However, in countries where iodine intake is adequate, chronic autoimmune thyroiditis is recognized as the most common cause of maternal thyroid insufficiency.[2]

The relationship between ID and maternal thyroid insufficiency during pregnancy has been known for a long time. Changes in maternal thyroid economy lead to an increase of 50 to 70% in daily iodine requirements. When the daily iodine intake is not sufficiently adequate to maintain the intrathyroidal iodine pool, the pool will gradually reduce and become depleted, leading to the inability of the maternal thyroid to meet the higher demands imposed by pregnancy and resulting in maternal hypothyroidism. The pathogenesis of ID-related maternal thyroid failure is more thoroughly discussed in Section 27.4.

Women with chronic autoimmune thyroiditis are at risk of gestational hypothyroidism because their thyroid function capacity is inadequate to meet the growing demand for hormone production imposed by pregnancy. Compared to gestational hypothyroidism due to ID, unless the latter is severe, hypothyroidism from autoimmune disease usually occurs earlier, because the integrity of the gland is already impaired before the establishment of pregnancy. Of course, women with autoimmune thyroid disease who are exposed to nutritional iodine deficiency have even higher risks of becoming hypothyroid than women with only one of these risk factors.[5]

Less commonly, gestational hypothyroidism can result from poor LT_4 replacement doses in women with hypothyroidism due to thyroidectomy or radioiodine ablation. The need for thyroxine increases very early during pregnancy. If replacement doses of LT_4 are not readily increased, these women, although euthyroid before pregnancy, may soon become overtly or subclinically hypothyroid.

Other causes, even more rare, include lymphocytic hypophysitis occurring during pregnancy[6] and hypothyroidism due to TSH receptor-blocking antibodies in women with autoimmune thyroid disorders.[3]

TABLE 27.2
Causes of Hypothyroidism

Primary Hypothyroidism

Congenital hypothyroidism (CH)	Thyroid dysgenesis or dyshormonogenesis
	Severe iodine deficiency
	Iodine excess (transient CH)
	Transplacental passage of TSH receptor-blocking antibodies (transient CH)
Acquired hypothyroidism	
Due to functional defects in thyroid hormone biosynthesis	Iodine deficiency
	Iodine excess
	Drugs (lithium, thionamides, perchlorate)
	Natural and chemical goitrogens
Due to reduced functional thyroid tissue	Chronic autoimmune thyroiditis
	Thyroid ablation (thyroidectomy, ^{131}I therapy, external irradiation)
	Degenerative or infectious disorders (Riedel's thyroiditis, de Quervain's thyroiditis, other rarer causes)
	Atrophic thyroiditis

Central Hypothyroidism

Pituitary causes (secondary hypothyroidism)	
Due to functional defects in TSH biosynthesis	Drugs
	Genetic defects in TSH biosynthesis (CH)
Due to reduced functional pituitary tissue	Developmental defects of pituitary (CH)
	Tumors
	Surgery
	Vascular, autoimmune, infiltrative, and infectious causes
Hypothalamic causes (tertiary hypothyroidism)	Hypothalamic disorders causing impaired TRH production or transport

Peripheral Hypothyroidism

Genetic defects that cause reduced sensitivity to thyroid hormone	Generalized resistance to thyroid hormone (Refetoff's syndrome)
	Thyroid hormone cell transport defect (Allan-Herndon-Dudley syndrome)
	Thyroid hormone metabolism alterations

27.3.1.4 Diagnosis

Medical history, signs, and symptoms—The clinical presentation can vary greatly, depending on length and severity of iodine deficiency and the degree of functional impairment associated with autoimmune thyroid disease. Usually, however, the signs and symptoms of hypothyroidism during pregnancy are very mild or absent, or remain unknown because they are erroneously attributed to the pregnancy state (weight gain, tiredness, drowsiness, constipation). Some elements in a medical history may, however, raise a diagnostic suspicion: among them, a family or personal history of thyroid or autoimmune diseases, a personal history of miscarriage, preterm delivery, infertility, and prior therapeutic head or neck radiation, are the most important risk factors for gestational hypothyroidism. As indicated in the recommendations by the Endocrine Society[2] and in the latest recommendations by American Thyroid Association,[3] the presence of even one of these factors should require testing of thyroid function parameters before pregnancy when possible or at the first prenatal visit.

Laboratory diagnosis—The diagnosis of thyroid insufficiency can be confirmed only by a thyroid function test. Measurement of TSH is the first level of investigation. In the presence of TSH levels above the reference range for gestational age, serum free T_4 measurement will distinguish overt hypothyroidism (high TSH and low free T_4 levels) or subclinical (high TSH and normal free T_4 levels). The subsequent detection of antithyroglobulin and antithyroid peroxidase antibodies (Tg-Abs and TPO-Abs, respectively) will provide information on the possible autoimmune origin of the disease.

For the purposes of laboratory diagnosis, it is important to emphasize that normal TSH and FT_4 values consulted should be those that apply to pregnant women and not those for the general population. In fact, pregnancy induces marked changes that invalidate the reference limits of the general population as a means to diagnose thyroid dysfunction during pregnancy. During the first trimester, the stimulatory effect of hCG on thyrocytes induces a transient increase in FT_4 levels mirrored by a lowering of TSH concentrations. Following this period, serum FT_4 concentrations decrease slightly (10 to 15% on average), and serum TSH values steadily return to normal. In line with these changes, the reference ranges of both FT_4 and TSH change during pregnancy, according to gestational age. In view of these changes, the use of "trimester-specific" reference ranges for free thyroid hormone and TSH measurements has been proposed, provided that the women recruited to derive such ranges have iodine intakes that are known to be appropriate to the needs of pregnancy.[2,3]

Instrumental diagnosis—Thyroid ultrasonography (US) is a second level investigation, in that it may be helpful in confirming a diagnosis of autoimmune thyroid disease (specific US features commonly found in non-pregnant adults with Hashimoto's thyroiditis), and can disclose the presence of goiter.

27.3.1.5 Treatment

Levothyroxine treatment—Regardless of the cause, maternal thyroid insufficiency should be promptly corrected by administering levothyroxine (LT$_4$) to achieve and maintain normal free T_4 and TSH levels throughout pregnancy. Pregnant women usually require larger LT$_4$ replacement doses than non-pregnant patients, so that the full daily replacement thyroxine dose is 2.0 to 2.4 µg/kg body weight. Women with severe hypothyroidism should be given for the first few days LT$_4$ doses twice the final daily estimated replacement dose to normalize maternal thyroid hormone levels as rapidly as possible.[2,3]

A large proportion (50 to 85%) of women who are already on treatment with LT$_4$ before conception often require adjustment of their daily thyroxine doses from the very first weeks of gestation. The average increase in the dose of levothyroxine during pregnancy is about 30 to 50%, but the magnitude of this increase varies according to several factors such as preconception TSH values and the etiology of hypothyroidism, among others.

In principle, women with hypothyroidism secondary to total thyroidectomy or radioiodine ablation require greater increases in their daily doses of LT_4 than women with autoimmune thyroiditis, because of some residual functional reserve in the latter. In all circumstances, the dose of LT_4 should be titrated to achieve a serum TSH level <2.5 mIU/L. The adequacy of the dose of thyroxine should be tested by measuring serum free T_4 and TSH levels within 30 days after initiation of treatment, after which thyroid function parameters should be tested every 4 weeks through mid-pregnancy, and every 6 to 8 weeks thereafter. Most patients need to decrease their daily doses of thyroxine about 4 weeks after giving birth.

Finally, because the increased requirements for exogenous T_4 usually appear as early as 4 to 6 weeks of pregnancy, women with known hypothyroidism can be advised to independently increase their doses of LT_4 by 25 to 30% upon a missed menstrual cycle to effectively prevent maternal hypothyroidism during the first trimester.[3]

Concerning autoimmune thyroiditis, euthyroid women with autoimmune thyroid disease face increased risks of miscarriage.[4] It has been reported that intervention with LT_4 may decrease the rate of miscarriage also in euthyroid patients, although the level of evidence is insufficient to recommend LT_4 therapy in antithyroid antibody-positive euthyroid women during pregnancy.[3]

Iodine—In addition to levothyroxine, hypothyroid pregnant women whose iodine intake is insufficient to meet the increased requirements for pregnancy should take daily iodine supplements. According to the latest recommendations for the control of iodine deficiency disorders (IDDs) in pregnancy set by a WHO expert panel, the recommended nutrient intake (RNI) for iodine during pregnancy and breast feeding should range between 200 and 300 μg/day, with an average of 250 μg/day. This goal is achievable through universal salt iodization (USI), provided that this measure is effective for at least 2 years. Otherwise, pregnant women should receive additional daily iodine to obtain the recommended dose of at least 250 μg I/day.[7]

Iodine supplementation can be provided in the form of potassium iodide (~100 to 200 μg/day) or prenatal preparations that usually contain 125 to 150 μg iodine. Importantly, the provision of adequate amounts of iodine before and during pregnancy is not an alternative to LT_4 therapy to correct maternal thyroid hypofunction. Adequate iodine is essential to *prevent* gestational thyroid insufficiency and provide the fetus with enough substrate to draw on for its own thyroid hormone synthesis.

27.3.1.6 Prognosis

Untreated or undertreated maternal hypothyroidism is associated with increased risks for obstetrical and fetal complications (Table 27.3). In addition, the offspring of these mothers face significantly increased risks of impaired neurodevelopment and mental and cognitive abilities.[8] The severity of obstetric complications and fetal brain damage varies widely, depending on several factors, from the degree of impaired maternal thyroid function to the timing and duration of its occurrence, among others. In general, the earlier the occurrence of maternal thyroid insufficiency, the more

---

TABLE 27.3

Maternal and Fetal Complications Reported in Association with Maternal Thyroid Hypofunction

Maternal Complications

Anemia

Postpartum hemorrhage

Gestation-induced hypertension and preeclampsia

Placental abruption

Increased risk of Caesarean section

Fetal Complications

Fetal death

Prematurity

Low birth weight

Fetal distress in labor

Congenital anomalies

Stillbirth

Perinatal death

---

severe (and irreversible) the consequences for both mother and fetus. Therefore, any delay in diagnosing and treating maternal hypothyroidism will result in a more severe prognosis.

27.3.2 THYROID HYPERFUNCTION DURING PREGNANCY

27.3.2.1 Definition

Gestational hyperthyroidism is defined by TSH values below the lower normal limit for gestational age and FT_4 values within (subclinical hyperthyroidism) or above (overt hyperthyroidism) the normal range for the pregnant state.[2]

As in the case of hypothyroidism, thyroid hyperfunction in some women may already be present before pregnancy or may develop during pregnancy as is the case with gestational transient thyrotoxicosis (GTT). This specific form of gestational hyperthyroidism occurs transiently near the end of the first trimester and is often mildly symptomatic unless associated with hyperemesis.

27.3.2.2 Epidemiology

Hyperthyroidism during pregnancy is much less frequent than hypothyroidism. Graves' disease occurs in 0.1 to 1% of all pregnancies, as overt (0.4%) or subclinical (0.6%) hyperthyroidism. Depending on the geographic area, the reported prevalence of hyperthyroidism due to GTT ranges from 0.3% (Japan) to 11% (Hong Kong). In Europe the prevalence is estimated between 2 and 3%.[2]

27.3.2.3 Etiopathogenesis

The two most common causes of hyperthyroidism in pregnant women are Graves' disease, which is responsible for over 85% of overt hyperthyroidism in pregnancy, and gestational transient thyrotoxicosis (GTT).

The pathogenesis of hyperthyroidism due to Graves' disease in a pregnant woman is the same as for a non-pregnant patient: it results from overstimulation of the thyroid by thyrotropin receptor stimulating antibodies (TR-Abs). Because thyroid autoantibody levels usually decline during pregnancy, Graves' disease typically improves with the progression of pregnancy and antithyroid therapy can commonly be discontinued in the third trimester. Due to the same immunological changes, Graves' disease very rarely arises de novo during pregnancy.[9]

GTT is a hyperthyroidism condition of non-autoimmune origin. For that reason, it is also called non-autoimmune gestational hyperthyroidism. GTT occurs transiently near the end of the first trimester of gestation and is frequently associated with hyperemesis. It is characterized by elevated free T_4 and T_3 levels, suppressed TSH, usually mild symptoms and signs of hyperthyroidism, and minimal or absent thyroid enlargement. The pathogenesis of this condition is related to the direct stimulatory activity of human chorionic gonadotropin (hCG) on thyroid function. In particular, a condition of overt hyperthyroidism may occur when hCG levels are particularly high (as in the case of twin pregnancies), in some cases of long-lasting hypersecretion of hCG, or when molecular isoforms of hCG with longer half-lives or more potent thyrotropic activities are produced. Finally, a mutant TSH receptor with increased sensitivity to hCG was reported to be responsible for a unique form of familial gestational thyrotoxicosis.[10]

Other causes of hyperthyroidism in pregnancy are rarer and include multinodular toxic goiter, toxic adenoma, subacute or silent thyroiditis, iodide-induced thyrotoxicosis, thyrotoxicosis factitia, hydatidiform mole, and hyperplacentosis.

27.3.2.4 Diagnosis

Medical history, signs, and symptoms—Women with histories of hyperthyroidism already known before pregnancy obviously pose no problem from a diagnostic view. However, recognition of a condition of hyperthyroidism that had not been diagnosed before pregnancy or occurring for the first time during pregnancy may be very difficult for several reasons. First, hyperthyroidism due to Graves' disease usually improves during pregnancy, although a transient worsening during the first trimester (likely related to the thyroid-stimulating activity of high levels of hCG) may be observed. Second, when present, symptoms such as palpitations, anxiety, nervousness, insomnia, heat intolerance, and sweating, may remain unknown because they are somewhat non-specific or attributed to the pregnancy.

Clinical findings that more usefully may raise a clinical suspicion of hyperthyroidism are a failure to gain weight (clear weight losses are rare), thyroid enlargement, or extrathyroidal manifestations of Graves' disease such as orbitopathy or dermopathy. Finally, when hyperthyroidism is due to gestational transient thyrotoxicosis, symptoms and signs are even more blurred and not routinely detectable due to the transient course of the disease that usually recovers spontaneously with decreases in hCG concentrations. Unlike hyperthyroidism due to Graves' disease, GTT is frequently associated with excessive vomiting, especially in women with more pronounced elevations in thyroid hormone concentrations.

Laboratory diagnosis—Clinical diagnosis of hyperthyroidism may be confirmed only by findings of elevated serum FT_4 concentrations and suppressed serum TSH levels. Measurement of thyroid receptor antibodies (TR-Abs) is a second level investigation parameter in that the presence of TR-Abs discriminates Graves' disease from other causes of gestational hyperthyroidism. However, it should be noted that the production of TR-Abs tends to decrease during the second half of pregnancy, and thus the interpretation of the results of a TR-Ab assay depends on gestational age.[10]

Beyond diagnostic utility, the determination of these antibodies has clear prognostic significance for the fetus. In fact, TR-Abs can cross the placenta and induce abnormal fetal thyroid gland stimulation, similar to that occurring in the mother.[11] In general, the risk of fetal or neonatal thyrotoxicosis is greater in infants born to mothers with Graves' disease of recent onset, in whom TR-Ab titers are usually higher than in those with less recent illness or in those who previously underwent ablative therapy (radioiodine or thyroidectomy). The latter, however, may have TR-Ab titers persistently elevated even long after ablative therapy, and the recommendation is to measure maternal TR-Abs in the first trimester in these women.[12] In all circumstances (current or past history of Graves' disease), if high TR-Ab titers in the first trimester are found, they must be re-tested in the last trimester because the risk of fetal or neonatal thyrotoxicosis is directly related to elevated levels of maternal antibodies.

When gestational transient hyperthyroidism is diagnosed, monitoring of thyroid hormones and TSH usually shows a gradual normalization of these indices that occurs in most cases occurs by mid-gestation. The finding of low or suppressed TSH levels in the absence of concomitant elevation of thyroid hormones beyond the limits of normality should not be interpreted as indicative of subclinical hyperthyroidism because the lowering in TSH levels during pregnancy may be normal.

Instrumental diagnosis—Thyroid radionuclide scans and radioiodine (^{131}I or ^{123}I) uptake tests are contraindicated in pregnancy and should never be performed. Thyroid ultrasonography can be helpful in cases of Graves' disease in which pathognomonic clinical and laboratory signs are lacking or when other causes of hyperthyroidism (subacute or silent thyroiditis, multinodular toxic goiter, or toxic adenoma) are suspected. The thyroid gland is typically normal in GTT women.

27.3.2.5 Treatment

Management of hyperthyroidism in pregnant women is particularly challenging for a physician because of the maternal and fetal complications related to maternal hyperthyroidism or the medications used to control thyroid hyperfunction. Also, treatment options during pregnancy are limited because some methods for treating hyperthyroidism (e.g., radioiodine) are contraindicated and others such as thyroidectomy should be reserved in very specific cases. In fact, antithyroid drugs are the mainstays of treatment of hyperthyroidism in pregnant women.[13]

27.3.2.5.1   Treatment of Graves' Disease in Pregnant Women

Medical treatment—As noted above, drug therapy is the treatment of choice for hyperthyroidism during pregnancy. All antithyroid drugs [methimazole (MMI), carbimazole (CBM), and propylthiouracil (PTU)] can cross the placenta, and therefore have the potential to cause fetal hypothyroidism.[14] For this reason, the lowest doses of antithyroid drugs should be used and the treatment goal should be to maintain maternal thyroid hormone levels in the upper non-pregnant reference range.[2] This strategy is believed to limit the risk of iatrogenic fetal hypothyroidism. The initial recommended dosage is 100 to 200 mg daily in three doses for PTU or 10 to 20 mg daily in a single dose for MMI. Thereafter the dose of PTU or MMI should be gradually adjusted in response to changes in maternal thyroid hormone levels that should be checked every 2 to 4 weeks. In most cases, antithyroid drugs can be discontinued during the third trimester because of normalization of maternal thyroid function by that time.

Recently, isolated reports of maternal liver injury related to the administration of PTU in pregnancy raised concern about the use of this drug. On the other hand, malformations associated with MMI, although rare, have been reported. In view of these considerations, the recommendation is to limit the use of PTU to the first trimester of pregnancy and switch to MMI thereafter.[3]

Finally, combined administration of antithyroid drugs and LT_4 should be avoided because the placental permeability for antithyroid drugs is high, whereas it is negligible for LT_4.

Surgical treatment—Surgical therapy for Graves' disease in pregnancy is indicated only in selected cases (severe antithyroid drug-related side effects, noncompliance with antithyroid drug therapy, and uncontrolled hyperthyroidism requiring high doses of antithyroid drugs). When deemed necessary, subtotal thyroidectomy should be performed in the second trimester due to the lower risk of teratogenic effects of anesthetic drugs in this period and the reduced placental permeability at this stage that increases later in pregnancy. Propranolol (10 to 40 mg/day in three doses) and potassium iodide (50 to 100 mg/day) can be both temporarily (10 to 14 days) used for preoperative preparation.

Radioiodine treatment—The use of radioactive iodine in pregnancy is *proscribed*, especially for the significant effects of radiation on the fetal thyroid that lead to destruction of the fetal thyroid, fetal hypothyroidism, and subsequent possible neurological damage.

27.3.2.5.2   Treatment of Gestational Transient Thyrotoxicosis

In most cases, GTT does not require treatment because of its spontaneous recovery within a few weeks. In selected cases, when thyroid hormone levels are unusually high, antithyroid drugs can be administered for a few weeks.[2] In such cases, maternal thyroid function should be kept strictly under control and antithyroid drugs discontinued as soon as maternal thyroid function reverts to normal. When GTT is associated with severe hyperemesis (more than 5% weight loss, dehydration, and ketonuria), in addition to treatment with fluids and electrolytes, propranolol may be transiently used because of its efficacy in reducing hyperemesis and symptoms of thyrotoxicosis. Although this drug has no teratogenic effects, its use should be limited because an association with intrauterine growth restriction has been reported.

27.3.2.6 Prognosis

Uncontrolled or poorly controlled maternal hyperthyroidism is associated with increased risk of maternal and fetal or neonatal complications (spontaneous abortion, congestive heart failure, thyrotoxic storm, preeclampsia, prematurity, low birth weight, and stillbirth). In contrast, pregnancy outcome is unaffected when maternal hyperthyroidism is adequately treated. In addition to the control of hyperthyroidism, prognosis in newborns of mothers with Graves' disease is affected by the possible transplacental passage of TR-Abs and antithyroid drugs.

In women with positive TR-Abs, the risk of fetal or neonatal thyrotoxicosis depends on TR-Ab titers during the second half of gestation. Rarely, a high titer of TR-Ab with blocking activity may be present and subsequently cause fetal or neonatal hypothyroidism. In turn, this condition may be responsible for irreversible neurological damage, the severity of which depends on the time of onset, degree, and length of thyroid insufficiency. Antithyroid drugs crossing the placenta may cause fetal hypothyroidism as well.[15]

27.4 THYROID DISEASES NOT ASSOCIATED WITH ALTERED THYROID FUNCTION

27.4.1 NON-TOXIC NODULAR THYROID DISEASE

27.4.1.1 Epidemiology

Nodular thyroid disease is a common clinical problem. Epidemiological studies in iodine-sufficient areas revealed prevalences of clinically detectable nodules in 5% and 1% of women and men, respectively. When thyroid ultrasonography is performed, however, these figures increase up to 50%.[16] On the whole, the prevalence of thyroid nodules is higher in women living in areas of iodine deficiency, increases with age, and is higher in women with prior pregnancies compared to nulliparous women. Data from studies of thyroid nodules during pregnancy reported prevalences in mildly to moderately iodine-deficient areas ranging from 3 to 21%.[3]

Depending on gender, age, family history, previous exposure to ionizing radiation, and other risk factors, 5 to 15% of nodules may be malignant, with differentiated thyroid carcinoma as the most frequent malignancy. Although data are limited, the prevalence of malignancy in thyroid nodules detected during pregnancy seems to be similar to that observed in the general population.[2]

27.4.1.2 Etiopathogenesis

The etiology of nodular thyroid disease in pregnancy does not differ from that in the non-pregnant population. Several studies revealed that in areas of mild iodine deficiency (or borderline iodine sufficiency), thyroid nodules definitely trended toward an increase in size during pregnancy, and new appearance of thyroid nodules was reported in about 15% of women with preexisting nodular thyroid disease.

Both events are likely related to changes in maternal thyroid economy typically associated with pregnancy under conditions of insufficient iodine intake. In such circumstances, the reduced production of thyroid hormone leads to a progressive increase in TSH concentrations, usually found to be about twice as high at pregnancy term than in early gestation. Thus, the chronic stimulation of follicular cells by TSH may be an important factor in determining increases in the volumes of nodules in pregnant women exposed to iodine restriction or overt iodine deficiency.[17]

27.4.1.3 Diagnosis

Medical history, signs and symptoms—As is the case outside of pregnancy, thyroid nodules are usually asymptomatic and discovered by chance after a patient finds a neck lump or because a physician discovers it during a routine examination. It is unusual for these nodules to reach sufficient size to cause significant symptoms such as dysphagia, dysphonia, and stridor. Bleeding in a nodule can cause a sudden increase in size and local pain and tenderness.

Physical findings in pregnant women have no particular distinguishing features compared with findings in non-pregnant patients (more extensively treated elsewhere in this text). In short, a benign thyroid nodule on physical examination can be appreciated as a discrete prominence in the context of an otherwise normal gland, it moves together with the thyroid gland during swallowing, and can be separated from overlying layers to some extent. When a lesion fluctuates, it is generally a cyst that is usually benign. Features such as fixation of the nodule to strap muscles or the trachea or enlargement of cervical lymph nodes are alarming in that they may suggest malignancy.

It should be noted that a moderate degree of thyroid enlargement is a relatively common finding in pregnant women since pregnancy acts as a strong goitrogenic stimulus even in areas with only moderate iodine restriction.[1]

Laboratory diagnosis—Thyroid function tests in pregnant women with nonfunctioning thyroid nodules do not provide specific information. FT_3, FT_4, and TSH determinations, however, should be performed to ascertain maternal thyroid status as part of a routine assessment. Determination of thyroglobulin levels is not useful because the concentrations of this glycoprotein may be not-specifically elevated, as in other goitrous conditions. Finally, calcitonin measurement as a standard procedure for evaluation of nodules is controversial unless a family history of medullary thyroid carcinoma or MEN2 is known.

Instrumental diagnosis—The use of radioactive iodine is contraindicated during pregnancy. Thyroid ultrasound (US) is the first level instrumental investigation in the diagnosis of thyroid nodules in pregnancy. It allows a precise characterization of clinically detectable nodules (size, echogenicity, vascularity pattern, etc.) and also the identification of other non-palpable nodules or suspicious lymph nodes. In addition, thyroid ultrasound is extremely useful for monitoring nodules throughout pregnancy because abnormal growth of a nodule may modify the therapeutic approach (see Section 27.4.1.4).

Nodules that have two or more suspicious features on US (hypoechoic pattern, irregular margins, intranodular vascular spots, microcalcifications, etc.) should be further evaluated by fine needle aspiration biopsy (FNAB), regardless of gestational age. If ultrasound shows no suspicious features, FNAB is not mandatory and may be deferred until after delivery according to the preferences of patients. This diagnostic tool has been shown to be safe and diagnostically reliable during pregnancy.

27.4.1.4   Treatment

Benign thyroid nodules—Medical treatment, in particular semisuppressive LT_4 therapy, is not recommended for benign thyroid nodules diagnosed during pregnancy. No consensus indicates this treatment is beneficial in terms of reduction or stability of nodular volume. However, several randomized studies carried out in regions with borderline or low iodine intakes demonstrated that, at least in the general population, LT_4 therapy in doses that lowered TSH to subnormal levels may result in a decrease in nodule size and/or prevent the appearance of new nodules. Surgery may be considered in cases that show rapid growth, even in the absence of suspicious features on repeated FNAB.

Suspicious and malignant thyroid nodules—When cytological findings are suspicious for malignancy, the current recommendation is close clinical and instrumental monitoring of the patient and refraining from medical or surgical treatment unless a rapid growth in nodule volume occurs or lymph node metastases appear. In the latter cases, surgery may be indicated during pregnancy, provided that it is done during the second trimester or, alternatively may be postponed until after delivery.

The management of pregnant women with cytological diagnoses of papillary thyroid carcinoma should take into account a number of clinical and prognostic factors. The most significant are gestational age and the extent of disease (disease limited to the thyroid gland or with extrathyroidal extension) at diagnosis. Since thyroidectomy should be performed during the second trimester, if papillary thyroid carcinoma is diagnosed beyond this period, surgery should be postponed until after delivery, regardless of the presence of other factors.

When papillary thyroid cancer is detected early in pregnancy, the therapeutic approach depends on both the growth of the nodule evaluated by ultrasound and the extent of the disease. In the case of rapid and significant growth (50% by volume and 20% in diameter in two dimensions), and/or the appearance of lymph node metastases prior to mid-gestation, thyroidectomy should be performed during the second trimester. The same therapeutic approach should be adopted if at the time of diagnosis (early pregnancy) evidence indicates extrathyroidal extension of the disease. Conversely, if a nodule remains stable and the disease is limited to the thyroid gland, surgery may be performed after a woman gives birth. When surgery is postponed until completion of pregnancy, women should receive LT_4 therapy in doses appropriate to maintain their TSH values in a low or semisuppressed range.[3]

Finally, women treated for thyroid cancer before becoming pregnant should continue their treatment with LT_4 during pregnancy, keeping the treatment goal set before conception on the basis of risk stratification. Of course, this requires a careful assessment of thyroid function (every 4 weeks), especially if changes are made to therapy. In addition, ultrasound and Tg monitoring should be performed in women with evidence of persistent disease before pregnancy.

27.4.1.5 Prognosis

Prognosis of benign thyroid nodules is favorable and not affected by pregnancy. Even in cases of malignant thyroid nodules diagnosed during pregnancy, the prognosis is no different from prognoses among the non-pregnant population. In particular, deferring thyroidectomy until after delivery does not adversely affect prognosis in women with differentiated thyroid cancer. Rather, a higher rate of complications in pregnant women undergoing thyroid surgery compared with non-pregnant women has been reported.

REFERENCES

1. Glinoer, D. 1997. The regulation of thyroid function in pregnancy: pathways of endocrine adaptation from physiology to pathology. *Endocr Rev* 18: 404–433.
2. Abalovich, M., Amino, N., Barbour, L.A. et al. 2007. Management of thyroid dysfunction during pregnancy and postpartum: an Endocrine Society clinical practice guideline. *J Clin Endocrinol Metab* 92: S1–S47.
3. Stagnaro-Green, A., Abalovich, M., Alexander, E. et al. 2011. Guidelines of the American Thyroid Association for the diagnosis and management of thyroid disease during pregnancy and postpartum. *Thyroid*. Jul 25 [Epub ahead of print].
4. Krassas, G.E., Poppe, K., and Glinoer, D. 2010. Thyroid function and human reproductive health. *Endocr Rev* 31: 702–755.
5. Moleti, M., LoPresti, V.P., Mattina, F. et al. 2009. Gestational thyroid function abnormalities in conditions of mild iodine deficiency: early screening versus continuous monitoring of maternal thyroid status. *Eur J Endocrinol* 160: 611–617.
6. Caturegli, P., Newschaffer, C., Olivi, A. et al. 2005. Autoimmune hypophysitis. *Endocr Rev* 26: 599–614.
7. WHO Secretariat. 2007. Prevention and control of iodine deficiency in pregnant and lactating women and in children less than 2-years-old: conclusions and recommendations of the technical consultation. *Public Health Nutr* 10: 1606–1611.
8. Morreale de Escobar, G., Obregon, M.J., and Escobar del Rey, F. 2004. Maternal thyroid hormones early in pregnancy and fetal brain development. *Best Pract Res Clinical Endocrinol Metab* 18: 225–248.
9. Weetman, A.P. 2010. Immunity, thyroid function and pregnancy: molecular mechanisms. *Nat Rev Endocrinol* 6: 311–318.
10. Rodien, P., Jordan, N., Lefèvre, A. et al. 2004. Abnormal stimulation of the thyrotrophin receptor during gestation. *Hum Reprod Update* 10: 95–105.
11. Laurberg, P., Nygaard, B., Glinoer, D. et al. 1998. Guidelines for TSH-receptor antibody measurements in pregnancy: results of an evidence-based symposium organized by the European Thyroid Association. *Eur J Endocrinol* 139: 584–596.
12. Laurberg, P., Bournaud, C., Karmisholt, J. et al. 2009. Management of Graves' hyperthyroidism in pregnancy: focus on both maternal and foetal thyroid function, and caution against surgical thyroidectomy in pregnancy. *Eur J Endocrinol* 160: 1–8.
13. Mestman, J.H. 2004. Hyperthyroidism in pregnancy. *Best Pract Res Clin Endocrinol Metab* 18: 267–288.
14. Rivkees, S.A. and Szarfman, A. 2010. Dissimilar hepatotoxicity profiles of propylthiouracil and methimazole in children. *J Clin Endocrinol Metab* 95: 3260–3267.

15. Nero, R., Beck-Peccoz, P., Chiovato, L. et al. 2011. Hyperthyroidism and pregnancy: an Italian Thyroid Association (AIT) and Italian Association of Clinical Endocrinologists (AME) joint statement for clinical practice. *J Endocrinol Invest* 34: 225–231.
16. Mazzaferri, E.L. 1993. Management of a solitary thyroid nodule. *New Engl J Med* 327: 553–559.
17. Wémeau, J.L. and Do Cao, C. 2002. Thyroid nodule, cancer and pregnancy. *Ann Endocrinol* 63: 438–442.

28 Iodine Deficiency in Pregnancy

Mariacarla Moleti, Francesco Vermiglio,
and Francesco Trimarchi

CONTENTS

Key words: iodine deficiency and pregnancy, maternal hypothyroxinemia, hypothyroidism in pregnancy, iodine deficiency-related neurological disorders.

28.1 INTRODUCTION AND DEFINITION

Iodine is an inorganic substrate essential for thyroid hormone synthesis. At present, no other use apart from thyroid hormone synthesis is known in human biology. Thyroid hormones are essential for normal progression of pregnancy and neurointellectual development of the fetus.

Recommended iodine intake in pregnancy based on a technical consultation on behalf of the World Health Organization (WHO) is 250 µg/day, roughly corresponding to a urinary iodine excretion (UIE) of 185 µg/L.[1] When this goal is not achieved, iodine intake is considered insufficient for the increased maternal and fetal thyroid needs. In fact, pregnancy represents the most vulnerable period of life if daily dietary iodine intake is inadequate because both mother and fetus are simultaneously exposed to the potentially severe consequences of iodine deficiency (ID). Different degrees of deficiency of this micronutrient during gestation can result in fatal events such as pregnancy interruptions or, when pregnancy progresses, in brain damage leading to irreversible major or minor neurointellectual disorders in the offspring.

28.2 EPIDEMIOLOGY

Iodine deficiency affects more than 2 billion people worldwide. In the latest evaluation of iodine deficiency disorders (IDDs), the WHO reported that only half of the countries from which data on UIE were available had optimal iodine nutrition status. Pregnant women from populations exposed to iodine deficiency are potentially at risk of suffering major iodine disorders. Also, pregnant women living in regions where iodine intake is considered sufficient for the general population may theoretically be at risk of suffering from the consequences of iodine deficiency (only transient and limited to gestational period) because of iodine intake that is not adequate to meet the increasing needs imposed by pregnancy.

28.3 IODINE HOMEOSTASIS IN PREGNANCY

Iodine requirements during pregnancy increase because of (1) possible iodide loss through the kidneys as the result of an increased renal clearance of iodide, (2) increased iodide consumption needed for the increased synthesis of thyroxine by the maternal gland, and (3) transfers of iodine from mother to fetus. All these factors contribute to the progressive and critical reduction of the maternal iodide pool and may adversely affect fetal iodide pool repletion if iodine intake is not adequately increased. An attempt to roughly quantify the losses of iodine resulting from these factors was made.

28.3.1 Possible Iodide Loss through Kidneys

This is the most controversial point since the studies on this issue report no differences, increases, and even reductions in UIE in pregnant women compared with non-pregnant women and the general population. Therefore, an increase in urinary excretion of iodine is neither proven nor quantitatively assessed.

28.3.2 Increased Iodide Consumption for Increased Synthesis of Thyroxine by Maternal Gland

The increased iodide consumption is due to the increased organification of this micronutrient in two tyrosines, monoiodotyrosine (MIT) and diiodotyrosine (DIT), the coupling of which generates thyroid hormones. The increase in maternal T_4 production, roughly estimated to exceed by 50% the normal hormone synthesis in the non-pregnant population, is aimed to guarantee the metabolic needs of the mother and the transfer of T_4 and iodide from the mother to the fetus. Consequently, additional 50 to 100 µg of iodine/day are needed to guarantee this increased output of thyroxine in pregnant women. This figure has been estimated on the basis of the 50% increase in the dose of LT_4 to be administered to maintain euthyroidism in hypothyroid women during gestation.

28.3.3 Transfer of Iodide from Mother to Fetus

The transfer of iodide from mother to fetus should provide a substrate for the production of thyroid hormones by the onset of fetal thyroid function in the second half of gestation and possibly to create (in the first half of gestation) a fetal iodide pool (placental iodide pool?) for the future needs of the fetal gland. This transfer has been estimated at about 50 µg/day. Also, this figure derives from objective data and from inferences such as the measure of the iodide accumulated in the fetal thyroid over gestation, the proportion of iodide content in overall fetal hormone production, and the substitutive doses of LT_4 to be administered to hypothyroid neonates.

Considering all these factors, the overall additional dose of iodine during gestation needed to provide an adequate substrate for both maternal and fetal needs is 150 µg/day. This supplement must be added to the usual dietary dose, thus reaching an overall daily dietary intake of 250 to 300 µg/day.[2]

28.4 CONSEQUENCES OF REDUCED AVAILABILITY OF IODINE ON MATERNAL THYROID

As a result of reduced availability of iodine, the first event is a decrease in T_4 production by the maternal gland. All the functional and morphological changes occurring

TABLE 28.1

Autoregulatory Thyroid Mechanisms of Adaptation to ID

Mother	Fetus
Increase in vascularity	No autoregulatory thyroid mechanisms
Increase in blood flow	Decreased synthesis of both T_4 and T_3
Iodine trapping	Increase in circulating TSH
Acinar cell height	
Hyperplasia	
Preferential production of T_3 over T_4	

in the maternal thyroid thereafter depend on this event and consist of a series of mechanisms to adapt to iodine deficiency (Table 28.1). Following the progressive decline of serum FT_4 throughout gestation, TSH increases to stimulate maternal thyroid function.

The extent of FT_4 decline and TSH increase closely depends on the severity of iodine deficiency. The more severe the deficiency, the higher the FT_4 decline and TSH increase. As a result of maternal thyroid stimulation by TSH and hCG as well, an enlargement of the maternal thyroid may lead to a transient gestational goiter that is only partially reversible after delivery.

Iodine deficiency then triggers goitrogenesis in the mother (and fetus) as an additional adaptive mechanism to this condition. Gestational goitrogenesis well correlates with the progressive increase in serum thyroglobulin (Tg) observed over the course of pregnancy so that Tg is considered a useful prognostic marker of thyroid enlargement and its prevention by iodine prophylaxis. Preferential secretion of T_3 by the maternal gland is another adaptive mechanism mainly aimed to save iodine. It is reflected by an elevated total T_3-to-T_4 molar ratio and is mainly due to the partial switch of the maternal thyroid hormone production from T_4 to T_3.[3]

28.5 CONSEQUENCES OF REDUCED AVAILABILITY OF IODINE ON FETAL THYROID

Around week 13 of intrauterine life, fetal thyroid development is completed and the fetal gland becomes fully operative around the 16th week of gestation. Thus, fetal neurodevelopment during the first trimester and part of the second trimester exclusively relies on the transfer of maternal T_4. Thereafter, the contribution of maternal T_4 to the fetus declines to roughly 40%, accounting for a 60% contribution of fetal hormone production to the entire fetal T_4 pool.

Unlike his mother, a fetus cannot rely on autoregulatory mechanisms such as preferential thyroidal secretion of T_3 to face the scarce availability of iodine. As a result, apart from adequate dietary iodine intake the transfer of maternal T_4 to a fetus represents the only compensatory system known at present to mitigate the consequences of fetal hypothyroidism.

TABLE 28.2
Clinical and Biochemical Patterns of Maternal and Fetal/Neonatal
ID-Related Thyroid Insufficiencies

Insufficiency	Pattern
Maternal isolated hypothyroxinemia	Serum FT_4 levels below and TSH within trimester-specific reference range
Maternal subclinical hypothyroidism	Serum FT_4 levels within and TSH above trimester-specific reference range
Maternal overt hypothyroidism	Serum FT_4 levels below and TSH above trimester-specific reference range
Fetal hypothyroidism	Indirectly suggested by fetal goiter, maternal thyroid insufficiency, or neonatal thyroid function deficiency
	Directly confirmed during gestation by serum FT_4 and TSH measurements in blood samples obtained via cordocentesis
Neonatal goiter, hypothyroxinemia, and hypothyroidism	Directly confirmed by clinical and instrumental evaluation and by serum FT_4 and TSH measurements; suggests previous ID-related fetal hypothyroidism

28.6 CLINICAL PICTURES OF IODINE DEFICIENCY IN PREGNANCY

Iodine deficiency (ID) in pregnancy can result in certain maternal, fetal, and neonatal thyroid diseases (Table 28.2):

Maternal
  Goiter
  Isolated hypothyroxinemia
  Subclinical hypothyroidism
  Overt hypothyroidism
Fetal
  Fetal goiter and hypothyroidism
Neonatal
  Neonatal goiter, hypothyroxinemia, and hypothyroidism

ID-related maternal thyroid deficiencies will affect both the mother and the fetus by compromising pregnancy outcome and affecting fetal neurointellectual development. Fetal hypothyroidism will affect the fetus only. The combination of maternal and fetal thyroid failure, as the result of severe iodine deficiency, leads to endemic cretinism.

28.6.1 MATERNAL GOITER

28.6.1.1 Definition

Maternal goiter is a thyroid enlargement clinically and/or ultrasonographically detected in a pregnant woman.

28.6.1.2   Epidemiology

An increase of 20 to 35% in thyroid volume has been reported in pregnant women living in regions of low iodine intake. Many of these women exhibited a doubling in thyroid size between early gestation and term.[4,5] The appearance of goiter in pregnancy should therefore suggest the risk of an ID-related thyroid dysfunction and biochemical evaluation of thyroid function is mandatory.

28.6.2   ISOLATED HYPOTHYROXINEMIA

28.6.2.1   Definition

Isolated hypothyroxinemia refers in this chapter to a condition characterized by serum TSH levels within the trimester-specific reference range and maternal free thyroxine concentrations below the trimester-specific reference range (Table 28.2).

Analysis of published studies dealing with isolated hypothyroxinemia reveals that the biochemical criteria on which diagnosis is based are very variable. This is mainly because the lower FT_4 limit below which isolated hypothyroxinemia is diagnosed is indicated by some authors in the 2.5th to 3rd percentiles and by others in 10th percentile. More recently, in the latest guidelines of the American Thyroid Association for the diagnosis and management of thyroid disease during pregnancy and postpartum, isolated hypothyroxinemia has been defined as "a normal maternal TSH concentration in conjunction with FT_4 concentrations in the lower 5th or 10th percentile of the reference range."[6]

Moreover, in some studies, the adopted reference ranges for FT_4 are the same as those used for general population; others cite pregnancy-specific intervals. Whatever the lower reference limit, the definition of maternal isolated hypothyroxinemia should fulfill the criteria of trimester-specific reference limits calculated in iodine-sufficient pregnant women.

28.6.2.2   Epidemiology

Epidemiological data on the prevalence of this mild maternal thyroid insufficiency are quite variable and range from 1.3 to 2.3% in the United States and above 20% in mildly iodine-deficient areas.[7] Apart from the different iodine nutrition status in the studied areas, this great variability in the prevalence of hypothyroxinemia probably arises from the lack of systematic data about changes of FT_4 levels over the course of pregnancy. Indeed, most studies dealing with this issue refer to single (often early) FT_4 determination. As a result, the actual prevalence of isolated hypothyroxinemia may be underestimated.

The few studies[8,9] evaluating longitudinal changes in FT_4 concentrations over an entire pregnancy suggest that this mild maternal thyroid failure frequently occurs late in gestation, starting from the second trimester onward. This trend toward a late-onset occurrence of maternal hypothyroxinemia may be the result of a failure of the maternal thyroid to keep up with sustained hormone demand due to a progressive depletion of iodine stores and inadequate daily iodine supplies.[10]

28.6.3   SUBCLINICAL HYPOTHYROIDISM

28.6.3.1   Definition

Subclinical hypothyroidism is the first stage of thyroid insufficiency. The transition from euthyroidism to hypothyroidism is indeed first detected by a slight increase in TSH value as the pituitary response to even a small decline in the production of T_4 that still remains within the reference range. As a result, subclinical hypothyroidism in pregnancy deals with serum TSH values above the trimester-specific reference range upper limit and FT_4 levels within the trimester-specific reference range. As a general rule, the reference range upper limit for serum TSH should not exceed 2.5 to 3.0 mIU/L according to most of the epidemiological data now available about trimester-specific reference ranges in iodine-sufficient pregnant women.[6]

28.6.3.2   Epidemiology

The prevalence of ID-related subclinical hypothyroidism is not firmly established due to the lack of systematic data that actually separate autoimmune from ID-related subclinical hypothyroidism, which closely depends on the severity of iodine deficiency.

28.6.4   OVERT HYPOTHYROIDISM

28.6.4.1   Definition

Overt hypothyroidism in pregnancy refers to a biochemical pattern characterized by serum FT_4 below and TSH above their respective trimester-specific reference ranges. As previously stated, the serum TSH trimester-specific reference range upper limit should not exceed 2.5 to 3.0 mIU/L.

28.6.4.2   Epidemiology

The prevalence of ID-related overt hypothyroidism is not firmly established due to the lack of systematic data that actually distinguish autoimmune from ID-related overt hypothyroidism, which closely depends on the severity of iodine deficiency.

28.6.5   FETAL GOITER AND HYPOTHYROIDISM

28.6.5.1   Definition and Epidemiology

A definition of fetal hypothyroidism is lacking because fetal thyroid failure is difficult to ascertain and is only suggested indirectly by the presence of fetal goiter or directly by reduced fetal thyroid hormones. Evaluation of fetal thyroid hormones requires cordocentesis, an invasive procedure charged by a not-negligible risk of fetal loss. This is the main reason why we do not have at our disposal a definite nosography or updated prevalence of this condition.

Fetal hypothyroidism is a potentially harmful consequence of prolonged iodine deficiency.

28.6.6 NEONATAL GOITER, HYPOTHYROXINEMIA, AND HYPOTHYROIDISM

All these conditions may be easily evaluated by clinical and instrumental examination and by serum FT_4 and TSH determinations at birth. Their presence may suggest a previous condition of fetal hypothyroidism.

28.7 ETIOPATHOGENESIS OF MATERNAL AND FETAL ID-RELATED THYROID DEFICIENCIES

Reduced availability of maternal dietary iodine intake is the only cause of all the iodine deficiency-related maternal and fetal thyroid deficiencies cited above. The inadequacy of this inorganic substrate for the synthesis of thyroid hormones is responsible for a decline in thyroid hormone concentration leading to the various clinical and biochemical pictures reported. The occurrence of isolated hypothyroxinemia or of both maternal and fetal hypothyroidism depends on the severity and duration of iodine deficiency.

28.8 CLINICAL FEATURES

Goiter appearance in pregnancy is considered the hallmark of iodine deficiency.[3] Unless a pregnant woman is overtly hypothyroid, symptoms and signs (other than goiter) of maternal thyroid failure are usually absent or when present may be erroneously interpreted as non-specific features attributed to the pregnancy state (drowsiness, asthenia, constipation, malaise, etc.).

28.9 CLINICAL CONSEQUENCES

The complications of maternal iodine deficiency-related thyroid insufficiencies involve both the maternal and fetal sides and compromise pregnancy outcomes and mainly neurointellectual development of the fetus. The consequences of fetal hypothyroidism affect the fetal side only. Both maternal and fetal ID-related consequences are reported in Table 28.3.

TABLE 28.3
Clinical Consequences of Maternal and Fetal ID-Related Thyroid Insufficiencies

Maternal Side Complications	Fetal or Neonatal Side Complications
Abortion	Stillbirth
Preterm delivery	Increased perinatal mortality
Anemia	Congenital anomalies
Gestational hypertension	Endemic cretinism
Placental abruption	Psychomotor defects
Postpartum hemorrhage	Retarded mental and physical development

TABLE 28.4

Neuropsychiatric and Intellectual Deficits in Infants and School Children Born to Mothers Residing in Areas of Mild to Moderate Iodine Deficiency

Region	Tests	Main Findings
Spain	Bayley, McCarthy, Cattell	Lower psychomotor and mental development
Italy (Sicily)	Bender-Gestalt	Lower perceptual integrative motor ability; neuromuscular and neurosensorial abnormalities
Italy (Tuscany)	Wechsler, Raven	Low verbal IQ, perception, and motor and attentive functions
Italy (Tuscany)	WISC	Lower velocity of motor response to visual stimuli
India	Verbal, pictorial learning, and motivation tests	Lower learning capacity
Iran	Bender-Gestalt, Raven	Retardation in psychomotor development
Italy (Sicily)	WISC	Attention deficit hyperactivity disorder (ADHD)

Source: Modified from Glinoer, D. and Delange, F. 2000. *Thyroid* 10: 871–887. With permission.

28.10 NEURO-INTELLECTUAL CONSEQUENCES IN PROGENY

Thyroxine transfer from mother to fetus is essential for normal fetal neurogenesis, especially during the first half of gestation when maternal thyroid is the only source of thyroid hormone for the fetus. Iodine deficiency may result in various degrees of maternal thyroid failure as extensively reported elsewhere in this chapter. Due to systematic intervention via iodine prophylaxis all over the world and improved iodine nutrition as the result of the general improvement of the quality of life, endemic cretinism has almost disappeared and is confined to the few countries where severe endemia still exists.

Today, endemic cretinism is of historical interest only as the most severe expression of the combination of both maternal and fetal ID-related thyroid failure. Apart from this extreme condition, moderate and even mild maternal thyroid insufficiencies resulting from moderate and even mild iodine deficiency may be responsible for neurointellectual disorders in the progeny by compromising their neurological performances and intelligence quotients[11] (Table 28.4).

28.11 DIAGNOSIS

Due to the scarcity and non-specificity of signs and symptoms, the diagnosis of different degrees of both maternal and fetal thyroid insufficiency relies on serum FT_4 and TSH measurements.

28.12 TREATMENT

28.12.1 IODINE

First, maternal and fetal thyroid insufficiency should be avoided by iodine prophylaxis. Regular and long-lasting use of iodized salt is effective in reducing the risks of both maternal and fetal thyroid insufficiency.[8] Universal salt iodization (USI)—the addition of suitable amounts of potassium iodide to all salt for human and livestock consumption—is now indicated as the most common tool for effective eradication of IDDs.[6] During gestation, USI is supposed to guarantee adequate (200 and 300 µg/day; average of 250 µg/day) iodine intake provided that this measure is effective for at least 2 years. Otherwise, pregnant women should receive additional daily amounts of iodine to obtain the recommended dose of at least 250 µg/day.[7] Iodine supplementation can be provided in the form of potassium iodide (~100 to 200 µg/day) or prenatal preparations that usually contain 150 µg iodine.

28.12.2 LEVOTHYROXINE (LT$_4$)

Maternal thyroid insufficiency (isolated hypothyroxinemia and both subclinical and overt hypothyroidism) should be promptly corrected by LT$_4$ administration. Treatment by LT$_4$ must be tailored for each pregnant woman according to the severity of thyroid function deficit and gestational age, with the aim to restore as soon as possible a biochemical pattern characterized by normal TSH and serum FT$_4$ levels within the trimester-specific reference range. In all circumstances, the dose of LT$_4$ should be titrated to achieve a serum TSH level <2.5 mIU/L throughout gestation. The adequacy of the dose of thyroxine should be tested at least monthly up to week 24 and every 6 to 8 weeks afterward by measuring serum-free T$_4$ and TSH levels, starting within 30 days of initiation of treatment.

28.13 PROGNOSIS AND FOLLOW-UP

As extensively discussed in this chapter, iodine deficiency during gestation can result in fatal events such as pregnancy interruption; if pregnancy progresses, it can cause brain damage leading to major or irreversible minor neurointellectual disorders in the offspring. These disorders may be prevented easily by administering adequate iodine supplements (iodized salt and prenatal preparations containing at least 150 µg iodine) to iodine-deficient mothers along with close monitoring of maternal thyroid function throughout pregnancy in iodine-deficient areas and prompt correction of any insufficiencies by LT$_4$ and iodine. In clinical practice, maternal thyroid parameters should be tested at least once per trimester in cases of normal results and every 4 to 6 weeks if LT$_4$ treatment is needed.

REFERENCES

1. de Benoist, B. and Delange, F., Eds. 2007. Report of WHO technical consultation on prevention and control of iodine deficiency in pregnancy, lactation, and in children less than 2 years of age. *Publ Health Nutr* (Special Issue) 10: 1527–1611.
2. Delange, F. 2007. Iodine requirements during pregnancy, lactation and the neonatal period and indicators of optimal iodine nutrition. *Publ Health Nutr* 10: 1571–1580.
3. Glinoer, D. 1997. The regulation of thyroid function in pregnancy: pathways of endocrine adaptation from physiology to pathology. *Endocr Rev* 18: 404.
4. Pedersen, K.M., Laurberg, P., Iversen, E. et al. 1993. Amelioration of some pregnancy-associated variations in thyroid function induced by iodine supplementation. *J Clin Endocrinol Metab* 77: 1078.
5. Romano, R., Jannini, E.A., Pepe, M. et al. 1991. The effects of iodoprophylaxis on thyroid size during pregnancy. *Am J Obstet Gynecol* 164: 482.
6. Abalovich, M. et al. 2007. Management of thyroid dysfunction during pregnancy and postpartum: an Endocrine Society clinical practice guideline. *J Clin Endocrinol Metab* 92: S1–S47.
7. Krassas, G.E., Poppe, K., and Glinoer, D. 2010. Thyroid function and human reproductive health. *Endocr Rev* 31: 702–755.
8. Moleti, M., Presti, V. P. L., Campolo M. C. et al. 2008. Iodine prophylaxis using iodized salt and risk of maternal thyroid failure in conditions of mild iodine deficiency. *J Clin Endocrinol Metab* 93: 2616–2621.
9. Berbel, P., Mestre, J.L., Santamaría A. et al. 2009. Delayed neurobehavioral development in children born to pregnant women with mild hypothyroxinemia during the first month of gestation: the importance of early iodine supplementation. *Thyroid* 19; 511–519.
10. Moleti, M., LoPresti, V.P., Mattina, F. et al. 2009. Gestational thyroid function abnormalities in conditions of mild iodine deficiency: early screening versus continuous monitoring of maternal thyroid status. *Eur J Endocrinol* 160: 611–617.
11. Glinoer, D. and Delange, F. 2000. The potential repercussions of maternal, fetal, and neonatal hypothyroxinemia on the progeny. *Thyroid* 10: 871–887.

29 Thyroid in the Elderly

Stefano Mariotti

CONTENTS

Key words: amiodarone-induced thyrotoxicosis (AIT), antithyroid auto-antibodies (ATAs), free thyroxine (FT_4), free triiodothyronine (FT_3), non-thyroidal illnesses (NTIs), non-thyroidal illness syndrome (NTIS), reverse T_3 (rT_3), subclinical hyperthyroidism (SHyper), subclinical hypothyroidism (SHypo), thyroid hormone binding globulin (TBG), antithyroglobulin auto-antibodies (Tg-Abs), toxic multinodular goiter (TMNG), toxic nodule (TN), thyrotropin releasing hormone (TRH), thyroid stimulating hormone (TSH), thyroxine (T_4), total thyroxine (TT_4), triiodothyronine (T_3), total triiodothyronine (TT_3).

29.1 INTRODUCTION

The relationship between aging and thyroid function and thyroid diseases and aging has been the object of considerable interest for a long time.[1] Several reasons justify this interest, stemming from the observation that symptoms of aging and common age-associated diseases may be difficult to distinguish from true hypothyroidism, leading to the hypothesis (largely disproved) that decreased thyroid function is a biological hallmark of senescence.

Moreover, thyroid diseases are frequent in the elderly and reveal specific and often subtle clinical manifestations when compared to those observed in younger patients. They are vague, subtle, and often hidden by concurrent diseases. The presence of age-associated disease with the consequent intake of several drugs may further mask specific hyperthyroid or hypothyroid symptoms and complicate the interpretation of thyroid function tests.

Increased risk of complications and/or drug interactions may require particular attention by a physician to select the most appropriate therapy. This is particularly true for hyperthyroidism (including mild and subclinical thyrotoxicosis) which in the elderly always requires treatment to avoid increased cardiovascular morbidity and mortality. Mild hypothyroidism may be associated in the oldest old with increased survival and should not be treated.

29.2 THYROID FUNCTION IN THE ELDERLY

29.2.1 NORMAL PHYSIOLOGY OF HYPOTHALAMUS–PITUITARY–THYROID FUNCTION

Several studies conducted over several decades provide evidence that normal senescence is associated in humans with almost normal hypothalamic–pituitary–thyroid activity.[1] Several minor thyroid function abnormalities have been described in the elderly, but most of them are the consequences of concomitant non-thyroidal illness (NTI) as detailed in Section 29.3.

The low metabolic rate in the elderly, once attributed to reduced thyroid function, is presently explained by a decrease of lean body mass.[1] Although reduced iodine uptake and thyroxine (T_4) secretion have been documented in aged humans, the degradation rate of T_4 is also decreased and both total (TT_4) and free (FT_4) serum T_4 concentrations are substantially unchanged even in the oldest old.[1] A different behavior is observed with serum total (TT_3) and free (FT_3) triiodothyronine (T_3) that show age-dependent decreases up to 95 to 100 years of age only partially explained by concurrent NTI.[1]

In selected groups of healthy elderly up to 85 years of age, serum thyroid stimulating hormone (TSH) concentrations are no different from those of younger adults in basal conditions.[1,2] Studies on circadian TSH secretion in small groups of highly selected healthy subjects displayed reductions of the daily secretion rate with blunting and a 1- to 1.5-hour anticipation of the nocturnal peak.[3] The evaluation of TSH response to thyrotropin releasing hormone (TRH) in the elderly provides inconsistent results (reduced, unchanged, increased). The pharmacological nature of this test and the difficulty of excluding in the elderly the subtle forms of mild thyroid failure represent the most probable explanation of this finding.[1] All these data suggest that a mild form of central hypothyroidism is present in the oldest old subjects, independent of NTI.

More recently, this picture has been challenged by results obtained in epidemiological studies of wide cohorts from the general population that show that mean circulating TSH concentrations are significantly higher in subjects aged >80 years even after careful exclusion of individuals at risk for mild primary hypothyroidism (i.e., those with detectable serum antithyroid autoantibodies [ATAs] or thyroid ultrasound abnormalities suggestive of underlying thyroid autoimmunity).[4] Although the question remains unsettled, a reasonable explanation for this phenomenon may be the impossibility in epidemiological studies to apply the strict criteria to select healthy individuals among centenarians and other small groups of elderly subjects.

29.2.2 THE CONUNDRUM OF AGING, NTI, AND THYROID FUNCTION

The major problem encountered in studying "normal" thyroid functions in old subjects is the high prevalence in the elderly of acute and chronic NTIs, multidrug intakes, and mild to severe nutrition defects. Since all these conditions are associated with alterations in thyroid function tests (known as NTI syndrome or NTIS), the assessment of thyroid function in the elderly is not easy and may be misleading.

NTIS is associated with a wide spectrum of thyroid function test abnormalities (typically low serum T_3 with high reverse T_3 [rT_3], normal to low T_4, and low to elevated TSH), depending on the acute or chronic nature of the underlying diseases, associated complications, and drug actions.[5] There is a rough correlation of the magnitudes of functional abnormalities, disease severity, and poor prognosis. Low serum T_4 is particularly associated with reduced survival. Several mechanisms are involved in circulating thyroid hormones in NTIS. Low serum T_3 and increased serum rT_3 concentration result from decreased peripheral conversion of T_4 to T_3 (from decreased intracellular T_4 availability to tissue 5′-deiodinase and/or reduced activity of this enzyme).[5]

Decreased serum TSH and increased T_4 clearance for reduced serum thyroid hormone binding globulin (TBG) synthesis or binding capacity due to the presence of circulating inhibitors (such as free fatty acids) account for low serum T_4 concentration. The presence of circulating substances that can interfere with the binding of thyroid hormone to TBG and other carrier proteins accounts for the marked variability observed in free thyroid hormone concentrations noted by most of the commonly available one-step FT_4 and FT_3 assays. Serum TSH concentration may be reduced in NTIS, especially in acutely sick patients and those with low energy intake or concurrent glucocorticoid or dopamine treatment. However, due to the sensitivity of third-generation assays (<0.01/mU/L), most patients with NTIS have detectable TSH levels.[6]

It is important to recall that during the recovery phases of several NTIs, serum TSH may transiently rise up to 15 to 20 mU/L, a condition that should not be confused with primary mild hypothyroidism. Thyroid function test abnormalities typical of NTIS are common in aged patients with concomitant diseases and to a lesser degree may also be observed in euthyroid healthy elderly. Some clues to differentiate the two

TABLE 29.1

Thyroid Function Test Abnormalities Observed in Euthyroid Aging and Subjects with NTIS

Thyroid Function Test	Euthyroid Aging	Subjects with NTIS
TSH	$=, =/\downarrow$	$=/\downarrow, =, \uparrow$§
FT_4, TT_4	$=$	$=, \downarrow, \uparrow$§§
FT_3, TT_3	$=, =/\downarrow$	$\downarrow\downarrow$
rT_3	$=, =/\uparrow$	$\uparrow\uparrow$

Note: $=$:Normal; $=/\uparrow$: slightly increased; $\uparrow$: increased, $\uparrow\uparrow$: markedly increased. $=/\downarrow$: slightly decreased; $\downarrow$: decreased; $\downarrow\downarrow$: markedly decreased. § = Recovery phase of NTI. §§ = Depending on method employed for FT_4; some one-step methods may be unreliable in NTI.

conditions are reported in Table 29.1, but confirmation of suspected intrinsic thyroid conditions may require deferment of thyroid testing until the specific NTI subsides. From a practical view, the identification of thyroid dysfunctions in severely ill patients cannot rely only on serum TSH alone (as suggested by most clinical practice guidelines for adults without evidence of concurrent NTI). It requires at least the combined measurements of serum FT_4 and TSH and a confirmation after adequate follow-up.

29.2.3 Age-Associated Diseases and Thyroid Economy

Beyond the general concepts examined in the previous paragraph, from a practical view, the interference of associated NTIs in elderly patients is often mediated by the effects of drug intake and this issue deserves more detailed examination. Moreover, ATAs are often detectable in subjects aged over 60 to 65 years in the absence of even very mild abnormalities in thyroid function. Thus, before describing specific thyroid dysfunctions and diseases in the elderly, the next section focuses on the effects of drugs of common geriatric use and on the relationships between age and thyroid autoimmunity.

29.2.4 Thyroid Function and Drug Intake

A high percentage of geriatric patients take medications that may interact[7,8] with thyroid function, thyroid tests, and levothyroxine (LT_4) substitution therapy. A complete discussion of the effects of drugs on thyroid function and economy is beyond the purpose of this chapter and is reported in detail elsewhere in this book (Chapter 31).

In general, drugs may interfere with thyroid function via several mechanisms (1) altering the results of thyroid hormone and TSH measurements without altering thyroid status; (2) inducing hypo- or hyperthyroidism; and (3) influencing optimal substitution doses required in hypothyroid patients by interfering with LT_4 absorption and metabolism. A representative but not exhaustive list of the relevant drugs is

TABLE 29.2
Main Drugs Interfering with Thyroid Function Tests without Producing Significant Thyroid Dysfunction

Drugs Decreasing TSH Secretion	Drugs Increasing TBG Concentration	Drugs Decreasing TBG Concentration	Drugs Interfering with Thyroid Hormone Binding to TBG	Drugs Decreasing T_4 to T_3 Conversion
Glucocorticoids	Estrogens (oral)	Androgens	Furosemide	Amiodarone
Dopamine	Tamoxifen	Anabolic steroids	Salicylates	Iopanoic acid
Octreotide	Mitotane	Nicotinic acid	Fenflofenac	Propranolol
Lanreotide	Fluorouracil	Glucocorticoids	Mefenamic acid	Glucocorticoids
	Perphenazine	L-asparaginase	Phenytoin	
	Clofibrate		Carbamazepine	
			Heparin	

TABLE 29.3
Drugs Potentially Producing Hypothyroidism or Hyperthyroidism

Thyrotoxicosis	Hypothyroidism	Thyrotoxicosis and/or Hypothyroidism (Silent Drug-Induced Thyroiditis)
Amiodarone	Thionamides	Interferon-α
Iodine excess	Lithium	Interleukin-2
	Iodine excess	Granulocyte macrophage colony-stimulating factor
	Amiodarone	Lithium
	Aminoglutethymide	Multiple kinase inhibitors
	Resorcinol (topical use on abraded skin)	

reported in Tables 29.2 through 29.4. The tables also show the mechanisms responsible for the specific interference.

Among these drugs, particular attention to the frequency and relevance of thyroid functional effects should be given to amiodarone and other iodine-containing compounds, cytokines (interferon-α, interleukin-2) and other biological drugs, and lithium. Further details on the complex thyroid dysfunctions related to the use of these drugs will be reported later in this chapter and elsewhere in this book. Clinicians should recall that many drugs (sulfonamides, sulfanylureas, ethionamide, p-aminosalicylic acid, phenylbutazone, and nicardipine) although able to inhibit thyroid function, display antithyroid activity that is too weak to directly cause thyroid failure. Thus, underlying thyroid abnormality should be always suspected if primary hypothyroidism is clearly documented in patients taking these drugs.[7]

Another aspect of thyroid–drug interaction relates to the effects exerted by altered thyroid function on the pharmacokinetics of many drugs needed to treat concomitant

TABLE 29.4
Drugs Influencing LT_4 Efficacy in Hypothyroid Patients on Substitution Therapy

Mechanism	Drug	Final Effect on LT_4 Requirement
Decreased LT_4 absorption	Soybean	
	Cholestiramine	
	Colestipol	
	Sucralfate	
	Aluminum hydroxide	
	Ferrous sulfate	
	Phenytoin	
Increased non-deiodinating T_4 clearance	Rifampin	Increased requirement of LT_4
	Carbamazepine	
	Phenytoin	
	Phenobarbital	
Decreased T_4 to T_3 conversion	Amiodarone	
	Propranolol	
Increased TBG	Estrogens	
Decreased TBG	Androgens	Decreased requirement of LT_4

diseases.[7] Increased and decreased plasma half-lives of digoxin, morphine, glucocorticoids, and insulin are observed in hypothyroidism and hyperthyroidism, often requiring careful adjustment of maintenance doses. Of particular relevance in geriatric patients are the effects of thyroid function on vitamin K-dependent coagulation factors that show slower clearance and consequent resistance to the anticoagulant effect of dicoumarols in hypothyroid patients; the opposite effects are observed in hyperthyroidism.[9]

29.2.5   THYROID AUTOIMMUNITY AND AGING

Several serum autoantibodies including antithyroid autoantibodies (ATAs) are frequently detected in the elderly in the absence of overt clinical manifestations of corresponding autoimmune disease.[1,10] Limiting the present discussion to the thyroid gland, it should be noted that the prevalence of clinically overt autoimmune thyroid diseases (AITDs such as chronic autoimmune [Hashimoto's] thyroiditis or Basedow-Graves' disease) is not increased in the elderly although primary autoimmune hypothyroidism (both overt and subclinical) is more frequently observed after 55 years of age.[10] It has been speculated that this peculiar age-dependent incidence of AITD may be a consequence of preferential expression in aged subjects of destructive autoimmune mechanisms and/or increased target gland susceptibility.[10]

As discussed later in this chapter, thyroid autoimmunity and/or mild hypothyroidism have long been suspected as risk factors for common age-associated disorders, particularly coronary heart disease, but no evidence supporting this hypothesis was noted in recent studies.[11] In contrast to hospitalized or institutional elderly, where high prevalence of detectable serum ATAs has been reported, ATAs are rarely found in free-living healthy centenarians and other highly selected aged populations,[10] suggesting that age-associated thyroid autoimmune phenomena may be indirect markers of age-associated disease rather than consequences of aging.

This hypothesis, however, is not supported by recent epidemiological studies carried out on females in the general population. The studies show that the fraction of frail elderly is increased in subjects with undetectable antithyroglobulin antibodies (Tg-Abs) that seem to represent a protective factor.[12] While the biological meaning of this observation remains unknown and needs further studies, from a practical view we can conclude that serum ATA measurement is certainly useful, as in younger subjects, to identify the autoimmune pathogenesis of thyroid dysfunctions but still cannot be proposed as a parameter to be included in a multifunctional geriatric evaluation.

29.3 THYROID DISEASES IN THE ELDERLY

29.3.1 HYPOTHYROIDISM

29.3.1.1 Prevalence

The prevalence of overt primary hypothyroidism for individuals over 65 years of age is reported as 0.5 to 6% while subclinical or mild thyroid failure ranges from 4 to 20%.[1,4] Hypothyroidism is more frequent in Caucasian women, in hospitalized as compared to free-living subjects, and in iodine-rich rather than iodine-deficient regions. The latter finding is believed to be due to iodine-dependent exacerbation of thyroid autoimmunity.[13]

29.3.1.2 Etiology and Pathogenesis

In comparison to younger patients, primary hypothyroidism in the elderly is less frequently caused by autoimmune thyroiditis which, however, still remains the main etiologic factor. The second most common cause of hypothyroidism in the elderly is iatrogenic and results from thyroid surgery, administration of antithyroid drugs or radioiodine, or head and neck radiation for non-thyroidal conditions. In iodine-rich areas, excess iodine derived from drugs (most typically amiodarone) or iodinated radiographic contrast agents may produce transient or permanent hypothyroidism. In iodine-deficient populations, the same substances are more frequently responsible for thyroxicosis.[13] Iodine-induced hypothyroidism develops preferentially in glands with underlying subtle organification defects such as coexistent autoimmune thyroiditis or previous radioiodine administration.

29.3.1.3 Clinical Features and Diagnosis

Hypothyroidism develops insidiously and the clinical diagnosis is very difficult because symptoms of aging or common age-associated diseases (cold intolerance, fatigue, dry skin, constipation, poor appetite, pericardial effusions, mental deterioration, hearing loss) may be confused with symptoms of true hypothyroidism. Because thyroid failure in the elderly often lacks its classic clinical features,[7] as exemplified by the frequent loss rather than gain of weight resulting from reduced appetite.

Thus, individually taken, none of the above signs or symptoms is indicative of hypothyroidism in elderly patients. The clue to the diagnosis may be a cluster of signs including metabolic (unexplained increases in serum cholesterol and creatine phosphokinase levels), hematological (macrocytic anemia), gastrointestinal (severe constipation, loss of appetite), and cardiovascular (congestive heart failure with restrictive cardiomyopathy, pericardial effusion) disturbances. Arthritic complaints, neurological signs (cerebellar ataxia, carpal tunnel syndrome, peripheral neuropathy) are common.

Neuropsychiatric manifestations (depression, lethargy, memory loss and apathy) are sometime observed, while psychosis is rare, but severe (myxedema madness). Old hypothyroid patients may present dementia, which is often preexisting and rarely improves after correction of hypothyroidism. Elderly patients are at risk of myxedema coma that may be precipitated by concurrent NTI or cold exposure and suspected in patients showing hypothermia, hyponatremia, hypoglycemia, and neurological signs. The mortality of this complication is high, unless vigorous therapy (see below) is given immediately.

As in younger subjects, the single best diagnostic test for primary hypothyroidism is increased serum TSH concentration, although confirmation is often needed. As discussed earlier, serum TSH may show transient non-specific lowering and subsequent increase during several NTIs and their recovery phases. Moreover, old subjects with primary hypothyroidism may have significantly lower serum TSH concentrations (due to NTIs and/or drug interference) than younger hypothyroid patients, possibly leading to underscoring the severity of thyroid failure. As noted earlier, TT_4 and FT_4 may be low also in severe NTIs, but markedly reduced serum T_4 concentrations are seen only in hypothyroidism. As in the younger patients, detection of circulating ATAs and/or a thyroid hypoechogenic pattern on ultrasonography help identify autoimmune primary hypothyroidism due to chronic autoimmune (Hashimoto's) thyroiditis (see Chapter 4).

29.3.1.4 Treatment

Treatment of overt hypothyroidism is usually LT_4 at doses that stably maintain normal serum TSH concentrations. In young adults, the average daily replacement dose is about 1.6 µg/kg body weight. Elderly patients require lower doses.[8] The therapeutic range in the elderly is narrow and old hypothyroid patients require close monitoring of serum TSH to avoid under- and overtreatment that may be observed in nearly half of geriatric patients.[14] To avoid ischemic or arrhythmic heart complications, LT_4 therapy should be cautiously initiated with 12.5 to 25 µg/day, followed by progressive increments of 12.5 to 25 µg/day every 4 to 8 weeks, to reach the full replacement dose in several months.

Particular attention should be paid in patients with coexistent or suspected cardiac disease because LT_4 substitution may precipitate angina or myocardial infarction and, in some cases, a full normalization of circulating TSH cannot be safely obtained. Long-term LT_4 substitution does not reduce bone mineral density, provided that serum TSH concentration is not suppressed.[8]

Therapy of hypothyroid coma represents an endocrine emergency and, unlike other forms of long-standing hypothyroidism, requires rapid restoration of normal thyroid hormone concentration associated with the correction of accompanying respiratory, cardiovascular, and fluid electrolyte abnormalities. This may be achieved with a single large intravenous bolus dose (300 to 500 µg) of LT_4 followed by maintenance doses of 50 to 100 µg/day intravenously until oral therapy can be re-instituted.[8,15] The use of LT_3 alone or in combination with LT_4 has been proposed to obtain a more rapid onset of action and overcome the block of the conversion of T_4 to T_3 typical of critical illness,[15] but the advantage of this approach remains to be proven.

29.3.2 SUBCLINICAL HYPOTHYROIDISM

Subclinical hypothyroidism (SHypo) is a condition of mild thyroid failure conventionally defined by raised circulating TSH associated with serum TT_4 (and/or FT_4) or TT_3 (and/or FT_3) still within the normal range and frequently observed in old people. As for overt thyroid failure, most cases are of SHypo are due to autoimmune thyroiditis or previous treatments of hyperthyroidism. SHypo may progress to overt hypothyroidism, with serum TSH concentration and ATA titers representing the main risk factors. In elderly subjects with SHypo, the proportion of subjects progressing to overt thyroid failure is about 25%, while normalization of serum TSH is observed in over one-third of cases.[16]

While overt hypothyroidism is associated with hyperlipidemia and increased risk of coronary artery disease, the cardiovascular risk associated with SHypo is still debated. Recent meta-analyses provided evidence for a slight but significant increased risk of coronary artery disease conferred by SHypo in young and middle-aged adults while the effect was not significant in subjects aged above 65 years. Indications for LT_4 substitution therapy in SHypo remain controversial for all ages and replacement therapy is generally advised only when serum TSH concentration exceeds 10 mU/L and/or when serum TSH is lower (5 to 10 mU/L) but associated to high titer serum ATAs and/or hypercholesterolemia, and/or symptoms suggestive of mild thyroid failure.[16]

These recommendations do not necessarily apply to the elderly, especially the oldest old individuals. Meta-analysis of available studies suggests that SHypo represents a small but significant risk factor for ischemic heart disease and cardiac mortality only in subjects below 65 years of age.[17]

Moreover, in very old people, mild hypothyroidism may be associated with longer survival, suggesting that lower metabolic status may exert some protective effect.[18] As summarized in Figure 29.1, mild thyroid failure along with other genetic or environmental factors may contribute to increase cardiovascular and other disease risks up to about 65 years of age but have opposite effects on the oldest old population that are enriched in selected low-risk survivors.[18]

An additional important point to consider before starting LT_4 treatment in an elderly patient with any degree of hypothyroidism is a potential adverse effect such as worsening of an underlying myocardial ischemia. As a matter of fact, SHypo in subjects older than 85 years very rarely, if ever, requires treatment. In old patients with overt hypothyroidism who take LT_4 substitution therapy, the dose of thyroid hormone should be reduced often. It has been suggested that in subjects aged 80 to 85 years or older, the target serum TSH should probably be settled at a concentration of 4.0 to 6.0 mIU/L.[19]

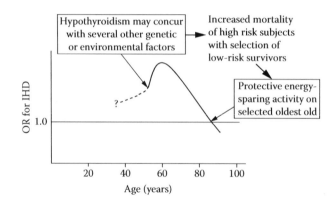

FIGURE 29.1   Hypothetical relationship between age and relative relevance of mild hypothyroidism as a risk factor for ischemic heart disease (IHD).

29.3.3   HYPERTHYROIDISM

29.3.3.1   Prevalence and Pathogenesis

Hyperthyroidism is a rather frequent disease in the elderly, with a prevalence ranging from 0.5 to about 2.3%.[13] As in younger patients, the most frequent causes are Graves' disease, toxic multinodular goiter (TMNG), and solitary toxic nodules (TNs), but the relative frequency of TMNG and TN is higher, especially in iodine deficiency areas where the prevalence in the general population of nodular goiter is high.[13]

In aged patients, hyperthyroidism due to drug intake is also more frequently observed, although overt hyperthyroidism is rare. Errors or inadequate compliance in thyroid hormone intake are frequently responsible for subtle or mild forms of iatrogenic thyrotoxicosis and require frequent checking of serum TSH concentrations. Iodine-induced hyperthyroidism is also not infrequent in geriatric patients due to the use of iodine-containing medications (e.g., amiodarone) or radiographic contrast media.

Amiodarone-induced thyrotoxicosis (AIT) may be observed in about 10% of patients residing in iodine-deficient areas and is less frequent in areas with normal or high iodine intakes where the predominant thyroid dysfunction produced by amiodarone is hypothyroidism.[20] AIT may produce sustained hypothyroidism in patients with preexisting thyroid autonomy (nodular goiter or preclinical Basedow-Graves' disease: type I AIT), or transient destructive thyrotoxicosis (type II AIT), but a precise distinction between the two types of AIT is not always possible because a single patient may have both conditions.[20]

29.3.3.2   Clinical Features and Diagnosis

Elderly hyperthyroid patients typically display fewer signs and symptoms, hence the term *apathetic* or *masked hyperthyroidism* has been suggested. Eye signs are often lacking, but Graves' ophthalmopathy, when present, is usually worse.[7] Tachycardia is less common, although it may be found in more than 50% of older patients. Presenting symptoms of thyrotoxicosis in the elderly frequently relate to heart complications including refractory congestive heart failure and angina. A high prevalence (about 10 to 35%) of atrial fibrillation is found in thyrotoxic patients, with the highest percentages seen in elderly males who also show high rates of arterial embolism (10 to 40%), perhaps due to a procoagulation state induced by hyperthyroidism.[7,9]

Weight loss is severe and may be associated with muscle wasting and weakness since hyperthyroidism in the elderly is often characterized by anorexia rather than increased appetite. Neurologic symptoms including depression up to lethargy, agitation and anxiety, dementia, and confusion are often present and may dominate the clinical picture. Accelerated bone loss caused by excess thyroid hormone is responsible for a further increase of the risks of osteoporosis and bone fracture typical of old age.[7]

With the exception of the very rare TSH-secreting adenomas, the diagnosis of overt hyperthyroidism is established on the basis of standard criteria (increased TT_4 or FT_4 and/or TT_3 or FT_3 and undetectable TSH measured by sensitive assays). As discussed earlier, several conditions (NTIs and drug intake) may cause reduction of serum TSH in elderly patients independent of hyperthyroidism, Although with appropriately sensitive (third generation) assays, serum TSH concentration is generally <0.01 mU/L in hyperthyroidism and in critically ill patients is between 0.01 and 0.1 mU/L, complete discrimination between the two conditions is not possible.[6]

Hence, biochemical diagnosis of overt hyperthyroidism must be confirmed always by increased circulating thyroid hormones, although inappropriately low serum T_3 and, more rarely, T_4 may be observed in severely ill patients. The diagnosis of the specific type of thyrotoxicosis is then based on thyroid scan, radioiodine uptake, and thyroid ultrasound; radioiodine uptake is particularly useful in differentiating hyperthyroidism from destructive or exogenous thyrotoxicosis.

29.3.3.3 Treatment

The high relapse rate after withdrawal and the increased incidence of adverse effects make thionamide antithyroid drugs (methimazole, carbimazole, and propylthiouracil) not recommended for long-term therapy.[21] Radioiodine (^{131}I) is often the treatment of choice for old hyperthyroid patients, since it produces a definitive cure and avoids the risks of surgery.[21] The main limits of ^{131}I therapy are represented by the time (2 to 12 weeks) needed to control hyperthyroidism and the transient worsening of thyrotoxicosis due to destructive radiation thyroiditis and/or antithyroid drug withdrawal.[21]

Stable euthyroidism should be therefore achieved with antithyroid drugs before ^{131}I administration and careful control of heart rate should be accomplished with beta blockers (or calcium channel blockers) as long as the patient remains thyrotoxic. In elderly patients, re-institution of thionamide therapy is often required to control thyroid function after ^{131}I administration: if possible, antithyroid drug resumption should be deferred at least 1 to 2 weeks to maintain treatment efficacy.

High doses of ^{131}I are recommended in old patients to avoid the risk of relapse or incomplete control of hyperthyroidism. Hypothyroidism may develop any time (generally within the first few months) after radioiodine therapy. Long-term follow-up of thyroid function is mandatory and overt thyroid failure should be corrected with minimal doses of LT_4 sufficient to maintain serum TSH in the desired range (see Sections 29.3.3.1 and 29.3.3.2).

Treatment of iodine-induced thyrotoxicosis and particularly AITs is difficult because iodine overload usually prevents the use of ^{131}I, thyroidectomy is hazardous in old patients with uncontrolled hyperthyroidism, and the response to conventional doses of antithyroid drugs is poor.[22] For a complete discussion of the therapeutic options in iodine-induced thyrotoxicosis, the reader is referred to Chapter 23 of this book.

29.3.4 SUBCLINICAL HYPERTHYROIDISM

Subclinical hyperthyroidism (SHyper), defined as low serum TSH and normal thyroid hormone concentrations, is caused by the same conditions responsible for overt hyperthyroidism. However, especially in aged populations, most cases arose from autonomous functioning uninodular or multinodular glands or exogenous thyroid hormone intake. The prevalence of subclinical hyperthyroidism is still incompletely known but is increased in the elderly and in populations living in iodine-deficient areas,[13] reaching about 10% if all subjects with serum TSH concentrations <0.4 mU/L are considered or 2 to 3% if the cut-off of serum TSH is set at <0.1 mU/L.

Iatrogenic thyrotoxicosis is still a frequent complication in the elderly. A recent U.S. survey found evidence of overtreatment in about one-half of old patients receiving LT$_4$ therapy, suggesting that more efforts should be made to reduce the impact of this avoidable complication.[14] It should be recalled that, with the exception of metastatic differentiated thyroid cancer, there is no indication for TSH-suppressive therapy with LT$_4$ in the elderly.[16] As discussed earlier, SHyper must be distinguished from other causes of low serum TSH such as NTIS.

Although most patients lack specific symptoms and the proportion progressing to overt hyperthyroidism is low (2 to 10%),[16] SHyper is clinically relevant in the elderly. Increased risk of atrial fibrillation has been clearly documented in male subjects aged over 60 years with low serum TSH concentration. Both endogenous and exogenous types of SHyper are significant risks for reduced bone density in postmenopausal women.[16] Based on these considerations and supported by the potential protective effects of mild thyroid failure in the oldest old subjects, there is general agreement that SHyper in the elderly deserves active treatment despite the lack of placebo-controlled longitudinal studies.[16]

29.3.5 NODULAR GOITER

Age-dependent increases in thyroid volume and nodularity have been documented by echography both in iodine-sufficient and iodine-deficient areas.[1] In non-endemic countries, the prevalence of clinically evident thyroid nodules is approximately 5% at 60 years of age, but pathological studies documented the presence of thyroid nodules in up to 90% of women and 60% of men over 70 to 80 years of age.[1] In areas of iodine deficiency, the ultrasonographic prevalence of nodular goiter after 60 years of age often exceeds 50%,[1] and is often associated with functional autonomy, with a full spectrum ranging from euthyroidism to overt hyperthyroidism.[13]

The diagnostic evaluation of nodular goiter in the elderly is similar to that in younger patients. Relevant nodules require fine needle aspiration cytology, although due to the increased prevalence of nodular goiter in the elderly, a thyroid nodule is less likely to be malignant in old than in young patients.[1,23] Most non-toxic nodular goiters are managed conservatively and surgery is indicated in the presence of strong suspicion of malignancy or significant airway obstruction. In old patients with contraindications to surgery, radioiodine has been successfully used to achieve partial reduction in thyroid size and relief of pressure symptoms. The effectiveness of this procedure may be increased by pretreatment with recombinant human TSH,[24] but the precise indication and procedure of ^{131}I therapy for non-toxic goiter in elderly patients remains to be settled. TSH-suppressive therapy with LT$_4$ in old patients with nodular goiter is contraindicated due to higher cardiovascular risks and the possibility of precipitating thyrotoxicosis when areas of functional autonomy are present.

29.3.6 THYROID CANCER

The overall annual age-specific incidence rate of clinical and occult differentiated thyroid carcinoma does not increase with age, but papillary carcinoma occurs more frequently during the third and the fifth decades and follicular cancer peaks in the late fifth decade. As a consequence, the ratio of papillary to follicular thyroid carcinoma is lower in the elderly (2:1) compared to the values (3 to 4:1) observed in younger patients.[1,7] Anaplastic thyroid carcinoma, the most lethal thyroid neoplasm, is almost exclusively observed in patients over 65 year of age as are other rare thyroid neoplasms such as sarcomas and primary thyroid lymphomas. As a consequence, the prevalence of differentiated thyroid carcinomas is lower in older than in younger patients, accounting only for 50 to 60% of all thyroid cancers in those over 60 years of age.

Age at the onset of disease is an important prognostic factor in differentiated thyroid carcinoma because these tumors are more aggressive in older patients, especially in males.[1,25] Early preoperative diagnosis using fine needle aspiration cytology and urgent aggressive therapy are therefore recommended.

The therapeutic approach for differentiated thyroid cancer is similar to that followed for younger persons, with total thyroidectomy and radioiodine ablation followed by LT$_4$ therapy. TSH-suppressive doses may be justified in old patients only in the presence of documented metastatic diseases. Ongoing studies show that multiple kinase inhibitors may be useful in arresting the substantial progression of metastatic differentiated and medullary thyroid carcinomas, but no specific data for elderly patients are presently available. External radiation and chemotherapy are used in thyroid lymphoma and anaplastic carcinoma, although in the latter condition, the outcome is in general rapidly fatal.

REFERENCES

1. Mariotti, S., Franceschi, C., Cossarizza, A. et al. 1995. The aging thyroid. *Endocr Rev* 16: 686–715.
2. Mariotti, S., Barbesino, G., Caturegli, P. et al. 1993. Complex alteration of thyroid function in healthy centenarians. *J Clin Endocrinol Metab* 77: 1130–1134.
3. van Coevorden, A., Laurent, E., Decoster, C. et al. 1989. Decreased basal and stimulated thyrotropin secretion in healthy elderly men. *J Clin Endocrinol Metab* 69: 177–185.

4. Surks, M.I. and Hollowell, J.G. 2007. Age-specific distribution of serum thyrotropin and antithyroid antibodies in the U.S. population: implications for the prevalence of subclinical hypothyroidism. *J Clin Endocrinol Metab* 92: 4575–4582.

5. Warner, M.H. and Becket, G.J. 2010. Mechanisms behind the non-thyroidal illness syndrome: an update. *J Endocrinol* 205: 1–13.

6. Franklyn, J.A., Black, E.G., Betteridge, J. et al. 1994. Comparison of second and third generation methods for measurement of serum thyrotropin in patients with overt hyperthyroidism, patients receiving thyroxine therapy, and those with nonthyroidal illness. *J Clin Endocrinol Metab* 78: 1368–1371.

7. Chiovato, L., Mariotti, S., and Pinchera, A. 1997. Thyroid diseases in the elderly. *Baillières Clin Endocrinol Metab* 11: 251–270.

8. Mandel, S.J., Brent, G.A., and Larsen, P.R. 1993. Levothyroxine therapy in patients with thyroid disease. *Ann Intern Med* 119: 492–502.

9. Marongiu, F., Cauli, C., and Mariotti, S. 2004. Thyroid, hemostasis and thrombosis. *J Endocrinol Invest* 27: 1065–1071.

10. Mariotti, S., Chiovato, L., Franceschi, C. et al. 1998. Thyroid autoimmunity and aging. *Exp Gerontol* 33: 535–541.

11. Wells, B.J. and Hueston, W.J. 2005. Are thyroid peroxidase antibodies associated with cardiovascular disease risk in patients with subclinical hypothyroidism? *Clin Endocrinol (Oxf)* 62: 580–584.

12. Wang, G.C., Talor, M.V., Rose, N.R. et al. 2010. Thyroid autoantibodies are associated with a reduced prevalence of frailty in community-dwelling older women. *J Clin Endocrinol Metab* 95: 1161–1168.

13. Laurberg, P., Cerqueira, C., Ovesen, L. et al. 2010. Iodine intake as a determinant of thyroid disorders in populations. *Best Pract Res Clin Endocrinol Metab* 24: 13–27.

14. Somwaru, L.L., Arnold, A.M., Joshi, N. et al. 2009. High frequency of and factors associated with thyroid hormone over-replacement and under-replacement in men and women aged 65 and over. *J Clin Endocrinol Metab* 94: 1342–1345.

15. Wartofsky, L. 2005. Myxedema coma. In *Werner and Ingbar's The Thyroid: A Fundamental and Clinical Text*, 9th ed., Braverman, L.E. and Utiger, R.D., Eds. Philadelphia: Lippincott-Raven, 850–855.

16. Biondi, B. and Cooper, D. S. 2008. The clinical significance of subclinical thyroid dysfunction. *Endocr Rev* 29: 76–131.

17. Razvi, S., Shakoor, A., Vanderpump, M. et al. 2008. The influence of age on the relationship between subclinical hypothyroidism and ischemic heart disease: a meta-analysis. *J Clin Endocrinol Metab* 93: 2998–3007.

18. Mariotti, S. 2008. Mild hypothyroidism and ischemic heart disease: is age the answer? *J Clin Endocrinol Metab* 93: 2969–2971.

19. Cooper, D.S. 2004. Thyroid disease in the oldest old: the exception to the rule. *JAMA* 292: 2651–2654.

20. Martino, E., Bartalena, L., Bogazzi, F. et al. 2001. The effects of amiodarone on the thyroid. *Endocr Rev* 22: 240–254.

21. Chiovato, L., Santini, F., and Pinchera, A. 1995. Treatment of hyperthyroidism. *Thyroid Int.* 2: 3–23.

22. Martino, E., Aghini-Lombardi, F., Bartalena, L. et al. 1994. Enhanced susceptibility to amiodarone-induced hypothyroidism in patients with thyroid autoimmune disease. *Arch Intern Med* 154: 2722–2726.

23. Boelaert, K., Horacek, J., Holder, R. L. et al. 2006. Serum thyrotropin concentration as a novel predictor of malignancy in thyroid nodules investigated by fine-needle aspiration. *J Clin Endocrinol Metab* 91: 4295–4301.

24. Fast, S., Nielsen, V.E., Bonnema, S.J. et al. 2009. Time to reconsider nonsurgical therapy of benign non-toxic multinodular goitre: focus on recombinant human TSH augmented radioiodine therapy. *Eur J Endocrinol* 160: 517–528.
25. Haymart, M.R. 2009. Understanding the relationship between age and thyroid cancer. *Oncologist* 14: 216–221.

30 Thyroid and Drugs

Salvatore Benvenga, Rosaria M. Ruggeri,
and Francesco Trimarchi

CONTENTS

Key words: thyroid homeostasis drug interference, drug-induced hypothyroidism, drug-induced hyperthyroidism, drug-induced thyroiditis, drugs and LT$_4$ pharmacokinetics, lithium, amiodarone, immune modulators, tyrosine kinase inhibitors, thyroid function testing drug interference.

30.1 INTRODUCTION

Over the years, several drugs used to treat non-thyroidal conditions have been shown to clinically modify thyroid status or simply alter serum thyroid function tests with no clinical consequences.[1,2] Most of these drugs are prescribed by specialists other than endocrinologists in many different clinical settings (Tables 30.1 and 30.2). For this reason, an accurate pharmacological history is necessary for any patient who presents with problems related to thyroid diseases or with altered functional tests that do not allow clear and immediate explanation.

In this chapter, we focus on drugs that cause clinically relevant thyroid dysfunction, influence LT$_4$ requirements, and impair absorption of exogenous LT$_4$ (Table 30.3). Information on drugs that interfere with thyroid function testing will be also provided (Table 30.4).

TABLE 30.1
Drugs (Used in Endocrinology) Interfering with Thyroid Homeostasis[a]

Drug	Indications
Aminoglutethimide	Cushing's syndrome
Androgens	Male hypogonadism
Antiandrogens	Hyperandrogenism, acne, male precocious puberty
Beta blockers	Thyrotoxicosis
Bile acid sequestants (i.e., cholestyramine)	Dyslipidemia
Calcium carbonate, citrate, acetate	Osteoporosis, hypocalcemia
Corticosteroids	Adrenal insufficiency, late onset congenital adrenal hyperplasia (LOCAH), Graves' ophthalmopathy
Dopamine and dopamine agonists (bromocriptine, cabergoline)	Hyperprolactinemia
Estrogens	Amenorrhea, oligomenorrhea, hirsutism, contraception, menopause, osteoporosis
Growth hormone (GH)	GH deficiency
Isoflavones with estrogenic activitiwa	Menopause
L-carnitine	Thyrotoxicosis
Somatostatin analogs (octreotide)	Acromegaly, neuroendocrine tumors (NETs)
Spironolactone	Hirsutism, hair loss, hyperaldosteronism
Sulfonylureas	Type 2 diabetes

[a] Drugs listed in alphabetical order.

TABLE 30.2
Drugs Commonly Used to Treat Non-Endocrine Diseases that Interfere with Thyroid Homeostasis

Specialty	Drugs	Disease or Test
Cardiology	Amiodarone	Atrial fibrillation, angina pectoris
	Beta blockers	Arrhythmia, hypertension
	Calcium channel antagonists	Hypertension, heart failure
	α-Methyldopa	Hypertension (gestational, etc.)
	Diuretics	Hypertension, congestive heart failure, edema
	Dopamine, dobutamine	Cardiogenic shock
	Heparin	Thrombosis
	L-carnitine	Myocardial infarction
	Iodinate contrast media	Coronary angiography
Dermatology	Antiseptics and disinfectants containing iodine or resorcinol	Psoriasis, hidradenitis suppurativa, erythematous eczema, acne
	Resorcinol	
	Antiandrogens, estrogens	Acne, hirsutism, hair loss
Gastroenterology	Dopamine antagonists (domperidone and metoclopramide)	Gastroesophageal reflux disease (GERD)
	Proton pump inhibitors, H2 receptor antagonist, sucralfate, aluminum hydroxide	Gastritis
	Interferon-α (plus ribavirin)	Chronic hepatitis C
Gynecology	Antiseptics and disinfectants containing iodine or resorcinol, vaginal lavages	
	Estrogens	Oligoamenorrea, contraception, menopause
	Isoflavones with estrogen activities	Menopause
	Danazol	Endometriosis
	Interferons	HPV-related condylomatosis
	α-Methyldopa	Gestational hypertension, preeclampsia
Hematology	Ferrous sufate, ferrous gluconate	Anemia
	GM-CSF	Leukopenia
	Alkylating agents (cyclophosphamide)	Lymphomas and leukemias
	Interferons	Lymphomas and chronic leukemias
	Thalidomide	Multiple myelomas
Infectious disease	Antipyretics, antiinflammatories (NSAIDs)	Herpes virus infection
		HIV
	Interferons	Tuberculosis
	Idoxuridine	
	Ritonavir, stavudine	
	Rifampin, rifabutin	
	Sulfonamides	

Continued

TABLE 30.2 (continued)
Drugs Commonly Used to Treat Non-Endocrine Diseases that Interfere with Thyroid Homeostasis

Specialty	Drugs	Disease or Test
Intensive care	Dopamine, dobutamine	Cardiogenic shock
	Glucocorticoids	
Neurology and psychiatry	Alemtuzumab, interferon-β	Multiple sclerosis
	Amphetamines	Abuse
	Antiepilepsy drugs	Epilepsy, trigeminal neuralgia
	Antidepressive tricyclics Sertraline	Depression
	Lithium	Bipolar depression
	Antipsychotics (phenothiazines, haloperidol)	Schizophrenia, mania, dementia
	Benzodiazepines	Anxiety, insomnia
Oncology	5-Fluorouracil	Lymphomas and leukemias
	Tyrosine kinase inhibitors	Breast and prostate cancer, adrenal
	Alkylating agents (cyclophosphamide)	cancer
	Aminoglutethimide	Breast cancer
	Androgens, tamoxifen	Prostate cancer
	Antiandrogens	Cutaneous T cell lymphomas
	Bexarotene	Breast cancer and soft-tissue sarcoma
	GM-CSF	Melanoma, renal carcinoma
	Interleukin-2	Kaposi's sarcoma, renal carcinoma
	Interferons	
Ophthalmology	Eye drops containing iodine	Glaucoma
	Acetazolamide	Herpes virus infection
	Idoxuridine	Uveitis
	Interferons	
Otolaryngology	Collutories containing iodine	
Pulmonology	Antipyretics, antiinflammatories, analgesics (NSAIDs and glucocorticoids)	
	Antibiotics (rifampim, rifabutin)	Tuberculosis
	Glucocorticoids	Asthma, sarcoidosis
Rheumatology	Antipyretics, antiinflammatories, analgesics (NSAIDs and glucocorticoids)	
	Interferons	
	Cyclophosphamide	
Radiology	Iodinate contrast media	
Surgery	Antiseptics and disinfectants containing iodine or resorcinol	
	Antipyretics, analgesics (NSAIDs)	
	Antibiotics (sulfonamides)	
	Somatostatin	Acute pancreatitis, gastroenteric hemorrhage
	Iodinate contrast media	Cholecystography

TABLE 30.2 (continued)
Drugs Commonly Used to Treat Non-Endocrine Diseases that Interfere with Thyroid Homeostasis

Specialty	Drugs	Disease or Test
Urology	Antiandrogens	Prostate cancer
General practice	Antipyretics, antiinflammatories, analgesics (NSAIDs and glucocorticoids)	
	Antibiotics (sulfonamides, rifampim, rifabutin)	
	Antiacids and antisecretory drugs	GERD, gastritis
	Dopamine antagonists (domperidone and metoclopramide)	GERD
	Beta blockers	Hypertension, tachycardia
	Diuretics	Hypertension, edemas
	Calcium carbonate	Osteoporosis
	Ferrous sulfate, ferrous gluconate	Anemia
	Heparin	Thrombosis

The effects of drugs whose fundamental purpose is to target the thyroid such as the thionamde antithyroid drugs, recombinant human TSH, and iodine will not be examined here. Due to space limitations, only representative papers can be cited in this chapter.

30.2   DRUG-INDUCED HYPOTHYROIDISM

30.2.1   LITHIUM

Lithium carbonate is used to treat bipolar depression. It is estimated that 1 in 200 persons receives lithium for treatment of bipolar disorders. Over the years, a large body of clinical knowledge has accumulated on the effects of lithium on thyroid physiology[1–3] and the association of lithium treatment and hypothyroidism, or less frequently hyperthyroidism (see below), is well documented. Lithium is concentrated by the thyroid, inhibits thyroid hormone release and, to a lower extent thyroid hormone synthesis, thus causing a compensatory increase in TSH levels. This may result in the development of goiter in up to 40% of cases and either subclinical or overt hypothyroidism in up to 35%.[3]

The presentation of subclinical or clinical hypothyroidism in lithium-treated patients is not different from presentations seen in other causes of hypothyroidism. Symptoms and signs of hypothyroidism may appear from weeks to years of starting lithium. Lithium-induced hypothyroidism occurs predominantly in females (female:male ratio = 5:1), especially at older ages, in patients taking lithium more than 2 years, and in those who test positive for serum thyroid antibodies.[3] A pre-existing autoimmune thyroid disease may be exacerbated by lithium treatment, as demonstrated by the increase in serum levels of thyroid antibodies during lithium

TABLE 30.3

Main Drugs Altering Hormone Indices of Thyroid Function and Thyroid Autoimmunity

Drugs	Mechanism	Biochemical				Clinical		Actions				Section Citing Details
								Withdraw Drug AND		Continue Drug AND		
		FT₃	FT₄	TSH	Ab	Hypo	Hyper	Do Not Treat TD	Treat TD	Do Not Treat TD	Treat TD	
Lithium	↓ TH synthesis and release ↑ Thyroid autoimmunity	→	→	←	↑+	✓					✓	30.2.1
	Cytotoxic effect ↑ Thyroid autoimmunity	=↑	←	→	-/↑+		✓				✓	30.4.2
Cytokines (IFNs, IL–2, GM–CSF)	↑ Thyroid autoimmunity	→	→	←	+/↑+	✓					✓	30.2.2
		=↑	←	→	+/↑+		✓				✓	30.4.3
	Cytotoxic effect	→	→	←	-	✓					✓	30.2.2
		=↑	←	→	-		✓			✓		30.4.3
Amiodarone	Iodine excess (AIH and type 1 AIT)	→↑	→←	←→	-	✓	✓		✓ ✓		✓ ✓	30.2.3 30.4.1
	Cytotoxic effect (type 2 AIT)	=↑	←	→	-		✓				✓	30.4.2
Tyrosine kinase inhibitors (TKIs)	Cytotoxic effect (sunitinib and sorafenib)	→↑	→←	←→	-	✓	✓		✓		✓ ✓	30.2.4 30.4.4

Cytotoxic effect ↑Thyroid autoimmunity (nilotinib)	↓ =↑	→↓ ←↑	↑ ↓	-/+ -/+	✓	✓ ✓		30.2.4 30.4.4
↑Metabolic clearance rate (imatinib, sorafenib)	=	→	↑			✓		30.3.2.1
Flavonoids, resorcinol: ↓TH synthesis	→	→	↑	–	✓			30.2.5 30.2.6
Antacids,[a] calcium and ferrous formulations, cholestyramine: ↓LT$_4$ absorption / ↑LT$_4$ requirement in hypothyroid patients	=	→	↑	–		✓		30.3.1
Estrogens: ↑TBG / ↑LT$_4$ requirement in hypothyroid patients	=	→	↑	–		✓		30.3.2.1
Rifampicin, rifabutin, antiepilepsy drugs: ↑Metabolic clearance rate / ↑LT$_4$ requirement in hypothyroid patients	=	→	↑	–		✓		30.3.2.1
Alemtuzumab: ↑Thyroid autoimmunity	←	←	→	+		✓	✓	30.4.5
Bexarotene: ↓TSH synthesis	=↓	→	↓	–		✓		30.7.1
Aminoglutethimide: ↓TH synthesis and release	→	→	↑	–		✓		30.7.2

Note: Ab = thyroid autoantibodies. AIH = amiodarone-induced hypothyroidism. AIT = amiodarone-induced thyrotoxicosis. FT$_3$ = free T$_3$, FT$_4$ = free T$_4$. GM-CSF = granulocyte–macrophage colony-stimulating factor. IFNs = interferons. IL-2 = interleukin-2. TD = thyroid dysfunction. =: unchanged. =↑: trendwise increased. ↑: increased. =↓: trendwise decreased. ↓: decreased. –: absent or negative. +: de novo appearance. ↑+: further increase.

[a] Proton pump inhibitors, H$_2$ receptor antagonists, sucralfate, aluminium hydroxide.

TABLE 30.4
Drugs Interfering with Thyroid Function Testing

Drug	Mechanism	Laboratory Findings[a]
Dopamine and dopamine agonists, Somatostatin analogs (octreotide)	↓ TSH synthesis	FT_4 = or =↓, TSH ↓
Dobutamine, Amphetamines, IFNα	↓ TSH synthesis	FT_4 = or =↓, FT_3 = or =↓, TSH ↓
Bexarotene	↓ TSH synthesis	FT_4=, FT_3 =↓ or ↓, TSH ↓
Glucocorticoids	↓ Peripheral conversion of T_4 to T_3 ↓ TBG synthesis	
Domperidone, metoclopramide hydrochloride, Antipsychotics (phenothiazines and haloperidol) Antidepressive tricyclics, α-methyldopa	↑TSH synthesis and release	FT_4=, FT_3 =, TSH ↑
Aminoglutethimide	↓ Thyroid hormone synthesis and release	FT_4=↓ or ↓, FT_3 =↓ or ↓, TSH↑
Antiepilepsy medications, antibiotics (rifampim, rifabutin), Ritonavir, imatinib, sorafebin, sertraline hydrochloride	↑Metabolic clearance rate	FT_4 ↓, FT_3 =, TSH ↑
Estrogens, antiandrogens, SERMs, Drugs of abuse (heroin, methadone), 5-fluorouracil	↑ TBG synthesis	FT_4= or =↓, FT_3 = or =↓, TSH ↑
Androgens	↓ TBG synthesis ↓ TSH synthesis	FT_4 =, FT_3 =, TSH ↓
NSAIDs, furosemide, heparin, sulfanylureas Antiepilepsy drugs Benzodiazepines	Displacement of thyroid hormones from TBG	FT_4=↑ or ↑, FT_3 =↑ or ↑, TSH =↓ or ↓
L-carnitine	Peripheral antagonism of thyroid hormones	FT_4 =, FT_3 =, TSH =

*Note:*NSAIDs = non-steroidal antiinflammatory drugs. SERM = selective estrogen receptor modulators.
[a] FT_3: free T_3. FT_4: free T_4. TBG: thyroxine-binding globulin. =: unchanged. =↑: trendwise increased. ↑: increased. =↓: trendwise decreased. ↓: decreased.

treatment, but the ability of lithium to induce thyroid autoimmunity *de novo* has not been demonstrated.

In consideration of the high incidence of lithium-induced hypothyroidism, it is reasonable to assay thyroid function indices (FT_3, FT_4, TSH) and thyroid antibodies (Tg-Abs, TPO-Abs) of all patients regardless of age and gender prior to lithium therapy. A preexisting thyroid disease is not, however, a contraindication to lithium treatment. The same assays should be repeated regularly every 6 months while a patient is on treatment, especially older women who are thyroid antibody-positive. Lithium therapy should not be stopped nor the dose modified if hypothyroidism develops. In such cases, LT_4 supplementation takes care of hypothyroidism and prevents further growth of goiter if present. Goiter and/or hypothyroidism do not always resolve after lithium is stopped.

30.2.2 IMMUNE MODULATORS (CYTOKINES)

30.2.2.1 Interferons

Interferons (IFNs) are employed to treat several neoplastic and non-neoplastic diseases (chronic hepatitis B and C, condylomatosis caused by human papilloma virus, Kaposi's sarcoma, some lymphomas and chronic leukemias, and renal carcinoma) and also to treat some autoimmune diseases (multiple sclerosis, Sjögren's syndrome, discoid lupus erythematosus, Behçet's disease, uveitis, and others). However, IFN administration may act as a strong stimulus on the immune system, thus exacerbating or inducing the onset of autoimmune reactions in various organs including the thyroid.[1,2]

Interferon-α (IFNα) is a human recombinant cytokine employed in the treatment of several malignant and infectious diseases, especially chronic hepatitis C. Thyroid dysfunction during IFNα therapy is quite common. Prospective studies have shown that up to 40% of hepatitis C virus (HCV) patients receiving IFNα develop serum thyroid antibodies, of whom 15% develop hypothyroidism.[1,2,4] These rates are greater when IFNα is combined with ribavirin in patients with hepatitis C.[2]

Approximately one half of patients developing hypothyroidism while on IFNα treatment present with a classical Hashimoto's thyroiditis, with positive serum TPO-Abs and/or Tg-Abs, and often with goiter. In the other half, transient or permanent hypothyroidism follows transient thyrotoxicosis due to destructive thyroiditis with negative thyroid antibodies. The etiology of such IFNα-induced thyroid dysfunctions is unknown and may be secondary to immune modulation by IFNα in the former type and/or direct toxic effects of interferon on thyrocytes in the latter.

Recent evidence suggests that genetic factors, gender, preexisting thyroid autoimmunity, and hepatitis C virus infection may contribute to the susceptibility to IFNα-induced thyroid disease.[4] Depression is a frequent side effect of IFN therapy in HCV patients and also a common symptom of hypothyroidism. However, in IFNα-treated HCV patients, no difference in FT_4 or TSH serum levels between the group who developed depression and those who did not was apparent.

Interferon-β (IFNβ) is employed to treat multiple sclerosis. It causes alterations in thyroid function that overlap those caused by IFNα in terms of frequency, pathogenesis, and clinical manifestations.[2]

Based on most published studies, preexisting thyroid disease or the development of thyroid dysfunction during treatment with IFNs does not represent an absolute contraindication to start or continue IFN treatment. In all patients who start IFN therapy, serum free thyroid hormones and TSH, TPO-Abs, and Tg-Abs should be measured before and periodically (every 3 months) during and after treatment with IFNs. In cases of hypothyroidism, patients are treated with LT_4, and the cycle of IFN therapy may be started or completed. In approximately half of the patients treated with IFNs, hypothyroidism is transient and thus reversible upon discontinuation of therapy. In the remainder of IFN-treated patients, hypothyroidism is permanent so that LT_4 replacement therapy should be lifelong.

30.2.2.2   Other Cytokines

Interleukin-2 (IL-2) is used, alone or in association with IFNα or lymphokine-activated killer cells in the treatment of metastatic melanoma and renal cell carcinoma. IL-2 therapy, alone or in combination with other drugs, may induce hypothyroidism in 20 to 50% of patients, likely by autoimmune mechanisms as suggested by the appearance of circulating TPO-Abs and/or Tg-Abs.[1,2] Hypothyroidism is usually transient and reversible upon discontinuation of therapy. Preexisting thyroid autoimmunity increases the risk of developing hypothyroidism. For this reason, serum assay of thyroid function and thyroid autoimmunity should be performed regularly before and during IL-2 treatment. As with IFN-induced disorders, hypothyroidism is easily treated with LT_4 without discontinuing IL-2 therapy.

Administration of granulocyte–macrophage colony-stimulating factor (GM-CSF) to patients with advanced breast cancer and soft-tissue sarcoma (or to patients with leukopenia) induces or exacerbates thyroid autoimmunity, most likely due to stimulation of antigen-presenting cells by GM-CSF.[1,2] In most cases, GM-CSF therapy elicited only the appearance or an increase of serum thyroid autoantibody levels. However, in approximately 10% of patients, thyroid dysfunction developed in the form of hypothyroidism alone or hypothyroidism preceded by transient hyperthyroidism.

Such thyroid dysfunction may also occur in the absence of thyroid autoantibodies, probably due to a direct toxic effect of the drug on thyrocytes. In all cases, thyroid dysfunction disappeared after cessation of GM-CSF. Patients scheduled to receive GM-CSF must be screened for serum thyroid autoantibodies because a positive result confers a high risk of developing a clinically relevant thyroid dysfunction. After GM-CSF therapy is started, serum thyroid antibodies and thyroid function indices (FT_3, FT_4, TSH) should be measured regularly (every 3 to 6 months) during treatment.

A similar picture of transient autoimmune hypothyroidism has been described in patients who developed hypersensitivity reactions to sulfonamides and antiepilepsy drugs, but the underlying mechanism is not well understood.

30.2.3   AMIODARONE

Amiodarone, a benzofuranic iodine-rich derivative with a structural resemblance to thyroid hormones, is a class III antiarrhythmic drug used widely to manage atrial fibrillation and other cardiac conditions. One amiodarone molecule contains two atoms of iodine (37% of its weight). A daily dose of 200 mg of amiodarone provides 75 mg of iodine, of which about 10% is available as inorganic iodine through deiodination of the drug, exposing patients to an iodine load 40 to 100 times greater than the normal daily intake of 150 μg.

The thyroid adapts to the iodine excess by acute inhibition of the iodine organification (Wolff-Chaikoff effect). Consequently, T_4 and T_3 production rates decrease and TSH increases. After a few weeks, the thyroid escapes from the Wolff–Chaikoff effect through the down-regulation of the NIS symporter. Iodine uptake by the

TABLE 30.5
"Obligatory" Effects of Amiodarone on Thyroid Homeostasis

	Early Effects (Transient)	Late Effects (Permanent for Duration of Therapy)[a]
Acute inhibition of iodine organification due to iodine excess (Wolff-Chaikoff effect)	↑24-hour urinary iodine excretion ↑TSH (but not exceeding 20 mU/L) ↓ T_4 and T_3 production	TSH ↓
Inhibition of types 1 and 2 5'-deiodinases		T_3 ↓, reverse T_3 ↑
Inhibition of T_4 transport into liver, resulting in decreased T_3 metabolic clearance rate		T_4 ↑, FT_4 ↑
Inhibition of T_3 binding to its nuclear receptor		
Changes in serum levels		FT_4 ↑, T_3 ↓, FT_3 ↓, TSH ↓

[a] Within 3 months of drug initiation. FT_3: free T_3. FT_4: free T_4. ↑: increased. ↓: decreased.

thyroid (although remaining high) decreases and serum TSH returns to baseline values. In addition, amiodarone inhibits type 1 deiodinase, resulting in serum T_3 and FT_3 decreases and a serum reverse T_3 increase.

Amiodarone also inhibits T_4 transport into the liver, causing a decreased T_4 metabolic clearance rate and increases of serum T_4 and FT_4. These changes in serum levels of thyroid hormones and TSH are to be expected in almost every patient taking amiodarone (Table 30.5), and clinicians need to be familiar with them. In such conditions, no therapy is required. After amiodarone discontinuation, serum TSH and thyroid hormones normalize within 2 months or longer.

In 15 to 20% of patients, however, amiodarone causes clinically significant thyroid dysfunction (thyrotoxicosis or hypothyroidism).[1,2,5,6] The relative proportion of amiodarone-induced thyrotoxicosis (AIT) and amiodarone-induced hypothyroidism (AIH) depends mainly on environmental iodine intake because AIT and AIH are relatively more frequent in iodine-deficient and iodine-sufficient areas, respectively. In contrast to AIT, which is a difficult condition to manage, AIH poses no particular problem.[2,5] AIH is likely due to an inability of the thyroid gland to escape from the Wolff-Chaikoff block. Persistent inhibition of organification then causes hypothyroidism.

Beside living in iodine-sufficient areas, other risk factors for AIH include female gender, older age, and preexisting positive thyroid antibodies (Table 30.6). De novo development of antithyroid antibodies during amiodarone use has not been reported.[5] No clear relation has been demonstrated between the development of AIH and daily or cumulative dosages of amiodarone or the duration of therapy, although most cases develop AIH between 6 and 18 months after starting amiodarone therapy. Rarely, AIH may occur late and even within the first year after drug withdrawal because of amiodarone's long half-life (40 to 55 days) and sequestration in adipose tissue.

Hypothyroidism may be difficult to recognize on clinical ground because some symptoms and signs (i.e., bradycardia and constipation) are also intrinsic common

TABLE 30.6

Risk Factors for Amiodarone-Induced Hypothyroidism (AIH)

Female gender

Older age

Iodine deficiency

Preexisting antithyroid antibodies

Autoimmune thyroiditis (such as Hashimoto's disease)

History of postpartum thyroid disease or painless thyroiditis

Previous thyroid disease (i.e., subacute thyroiditis)

Partial thyroidectomy

History of radioactive iodine administration

Family history of thyroid disease

side effects of amiodarone. Thus, AIH should be confirmed by thyroid function tests. Appearance of goiter is rare.

In cases of AIH, amiodarone withdrawal is not mandatory. If amiodarone cannot be discontinued from a cardiological view, LT_4 replacement therapy should be started. The dose of LT_4 required for adequate correction of hypothyroidism may be higher than in conventional hypothyroid patients, probably due to amiodarone-induced inhibition of pituitary type 2 5′-deiodinase, an inhibition that causes decreased intrapituitary production of T_3. LT_4 replacement should be maintained as long as amiodarone is continued.

If amiodarone can be discontinued, spontaneous regression of AIH in 2 to 3 months occurs in approximately 60% of the patients. In the remaining 40%, hypothyroidism is prolonged (up to 5 to 8 months) or permanent, especially if TPO-Abs are present. Consequently, LT_4 replacement therapy is often necessary even if amiodarone is stopped. After 6 to 12 months, L T_4 supplementation can be stopped to evaluate the need for continued therapy.

In consideration of the relevance of thyroid dysfunctions during amiodarone therapy, measurements of serum TSH, FT_4, FT_3, TPO-Abs, and Tg-Abs should be performed before starting therapy, to detect preexisting thyroid dysfunctions. Serum TSH, FT_4, and FT_3 testing should be repeated after 3 months of therapy, and these results should be considered baselines for a patient on amiodarone (Table 30.5). Thyroid function assays should be repeated every 3 to 6 months during amiodarone use and even within the first year after drug discontinuation.

30.2.4 TYROSINE KINASE INHIBITORS

Tyrosine kinase inhibitors (TKIs) are novel chemotherapeutic drugs employed to treat several types of malignancies. The main pharmacological effect of TKIs is the inhibition of a variety of receptors with tyrosine kinase activities. These activities are signals involved in carcinogenesis, cell proliferation, and neoangiogenesis. Some (but not all) TKIs may affect thyroid function in two distinct ways: (1) by increasing LT_4 requirements in hypothyroid patients on replacement therapy (i.e., imatinib and sorabefin) or (2) by causing primary hypothyroidism in previously euthyroid patients (i.e., sunitinib, sorabefin, nilotinib, dasatinib).[2,7,8] We will discuss the effects of TKIs on euthyroid patients here; the effects of TKIs on patients under LT_4 replacement therapy will be discussed below.

Sunitinib, a multitargeted TKI approved to treat metastatic renal cell carcinoma and gastrointestinal stromal tumors, has been reported to induce subclinical or overt hypothyroidism. Based on retrospective or prospective studies, sunitinib can induce hypothyroidism in 53 to 85% or 36 to 71% of patients, respectively.[7] The mechanism by which sunitinib-induced hypothyroidism occurs is unknown. The evidence available suggests that sunitinib exerts a direct toxic effect on the thyroid gland, inducing a destructive thyroiditis in which follicular cells are induced to apoptosis. In its most severe form, a transient hyperthyroidism may precede the onset of hypothyroidism, but more commonly hypothyroidism alone occurs.

An effect of sunitinib on iodine uptake has been also postulated, but not confirmed by in vitro studies. More recently, observations of reduced thyroid blood flow, thyroid volume shrinkage, and hypothyroidism were interpreted as a direct inhibition of vascular endothelial growth factor receptor in the thyroid by the drug. The absence of circulating thyroid autoantibodies in patients who develop sunitinib-induced hypothyroidism excludes autoimmune mechanisms.[2]

Sorafenib is another multitargeted TKI used to treat several solid tumors and (based on different studies) cause subclinical or overt hypothyroidism in 18% to 68% of patients. In a number of such patients, hypothyroidism is preceded by a phase of mild, transient hyperthyroidism. Similar to sunitinib, sorafenib may affect thyroid function through a destructive mechanism involving a direct toxic effect on thyrocytes.[2] An enhanced peripheral metabolism of thyroid hormones, likely due to activity of type 3 deiodinase, may contribute to hypothyroidism.[9]

A high frequency of thyroid abnormalities (hypothyroidism or hyperthyroidism) is reported also in patients with chronic myeloid leukemia under treatment with the second-generation nilotinib and dasatinib TKIs (55 and 70% of patients, respectively).[8] Although the mechanism is still unclear, it is noteworthy that 4 of the 55 patients treated with nilotinib developed circulating thyroid autoantibodies, indicating that this TKI may induce autoimmune thyroiditis.[8]

While risk factors for TKI-induced hypothyroidism are still unclear, close monitoring of thyroid function tests is recommended in all patients on these medications. In all cases reported in the literature, correction of TKI-induced hypothyroidism was achieved with LT_4 therapy at standard doses, with no need to discontinue TKI therapy. In the few patients in whom the drug was discontinued, spontaneous returns to euthyroidism were observed. However, the literature reports cases of ultrasonographically confirmed thyroid atrophy, suggesting a permanent hypothyroidism as a possible outcome.[2]

30.2.5 FLAVONOIDS

Flavonoids are present in fruits, vegetables, beverages derived from plants (tea, red wine), and in many dietary supplements or herbal remedies including ginkgo biloba and soy isoflavones with estrogenic activities. Flavonoids exert antithyroid effects by inhibiting thyroid peroxidase (TPO).[10] Moreover, flavonoids acting on iodothyronine deiodinase enzymes also inhibit the peripheral metabolism of thyroid hormones. Thus, a high consumption of pharmaceutical or dietary products containing flavonoids may lead to goiter and hypothyroidism. Iodine deficiency greatly increases such antithyroid effects, whereas iodine supplementation is protective.

Based on in vitro and animal data, a remaining theoretical concern is that in individuals with compromised thyroid function and/or whose iodine intake is low, soy derivatives may increase risks of developing clinical hypothyroidism.[10] Moreover, soy derivatives may affect LT_4 absorption (see below) in hypothyroid patients on replacement therapy.

30.2.6 RESORCINOL

Resorcinol is a phenolic derivative used by dermatologists as an antiseptic and disinfectant. Moreover, it is used (5 to 10%) in ointments for the treatment of chronic skin diseases such as psoriasis, hidradenitis suppurativa, and erythematous eczema. It is present in topical acne treatments at a concentration of 2% or less, and may be present as an antidandruff agent in shampoos and sunscreen cosmetics. It is also present in vaginal lavages.

Resorcinol has been demonstrated to cause hypothyroidism by inhibition of TPO and consequent reduction of thyroid hormone biosynthesis.[1] In cases of hypothyroidism, administration of medications containing resorcinol should be discontinued. Hypothyroidism is always transient and regresses with discontinuation of the drug.

30.2.7 THALIDOMIDE

Thalidomide, a hypnotic drug well known for its teratogenic properties, has been reevaluated for its therapeutic effects in cancer (multiple myeloma). Studies on over 150 patients treated with thalidomide in association with chemotherapy have shown a significant incidence of hypothyroidism (TSH >5 µIU/l in 20% of patients and >0 µIU/l in 7% of patients) compared to patients treated with chemotherapy alone.[1] The mechanism by which the drug induces hypothyroidism is unclear.

30.3 DRUGS AFFECTING THYROID HORMONE REPLACEMENT THERAPY

Several drugs have been shown to affect the efficacy of thyroid hormone replacement therapy by impairing absorption of exogenous LT_4 or influencing LT_4 requirement.[1,2]

30.3.1 DRUGS IMPAIRING LT_4 ABSORPTION

Normally, 50% or more of oral LT_4 is absorbed, and most of this absorption occurs within the first 2 hours.[11] A patient should take LT_4 on an empty stomach for optimal absorption[12] in the duodenum and jejunum, and it requires stomach acidity, as demonstrated by impaired absorption in patients with chronic gastritis and achlorhydria.[13]

Absorbable antacids (such as proton pump inhibitors [PPIs] and H2 receptor antagonists), non-absorbable antacids (such as sucralfate, aluminium and magnesium hydroxides), and calcium formulations (calcium carbonate, citrate, and acetate) may decrease the intestinal absorption of LT_4 to a variable extent because of an increase in gastric pH or direct sequestration of the LT_4 into insoluble complexes. The same sequestration is operated by ferrous sulfate or ferrous gluconate and bile acid sequestrants such as cholestyramine. Bile acid sequestrants also interfere with the enterohepatic circulation of LT_4, further reducing its absorption.[1,2]

Table 30.7 lists drugs that may affect LT_4 absorption. The list is growing and includes new medications such as sevelamer hydrochloride (a phosphate-binding compound used to treat hyperphosphatemia), chromium picolinate (an over-the-counter nutritional supplement), sodium polystyrene sulfonate (a polyanion effective in reducing serum potassium levels), and soy protein derivatives.

To maintain euthyroidism, hypothyroid patients should take levothyroxine at least 4 hours before taking any medication that might interfere with absorption to minimize interactions. Sometimes, levothyroxine dosage may need to be increased by 20 to 30% (up to 100% in the cases of resin binders). Unpublished data by Benvenga et al. indicate the problem of LT_4 malabsorption caused by PPI can be solved by switching the conventional LT_4 tablets with other LT_4 formulations (soft gel capsules or ethanol solution). Indeed, in vitro experiments showed that the release of LT_4 from a soft gel capsule under a wide range of pH values is more consistent compared to branded or generic tablet formulations.[14]

TABLE 30.7
Drugs Interfering with LT_4 Absorption

Drug	Indications
Aluminium hydroxide	Gastroesophageal reflux disease (GERD), gastritis
Bile acid sequestants (i.e., cholestyramine)	Dyslipidemia, type 2 diabetes
Calcium carbonate	Osteoporosis, hypocalcemia
Ferrous sulfate, ferrous gluconate	Anemia
Chromium picolinate	Nutritional supplement
H_2 receptor antagonist (cimetidine, ranitidine, etc.)	GERD, gastritis
Isoflavones with estrogenic activities	Menopause
Protonic pump inhibitors (PPIs)	GERD, gastritis
Sevelamer hydrochloride	Hyperphosphatemia
Sodium polystyrene sulfonate	Hyperkalemia
Sucralfate	GERD
Soy derivatives	Nutritional and dietetic supplements

30.3.2   Drugs Affecting LT$_4$ Requirements

30.3.2.1   Drugs Interfering with Thyroid Hormone Transport

A number of drugs are capable of inducing changes in circulating levels of thyroid hormones, interfering with their plasma transport.[1,2] In most cases, this interference occurs if serum levels of total T$_4$ and/or total T$_3$ are assayed (an unlikely situation now, since serum levels of FT$_4$ and/or FT$_3$ are the usual assays nowadays).

Some drugs (such estrogens, androgens, antiandrogens, selective estrogen receptor modulators [SERMs], corticosteroids, 5-fluorouracil, and drugs of abuse) interfere with the synthesis and/or glycidic composition of the carrier proteins (mainly thyroid-binding globulin [TBG]), causing increases or reductions in their concentrations.[1]

In cases of therapy with oral estrogens that increase serum TBG, adjustments of LT$_4$ dosage may be required in hypothyroid patients. This effect is not observed with transdermal estrogen administration because of the absence of the liver first-passage of the drug. In contrast, androgens reduce the sialylation or synthesis of TBG and consequently its serum concentration. Androgen treatment of hypothyroid women receiving LT$_4$ replacement therapy may require a dose reduction of LT$_4$ to half the initial dose.

Other drugs (non-steroidal antiinflammatory drugs [NSAIDs], furosemide, heparin, sulfonylureas, antiepilepsy drugs such as phenobarbital, diphenylhydantoin, phenytoin, and carbamazepine) can displace thyroid hormones from carrier proteins and transiently elevate FT$_4$ and FT$_3$ concentrations and depress TSH levels.[1,2] The effects of these drugs most often result in transient and asymptomatic changes of thyroid function tests that may have clinical relevance in hospitalized patients receiving polytherapy due to a complex interplay of multiple drugs or medical conditions.

Knowledge of these interactions (often not listed on data sheets) is therefore very important. These effects are dose-dependent (i.e., >2 g for NSAIDs, >80 to 100 mg for furosemide, and >2.000 U for heparin) and largely related to the half-lives of the drugs. Unlike other drugs, the action of heparin is not direct; it is mediated by the increased serum concentrations of free fatty acids for activation of lipoprotein lipase. Therefore, to avoid laboratory interference with test results, FT$_4$ levels should be measured 1 hour or more after intravenous administration or 10 hours or more after administering low molecular weight heparin.

30.3.2.2   Drugs Altering LT$_4$ Metabolism

Several drugs may alter the metabolic clearance rate of absorbed LT$_4$,[1,2] for example, in the deiodinase system, liver cytochrome P450 metabolizes thyroid hormones. Consequently, drugs activating this system (rifampim, rifabutin, and antiepilepsy drugs) increase the metabolic clearance rate of T$_4$ by about 20%. This metabolic alteration is not clinically important in euthyroid subjects, resulting only in mild thyroid function test abnormalities.

However, hypothyroid subjects on LT$_4$ replacement therapy may need higher dosages to maintain euthyroidism (up to 100% of the dose in patients receiving rifampim—the most potent in this group of drugs). Ritonavir, a potent P450 mixed hepatic enzyme inhibitor and inducer, can increase thyroxine glucuronidation, thus requiring an up to twofold increase of the daily dosage of LT$_4$. Administration of imatinib and sorafenib, novel chemotherapeutic agents belonging to the TKI group, has been reported to require an increment of LT_4 dosages in patients under replacement therapy, likely due to increased liver metabolism of thyroid hormone. Serotonin reuptake inhibitors, such as sertraline hydrochloride, are thought to induce an increase of LT_4 requirements through a similar mechanism of action.

30.4 DRUG-INDUCED HYPERTHYROIDISM

30.4.1 AMIODARONE

The effects of amiodarone on thyroid homeostasis have been reported in detail in Section 30.2.3 and Tables 30.3 and 30.5. As stated earlier, the use of this antiarrhythmic drug may be complicated by the occurrence of hyperthyroidism (AIT) in about 10% of patients.[5,6] AIT preferentially occurs in geographic areas with insufficient iodine intake and in males.

Thyroid autoimmunity is not involved in the pathogenesis of and does not represent a risk factor for developing AIT. No *de novo* occurrence of TSH receptor stimulating antibodies has been observed in amiodarone-treated patients. Two main mechanisms can lead to AIT (Table 30.3). Type 1 AIT is a form of iodine-induced hyperthyroidism in patients with preexisting nodular goiter or latent Graves' disease. Type 2 AIT is a form of destructive thyroiditis, likely due to a direct toxic effect of amiodarone or its high iodine content that generally develops in patients without preexisting clinical, biochemical, and morphological evidence of thyroid disease.[5,6] However, the two mechanisms may appear in the same patient (mixed or indefinite AIT).

Distinction between the two forms of AIT is crucial because it affects the therapeutic approach. The main features distinguishing the two forms of AIT are summarized in Table 30.8. The relative frequency of type 1 AIT has decreased over recent decades, whereas the frequency of type 2 has increased.[5,6]

TABLE 30.8
Clinical and Pathogenic Features of Types 1 and 2 Amiodarone-Induced Toxicosis

Factor	Type 1	Type 2
Pathogenesis	Iodine-induced hyperthyroidism	Destructive thyroiditis
Preexisting thyroid disease	Yes	No
Physical examination	Diffuse or nodular goiter	Sometimes, firm painful goiter
Thyroid antibodies	Present or absent	Mostly absent
Thyroid ultrasonography, color Doppler sonography	Diffuse or nodular goiter Normal or increased vascularity	Heterogeneous pattern Decreased vascularity
Thyroidal ^{131}I uptake	Low, normal, or increased	Low or absent
Thyroid ^{99m}Tc Sestamibi scintigraphy	Clear thyroid detection	No thyroid uptake
Spontaneous remission	No	Likely
Preferred medical therapy	Thionamides and $KClO_4$	Glucocorticoids
Subsequent hypothyroidism	Unlikely	Possible

In consideration of the relevance of AIT, assessments of serum TSH, FT_4, FT3, and thyroid autoantibodies and neck ultrasound (US) are recommended before amiodarone treatment is started. Measurements of TSH, FT_3, and FT_4 should be performed every 3 to 6 months for patients on amiodarone therapy, even if the value of such controls is limited by the sudden onset of AIT.

AIT may occur at any time during amiodarone treatment and even several months after discontinuation due to the extensive tissue storage and long half-life of the drug. The onset of AIT is usually very rapid, often sudden and explosive. When AIT occurs, amiodarone should be discontinued, mostly in type 1 AIT, if feasible from a cardiological view. It should, however, be noted that the effects of amiodarone on thyroid function may last for several months after withdrawal, because of its long half-life. Thus, discontinuation of amiodarone does not resolve the hyperthyroidism or influence the response to medical therapy over the short term.

Type 1 AIT is best treated by antithyroid drugs (methimazole or propylthiouracil at high dosages). However, the efficacy of these drugs is reduced on an iodine-replete gland, and higher dosages and longer times are required to restore euthyroidism. To increase the sensitivity of the thyroid gland to thionamides, potassium perchlorate ($KClO_4$), which inhibits the NIS symporter and decreases thyroid iodine uptake, may be added for 2 to 6 weeks at doses of 1 g or less per day. This drug used by endocrinologists in Europe is not commonly available in the United States where most endocrinologists employ thionamides alone as first line treatment for type 1 AIT. In most case, thionamides plus $KClO_4$ restore euthyroidism in 2 months, even if amiodarone is continued. In AIT patients resistant to medical therapy and very severe cases, total thyroidectomy may become an option. To obtain a better (although transient) control of thyrotoxicosis before surgery in the past, a short course of iopanoic acid (in association with antithyroid drugs) was used (1 g iopanoic acid daily). Unfortunately, iopanoic acid is no longer manufactured and is now unavailable.[5,6]

Type 2 AIT is effectively treated with oral corticosteroids (prednisone, initial dose of 0.5 to 0.7 mg/kg body weight per day) and the treatment is usually continued for 3 months. Thionamides are not effective in type 2 AIT and discontinuation of amiodarone is probably not necessary. In most cases of type 2 AIT, the response to the treatment is dramatic and more than 50% of patients achieve control of hyperthyroidism within 4 to 6 weeks. The best treatment for the mixed or indefinite forms of AIT is a combination of thionamides (with or without potassium perchlorate) and oral corticosteroids.[5,6]

After euthyroidism has been restored and amiodarone discontinued for several months, thyroid ablation is commonly recommended for the underlying disorder in type 1 AIT, particularly if thyrotoxicosis recurs. In cases of type 2 AIT, periodic assessments of thyroid function should be performed despite the high incidence of hypothyroidism after type 2 AIT has been cured.[5,6]

If amiodarone must be restarted, prophylactic radioiodine or prophylactic thyroidectomy is usually recommended for type 1. Only monitoring is recommended for type 2 AIT. When amiodarone is again used, thyrotoxicosis may recur. However, few studies have shown that re-exposure to amiodarone may be followed by hypothyroidism. In this case, amiodarone does not have to be discontinued. The hypothyroidism is corrected using LT_4.[5,6]

30.4.2 LITHIUM

As reported in Section 30.2.1, the association between lithium therapy and hypothyroidism is well known. However, reports of lithium-associated hyperthyroidism also exist, but this complication is less well known, probably because it is overlooked. Recently, Carlè and coworkers reported that the prevalence of lithium-associated hyperthyroidism in the Danish population was 0.7%, similar to that of amiodarone-induced hyperthyroidism (0.8%).[11]

Lithium-associated hyperthyroidism usually presents as a transient, destructive thyrotoxicosis, resembling the clinical features of silent thyroiditis, but thyroid auto-antibodies are positive in up to 50% of patients. Several pathogenetic mechanisms have been proposed: an exacerbation or induction of thyroid autoimmunity, a direct toxic effect of lithium on thyrocytes, and a toxic effect of iodine, whose intrathyroidal concentration increases under lithium administration, because lithium reduces its release from the thyroid.

As noted in Section 30.2.1, due to the high incidence of lithium-induced thyroid abnormalities, serum thyroid function indices (FT_3, FT_4, TSH) and thyroid antibodies (Tg-Abs, TPO-Abs) should be checked before starting lithium therapy and repeated regularly every 6 months during treatment, especially in thyroid antibody-positive patients.

Lithium-associated thyrotoxicosis is usually self-limiting and mild, requiring only control of symptoms with beta blockers. There are no data available on treatment with corticosteroids, but such drugs should be avoided because they may increase the risk of manic episodes. Lithium therapy should not be stopped nor the dose modified if hyperthyroidism develops.

30.4.3 IMMUNE MODULATORS (CYTOKINES)

30.4.3.1 Interferons

The use of IFNs (Section 30.2.2) may be associated with the development of thyrotoxicosis by autoimmune or non-autoimmune mechanisms in 2 to 8% of patients.[1,2] In most cases, patients present with a form of destructive thyroiditis, likely due to a direct toxic effect of the drug on thyrocytes. Indeed, this form of destructive thyrotoxicosis resembles silent thyroiditis because of its transient clinical course and also the low radioiodine uptake on thyroid scintigraphy and the hypoechoic pattern on thyroid echography. However, in 20 to 25% of patients who develop hyperthyroidism, classic Graves' disease also occurs, sometimes associated with Graves' ophtalmopathy.[2]

IFN-induced thyrotoxicosis significantly impacts patients who often complain of other important non-thyroid-related side effects from IFNs. A specific treatment for destructive thyrotoxicosis is not available, but in most cases, symptom control may be achieved with beta blockers. In cases of Graves' disease, thionamides are effective in controlling hyperthyroidism.[2]

As cited in Section 30.2.2, neither preexisting thyroid disease nor the development of thyroid dysfunction during treatment with IFNs contraindicates starting or continuing IFNs. In all patients, serum free thyroid hormones, TSH, TPO-Abs, and

Tg-Abs should be measured before and periodically (every 3 months) during and after treatment with IFNs. IFN-induced thyrotoxicosis is generally transient. It may be followed by a phase of hypothyroidism, requiring LT_4 replacement. In patients who need prolonged and/or repeated cycles of IFN therapy, prophylactic radioiodine or prophylactic thyroidectomy may be proposed to prevent relapses of thyroiditis and/or Graves' disease.[2]

30.4.3.2 Other Cytokines

As reported above, IL-2 therapy may cause hypothyroidism in up to 50% of patients, mostly those with positive thyroid autoantibodies. An early phase of destructive thyrotoxicosis with variable degrees of hyperthyroidism may precede hypothyroidism and requires only control of symptoms with beta blockers. Thyroid dysfunction is usually transient and reversible after drug discontinuation.[2]

30.4.4 TYROSINE KINASE INHIBITORS

As reported in Section 30.2.4, sunitinib and sorafenib can cause hypothyroidism via a direct toxic effect on thyrocytes. In 20 to 24% of such patients, transient thyrotoxicosis of various degrees precedes the onset of hypothyroidism and may require prompt discontinuation of the drug or a dosage reduction if the symptomatology is severe.[2]

30.4.5 ALEMTUZUMAB

Alemtuzumab is a monoclonal antibody directed against the CD52 cell surface antigen expressed by lymphocytes and monocytes. Administration of alemtuzumab induces complement-mediated lysis of CD52 cells. This mechanism is the basis for its use in treating several autoimmune disorders including multiple sclerosis (MS) and rheumatoid arthritis, as well as chronic lymphocytic leukaemia and HIV infectious disease. It has been reported that alemtuzumab induces the onset of a classic Graves' disease with or without ophthalmopathy in up to 33% of patients with MS. These patients develop TSH receptor antibodies *de novo*.[2] The clinical presentation and antithyroid drug-based management of alemtuzumab-induced hyperthyroidism are no different from presentation and management of classic Graves' disease.

Note that the occurrence of Graves' disease has not been reported in patients in whom the drug was used to treat disorders other than MS, such as rheumatoid arthritis or chronic lymphocytic leukemia. Thus, for reasons that remain unclear, MS patients are peculiarly susceptible to this complication.[2]

As with IFN therapy, the development of thyroid dysfunction does not represent a contraindication to treatment, but the risks and benefits of the treatment must be assessed.

30.5 DRUG-INDUCED THYROIDITIS

As noted above and summarized in Table 30.3, several drugs such as lithium, amiodarone, immune modulators (IFN, IL-2, and GM-CSF), and TKIs are capable of inducting autoimmune or non-autoimmune thyroiditis, leading to clinically relevant thyroid dysfunction (hyperthyroidism, hypothyroidis, or both) in a significant number of patients.[1,2,5-9] In most cases, thyroid dysfunction is transient and reversible after drug withdrawal. Drug-induced thyroid dysfunction and preexisting thyroid disease do not contraindicate such therapies, but the risks and benefits of the treatment must be assessed. Close monitoring of thyroid function and autoimmunity is recommended.

30.6 DRUG-INDUCED THYROID TUMORS

To the best of our knowledge, a possible association between administration of a particular drug and thyroid cancer has not been demonstrated yet.

30.7 DRUGS INTERFERING WITH THYROID FUNCTION TESTING

Several medications may induce transient and asymptomatic changes in thyroid functioning tests in euthyroid patients without causing clinically evident thyroid dysfunction and without need for treatment.[1] Administration of such drugs may interfere with the proper interpretation of thyroid function test results and lead clinicians to inappropriate therapy. The main drugs that can affect the thyroid function tests are listed in Table 30.4. However, exceptions such as bexarotene exist.

30.7.1 Drugs Interfering with TSH Synthesis and Secretion

Dopamine and dopamine agonists (bromocriptine, cabergoline), somatostatin analogs (octreotide), dobutamine, amphetamines, and corticosteroids can decrease serum TSH.[1] Patients who take these medications over long periods do not have sustained reductions of FT_4; consequently, secondary hypothyroidism does not develop.

Bexarotene, a retinoid X receptor agonist used to treat cutaneous T cell lymphomas, inhibits the synthesis of TSH in the pituitary, causing an asymptomatic reduction of TSH levels in more than 90% of patients when administered at low dosage (6.5 mg/m^2/day). Transient central hypothyroidism requiring LT_4 replacement occurs in up to 50% of patients when bexarotene is administered at high dosages (>300 mg/m^2/day).[1]

IFNα can acutely suppress TSH levels, probably due to the concomitant rise in serum IL-6 concentrations. On the other hand, dopamine antagonists (antipsychotics such as phenothiazines and haloperidol, domperidone, metoclopramide hydrochloride, and cimetidine), antidepressive tricyclics and α-methyldopa that reduce dopamine synthesis can produce slight elevations in TSH levels but usually not greater than 10 mIU/L without altering thyroid function.[1,2] Spironolactone, an aldosterone antagonist used to treat primary hyperaldosteronism and hypertension along with hirsutism and hair loss may negligibly increase TSH levels, without clinical consequences.[1]

30.7.2 Drugs Interfering with Thyroid Hormone Synthesis and Secretion

Aminoglutethimide is an inhibitor of the aromatase enzyme used to treat metastatic breast cancer, advanced prostate cancer, and Cushing's syndrome. Due to interference with the synthesis and secretion of thyroid hormones, treatment with aminoglutethimide frequently results in reduction of serum FT_3 and FT_4 and increased TSH, without obvious clinical manifestations. The occurrence of goiter and hypothyroidism has been reported rarely, mainly in thyroid antibody-positive patients.[1]

30.7.3 Drugs Interfering with Thyroid Hormone Transport

As reported in Section 30.3.2.1, several drugs may interfere with the plasma transport of thyroid hormones. In euthyroid patients, treatment with such drugs may cause abnormal results of thyroid function tests without clinical consequences. Moreover, during continued administration of such drugs, FT_4, FT_3, and TSH levels return spontaneously to normal.[1,3]

Some drugs (NSAIDs, furosemide, heparin, sulfonylureas, and antiepilepsy drugs) may displace thyroid hormones from the carrier proteins (mainly TBG), thus increasing FT_4 and FT_3 levels and lowering TSH levels.[1,2] With sulfonylureas, carbamazepine, and phenytoin, these effects occur at doses well above therapeutic range. Other drugs interfere with the synthesis and/or glycidic compositions of the carrier proteins (estrogens, androgens, antiandrogens, tamoxifen, corticosteroids, 5-fluorouracil, drugs of abuse, propranolol at a dosage of >160 mg/day). Again, in most cases, changes in serum concentrations of thyroid hormones have no clinical significance.

30.7.4 Drugs Interfering with Thyroid Hormone Metabolism

As noted in Section 30.2.2, several drugs can alter the metabolism of thyroid hormones by acting on the deiodinases or on the hepatic glucuronidation enzymes.[1,2] Some drugs (i.e., antiepilepsy medications and antibiotics such as rifampim, rifabutin) increase the metabolic rates of thyroid hormones via the cytochrome P450 system, lowering FT_4 levels and increasing TSH levels.

Other drugs (amiodarone, iodinated contrast media, cyclophosphamide, propranolol, corticosteroids, and propylthiouracil) inhibit the deiodinases. Amiodarone and iodinated contrast media, as well as several iodinated pharmaceutical preparations with antiseptic or cosmetic indications (Table 30.9) can inhibit the conversion of T_4 to T_3 both in the peripheral circulation and in the pituitary and can produce elevations in FT_4 levels, reductions in total T_3 levels, and transient rises in TSH levels. These effects add to the well known inhibition of iodine organification (Wolff-Chaikoff effect).

Alkylating agents such as the cyclophosphamide lead compound may induce increases of serum total and free T_4 and reduction (until suppression) of TSH. Beta blockers and corticosteroids also inhibit the peripheral conversion of T_4 to T_3.

TABLE 30.9
Common Iodine-Containing Drugs and Products

Amiodarone

Iodinate contrast media

Antiseptics and disinfectants containing iodine, vaginal lavages

Cosmetics and dietary supplements

Propranolol hydrochloride (>160 mg/day), atenolol, and metoprolol tartrate produce small reductions in total and freeT_3 levels. Similarly, large doses of corticosteroids (e.g., >4 mg dexamethasone) produce small reductions in total T_3 levels. Most patients on these medication do not develop overt thyroid dysfunction (hyperthyroidism or hypothyroidism).

Recombinant human growth hormone (rhGH) therapy given to both children and adults with GH deficiencies is associated with a small but significant decrement of serum FT_4 and increase of serum T_3 levels. These changes are independent of TSH and result from increased peripheral conversion of T_4 to T_3. However, the incidence of hypothyroidism is low.[15] Monitoring of thyroid function during rhGH therapy is wise, particularly in the first 6 to 12 months of therapy when the largest decrease in FT_4 occurs.

30.7.5 Drugs Interfering with Interactions of Thyroid Hormones and Target Tissues

L-carnitine is a quaternary amine used to treat rare conditions of primary deficiency and in the two known conditions of secondary tissue deficiency (i.e., myocardial infarction and chronic renal failure on hemodialysis). L-carnitine is also used to protect against the toxic effects of some drugs (valproate, adriamycin, Zivoduline) and as a dietary supplement. It antagonizes the peripheral effects of thyroid hormones without altering their plasma concentrations.[16] This effect is clinically significant allowing L-carnitine to be used to alleviate the symptoms of thyrotoxicosis. Effects similar to those of carnitine at the cellular level have been reported for other drugs: benzodiazepines (lormetazepam), diphenylhydantoin, some NSAIDs, calcium channel blockers (verapamil and nifedipine), and desethyl-amiodarone, the major metabolite of amiodarone.[1]

REFERENCES

1. Meier, C.A. and Burger, A.C. 2005. Effects of drugs and other substances on thyroid hormone synthesis and metabolism. In *Werner and Ingbar's The Thyroid: A Fundamental and Clinical Text,* 9th ed., Braverman, L.E. and Utiger, R.D., Eds. Philadelphia: Lippincott Williams & Wilkins, 229.
2. Barbesino, G. 2010. Drugs affecting thyroid function. *Thyroid* 20: 763–770.
3. Lazarus, J.H. 2009. Lithium and thyroid. *Best Pract Res Clin Endocrinol Metab* 23: 723–733.
4. Mandac, J.C., Chaudhry, S., Sherman, K.E. et al. 2006. The clinical and physiological spectrum of interferon-α-induced thyroiditis: toward a new classification. *Hepatology* 43: 661–672.
5. Eskes, S.A. and Wiersinga, W.M. 2009. Amiodarone and thyroid. *Best Pract Res Clin Endocrinol Metab* 23: 735–751.
6. Bogazzi, F., Bartalena, L., and Martino, E. 2010. Approach to the patient with amiodarone-induced thyrotoxicosis. *J Clin Endocrinol Metab* 6: 2529–2535.
7. Torino, F., Corsello, S.M., Longo, R. et al. 2009. Hypothyroidism related to tyrosine kinase inhibitors: an emerging toxic effect of targeted therapy. *Nat Rev Clin Oncol* 6: 219–228.

8. Kim, T.D., Schwarz, M., Nogai, H. et al. 2010. Thyroid dysfunction caused by second-generation tyrosine kinase inhibitors in Philadelphia chromosome-positive chronic myeloid leukemia. *Thyroid* 20: 1209–1214.

9. Abdulrahman, R.M., Verloop, H., Hoftijzer, H. et al. 2010. Sorafenib-induced hypothyroidism is associated with increased type 3 deiodination. *J Clin Endocrinol Metab* 95: 3758–3762.

10. Messina, M. and Redmond, G. 2006. Effects of soy protein and soybean isoflavones on thyroid function in healthy adults and hypothyroid patients: a review of the relevant literature. *Thyroid* 16: 249–258.

11. Benvenga, S., Bartolone, L., Squadrito, S. et al. 1995. Delayed intestinal absorption of levothyroxine. *Thyroid* 5: 249–253.

12. Centanni, M., Gargano, L., Canettieri, G. et al. 2006. Thyroxine in goiter, *Helicobacter pylori* infection, and chronic gastritis. *New Engl J Med* 354: 1787–1795.

13. Pabla, D., Akhlaghi, F., and Zia, H. 2009. A comparative pH-dissolution profile study of selected commercial levothyroxine products using inductively coupled plasma mass spectrometry. *Eur J Pharm Biopharm* 72: 105–110.

14. Carlé, A., Pedersen, I.B., Knudsen, N. et al. 2011. Epidemiology of subtypes of hyperthyroidism in Denmark: a population-based study. *Eur J Endocrinol* 164: 801–809.

15. Losa, M., Scavini, M., Gatti, E. et al. 2008. Long-term effects of growth hormone replacement therapy on thyroid function in adults with growth hormone deficiency. *Thyroid* 18: 1249–1254.

16. Benvenga, S., Ruggeri, R.M., Russo, A. et al. 2001. Usefulness of L-carnitine, a naturally occurring peripheral antagonist of thyroid hormone action, in iatrogenic hyperthyroidism: a randomized, double-blind, placebo-controlled clinical trial. *J Clin Endocrinol Metab* 86: 3579–3594.

31 Thyroid Disruptors

Marco Centanni and Susanna Carlotta Del Duca

CONTENTS

Key words: endocrine disruptors, pollutants, brain development, organochlorine compounds, cosmetics, phthalates.

31.1 DEFINITION

An endocrine disruptor is defined as an exogenous agent that interferes with synthesis, secretion, transport, metabolism, binding action, or elimination of natural bloodborne hormones in the body that are responsible for homeostasis, reproduction, and developmental processes.[1] Endocrine disruptors are also called xenobiotics. When they interfere with thyroid homeostasis, they are designated thyroid disruptors (TDs). In a broad sense, those conditions eliciting disruption by xenobiotics (e.g., iodine deficiency) may be included as thyroid disruptors or at least co-disruptors.

31.2 EPIDEMIOLOGY

Epidemiological data (incidence and/or prevalence) about the impacts of xenobiotics on human public health are limited. This is because of genetic differences, varying exposures of different populations, and the asymmetrical distribution of pollutants in terms of geographic areas, heterogeneous national policies, and prevailing industrial or rural development.

31.2.1 Exposed Populations

Genetic susceptibility to xenobiotics (e.g., polymorphisms in detoxification genes) and personal behaviors such as smoking and nutritional habits may modify individual resistance to toxics.[2] Hence, some categories of people may be at particularly high risk for exposure to TDs; workers in chemical industries and those working with pesticides are important examples.[1] Industrialized areas are characterized by higher levels of contamination from chemicals that may leak into the soil, thus entering the food and water chains. Exposure even occurs in subjects who breathe contaminated air containing dust or come into contact with polluted soil (Figure 31.1).

The fetal and early postnatal developmental periods seem to be very vulnerable to exposure. In fact, xenobiotics are readily transferred from the placenta to the fetus and from breast milk to a newborn. Disruptors may interact with the neurological, immune, and endocrine networks of the fetus.[3] Hence, every embryo, fetus, and infant must be considered at high risk of contamination damage because of their fast growth rates and small weights as compared with the relatively high levels of some TDs (particularly organochlorine pollutants) across the placenta or ingested through breast milk. The set point for fetal thyroid axis seems to be modulated by the

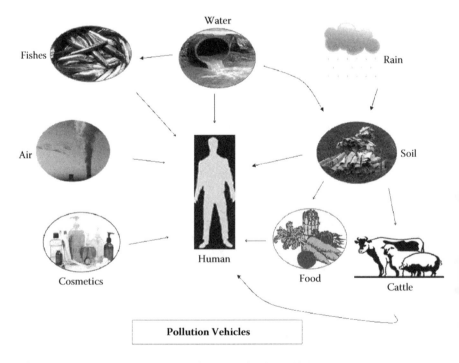

FIGURE 31.1   Thyroid disruptors: main contamination vehicles.

maternal environment surrounding the fetus, as already shown, i.e., for body weight regulation and obesity.[4] Hence, maternal exposure to TDs seems to play a key role for thyroid disruption.

31.2.2 SOURCES OF THYROID DISRUPTORS

Several classes of compounds may be classified as thyroid disruptors. Some are natural pollutants, some are drugs, and most are synthetic chemical compounds. Table 31.1 is a tentative list of these substances; they are divided into naturally occurring and synthetic disruptors.

TABLE 31.1
Main Thyroid Disruptors and Their Sources

Natural Pollutants

Perchlorate	Propellants and rockets, fireworks, matches, airbag systems, fertilizers
Thiocyanate	Cigarette smoke, vegetables
Flavonoids	Soy, peanuts, millet
Heavy metals (lead, cadmium, and methylmercury)	Hydraulic devices, fuel combustion materials, paints, alloys, batteries, lamps, thermometers, dental amalgams, seafood

Synthetic Pollutants

Polybrominated diphenyl ethers (PBDEs), tetrabromobisphenol A (TBBA), polybrominated biphenyls (PBBs)	Flame retardants in furniture, computers, televisions, textiles
Polychlorinated biphenyls (PCBs)	Hydraulic fluids, paints, inks, carbonless copy paper, heat insulation
Bisphenol A (BPA)	Polycarbonate and plastic products (food can linings, adhesives, dental sealants, compact discs)
Dioxin	Herbicides, industrial burning processes
Phtalates	Polyvinylchloride (PVC), food packaging, toys, emollients, additives
Benzophenones	UV filters, cosmetics
Dichlorodiphenyltrichloroethane (DDT), linuron, procymid	Indoor sprays, pesticides
Paraben	Cosmetics and nail products
Perfluorinated chemicals	Stains and oil-resistant coatings

Drugs

Methimazole, propylthiouracil	Antithyroid drugs
Amiodarone	Antiarrythmic drugs
Phenobarbital, phenytoin	Anticonvulsant and antiepileptic drugs
Fenamate	Anti-inflammatory drugs
Diethylstilbestrol	Synthetic estrogen preparations

Among the naturally occurring TDs, perchlorate is an oxidant representing one of the more pervasive contaminants in drinking and irrigation waters and in foods. Ubiquitous exposure to perchlorate makes it one of the more relevant pollutants. It is contained in fireworks, matches, airbag operation systems, and fertilizers but notably as a component of rocket propellants. Low levels of perchlorate have been measured in rainwater, snow, and groundwater. Several vegetables (tomatoes, cucumbers, lettuce, and soybeans), tobacco, eggs, and cow's milk have been shown to be contaminated with variable concentrations of perchlorate.[5]

Thiocyanates represent byproducts of the enzymatic hydrolysis of thioglucosides. Mostly found in vegetables of the Brassicaceae family (cabbage, turnips, mustard, sprouts, kale), they are also contained in cassava, sweet potatoes, corn, apricots, cherries, and almonds and in cigarette smoke as well.[6]

Additional natural TDs are heavy metals (lead, cadmium, and methylmercury) and the important polyphenols (simple phenols, flavonoids, catechins, and tannins), well known for their antioxidant capacities and protective effects against cardiovascular diseases, some forms of cancer, and menopausal symptoms and discomfort. Wine, coffee, tea, millet, and soy plants may contain significant amounts of polyphenols.

Flavonoids are widely distributed in fruits and vegetables, and possess several biological activities, including antioxidant and potent antithyroid properties, especially in iodine deficiency conditions. Isoflavones (genistin, daidzin, glycitin) are soy-derived, cognate substances showing goitrogenic effects, besides their characteristic estrogen-like activities.[7]

Among synthetic chemicals, widespread industrial products often structurally similar to thyroxine are the organochlorine (OC) compounds and their by-products. These organohalogenated pollutants include dioxin, fire retardants (PBDEs, TBBPA, PBBs) and polychlorinated biphenyls (PCBs). These latter are used in several industrial processes (e.g., production of paints, inks, hydraulic fluids, heat insulation). Their production and use were stopped in the mid-1970s but the materials persist in the environment, due to their slow degradation.[3]

Similarly, the use of other OC compounds (the pesticides) was banned by the United States and many other countries between 1970 and 1980. In the past, however, dichlorodiphenyltrichloroethane (DDT) and its dichlorodiphenyldichloroethylene (DDE) metabolite, commonly used in agricultural settings were used to fight malaria in endemic areas. Unfortunately, these pesticides are highly persistent in the environment, so that higher levels of their metabolites have been detected in agriculture workers' biological fluids. In particular DDE, a relevant breakdown product of DDT, is extremely stable (half-life of 7 to 11 years). It is not further processed by organisms or by the environment and progressively accumulates in fat. Hence, the general population is still exposed through food, although occupational exposure through inhalation and dermal contact has stopped.[2]

Some plastic products may contain phthalates or bisphenol A (BPA), both able to alter thyroid homeostasis. Phthalates can be considered ubiquitous due to their ability as inductors of flexibility and also as denaturants or solvents in personal care products (perfumes, cosmetics, shampoos) and medication coatings.[8] Bisphenol A is an organic compound used to make polycarbonate plastics, epoxy resins, and plastic products such as compact discs, adhesives, dental sealants, powder paints, and food can linings.[9]

Contradictory results surround the role of paraben, a preservative of cosmetics and foods, banned in Denmark as a TD. Convincing activity was described also for benzophenone-2 used for ultraviolet (UV) filters, and perfluorooctanoic acid, a stable compound that contaminates stain- and water-resistant coatings for carpets and hydraulic fluids.

Some drugs also act as disruptors. Beside the well known antithyroid drugs, the most common are amiodarone (antiarrhythmic), phenobarbital, and phenytoin (anticonvulsant and antiepileptic), diethylstilbestrol (synthetic estrogen), fenamate (anti-inflammatory).

31.3 PATHOPHYSIOLOGY OF TDS

31.3.1 BIOCHEMICAL CHARACTERISTICS AND DISTRIBUTION

Several pollutants possess physical and chemical properties similar to those of thyroid hormones. As a result, they may behave like "hormone mimics," as described for toxic halogenated aromatic compounds that are widely distributed in the environment and used in industrial chlorination. Among these chemicals, polychlorinated biphenyls (PCBs), polybrominated diphenyl ethers (PBDEs), and tetrachlorodibenzodioxin (TCDD) show the closest structural relationships with T_4.[10]

In general, these compounds are diphenyls with one sterically accessible and polarizable aromatic ring and some hydrophobic lateral substituents (usually halogens) linked to the opposite adjacent ring. The described structure is essential for the molecular recognition of these compounds from specific binding sites (Figure 31.2). Most thyroid disruptors, like other endocrine disruptors, have low water solubilities and extremely high fat solubilities, and thus accumulate in adipose tissues. They are often by-products of chemical industries or natural pollutants that readily contaminate soil and groundwater. Regulatory policies covering these chemicals vary widely

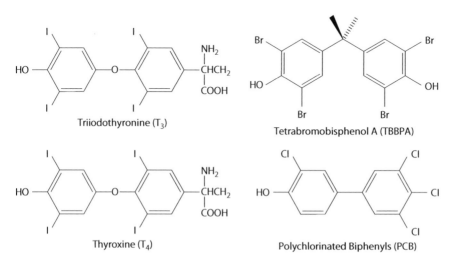

Triiodothyronine (T_3)

Tetrabromobisphenol A (TBBPA)

Thyroxine (T_4)

Polychlorinated Biphenyls (PCB)

FIGURE 31.2 Structural analogy between thyroid disruptors and iodothyronines.

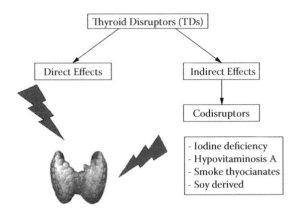

FIGURE 31.3 Mode of action of thyroid disruption.

among countries and even their reference exposure levels may vary greatly. These compounds enter the human body through breathing, ingesting food, drinking water, or simply by contact.[1] Hence, two consequences may ensue: (1) asymmetrical distribution of disruptors among different countries and (2) asymmetrical contamination of people, depending on their jobs and/or exposure, dietary and living habits, and other factors.

Although the production of some chemicals was banned several years ago, they have long half-lives, do not decay easily, may not be metabolized, or may be transformed into more toxic molecules. Some of these substances remain highly concentrated in the environment for decades. More important, human beings are continuously exposed to mixtures of pollutants whose effects can be additive or synergistic, leading to unexpected results that are different from results of exposure to the individual substances.[1]

Thyroid gland homeostasis, however, is maintained by a redundant control system that provides enormous adaptive ability to withstand adverse effects of TDs. Unfortunately, most of these systems are effective only when iodine supply is adequate, which is not the case for about 2 billion people around the world who are exposed to mild to severe iodine deficiencies.[4] In this situation, TDs may exert their own effects or unveil or aggravate effects caused by iodine deficiency. Hence, two different and not independent detrimental effects may be exerted by thyroid disruptors: (1) a direct interaction with the hypothalamus–hypophysis–thyroid (HPT) axis and thyroid homeostasis and (2) a mediated interaction via mutual enhancement of iodine deficiency and environmental goitrogens like a soy diet and smoke cyanide[4] (Figure 31.3).

Marginal hypovitaminosis A may enhance susceptibility to thyroid disruption as demonstrated in several studies in animals.[10] However, it remains difficult to establish a definite relationship between exposure to pollutants and adverse effects on the human thyroid axis due to the subtle but long-lasting effects of these compounds.

31.3.2 MECHANISMS OF ACTION OF TDS

The growing number of TDs led to several in vitro and animal studies focused on the potential mechanisms of action exerted by various disruptors. A tentative,

TABLE 31.2
Thyroid Disruptors: Mechanisms Perturbing Thyroid Homeostasis and Their Effects

Effect	Mechanisms	Thyroid Disruptors
	Blocking uptake of iodide by sodium–iodide symporter	Perchlorates, thiocyanate, phthalates, nitrates, bromates, propylthiouracil
Decreased synthesis of T_3 and T_4	Inhibition of TPO activity	Soy isoflavones, benzophenone-2, amitrole, methimazole, ethylenethiourea, thiocyanate
	Inhibition of TSH receptor	PCBs
Decreased fetal brain T_4 levels	Competitive binding to thyroid transport protein	PCBs, flame retardants, phenols, phthalates
Altered thyroid hormone-responsive genes	Altering binding to thyroid receptor	OH-PCBs, BPA, flame retardants
Decreased peripheral T_3 production	Inhibition of deiodinase activity	PCBs, PBDEs, heavy metals, octylmethoxycinnamate
	Inhibition of sulfation	PCBs, triclosan, pentachlorophenol, dioxin
Increased biliary iodothyronine catabolism	Enhanced hepatic metabolism	Acetochlor (herbicide), PCBs, BPA, dioxin
	Decreasing transporter activity across cell membrane	Dioxin, flame retardants, BPA, PCBs

comprehensive but not exhaustive summary is reported in Table 31.2. Chemical pollution may disrupt thyroid homeostasis through all the physiological steps of the hypophysis–thyroid–target cell axis. In fact, they have been proven to interfere with iodine uptake, intrathyroid iodine metabolism, binding to transport proteins, cellular uptake, thyroid hormone (TH) metabolism, and TH receptor interaction[1,6,8] (Figure 31.4).

In particular, the key processes subject to interference are iodide uptake by the sodium–iodine symporter (NIS), iodide organification by thyroid peroxidase (TPO), binding of thyroxine (T_4) to its transporters, peripheral metabolism of iodothyronines, and interaction of T_3 with thyroid response elements (TREs). More than one level may be the target of a single disruptor and multiple disruptors may act at a single level.

31.3.2.1 Effects of TDs on Iodine Uptake and Intrathyroid Iodine Pool

The most common mechanisms of disrupting thyroid homeostasis involve iodine uptake and metabolism. The first step of iodothyronine synthesis is iodine uptake through the cell membrane symporter (NIS). The effect of TDs on NIS protein has been shown for phthalates, nitrates, bromates, perchlorates, and thiocyanates. The latter compounds show 30 times higher binding affinity for NIS than iodide, thus competing with iodine and inhibiting it from entering follicular cells.

Perchlorate uptake occurs in a dose-dependent manner through NIS and its exposure may be evaluated by its urinary levels; in humans, its metabolism is negligible.[5]

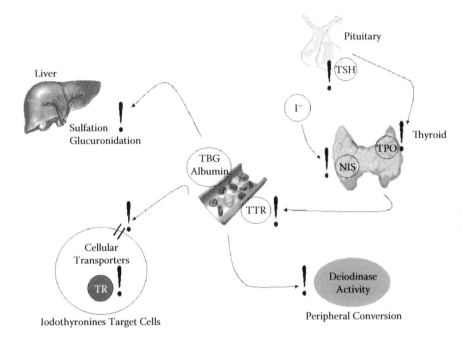

FIGURE 31.4 Main sites of thyroid homeostasis disruption.

Despite low perchlorate estimates in the adult population,[6] the possible interaction of perchlorate with other thyroid disruptors should also be investigated.

Dose-dependent and synergistic effects of different TDs having the same NIS inhibitory actions have been described in smokers. Preformed thiocyanate in cigarette smoke can block iodine uptake into mammary tissue. The iodine content found in breast milk from smoking mothers was half the content found in non-smoking mothers.[5,6]

Perchlorate exerts greater effects in smokers than in non-smokers and this finding supports the mutual enhancement of these two disruptors. The evidence that NIS protein is underexpressed in thyroid carcinomas sheds light on a possible relation between TD effects on NIS activity and carcinogenesis.[6]

A second, more important, disruption of iodothyronine synthesis occurs through the inhibition of thyroid peroxidase that causes interference with thyroglobulin iodination. This effect was shown for several classes of chemicals such as benzophenones, polyphenols, and some herbicides and fungicides. These TDs were shown to inhibit TPO formation and thus the iodination and coupling of iodothyrosil residues, thereby reducing T_4 and T_3 release, even in the presence of adequate iodide and effective NIS activity.[1,6]

31.3.2.2 Interference with Protein and Cellular Binding

Xenobiotics may impair the blood transport of thyroid hormones and also inside–out cellular trafficking. TDs interfere with transport proteins via a competitive mechanism that decreases binding to carriers for transport and cellular uptake of endogenous iodothyronines. No environmental chemicals have been demonstrated to compete with thyroid hormones for binding to thyroxine binding globulin (TBG) or albumin with significant strength. On the contrary, many compounds such as PCBs, flame retardants, phenols, and phthalates, bind to transthyretine (TTR) with higher affinity than T_4 does.

Although the quantitative transport of thyroid hormone by TTR in humans is not predominant, TTR is critical to crossing the blood–brain barrier by thyroid hormone in humans. The competitive binding to TTR by environmental pollutants may mediate on one side the entry of TDs into various tissues such as placenta and the fetal compartment. On the other side, they may decrease fetal brain T_4 levels.[1]

Animal studies revealed that phthalates and chlordanes may inhibit T_3 uptake and other xenobiotics may reduce mRNA and protein levels of organic anion-transporting polypeptides (OATPs). This may reduce TH influx into the brain and liver by decreasing transporter activity. The bioavailability of thyroid hormones to nuclear receptors may also become compromised if TDs alter the expression of cellular proteins important for hormone transport into and out of cells. The changes in the activities of these transporter proteins may enhance other disruptions exerted by TDs, thus exacerbating hormone homeostasis impairment.[11] One report also suggested a further interference of PCBs with the binding of TSH to its receptor.

Intracellular metabolism may be affected by TDs, and in particular by PCBs, PBDEs, and heavy metals like cadmium and methyl mercury. These TDs modify deiodinase activity inside cells. In fact, a mixture of PCBs has been shown to enhance brain type II deiodinase activity,[1,6,11] while short term exposure to a UV inhibitor (octyl-methoxycinnamate) decreased the activity of hepatic type I deiodinase.

In addition to deiodination, iodothyronines may be metabolized by conjugation with sulfate or glucuronic acid by diphosphoryl glucuronosyltransferase (UGT) or sulfotransferase (SULT) isoenzymes in the liver and kidneys. Sulfotransferase activities are downregulated and UGT hepatic catabolism upregulated by several TDs such as PCBs, triclosan, dioxins, and pentachlorophenol, with overall increases of biliary T_3 and T_4 clearance.[6]

31.3.2.3 Nuclear Interactions of TDs

Little evidence is available about the mechanisms of thyroid disruptors that affect TH-stimulated gene transcription. TDs seem to exert their effects as partial agonists and antagonists of thyroid hormones by modulating co-stimulatory and co-repressor proteins. PCBs modulate the expression of TH-responsive genes by favoring the dissociation of the thyroid receptor (TR)–retinoid X heterodimer complex from the thyroid response element (TRE).[6,9]

The re-expression of T_3-suppressed genes seems to be triggered by bisphenol A, which instead suppresses T_3-mediated gene activation through thyroid receptors α and β. This effect is dose-dependent and requires the recruitment of co-repressor proteins, indicating that bisphenol A operates as a pure T_3 antagonist. In fact, animal studies have shown that thyroid receptor β levels in oligodendrocytes and their precursor cells decreased significantly after bisphenol A exposure, suggesting a suppression of T_3-induced differentiation of these neuronal cells.

Furthermore, bisphenol A acts as disruptor in other endocrine processes by suppressing DNA methylation, producing epigenetic and conformational changes. However, whether such mechanism operates in thyroid disruption is not proven. In vitro studies demonstrate that phthalates and phenols inhibit the expression of the thyroid receptor β gene and that synthetic isoflavonoids exert pure antagonistic effects on T_3-induced DIO1 gene expression.[12]

31.4 CLINICAL ASPECTS

The complex interactions of TDs with the redundant pathophysiology of iodothyronines prevented the recognition of their burden effects in a single patient. However, animal and human studies revealed potential additive hidden effects on the HPT axis. Chemical disruption impairing thyroid homeostasis during development may result in brain damage with mental retardation and neurological defects.[7] This is due to a disturbance of the iodothyronine-controlled processes such as migration, dendrite-, and synapto-genesis. Impairment of T_3- dependent oligodendrocyte development has been described in BPA-exposed rats.

Hearing impairment and cochlear defects may also be clinical features of TD exposure during pregnancy. Impaired cognitive functions have been described after PCB exposure in different countries. Indeed, different IQs in siblings have been measured and lower IQs in those born after PCB exposure of their mothers.[9]

Environmental inhibitors of NIS may decrease iodine availability in the thyroid gland. This is especially dangerous if the exposure occurs during the gestational period, interfering with the placental and fetus iodine pools. This is demonstrated for perchlorate, but other TDs interfering with NIS have been found in measurable quantities in human amniotic fluid.

However, estimated daily perchlorate below the Environmental Protection Agency (EPA) reference dose (0.7 µg/Kg/day) in the adult population has been reported. A lifetime exposure to these levels of perchlorate is devoid of appreciable risks of adverse effects. Synergistic effects with other NIS inhibitors such as thiocyanates, phthalates, and herbicides then become crucial for the dose-dependent NIS blocking action to occur. Again, this demonstrates the pitfalls of a safe reference dose for a single disruptor.[6,8]

The World Health Organization designates a median lower limit of urinary iodine <100 µg/L as mirror of increased risk of goiter in a population due to dietary iodine deficiency. In these subjects, increasing levels of urinary perchlorate may be predictive of low serum T_4 and high serum TSH levels. In women with urinary iodine levels >100 µg/L, rising levels of urinary perchlorate may predict high levels of TSH without FT_4 anomalies.[6] In subjects living in OC-polluted areas who had high blood OC levels and optimal urinary iodine levels, thyroid volumes appeared significantly enlarged. Some authors suggested that the presence of goiter in iodine-sufficient areas may be a sign of toxic effects of OCs.

A number of chemicals may alter circulating iodothyronines based on animal studies. However, evidence of changes of iodothyronines in humans upon exposures to different disruptors is not unequivocal. PBDE exposure decreases total and free T_4 and increases TSH in animals while these effects in humans are less clearly defined. PBDE effects on animal thyroid homeostasis represent further examples of co-disruption (Figure 31.3). In fact, these flame retardants also modify retinol circulating levels. Some authors suggested that even a marginal vitamin A deficiency, like the one described for marginal malnutrition and other causes of reduction of retinol circulating complex (RCC), may cooperate in lowering iodothyronines upon PBDE exposure.

The target of these xenobiotics is the cross-talk between thyroid homeostasis and the retinol network.[10] Serum FT_4 level may be an appropriate measure of OC effects on thyroid hormone levels in blood. However, long exposure to high PCB levels may increase FT_4 displacement from its TTR binding site but this in turn leads to increased cellular uptake of FT_4 and raised intracellular T_4 to T_3 deiodinase conversion and glucuronidation.

These mechanisms have not been associated with clear-cut changes of circulating iodothyronines, perhaps due to the multiple actions of TDs and the individual steady state thyroid homeostasis. This issue is therefore still controversial.

More reliable is the evidence that a dioxin derivative (TCDD) may reduce serum total T_4 without affecting T_3 in rats, where it inhibits liver D1 activity and increases brown adipose tissue D2 activity. It has been suggested that changes in deiodinase activity induced by xenobiotics may modify peripheral iodothyronine homeostasis in a way that resembles euthyroid sick syndrome.[7] Exposure to bisphenol A, a selective thyroid receptor β antagonist has been associated with effects mimicking thyroid resistance syndrome in which the receptor is defective, leading to increased serum T_4 and slightly elevated TSH.

Attention deficit hyperactivity disorder (ADHD) was described in association with thyroid resistance in humans and rats and BPA-exposed rats showed ADHD-like symptoms. Since BPA exposure may modify cortical histogenesis, it has been suggested that early impairment of cortex development occurs in BPA-exposed animals, perhaps due to its effect on TH signalling.[9]

31.4.1 Disruptors and Thyroid Immune Response

A substantial body of evidence supports a disrupting action of environmental toxins on immune systems. Prenatal OC exposure has been correlated with thymocyte destruction, increased prevalence of autoimmune and/or infectious diseases, decreased vaccine responses, and altered or impaired function of leukocytes and/or immunoglobulins. Also, the polyhalogenated biphenyl compounds seem to possess immunotoxic properties.

Environmental disruptors seem to contribute to the increased prevalence of autoimmune diseases through the activation of Th17 cells. The pathogenesis of autoimmune thyroid disease (ATD) is a composite and multistep process. It is triggered in genetically predisposed individuals with impaired immune responses by different stress events. Human Th17 cells possess inflammatory properties and enhance autoimmune processes including ATD.

The aryl hydrocarbon receptor (AhR), a ligand-dependent transcription factor known for mediating the toxicity of dioxin, is expressed in these lymphocytes and enables the transmission of different environmental signals through interaction with the so-called xenobiotic responsive element (XRE). Activation of AhR

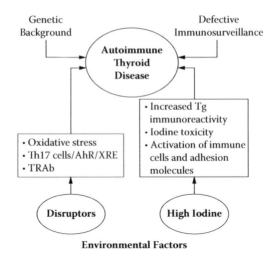

FIGURE 31.5 Disruptors and thyroid autoimmunity. AhR = aryl hydrocarbon receptor. XRE = xenobiotic responsive element. TRAb = anti-TSH receptor antibody.

by high-affinity ligands such as OCs can stimulate Th17 differentiation and their production of cytokines, thus exacerbating Th17-mediated autoimmunity.[13] This is not, of course, the only suggested mechanism of disruption.

Actually, polyhalogenated biphenyls seem to interfere also by inducing oxidative stress and impairing thyrocyte iodine syntransport. Increased concentrations of thyroperoxidase (TPO-Ab), thyroglobulin (Tg-Ab) and TSH receptor stimulating (TR-Ab) antibodies have been detected in highly PCB-exposed personnel as compared with individuals living in the same area and not exposed.

The thyrotropin receptor is also a target of the disruption observed in the smoking-dependent worsening of Graves' disease and orbitopathy. Retro-orbital tissues, in fact, strongly react with thyrotropin receptor-stimulating antibodies because smoking makes thyrotropin receptors more immunogenic.

Even iodine excess has been implicated in inducing or precipitating thyroid autoimmunity, based on the increased immunogenicity of highly iodinated Tg, the direct toxic effect due to the production of free oxygen radicals in thyroid cells, and the direct stimulation of immune cells by iodine (Figure 31.5).

After monitoring iodine prophylaxis in various populations, a high incidence of ATD was observed in countries where iodine supplementation was adequate. Coal pollution, agricultural fungicides, dust and gas released from cars and heavy industry are also involved in the pathogenesis of ATD, but whether the described mechanisms were involved in the disrupting activity is not known.[13]

31.4.2 TDs AND THYROID CANCER

Some two decades ago, fetal exposure to the diethylstilbestrol synthetic estrogen led to the development of vaginal carcinomas or genital tract malformations. That early experience suggested focusing on endocrine disruptors as promoters of cancer.[14] As to the concern about thyroid cancer, the best described disruptor is the exposure to high doses of radioiodine as in nuclear plant accidents. Because the uptake of ^{131}I occurs only in cells that actively transport iodide, thyroid cells are obviously the major targets.

As a matter of fact, the incidence rate of differentiated papillary and follicular thyroid cancers has increased continuously since 1988. Studies following the nuclear catastrophe in Chernobyl have shown that exposure of cells to ionizing radiation may cause double strand DNA breaks at fragile sites. This, in turn, may create gene rearrangements that trigger neoplastic transformation.

In particular these rearrangements may downregulate DNA repair processes or activate unregulated transcriptional and transductional events. Two oncogenes are alternatively recognized in papillary thyroid carcinoma (PTC). They are RET and more recently, B-RAF. The MAP kinase pathway, whose role in the pathogenesis of PTC is crucial, is activated by both these genes. RET and PTC rearrangements characterizing papillary thyroid cancer have been identified in children from the Chernobyl area. However, differentiated thyroid cancer is a multistep process that may involve additional environmental and hormonal cofactors.

In animal models, exposure to several pesticides (toxaphene, lofentezine, fipronil, fenbuconazole, and others) induced follicular thyroid carcinoma apparently by interfering with "transcriptional" machinery through epigenetic mechanisms. Animal studies have also shown that exposure to other xenobiotics (sulfonamides, lithium, perchlorate, thiocyanate, etc.) that disrupt thyroid homeostasis at different levels (e.g., iodothyronine biosynthesis, secretion and/or peripheral T_4 to T_3 conversion), may lead to a chronic increase of TSH.

Evidence also indicates that a possible crucial step in thyroid cell carcinogenesis is the impairment of the pituitary–thyroid axis with increased stimulation of thyroid cell growth by TSH. This action of TSH on follicular cells is physiological but such an increase, when prolonged, is associated with higher incidence of thyroid tumors. Whether xenobiotics affecting thyrocyte growth may act also as cocarcinogens in human thyroid cancer is difficult to establish. Again, a cooperative effect of exposure to pollutants and other permissive mechanisms (e.g., TSH-dependent growth signals) may unveil the effect of an otherwise hidden disruption.

31.5 DIAGNOSIS

The detection of thyroid disruption effects is fairly complex. In fact, the nature of thyroid disruption and the modes of action of TDs based on subtle changes of iodothyronine pathophysiology are unfavorable for identifying specific cause-and-effect links. Even more difficult is discriminating the effects when more than one xenobiotic is involved.

Further diagnostic problems stem from the lag time between exposure to TDs and measurable effects that depend on the age at and the duration of exposure. Also, most thyroid disruptors cannot be evaluated easily and when measured show no clear relationship with clinical effects. One possible exception is perchlorate, which has been related to lower levels of iodine in breast milk. In fact, due to widespread food and water contamination, perchlorate exposure may be assessed by urinary levels and during lactation by breast milk, using ion chromatography and tandem mass spectrometry. Another example is iodine deficiency or excess that may be measured routinely as urinary iodine. However, these measures are "drops in the sea," considering that the number of thyroid disrupting agents may exceed 150.

31.6 PROPHYLAXIS

The ubiquitous distribution of disruptors and the lack of specific treatments make prophylaxis the only possible defense against pollutants. The best example of prophylaxis is the one operating in cases of nuclear plant accidents. Iodine prophylaxis is, in fact, the way to protect the thyroid gland from possible radiation injury. This effect is supported by the ability of iodine to prevent binding of radioiodine through saturation of active iodine transport by NIS and the Wolff-Chaikoff phenomenon.

In adults and adolescents radioiodine uptake by the thyroid gland is prevented by administration of 100 mg of iodine, or 130 mg of potassium iodide (KI), or 170 mg of potassium iodate (KIO_3), according to the WHO guidelines for iodine prophylaxis in cases of nuclear accidents. In particular KI is highly effective in blocking uptake of radioiodine if taken shortly before or shortly after exposure, particularly for infants, children, and pregnant or nursing women (Table 31.3).

When prophylaxis is not feasible, we advise the "precautionary principle" according to the Endocrine Society scientific statement (Table 31.4). Accurate control of chemical industries, the use of so-called biological agriculture that limits or prevents the use of pesticides, and accurate medical surveys of routinely exposed workers are useful attempts to reduce pollution effects in well-developed countries. In particular, careful iodine prophylaxis should be implemented prior to pregnancy and exposure to TDs during pregnancy must be avoided.

TABLE 31.3
WHO Recommendations for Iodine Prophylaxis after Nuclear Accidents

Age Group	Iodine (mg)	KI (mg)	KIO_3 (mg)	Fraction of 100 mg Tablet
Adults and adolescents (over 12 years old)	100	130	170	1
Children (3 to 12 years)	50	65	85	1/2
Infants (1 month to 3 years)	25	32	42	1/4
Neonates (birth to 1 month)	12.5	16	21	1/8

TABLE 31.4
Recommendations to Reduce TD Exposures

Identify clusters of patients at high risk of contamination from occupational exposure to TDs

Keep informed and inform people about chronic pollution

Inform patients about environmental sources and potential risks of exposure to TDs

When an unforeseen disorder occurs in a defined geographic area, consider possible local contamination by TDs

Avoid acute exposure of pregnant patients to TDs to prevent interference with central nervous system development of fetus

Avoid ingesting fruits and vegetables from known or suspected pollutant areas

REFERENCES

1. Diamanti-Kandarakis, E., Bourguignon, J.P., Giudice, L.C. et al. 2009. Endocrine-disrupting chemicals: an Endocrine Society scientific statement. *Endocr Rev* 30: 293–342.
2. Lacasana, M., Lopez-Florez, I., Rodriguez-Barranco, M. et al. 2010. Association between organophosphate pesticides exposure and thyroid hormones in floriculture workers. *Toxicol Appl Pharmacol* 243: 19–26.
3. Crinnion, W.J. 2009. Maternal levels of xenobiotics that affect fetal development and childhood health. *Altern Med Rev* 14: 212–222.
4. Schmutzler, C., Gotthardt, I., Hofmann, P.J. et al. 2007. Endocrine disruptors and the thyroid gland: a combined in vitro and in vivo analysis of potential new biomarkers. *Environ Health Perspect* 115: 77–83.
5. Leung, A.M., Pearce, E.N., and Braverman, L.E. 2010. Perchlorate, iodine and the thyroid. *Best Pract Res Clin Endocrinol Metab* 24: 133–141.
6. Lyn, P. 2009. Thyroid disruption: mechanisms and clinical implications in human health. *Altern Med Rev* 14: 326–346.
7. Mastorakos, G., Karoutsou, E.I., Mizamtsidi, M. et al. 2007. The menace of endocrine disruptors on thyroid hormone physiology and their impact on intrauterine development. *Endocrinology* 31: 219–237.
8. Jugan, M.L., Levi, Y.P., and Blondeau J. 2010. Endocrine disruptors and thyroid hormone physiology. *Biochem Pharmacol* 79: 939–947.
9. Zoeller, T.R. 2010. Environmental chemicals targeting thyroid. *Hormones* 9: 28–40.
10. Talsness, C.E. 2008. Overview of toxicological aspects of polybrominated diphenyl ethers: a flame retardant additive in several consumer products. *Environ Reser* 108: 158–167.
11. Crofton, K.M. 2008. Thyroid disrupting chemicals: mechanisms and mixtures. *Int J Androl* 31: 209–223.
12. Hofmann, P.J., Schomburg, L., and Köhrle, J. 2009. Interference of endocrine disrupters with thyroid hormone receptor dependent transactivation. *Toxicol Sci* 110: 125–137.
13. Duntas, L.H. 2008. Environmental factors and autoimmune thyroiditis. *Nat Clin Pract Endocrinol Metab* 4: 454–460.
14. Soto, A.M. and Sonnenschein, C. 2010. Environmental causes of cancer: endocrine disruptors as carcinogens. *Nat Rev Endocrinol* 6: 363–370.

Index